MUSCLE *and* SENSORY TESTING

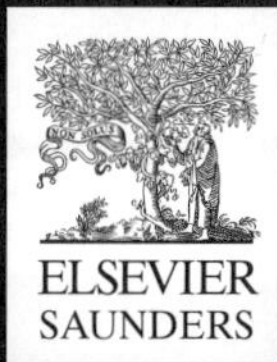

evolve

∴ To access your Student Resources, visit the Web address below:

http://evolve.elsevier.com/Reese/muscle/

- **Pediatric Handheld Dynamometry Tests**
  Video segments on 7 pediatric handheld dynamometry tests for shoulder abduction, elbow flexion, elbow extension, hip flexion, hip abduction, knee extension, and knee flexion.
- **Data on Pediatric Values**
- **WebLinks**
  An exciting resource that lets you link to hundreds of websites carefully chosen to supplement the content of the textbook. The WebLinks are regularly updated, with new ones added as they develop.

MUSCLE *and* SENSORY TESTING

SECOND EDITION

Nancy Berryman Reese, PhD, PT

Professor and Chairperson
Department of Physical Therapy
University of Central Arkansas
Conway, Arkansas

Adjunct Assistant Professor
Department of Neurobiology and Developmental Sciences
University of Arkansas for Medical Sciences
Little Rock, Arkansas

CONTRIBUTORS

Venita Lovelace-Chandler, PhD, PT, PCS
Chairperson,
Department of Physical Therapy
Chapman University
Orange, California
Techniques of Pediatric Muscle Testing

Gary L. Soderberg, PhD, PT, FAPTA
Professor and Director
Physical Therapy Research
Program in Physical Therapy
Southwest Missouri State University
Springfield, Missouri
Handheld Dynamometry for Muscle Testing

Reta J. Zabel, PhD, PT, GCS
Associate Professor of Physical Therapy
Conway, Arkansas
Techniques of Functional Muscle Testing

PHOTOGRAPHER

Michael A. Morris, AGM, FBCA
University of Arkansas for Medical Sciences
Media Services
Little Rock, Arkansas

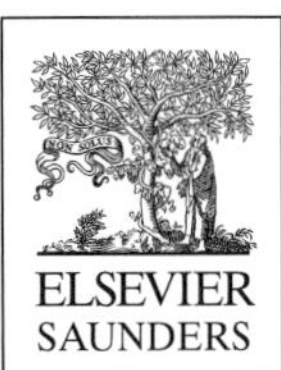

ELSEVIER
SAUNDERS

11830 Westline Industrial Drive
St. Louis, Missouri 63146

MUSCLE AND SENSORY TESTING, SECOND EDITION ISBN 0-7216-0337-8

Previous edition copyrighted 1999

Library of Congress Cataloging-in-Publication Data

Application Submitted.

or

International Standard Book Number 0-7216-0337-8

Acquisitions Editor: Marion Waldman
Developmental Editor: Marjory I. Fraser
Publishing Services Manager: Melissa Lastarria
Senior Project Manager: Joy Moore
Designer: Julia Dummit

Printed in the United States of America

Last digit is the print number: 9 8 7 6 5 4 3 2 1

To David, Elizabeth, and Nicole,
who have blessed my life with their presence

PREFACE TO THE FIRST EDITION

Muscle and Sensory Testing is designed for students and professionals in health care disciplines who employ the techniques of muscle strength testing and neurologic screening in the course of patient examination. Rarely does a health care practitioner perform a physical examination that includes the testing of muscle strength without also including some other component of the neurologic examination (sensation testing, reflex testing, etc.). Indeed, muscle strength testing is an integral component of the basic neurologic examination. However, most muscle testing texts do not include techniques for the remainder of the neurologic examination, and most texts that discuss the neurologic examination fail to include comprehensive techniques for testing muscle strength. This text fills that void by providing comprehensive coverage of muscle strength testing and the neurologic screening examination. The use of observational gait analysis as a screening tool for muscle testing also is included.

The first six chapters of *Muscle and Sensory Testing* address muscle strength testing from birth through adulthood, using both manual and dynamometric techniques. Chapter 1 deals with the history of manual muscle testing and provides basic guidelines for performing the manual muscle test. Chapters 2, 3, and 4 cover manual muscle testing for the extremities, head, neck, and trunk. Techniques of manual muscle testing for the pediatric population are discussed in Chapter 5, and the use of the handheld dynamometer for examining muscle strength is discussed in Chapter 6. Techniques of the neurologic screening examination, including interpretive comments, are detailed in Chapters 7 and 8. The final chapter discusses the use of observational gait analysis as a screening tool for muscle testing. The authors assume that those using this book have completed courses in human anatomy and neuroanatomy and have a basic understanding of kinesiology. In Chapters 2, 3, and 4, pertinent anatomic information regarding muscular attachments, innervation, and actions has been included, as appropriate. Unless otherwise indicated, all anatomic information was derived from the 30th American edition of *Gray's Anatomy,* Carmine D. Clemente, editor (Philadelphia, Lea and Febiger, 1985).

Research for this book revealed very little consensus among practitioners regarding muscle testing techniques. Many practitioners appear to be "married" to a particular muscle testing technique for one reason or another. As a case in point, two separate reviewers of this text expressed totally opposing opinions regarding the correct technique for testing the tensor fasciae latae muscle. In instances in which there is a wide divergence in opinion regarding the manual testing of a particular muscle, more than one technique is included, and the reader may choose the most appropriate approach.

Although manual muscle testing has been criticized as being subjective and nonquantitative, it remains a valid and reproducible method of examining muscle strength if used appropriately.

Manual muscle testing is the most convenient and inexpensive method of examining muscle strength, and may be the only method of accurately examining strength in a very weak muscle. However, in cases in which quantitative assessment of muscle strength is vital, and when muscle strength approaches normal, other methods of strength testing may be preferable. For this reason, both manual and dynamometric muscle strength testing are included in this text. Practitioners who routinely test muscle strength should be familiar with both methods.

None of the components of the neurologic examination, especially muscle testing, can be learned quickly. Mastery of these techniques is accomplished only after repeated practice, first on individuals free of disease (so that the normal range of muscle strength and neurologic functioning can be appreciated), then on patients. Each of the techniques presented in this text is an essential part of the repertoire of examination tools for all practitioners who deal with patients with neuromusculoskeletal disorders. Mastery of the techniques presented herein will provide the clinician with a significant number of the tools needed to perform a thorough and efficient examination of the neuromusculoskeletal system.

Nancy Berryman Reese

PREFACE TO THE SECOND EDITION

Creation of this second edition of *Muscle and Sensory Testing* was undertaken to achieve three primary goals: to facilitate critical thinking in students in regard to muscle testing, to increase ease of use of the text, and to respond to feedback from educators and students. The first goal was addressed through the addition of case studies and clinical notes to several chapters in the text and through the addition of the most current information on muscle testing available in the literature. The case studies and clinical notes provide a basis for application of muscle testing and challenge the student to consider situations in which testing may need to be modified or additional testing undertaken based on individual patient scenarios. The most recent literature has been incorporated into all chapters for which new information was available.

The addition of a DVD to the second edition increases the ease of use of the text. The accompanying DVD contains a videotaped demonstration of all examination techniques in Chapters 2, 3, 4, 7, 8, and 9 so that the user can actually learn the techniques contained in these chapters independently. The DVD also contains examples of the use of handheld dynamometry in children, a feature not contained in any other muscle testing text.

Feedback from educators, clinicians, and students regarding the first edition resulted in several additional improvements to this text. A completely new chapter on Functional Muscle Testing (Chapter 5) has been added to this edition. This chapter contains a number of functional tests of muscle strength that are appropriate for a variety of individuals, but particularly for the older adult population. The line drawings that accompany each of the manual muscle tests in Chapters 2 through 4 have been updated to include a visual representation of the nerve innervating each muscle. In addition, Chapter 1 has been significantly expanded to include information regarding changes in muscle strength with age and sex, a discussion of various methods of muscle strength assessment and guidelines for their use, and several student exercises designed to instruct the student in the principles of muscle testing.

The alterations made to produce this second edition of *Muscle and Sensory Testing* have resulted in a text that is more comprehensive and more easily used for self-directed learning. In addition, the information contained in the second edition should challenge students to think more critically about muscle testing and its use in the examination and diagnosis of patient disorders.

Nancy Berryman Reese

ACKNOWLEDGMENTS

As with any project of this magnitude, the work of numerous individuals has contributed to the production of the second edition of *Muscle and Sensory Testing*. My sincere thanks goes to the editorial staff at Elsevier: Andrew Allen, Marion Waldman, and Marjory I. Fraser, all of whom have provided valuable support and encouragement desperately needed by the author. I am indebted to my contributing authors: Venita Lovelace-Chandler, PhD, PT, PCS, Gary L. Soderberg, PhD, PT, FAPTA, and Reta J. Zabel, PhD, PT, GCS, whose continuing scholarship and expertise provided an invaluable addition to this text. For this edition, as in all projects in which photography is involved, I again had the great good fortune to work with Michael A. Morris, AGM, FBCA, whose work is above reproach. Michael did all the beautiful photography in the text, and he, along with the very talented Lana Campbell and Dale Seidenschwarz, directed, edited, and produced the DVD that accompanies this edition. Secretarial and research support was provided by many individuals, including Amber Bates, Hannah Hix, Anguel Kehayov, and Betty Young. Their assistance was invaluable during this process. Special thanks go to my colleague, William D. Bandy, PhD, PT, SCS, ATC, for proofreading and advice and for being a wonderful support and sounding board. I am indebted to the many individuals who served as models for the photographs: Davis Allen, Joseph Beck, Nick Barnes, Richard Byrum, Ayana Rayanne Johnson, Kelly Kasserman, Laura LaMastus, Verdarhea Langrell, Morgan Mourot, Martye Murphy, Mackenzie Ann Powers, Frankie Pratt, Angela Raines, Elizabeth Reese, Nicole Reese, Sarah Runnells, David Smith, David Taylor, PhD, PT, Ann Winston, MS, PT, and especially Sherry Holmes and Myla Quiben, PT, DPT, who served as models for the examiner in the photographs for the book and DVD.

I would be particularly remiss were I to fail to thank the people who have provided me with emotional and financial support during the completion of this project. On a daily basis, I am the recipient of continuous encouragement and help from my colleagues in the Department of Physical Therapy at the University of Central Arkansas. Nowhere is there a more supportive group of faculty, and I consider myself privileged to be able to work with such outstanding individuals and even more privileged to be able to call them friends. Most important, I am eternally grateful to my family for their unending patience, tolerance, and love. I am truly fortunate to have a husband and children who have stood behind me through good times and bad, parents who taught me well, and an extended family that supports me in all my endeavors. I am grateful to God for all the wonderful blessings he has given me.

Nancy Berryman Reese

CONTENTS

1

OVERVIEW of MUSCLE STRENGTH ASSESSMENT

While attempts to quantify human muscle strength have been occurring for hundreds of years,[29] agreement on the definition of muscle strength is not evident in the literature. Some authors use the term *muscle strength* to refer to the ability of muscle to develop tension[84] or torque.[20] Other authors provide a more restrictive definition that limits strength to force generated over a single, unlimited episode against an immovable resistance[57] whereas still others advocate the use of muscle power as a substitute for muscle strength.[82] In recognition of the fact that human muscle must be capable of force generation in a static position and through a range of motion, the term *muscle strength* will be defined herein according to Knuttgen and Kraemer[55] as "the maximal force a muscle or muscle group can generate at a specified or determined velocity."

Tests of muscle strength have been, and continue to be, performed for many and varied reasons. Strength may be tested in relation to athletic performance, a practice common at least since the time of the ancient Greeks with the original Olympic games. In a health care setting, strength concerns are more often related to the diagnosis and treatment of disease and restoration of function. Muscle strength testing is an essential component of the examination of all patients, particularly those with musculoskeletal or neuromuscular pathology. Numerous such pathologies leave the patient with less than optimal muscle strength and control, and clues to diagnosing such disorders are often found during examination of muscle strength. For example, muscle testing is used in patients with spinal cord injury to help determine the level of the lesion and the degree of damage to the cord. Patterns of muscle strength loss may help differentiate between two possible diagnoses (e.g., C6 radiculopathy versus median nerve lesion). Strength testing may be used to determine a patient's ability to perform activities of daily living or to assess an injured athlete's ability to return to competition.

FACTORS AFFECTING MUSCLE STRENGTH: RELATIONSHIP OF MUSCLE STRENGTH WITH AGE AND SEX

Muscle strength does not remain constant over an individual's life span but demonstrates a pattern of gradual increase during childhood and into young adulthood followed by a gradual decline through the remainder of the person's life. Many researchers have examined muscle strength development in children. Many of these investigations report a strong relationship between the steady increases in muscle strength and increases in muscle size experienced during growth and development.[28,49,50,75,83,91] Among the most predictive factors of muscle strength in both sexes are muscle cross-sectional area,[28,49,50] height,[28,75,83,88] weight,[75,83,88,91], and age.[5,50,71,75,81,88] Muscle strength in boys is greater that that of girls from as early as age 9 or 10 years[88] and appears to be due, at least until puberty, to body mass and height, both of which are larger in males than females as a group.[28,80] However, longitudinal studies indicate that around the time of peak height velocity, the rate of increase in muscle strength in males becomes disproportionate to body mass and height increases, whereas the rate of muscle strength increase in females remains proportionate.[75,83] This disproportionately high increase in male strength has been attributed to plasma testosterone levels, which rise rapidly around the time of peak height velocity.[83]

Increases in muscle strength appear to continue until sometime between age 20 and 30.[3,4,10,22,72] Strength then shows slight declines until the fifth or sixth decade, when rates of decline in muscle strength increase.[4,21,22,72,90] Declines in muscle strength do not appear to be consistent between muscle groups[4,21,52,90] or between men and women.[48,72,78] Loss of isometric muscle strength from ages 20 to 80 has been reported to range from 32% to 52% in women[22,47,72,79,102] and from 34% to 60% in men,[22,72] with declines in muscle strength in women starting later than those in men.[22,63,90]

Although the reasons for declines in strength associated with aging have not been fully elucidated, possible mechanisms are varied. Total muscle mass declines with aging, with reductions estimated to be somewhere between 20% and 40% between the third and ninth decades,[36,37,52,61,92,94,102] although such declines may be ameliorated with physical activity.[8,54,69,95] Motor neurons in the spinal cord also are lost during the aging process, particularly after age 60, which may account for some of the declines in muscle force.[92] Additionally, the number and size of muscle fibers are apparently reduced with aging, contributing to a decline in the contractile capabilities of the muscle.[37,45,58,60,61,93]

APPROACHES TO MUSCLE STRENGTH TESTING

Using the definition of muscle strength as "the maximal force a muscle or muscle group can generate at a specified or determined velocity," one can measure muscle strength in a variety of ways, depending on the velocity of motion and type of resistance used in the test. Although a variety of methods of examining muscle strength exist, there are basically three different approaches to muscle strength testing that are described in the literature and used clinically: isotonic, isokinetic, and isometric testing.

Isotonic strength testing has traditionally been defined as the testing of strength using a constant external resistance.[17] However, the term *isotonic* (Greek, isos: equal and tonos: straining) is a misnomer in this situation, because isotonic properly refers to constant *muscle tension*, a situation that very rarely occurs in muscle, rather than constant external resistance. Regardless of the misuse of the term, isotonic strength testing typically involves the use of free weights or resistance machines and may use testing techniques such as the one-repetition maximum (1-RM), which is considered by many to be the "gold-standard" in muscle strength assessment.[56] However, such testing may prove overtaxing to the subject, because several repetitions of weight lifting normally are necessary as the examiner attempts to discover the maximum weight the subject can lift or move.[17] Additionally, such testing may be time-consuming, lack the portability of other muscle strength testing methods, cause injury, and tests gross strength of muscle groups rather than strength of individual muscles.[42]

Isokinetic strength testing was developed in the 1960s and involves measurement of muscle strength by having the subject provide resistance through the range of motion at a constant velocity.[74] Isokinetic dynamometers generate an isokinetic torque curve, and muscle strength is determined by measuring the highest point on the curve.[27] Because peak torque is normally used to define muscle strength when using isokinetic dynamometry, the result is measurement of strength at only one point in the range of motion (although isokinetic dynamometry is capable of providing strength data throughout the range of motion).[6,98] Reliability of isokinetic testing is high, provided testing protocols are followed strictly.[19,30] Like isotonic testing, isokinetic testing tests gross strength of muscle groups rather than strength of individual muscles. Isokinetic testing costs may be prohibitive, with the price of instruments estimated at $40,000.

Isometric (Greek, isos: equal and metron: measure) testing of muscle strength involves having the muscle generate force against an immovable resistance so that muscle length remains the same throughout the test. Thus, factors that can confound a muscle test, such as variability in muscle length and velocity of joint motion, are eliminated. The two most commonly used methods of isometric muscle testing, manual muscle testing (MMT) and handheld dynamometry (HHD), are highly portable and inexpensive, with MMT requiring no equipment other than the examiner's hands. A disadvantage of isometric strength testing is that, because muscle length is held constant, isometric testing provides muscle strength data at only one point in the range of motion.

SELECTION OF THE APPROPRIATE TESTING TOOL

No single method of examining muscle strength is appropriate in every situation. Therefore the examiner needs to have an arsenal of muscle testing tools available and the knowledge of the advantages and disadvantages of each method so that the optimal tool may be selected and the desired information may be obtained for each patient. In some cases, selection of the testing method may be limited by constraints such as the patient's condition, equipment availability, or other factors, and the data obtained may be less than perfect. For example, because children younger than 3 years do not have the ability to cooperate with complex testing situations such as those used with MMT, HHD, or isokinetic testing, muscle strength testing is best accomplished by observing functional activities (see Chapter 6) in such patients. However, these data obtained are not as quantifiable as those available with methods such as HHD or isokinetic dynamometry. Compromises such as these are frequently necessary in assessing muscle strength, and the examiner must make the judgment as to the best testing method in each situation.

Generally, the following guidelines will assist the examiner in choosing the best method of muscle strength assessment.

1. **Select the tool that is most appropriate for the patient's strength.** Patients with significant weakness are best assessed using MMT or functional muscle testing. HHD and other instrumented forms of muscle testing typically are not sensitive enough to detect very low levels of muscle strength. Conversely, patients with muscle strength levels in the range of 4 or 5 using MMT would optimally be tested using HHD or isokinetic dynamometry, because MMT does not allow clearly quantifiable discrimination between

gradations of muscle strength in these ranges (see Validity of Manual Muscle Testing).

2. **Select the tool that is most appropriate for the patient's age.** As mentioned previously, methods of muscle strength assessment requiring the following of complex instructions or concentrated attention are not useful in patients under the age of 3 or 4 as a rule, although cognitive and attention skills of the individual patient may expand or contract that age range. Additionally, elderly patients may not be able to tolerate certain positions or may lack the motor control or balance to perform certain tasks required of some testing methods. Such limitations must be considered in selection of the testing method.
3. **Select the tool that fits the testing environment.** Sophisticated equipment may not be available or practical in all situations. For example, in the home environment, the examiner is unlikely to have access to an isokinetic dynamometer whereas a handheld dynamometer may be readily available.
4. **Select the testing method for which the tools are available.** This rule goes almost without saying. Obviously, isokinetic dynamometry cannot be performed without access to an isokinetic dynamometer.
5. **When more than one reliable testing method is available, select the method that provides the most quantifiable data.** Many methods of muscle strength testing contain a large subjective component. Objective, quantifiable data are preferred when making assessments about a patient's strength or inferences about changes in patient status. Use of quantifiable methods of strength testing results in more reliable normative data upon which to base patient strength assessment.

Methods of assessing strength may seem almost as numerous as the reasons for testing. Most of this text is devoted to a description of noninstrumented and minimally instrumented methods of assessing muscle strength. Such testing methods are portable, economical, easily learned (with practice), and applicable to a wide range of patients. Strength testing methods that use more cumbersome or sophisticated instrumentation, although described briefly elsewhere in this chapter, are beyond the scope of this text. Readers are referred to sources cited at the end of this chapter for more in-depth discussions of these types of muscle testing.[44,56] Due to the complexity of testing techniques and the time required to perform comprehensive muscle strength testing, screening examinations for muscle strength often are used to reveal areas of weakness requiring further investigation. Manual muscle screening and some of the functional muscle tests described in Chapters 5 and 6 of this text are examples of screening examinations for muscle strength. In many instances, assessment of muscle strength occurs as part of an overall assessment of nervous system function. For this reason, techniques for assessment of other nervous system functions, such as peripheral sensation, reflex testing, and cranial nerve integrity, are included in Chapters 8 and 9. The remainder of this chapter, as well as Chapters 2 to 4, is devoted to a discussion of MMT, and Chapter 7 is devoted to handheld dynamometry.

NONINSTRUMENTED MUSCLE STRENGTH TESTING: MANUAL MUSCLE TESTING

Credit for the first published description of MMT in the United States is generally attributed to Wilhelmine Wright,[101] an assistant to orthopedic surgeon Robert W. Lovett, M.D. Lovett first used manual and then spring balance muscle testing in his treatment of patients with poliomyelitis in the early twentieth century.[64,66,70] Wright published and apparently was instrumental in developing the MMT techniques used by Lovett.[99] Initially, the system of grading muscle strength used by Lovett was based on three possible classifications: normal, partially paralyzed, or wholly paralyzed. Later, this grading system was modified to include the grades of normal, good, fair, poor, trace, and totally paralyzed.[65]

Since the time of Lovett, several individuals have contributed to and modified his muscle testing method. In a 1927 article in the *American Journal of Surgery*,[67] LeRoy Lowman, M.D., recommended a grading scale for muscle testing that included the use of numeric grades (0 to 9) and plus/minus designations for the grades of fair through normal. In the 1930s, the Kendalls (Henry O. and Florence P.) introduced the concept of percentages in grading manual muscle tests and published their work on muscle testing in a text that is now in its fourth edition and is widely used in the United States and other parts of the world.[51] In the 1940s, a second major manual of muscle testing was published, this authored by Daniels et al.[25] These authors included positions for testing the muscle both against gravity and with gravity "eliminated" and used a grading scale from zero to normal, much like the one used by Lovett. What has come to be commonly known as the Daniels and Worthingham method of muscle testing has most recently been published in a somewhat modified form by Hislop and Montgomery.[41]

Several individuals have examined the reliability and validity of MMT (see below) and have made strides toward improving the standardization of muscle testing techniques.[9,12,13,16,33-35,40,43,53,62,85-87,96] Concerns over the lack of quantifiable data available from MMT have led to the development of instrumented forms of muscle testing such as the handheld dynamometer and the isokinetic dynamometer.[6,27,76] These instruments are gaining wider acceptance clinically and are quite useful in certain situations (particularly when the patient's strength is in the good to normal range). However, MMT remains the method of choice for assessing the strength of patients whose muscle test grades fall below fair and is the most convenient and inexpensive method of strength assessment currently available.

MANUAL MUSCLE TESTING VERSUS MANUAL MUSCLE SCREENING

Performing a manual muscle test involves extensive time, effort, and attention to detail to ensure that the results obtained are as accurate as possible. The patient's positioning, along with the examiner's technique, must be standardized and adhered to to avoid biasing the results in a manual muscle test. Due to the extensive time and effort needed to perform a comprehensive manual muscle test, manual muscle screening frequently is used to provide a quick overview of the patient's muscle strength. The information thus obtained can help the examiner identify potential areas of strength deficit that then can be investigated further with more standardized methods of strength assessment. During manual muscle screening, muscle strength is assessed by placing the patient in positions of convenience, rather than in specific positions in which the muscles are working against, or outside the influence of, gravity. The strength of muscle groups then are tested through manual resistance supplied by the examiner, allowing rapid, although crude, assessment of muscle group strength. Screening of muscle strength is part of the upper and lower quarter screening examination and is useful as a survey of the overall strength of a patient prior to functional activity or training in activities of daily living.[68] Figures 1-1 to 1-4 demonstrate differences in the testing techniques used in manual muscle screening, versus MMT, of the triceps brachii (elbow extensor) and biceps femoris (knee flexor) muscles. Manual muscle screening is a valuable tool for the rapid survey of gross strength but does not provide data that are accurate or quantifiable enough for diagnosis of neuromuscular disease or for evaluation of patient progress in terms of strength gains.

Resisted movement testing, used to differentiate between contractile and noncontractile sources of musculoskeletal pain, also uses a form of MMT.[24,68] During resisted movement testing, the patient's joint is placed in a mid-range position, and isometric testing of muscle strength is performed to uncover any muscle weakness or pain that might be present with resisted motion. The presence of weakness with or without pain during isometric contractions performed in such neutral joint positions points to a muscular contribution to the musculoskeletal pathology. However, due to the lack of strict adherence to gravity-resisted versus gravity-eliminated positioning during resisted movement testing, the information obtained about muscle strength cannot be graded or quantified any further than application of the terms "strong" or "weak."

RELIABILITY OF MANUAL MUSCLE TESTING

A limited number of studies investigating the reliability of MMT have been performed. One of the earliest investigations occurred during the 1952 gammaglobulin field trials for the treatment of poliomyelitis.[62] Lilienfeld et al.[62] reported on the interrater reliability of a standardized protocol for MMT by comparing experienced examiners both with novice examiners and with other experienced examiners. Although only descriptive statistics were reported, the authors found complete agreement (assigning of the same MMT grade) between examiners in 60% to 66% of the tests and agreement within plus or minus one full grade in 91% to 95% of the manual muscle tests given. Similar results were reported by Blair[12] in a later study. However, in the studies of Lilienfeld et al.[62] and Blair,[12] the MMT scores were modified by

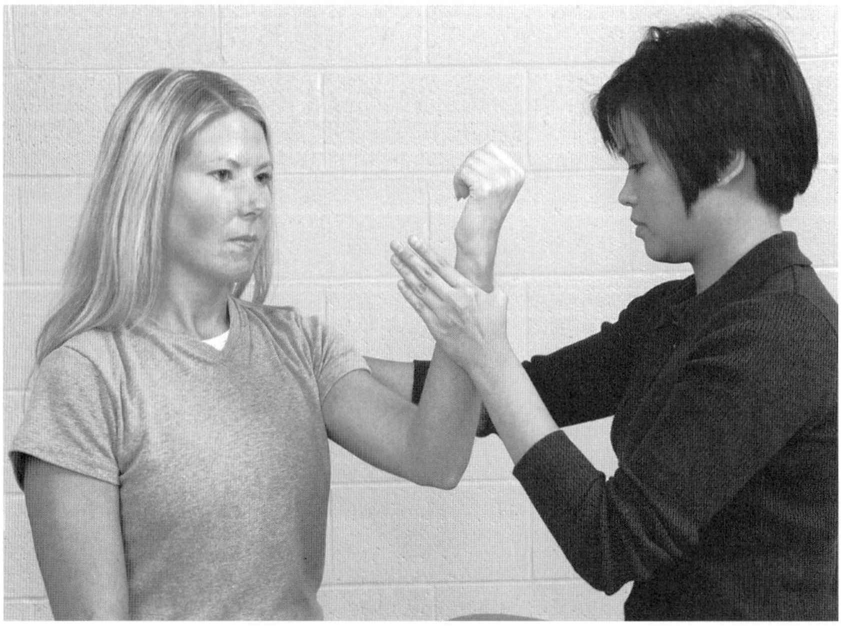

Fig. 1-1. Manual muscle screening of triceps brachii muscle. Note lack of specific patient positioning in regard to gravity.

Fig. 1-2. Manual muscle testing of triceps brachii muscle. Note positioning of patient so that muscle is acting against gravity.

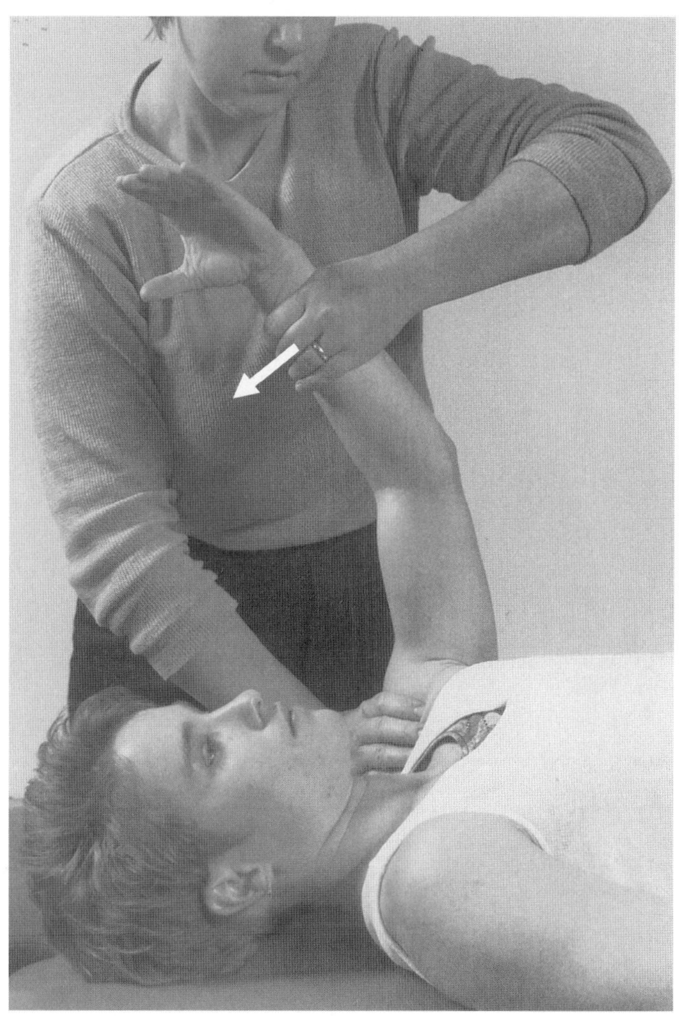

Fig. 1-3. Manual muscle screening of biceps femoris muscle. Note lack of specific patient positioning in regard to gravity.

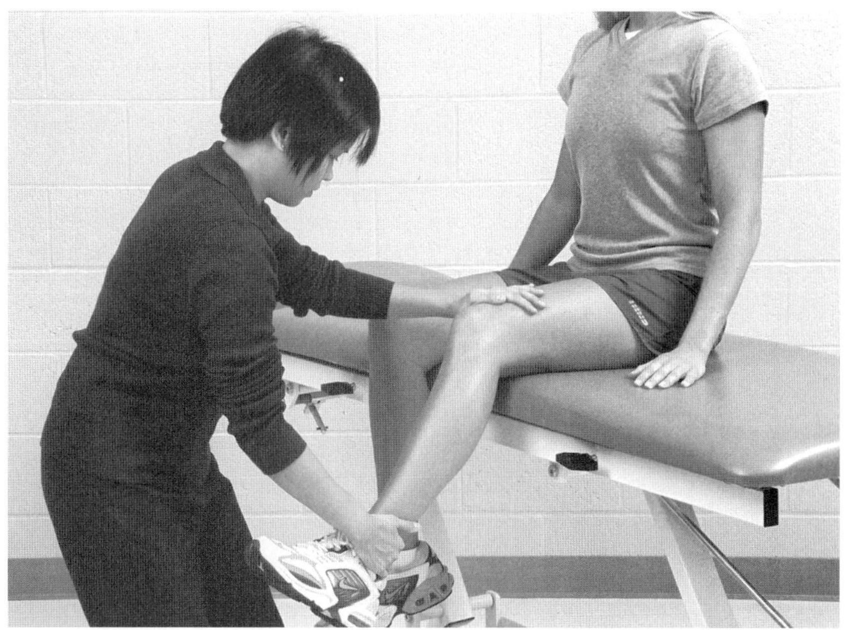

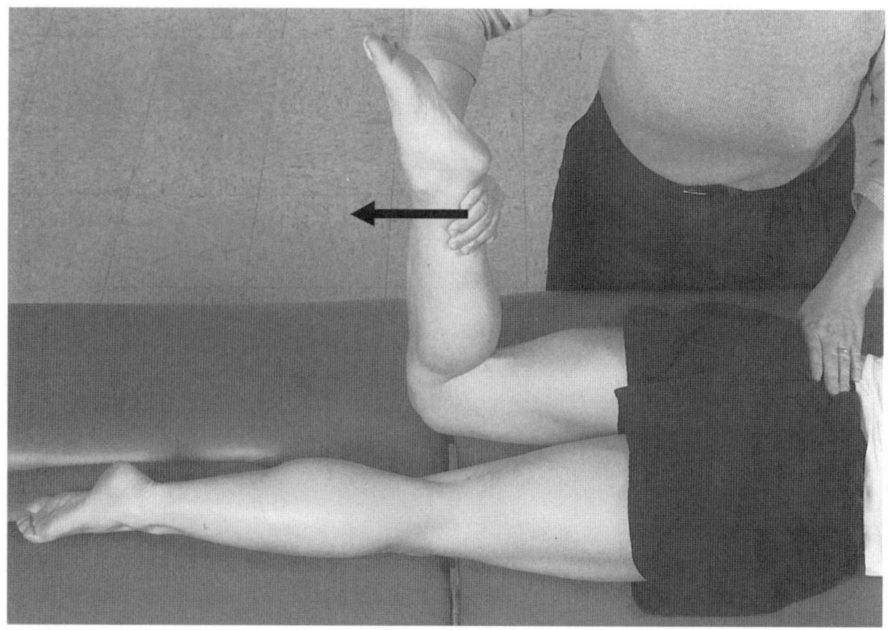

Fig. 1-4. Manual muscle testing of biceps femoris muscle. Note positioning of patient so that muscle is acting against gravity.

applying a weighting factor for muscle bulk, which makes comparison with later studies difficult.

Somewhat lower levels of reliability were reported by Iddings et al.[43] who examined both interrater and intrarater reliabilities of MMT. These authors reported levels of complete interrater agreement of 41% to 51% and agreement within plus or minus one full grade of 87% to 93%. Intrarater agreement was somewhat higher, with complete agreement occurring in 54% to 65% of the tests, whereas agreement within plus or minus one full grade was reported in 96% to 98% of the tests. The examiners in the study by Iddings et al.,[43] unlike those in the studies of Lilienfeld et al.[62] and Blair,[12] did not use a standard MMT protocol. Each examiner was allowed to use the MMT technique of his or her choice. No weighting for muscle bulk was included in this or any subsequent report on the reliability of MMT.

In a study designed to improve the standardization of MMT for use with patients with chronic renal disease, Silver et al.[87] examined the interrater reliability of a standardized protocol of MMT based on the techniques described by Daniels et al.[25] Like the previous authors, Silver et al.[87] reported their results only in terms of descriptive statistics and found complete agreement among examiners in 67% of the muscle tests performed, with agreement within a one-half grade occurring in 97% of the muscles tested. The apparently stronger reliabilities reported in this study (97% agreement within a one-half grade versus 95% within one full grade reported by earlier groups) may have been due to the strong emphasis placed by Silver et al.[87] on standardization of the technique of muscle testing and grading used.

At least three groups have used inferential statistics to analyze the reliability of MMT in the normal population. Wadsworth et al.[96] measured the intrarater reliability of MMT using five muscle groups: shoulder abductors, elbow extensors, wrist extensors, hip flexors, and knee flexors. Muscle testing protocols were standardized, and the examiner performing the testing had 8 years of clinical experience. Test-retest reliability coefficients were 0.63 for knee flexors, 0.74 for hip flexors, and 0.98 for shoulder abductors. Because grades on both test and retest for wrist and elbow extensors were the same, correlation coefficients for these muscle groups could not be calculated.

In an article published in the same year as the study by Wadsworth et al.,[96] Frese et al.[35] reported the interrater reliability of manual muscle tests of the gluteus medius and middle trapezius muscles. Interrater reliability coefficients ranged from 0.04 to 0.66, including muscle test grades below 3 (fair). Although one would expect somewhat lower interrater reliability than intrarater reliability, the reliabilities reported in the Frese et al.[35] study are quite poor. Differences in design between the studies by Wadsworth et al.[96] and Frese et al.[35] may account for much of the variation seen in the reported reliabilities. Examiners in the Frese et al.[35] study did not use standard techniques for muscle testing but were allowed to test each muscle using the technique with which the examiner was most comfortable. The muscle testing techniques of both Kendall et al.[51] and Daniels and Worthingham[25] were used, but the two techniques use different methods of positioning the patient and resisting the muscle, particularly for the middle trapezius. Additionally, the examiners participating in the Frese et al.[35] study had an average of 2.3 years of experience compared with the 8 years of experience possessed by the examiner in the other study by Wadsworth et al.[96] No mention was made in the Frese et al.[35] study of the establishment of intrarater reliability before the investigation of interrater reliability.

A study that examined both intrarater and interrater reliabilities of MMT in the healthy population was published by Brandsma et al.[16] in 1995. These researchers focused on reliability of MMT for the intrinsic muscles of the hand. Comparison was made of MMT scores obtained by one experienced examiner in a test-retest situation (intrarater reliability) and by two experienced examiners on the same group of patients (interrater reliability). Both intrarater and interrater reliabilities were calculated using Cohen's weighted kappa and ranged from 0.71 to 0.96 for intrarater and from 0.72 to 0.93 for interrater, results similar to these reported by Wadsworth et al.[96] and appreciably higher than those reported by Frese et al.[35]

Reliability of MMT in individuals with musculoskeletal and neuromuscular pathology has also been examined. In a study by Florence et al.,[34] physical therapists, all possessing 16 to 20 years of experience, performed manual muscle tests on 18 different muscle groups in males with Duchenne's muscular dystrophy. A standardized method of muscle testing was used, and a modified Medical Research Council (MRC) scale was used in grading the muscles. Intrarater reliability was calculated using Cohen's kappa, and results for individual muscle groups ranged from 0.65 to 0.93. The intrarater reliability of MRC grades 0 to 5 ranged from 0.80 to 0.99, with the highest reliabilities found in grades below 3 and the lowest reliabilities in grades 3+ (0.80), 4– (0.83), and 5– (0.83).

In a later study, another group of investigators examined the interrater reliability of performing MMT on a group of 12 children with varying types of muscular dystrophy.[33] Muscle testing was confined to those groups previously shown to be tested reliably,[34] namely shoulder abductors, elbow and hip flexors, knee extensors, and ankle dorsiflexors. All examiners (n = 12) underwent 3 days of training by an experienced tester, and a modified MCR scale was used to grade the muscle tests.[33] Examiners were divided into three groups of four testers for assessment of interrater reliability. Initially, reliability between the three groups ranged from 0.62 to 0.76, thus an additional training session was scheduled. Interrater reliability (intraclass correlation coefficients [ICCs]) averaged 0.90 subsequent to the additional training. Intrarater reliability was reported for one of the three groups of examiners and averaged 0.95 (ICC) over the 2 years of study.

A third study that examined reliability of MMT in individuals with pathology focused on a modified method of scoring muscle strength termed the MRC *sumscore*.[53] The MRC sumscore was defined by the authors as the "summation of the strength of six muscle groups tested on both sides according to the MRC scale." The six muscle groups included in the sumscore were the shoulder abductors, elbow flexors, wrist extensors, hip flexors, knee extensors, and ankle dorsiflexors. Manual muscle tests of these six muscle groups were performed bilaterally on a group of patients with Guillain-Barré syndrome, and then the MRC scores (0 to 5) for all muscle groups (six per side) were summed to achieve the MRC sumscore. Calculation of ICCs for interrater reliability for both more and less experienced examiners resulted in ICCs of 0.98 and 0.96, respectively, for the two groups of examiners.

Most of the studies cited above indicate good intrarater reliability for MMT. In instances where lower intrarater reliabilities are reported, the examiners failed to use a standardized protocol for MMT.[43] A similar observation can be made regarding the conflicting data reported for interrater reliability. Those studies reporting lower interrater reliabilities used a research protocol wherein each examiner was allowed to use his or her own method of MMT.[35,43] Higher interrater reliability was achieved when a uniform method of MMT was used by all examiners.[12,16,33,53,62,87] Clinicians should be aware that unless standardized methods of MMT are used, the reliability of MMT will suffer.

VALIDITY OF MANUAL MUSCLE TESTING

Validity has been defined as "the degree to which an instrument measures what it is purported to measure."[23] One method of assessing validity is to perform correlational studies in which two different tests are administered to the same group of patients.[73] Several researchers have compared MMT with muscle testing using HHD, strain gauge, or isokinetic dynamometer to determine whether a correlation exists between these forms of muscle testing.[1,2,9,13,15,32,40,86] Beasley[9] was the first to examine the correlation between MMT and HHD. He compared the two methods of muscle testing on the knee extensor muscles of a group of normal and postpolio children aged 9 to 12 years. The results of Beasley's study,[9] which included only children with knee extensor muscles of grade fair or higher, found poor correlations between MMT and HHD scores particularly in muscles with grades of normal or good. The children in Beasley's study with as much as a 50% reduction in knee extensor strength were assigned an MMT grade of normal, and the same MMT grade was assigned to muscles with as much as a 20% to 25% difference in strength as measured by HHD.[9]

Studies performed subsequent to Beasley's study[9] have demonstrated similar problems with correlation between MMT and HHD, MMT and strain gauge, and MMT and isokinetic dynamometry above an MMT grade of good (4).[1,2,13,15,32,77,86] However, for muscles with an MMT grade below 4, high correlations have been demonstrated between MMT and HHD[13,15,40,77,86] and between MMT and strain gauge.[1] Schwartz et al.[86] also demonstrated that specific MMT grades (from poor-plus to good) correspond to discrete ranges of myometry scores, indicating that "although MMT is a subjective measurement of strength, there are associated underlying objective parameters as represented by myometry data."

The high correlations exhibited between MMT and HHD for muscles with an MMT grade below 4 demonstrate that both methods of testing measure strength, a good indication of the validity of MMT. Additionally, MMT scores at 72 hours after spinal cord injury have been shown to be good predictors of functional muscle recovery at the zone of injury[18] and of functional status of patients with quadriplegia at rehabilitation discharge,[59] indicating that MMT possesses predictive validity.

In summary, MMT is a valid method of measuring muscle strength as substantiated by several groups of researchers. MMT is designed to measure the entire range of muscle strength, from 0 (no evidence of muscle contraction) through 5 (movement through the complete range of motion against gravity and maximum resistance). Other forms of muscle strength testing, such as HHD and isokinetic dynamometry, are limited in their ability to accurately assess the lower grades of muscle strength. However, when MMT scores exceed grade 4, the MMT loses much of its ability to discriminate between gradations of strength, whereas HHD and isokinetic dynamometry retain their sensitivities in these ranges. In instances in which documentation of strength levels is critical above an MMT grade of 4, the examiner might be well advised to use an alternative form of measuring muscle strength such as HHD or isokinetic dynamometry.[31]

CONSIDERATIONS IN THE PERFORMANCE OF THE MANUAL MUSCLE TEST

MMT is designed to measure muscle strength, which has been defined as the ability of the muscle to develop tension against resistance.[57,84] The amount of tension generated by a muscle in a given situation will vary according to a number of factors, including number and firing rate of motor units activated, length of the muscle at the time of the contraction, muscle cross-sectional area, fiber type composition of the muscle, point of application of resistance, stabilization techniques used, and motivational state of the subject.[7,11,38,46,89,97,100] Although the anatomic and physiologic factors influencing muscle strength cannot be controlled in a testing situation, many factors such as patient positioning, stabilization, point of force application, and use of motivation can and should be controlled. These factors should be standardized for each muscle test to maintain consistency and to optimize the validity and reliability of MMT.

Instructing and Motivating the Patient

Patients should be provided with explicit instructions before performing any examination technique, including strength testing. Studies have indicated that standardization of instructions may improve the reliability of the results of strength testing.[20] Such testing techniques require the full cooperation and best effort of the patient, factors that are likely to be enhanced as the patient's understanding of the purpose of the test increases.

Before beginning the procedure, describe to the patient exactly what will be taking place and why the measurement must be performed. If any testing apparatus is to be used during the procedure, show the patient the tool, and explain, in layperson's terms, its purpose and how it will be used. Instruct the patient in the position he or she is to assume, again using layperson's terms and avoiding terms such as *supine* or *prone*. Explain to the patient the necessity of exerting maximum effort during the examiner's resistance of each movement for the results of the testing to be meaningful. Detailed explanations of every step of the procedure should not be provided initially, as this will only confuse the patient. A brief, general explanation is best at this point, and further explanations may be given once the procedure is in progress, remembering to use layperson's terms with all explanations provided. An example of initial patient instructions is as follows:

> Ms. Bates, I need to measure how much strength you have in the muscles that straighten your elbow. This information will tell me how much your strength is improving and will give me an idea of what changes we need to make in your plan of care. At a certain point during the test, I will push against your arm and will ask you to try to keep me from bending your elbow. When I do that, I want you to try as hard as you can to keep me from bending your elbow. I will need you to lie on this table on your back so that I can test your muscles.

Patient Positioning

Proper positioning of the patient during muscle testing is essential in ensuring that the appropriate muscle is being tested and in preventing substitution by other muscles. The choice of a preferred patient position for each MMT is based on several criteria. For a position to be considered optimal, all criteria should be met. Although this is not an exhaustive list, the major criteria in selecting a preferred patient position for measurement of muscle strength are as follows:

1. **The distal joint segment should be placed in the desired position in relation to the pull of gravity.** Gravity plays an integral part in MMT, and the patient's ability or inability to move the designated part against gravity determines the position in which the patient should be placed for the muscle test. Patients who are able to move the appropriate joint actively through the complete range of motion against gravity are placed in the so-called gravity-resisted position for testing. That is, the patient is positioned so that the distal segment of the joint must move against gravity to complete the range of motion. An individual who is unable to move the distal segment of the tested joint through the complete range of motion against gravity is placed in the so-called gravity-eliminated position to test the muscle (see Clinical Comment: Gravity-Eliminated Testing Position).
2. **The patient should be positioned so that the proximal segment of the joint is most easily and optimally stabilized.** Stabilization of the proximal joint segment is of critical importance during MMT. Stabilization may be provided via several avenues, including use of a firm testing surface, patient positioning, muscle activity by the patient, and manual holds by the examiner.[97] The origin of the muscle being tested must be firmly fixed so that maximal contraction against the insertion can occur, although stabilization over the muscle belly being tested should be avoided. Failure to provide such fixation may cause underestimation of strength by the examiner due to the patient's inability to produce optimal force with the muscle or may result in substitutions by other muscles in an effort to compensate for an inability of the agonist to generate sufficient force.[39,84,89,97] The examiner should be consistent in the use and technique of stabilization each time a muscle test is performed.
3. **The patient should be positioned so that the motion to be performed is not restricted in any way.** Motion should not be blocked by external objects, such as the examining table, or by internal forces, such as muscle tightness in the antagonistic muscle group.
4. **The joint should be positioned at the beginning of the range of motion for the movement to be performed.** Such positioning allows observation of the movement through the complete range of motion, an observation that is necessary to accurate grading of muscle strength.

5. **The patient should be positioned so that the examiner's body mechanics are optimized during stabilization and application of resistance.** The examiner should not endure undue stress in providing stabilization of the proximal joint segment or while resisting the distal segment (gravity-resisted test only). Aids to patient positioning, such as the use of a hi-low examining table, a stool for the examiner, or other devices, may be needed to facilitate optimal body mechanics for the examiner.
6. **The patient must be able to assume the position.** In some cases, this criterion cannot be met (see Case 2-1, Chapter 2), and an alternative position must be used. In any instance in which an alternative position is used, the examiner should design the position so that it adheres to the previous five criteria as closely as possible.

CLINICAL COMMENT: GRAVITY-ELIMINATED TESTING POSITION

The term *gravity eliminated* has been commonly used with reference to MMT for many years. However, the term is rather misleading in that gravity is not *eliminated*, but the effects of gravity are *lessened* in this position. The examiner positions the patient so that movement of the distal joint segment is neither directly resisted nor directly assisted by gravity.

FURTHER EXPLORATION: PATIENT POSITIONING—GRAVITY-RESISTED VERSUS "GRAVITY-ELIMINATED"

The following activities are designed to help the student evaluate and design preferred and alternative patient positions for muscle strength testing.

1. Without looking at the specific manual muscle tests described in this text, design a testing position that would allow each of the muscles listed in item 2 to work in the following scenarios:
   a. Against gravity
   b. In a "gravity-eliminated" position
   c. With gravity (assisted by the pull of gravity)
2. The following muscles are to be tested:
   a. Biceps brachii
   b. Pectoralis major
   c. Semimembranosus
   d. Peroneus longus
3. Apply the criteria for positioning (listed in the previous section) to each of the positions you devised. How well does each position meet the criteria listed? Make modifications to your devised position as needed, so that it adheres more closely to the positioning criteria.

FURTHER EXPLORATION: PALPATING MUSCLE CONTRACTION

The following activities are designed to assist the student in detection of muscle contraction via manual palpation.

1. Ask a partner to sit in a comfortable chair without arms.
2. Position yourself in front of and to one side of your partner, with one hand on the superior aspect of your partner's shoulder and the other hand (fingertips) on the anterior aspect of your partner's arm (see Figure 2-86).
3. Ask your partner to strongly contract the elbow flexors (partner's elbow will flex) while you palpate the muscle contraction.
4. Now, ask your partner to contract the elbow flexors weakly, producing little or no movement of the elbow.
5. Have your partner repeatedly perform weak contractions of the elbow flexors while you palpate the entire length of the biceps brachii muscle. Determine where along the muscle the weak contraction is best detected.
6. Repeat the exercise for the knee extensors (see Figure 4-62), palpating the quadriceps muscles over the anterior aspect of the thigh.

CLINICAL COMMENT: MUSCLE PALPATION

An examiner should always confirm a contraction of the muscle being tested by palpating the muscle during the patient's active movement. Palpation is critical for very weak muscles, especially if little to no active movement is produced (grades below 2). Additionally, palpation of the muscle during active movement by the patient assists the examiner in ruling out the possibility of substitution by other muscles.

FURTHER EXPLORATION: STABILIZATION

The following activities are designed to help the student appreciate the effects of proper versus improper positioning on the muscle strength test.

1. Perform a gravity-resisted test of the muscle groups listed below, first including, and then excluding, the stabilization described. Refer to the page numbers provided for a description of each test.
   a. Elbow flexors, p. 99–101
   b. Shoulder horizontal adductors, p. 78–79
   c. Hip lateral rotators, p. 298–301
   d. Knee flexors, p. 310–314
2. As each muscle group is tested, observe the results of the test with and without stabilization. Answer the following questions.
   a. What differences do you observe in each situation?
   b. Is the patient able to generate a more forceful contraction with the proximal joint segment stabilized or unstabilized?
   c. Do substitutions by other muscle groups occur more often when the proximal joint segment is stabilized or unstabilized?
3. Would stabilization of the proximal joint segment be more, or less, important in a patient with muscle weakness? Why?

APPLICATION OF RESISTANCE

Testing muscles with MMT grades above 3 requires the application of manual resistance by the examiner. In this text, the "break test" is used to apply resistance. During a break test, the examiner applies resistance against the patient's body part, increasing the resistance applied until the patient's muscular contraction is overcome by the examiner (the patient "breaks") or until maximum resistance has been applied and held for 4 to 5 seconds.[14,20,89] Both "make" and "break" tests are used in MMT, and both have been found to be reliable, although more force appears to be produced by muscles tested under the "break" than under the "make" method.[14]

When applying resistance, the examiner should generally apply the force *perpendicular to the distal end of the distal segment of the joint being tested*. With the exception of a few cases, resistance should not be applied any further distally than the distal end of the bone on which the muscle being tested inserts (i.e., resistance for the deltoid should be applied over the distal end of the humerus). Although this technique may result in a shorter lever arm for the application of resistance, the possible confounding of the results that can occur when one applies resistance over weak distal joints is avoided.

For most muscle tests in this text, resistance is applied at the end of the gravity-resisted range of motion. In many cases, this is not the strongest point in the range of motion for the muscle being tested.[11,100] However, application of force at the end of the gravity-resisted range of motion provides a consistent point for the application of resistance and may help prevent the examiner from overestimating the patient's strength, a documented tendency in MMT grades above 4.[9] As maximum force generated by the muscle changes significantly with muscle length and joint angle,[7,38,89] the examiner must exercise extreme care to apply resistance at the same point in the range of motion each time the muscle is tested. To do otherwise would result in an unreliable muscle test.

FURTHER EXPLORATION: LEVER ARM LENGTH

The following activities are designed to help the student understand the effects of lever arm length on the perceived strength of the muscle contraction.

1. Perform a gravity-resisted test of the muscle groups listed below, using the two different points of resistance described. Refer to the page numbers provided for a description of the patient positioning and stabilization for each test.
   a. Shoulder abductors, p. 69–70
      i. Resistance just proximal to elbow
      ii. Resistance at wrist
   b. Scapular adductors (middle trapezius), p. 28–29
      i. Resistance on scapula
      ii. Resistance at wrist

CLINICAL COMMENT: USE OF RESISTANCE DURING MMT

If a patient is able to move through the complete range of motion when placed in a gravity-resisted position, one knows at that point that the muscle test grade is at minimum a 3. Manual resistance is then applied by the examiner and the muscle's strength is assessed according to the scale in Table 1–1.

Resistance is not applied to a muscle that is unable to move through the complete range of motion against gravity.

2. As each muscle group is tested, observe the results of the test for each resistance point utilized. Answer the following questions.
   a. Does the patient seem stronger or weaker when using the more proximal resistance point? The more distal point?
   b. Would changing the position of the intervening joint(s) make a difference in the results when the distal resistance point is used (e.g., flexing the elbow)?
3. Could pathology involving the intervening joint affect the results of the muscle test when the distal resistance point is used? If so, how?

GRADING SCALE

As discussed, a variety of methods have been used in grading the MMT. The scale used in this text is a modification of the MRC scale in that either numbers or word/letters can be used (Table 1-1). Plus and minus designations are included at some points, but extreme caution is advised when assigning plus or minus grades, especially when the testing is being performed by a novice examiner. The accurate use of plus/minus designations requires considerable skill and experience in the art of MMT.

Definitions for each grade are provided in Table 1-1 with the corresponding number/word designation. One should be aware that grades above 3 tend to be much more subjective than grades 3 or below due to the inability to precisely define the amount of force that constitutes "maximum," "moderate," or "minimal" resistance. Additionally, evidence indicates that there are serious questions regarding the ability to differentiate strength differences in the grades above 3 or to identify losses in muscle strength of up to 50%.[9,13,40,85,86,96]

Given the subjectivity of muscle grades above 3, one should be particularly careful regarding the method of application of manual resistance. To maintain consistency in testing, each individual examiner must *not* deviate from the amount of resistance that the examiner defines as maximal, moderate, and

Table 1-1. MUSCLE TEST GRADES

NUMBER (AND LETTER) GRADE	WORD GRADE	DEFINITION
0	Zero	No evidence of contraction by vision or palpation
1 (Tr)	Trace	Slight contraction; no motion
2– (P–)	Poor minus	Movement through partial test range in gravity-eliminated position
2 (P)	Poor	Movement through complete test range in gravity-eliminated position
2+ (P+)	Poor plus	Movement through complete test range in gravity-eliminated position and through up to one half of test range against gravity
3– (F–)	Fair minus	Movement through complete test range in gravity-eliminated position and through more than one half of test range against gravity
3 (F)	Fair	Movement through complete test range against gravity
3+ (F+)	Fair plus	Movement through complete test range against gravity and able to hold against minimum resistance
4 (G)	Good	Movement through complete test range against gravity and able to hold against moderate resistance
15 (N)	Normal	Movement through complete test range against gravity and able to hold against maximum resistance

minimal. One might be tempted to assign a grade of 5 to the triceps muscle of an elderly female who "breaks" under moderate resistance, rationalizing that this patient's strength is probably normal for someone of her age and gender. Such allowances and rationalizations result in poor reliability of MMT both in repeated tests by the same examiner (intrarater reliability) and between tests by different examiners (interrater reliability). By maintaining a consistent definition of each level of resistance an examiner is able to ensure that reliability in testing is maximized.

The use of numerals as grades for muscle testing should not lead one to think that muscle test grades are interval measures. Michaels[73] defines an interval scale as "one on which the categories are numerical units and the intervals between the units are assumed to be of equal size." The intervals between muscle test grades are not equal, and therefore the MMT grading scale is more appropriately classified as an ordinal scale. One should not then consider that the difference in strength between the muscle test grades of 5 and 4 is equivalent to the difference in strength between the muscle test grades of 4 and 3. Such assumptions are invalid and cannot be made regarding ordinal data.

Table 1-2 provides a format and rationale for performing a manual muscle test. The use of a standardized procedure for all muscle tests will assist the examiner in achieving consistency, which is critical in establishing reliability of MMT.

Table 1-2. FORMAT AND RATIONALE FOR MANUAL MUSCLE TEST

STEPS	RATIONALE
1. Explain purpose of procedure to patient.	Patient needs to be fully engaged in process to achieve accurate strength measurement.
2. Place patient in gravity-resisted position.	Assume patient can move against gravity unless patient is known to be unable to do so, then use gravity-eliminated position.
3. Stabilize proximal joint segment.	Proper stabilization of proximal muscle attachment allows tested muscle to produce optimal contraction and decreases likelihood of substitution by synergists.
4. Instruct patient in specific movement to be performed while passively moving distal segment through ROM.	Shows patient exact movement expected and allows assessment of patient's available ROM.
5. Return distal segment to starting position.	Patient must return to starting position so full movement can be performed actively.

Continued

CLINICAL COMMENT: RANGE OF MOTION

The criteria for assigning a strength grade during MMT are based in part on the patient's ability to perform the movement in question through the *complete range of motion. Complete range of motion* refers to the total range of movement possible for the joint being tested unless the patient has some structural impairment making complete movement at the joint in question impossible (i.e., loose body in the joint). In such a case, the patient's *available* range of motion becomes the complete range of motion for the joint.

Table 1-2. FORMAT AND RATIONALE FOR MANUAL MUSCLE TEST—cont'd

STEPS	RATIONALE
6. Ask patient to perform movement while muscle is being palpated and stabilization maintained.	Muscle is palpated to confirm presence of active muscle contraction.
7. Apply resistance (only if patient can complete ROM against gravity) by moving palpating hand to appropriate position for resisting the muscle.	**Resistance is applied only if patient is able to complete movement against gravity.** Since palpation is no longer necessary, palpating hand should be used to apply resistance.
	OR
8. Reposition patient in gravity-eliminated position (if patient is **unable** to complete ROM against gravity), and repeat steps 3-6. **Do not apply resistance**.	Patients unable to move against gravity should be retested in a position where the resistance of gravity on the movement is lessened. If patient is unable to complete movement against gravity, resistance is not appropriate.
9. Assign appropriate muscle grade.	Grade should be assigned based on scale in Table 1-1.

Rom, range of motion.

References

1. Aitkens S, Lord J, Bernauer E, et al. Relationship of manual muscle testing to objective strength measurements. *Muscle Nerve* 1989;12:173–177.
2. Andersen H, Jakobsen J. A comparative study of isokinetic dynamometry and manual muscle testing of ankle dorsal and plantar flexors and knee extensors and flexors. *Eur Neurol* 1997; 37:239–242.
3. Asmussen E, Heeboll-Nielsen K. Isometric muscle strength in relation to age in men and women. *Ergonomics* 1962;5:167–169.
4. Bäckman E, Johansson V, Hager B, et al. Isometric muscle strength and muscular endurance in normal persons aged between 17 and 70 years. *Scand J Rehab Med* 1995;27:109–117.
5. Baldauf KL, Swenson DK, Medeiros JM, et al. Clinical assessment of trunk flexor muscle strength in healthy girls 3 to 7 years of age. *Phys Ther* 1984;64:1203–1208.
6. Baltzopoulos V, Brodie DA: Isokinetic dynamometry: Applications and limitations. *Sports Med* 1989;8(2):101–116.
7. Bandy WD, Lovelace-Chandler V. Determinants of muscle strength. *Phys Ther Pract* 1992; 2:1–10.
8. Bassey EJ, Bendall MJ, Pearson M. Muscle strength in the triceps surae and objectively measured customary walking activity in men and women over 65 years of age. *Clin Sci* 1988; 74:85–89.
9. Beasley WC. Influence of method on estimates of normal knee extensor force among normal and postpolio children. *Phys Ther Rev* 1956;36:21–41.
10. Bemben MG, Massey BH, Bemben DA, et al. Isometric muscle force production as a function of age in healthy 20- to 74-yr-old men. *Med Sci Sports Exerc* 1991;23:1302–1310.
11. Bender JA, Kaplan HM. The multiple angle testing method for the evaluation of muscle strength. *J Bone Joint Surg* 1963;45A:135–140.
12. Blair L. The role of the physical therapist in the evaluation studies of the poliomyelitis vaccine field trials. *Phys Ther Rev* 1957;37:437–447.
13. Bohannon RW. Manual muscle test scores and dynamometer test scores of knee extension strength. *Arch Phys Med Rehabil* 1986;67:390–392.
14. Bohannon RW. Make tests and break tests of elbow flexor muscle strength. *Phys Ther* 1988; 68:193–194.
15. Bohannon RW. Measuring knee extensor muscle strength. *Am J Phy Med Rehabil* 2001; 80:13–18.
16. Brandsma JW, Schreuders TAR, Birke JA, et al. Manual muscle strength testing: Intraobserver and interobserver reliabilities for the intrinsic muscles of the hand. *J Hand Ther* 1995;8:185–190.
17. Brown LE, Weir JP. ASEP procedures recommendation, I: assessment of muscular strength and power. *J Exerc Phys* 2001;4:1–21.
18. Brown PJ, Marino RJ, Herbison GJ, et al. The 72-hour examination as a predictor of recovery in motor complete quadriplegia. *Arch Phys Med Rehabil* 1991;72:546–548.
19. Byl NN, Wells L, Grady D, et al. Consistency of repeated isokinetic testing: effect of different examiners, sites, and protocols. *Isokinetics Ex Sci* 1991;1:122–130.

20. Caldwell LS, Chaffin DB, Dukes-Dobos FN, et al. A proposed standard procedure for static muscle strength testing. *Am Ind Hyg Assoc J* 1974;35:201–206.
21. Christ CB, et al. Maximal voluntary isometric force production characteristics of six muscle groups in women aged 25 to 74 years. *Am J Hum Biol* 1992;4:537–545.
22. Clement FJ. Longitudinal and cross-sectional assessments of age changes in physical strength as related to sex, social class, and mental ability. *J Gerontology* 1974;29:423–429.
23. Currier DP. *Elements of Research in Physical Therapy*, 2nd ed. Baltimore: Williams & Wilkins, 1984.
24. Cyriax, J. *Textbook of Orthopaedic Medicine*, 8th ed. Philadelphia: Baillière Tindall, 1982.
25. Daniels L, Williams M, Worthingham C. *Muscle Testing: Techniques of Manual Examination.* Philadelphia: WB Saunders, 1947.
26. Daniels L, Worthingham C. *Muscle Testing: Techniques of Manual Examination*, 5th ed. Philadelphia: WB Saunders, 1986.
27. Delito A. Isokinetic dynamometry. *Muscle Nerve* 1990; S53–57.
28. De Ste Croix MBA, Armstrong N, Welsman JR, et al. Longitudinal changes in isokinetic leg strength in 10–14-year-olds. *Ann Hum Biol* 2002;29:50–62.
29. Duvall EN, Houtz SJ, Hellebrandt FA. Reliability of a single effort muscle test. *Arch Phys Med* 1947;April:213–218.
30. Dvir Z. Clinical applicability of isokinetics: a review. *Clin Biomech* 1991;6:133–144.
31. Dvir Z. Grade 4 in manual muscle testing: the problem with submaximal strength assessment. *Clin Rehabil* 1997;11:36–41.
32. Ellenbecker TS. Muscular strength relationship between normal grade manual muscle testing and isokinetic measurement of the shoulder internal and external rotators. *Isokinet Exerc Sci* 1996;6:51–56.
33. Escolar DM, Henricson EK, Mayhew J, et al. Clinical evaluator reliability for qualitative and manual muscle testing measures of strength in children. *Muscle Nerve* 2001;24:787–793.
34. Florence JM, Pandya S, King WM, et al: Intrarater reliability of manual muscle test (Medical Research Council scale) grades in Duchenne's muscular dystrophy. *Phys Ther* 1992;72:115–126.
35. Frese E, Brown M, Norton BJ. Clinical reliability of manual muscle testing: Middle trapezius and gluteus medius muscles. *Phys Ther* 1987;67:1072–1076.
36. Frontera WR, Hughes VA, Lutz KJ, et al. A cross-sectional study of muscle strength and mass in 45- to 78-yr-old men and women. *J Appl Physiol* 1991;71:644–650.
37. Frontera WR, Hughes VA, Fielding RA, et al. Aging of skeletal muscle: a 12-yr longitudinal study. *J Appl Physiol* 2000;88:1321–1326.
38. Gordon AM, Huxley AF, Julian FJ. The variation in isometric tension with sarcomere length in vertebrate muscle fibres. *J Physiol* 1966;184:170–192.
39. Hart DL, Stobbe TJ, Till CW, et al. Effect of trunk stabilization on quadriceps femoris muscle torque. *Phys Ther* 1984;64:1375–1380.
40. Herbison GJ, Issac Z, Cohen ME, et al. Strength post-spinal cord injury: myometer vs manual muscle test. *Spinal Cord* 1996;34:543–548.
41. Hislop HJ, Montgomery J. *Daniels and Worthingham's Muscle Testing*, 7th ed. Philadelphia: WB Saunders, 1995.
42. Hurley BF. Age, gender, and muscular strength. *J Gerontology Ser A* 1995;50A:41–44.
43. Iddings DM, Smith LK, Spencer WA. Muscle testing, II: reliability in clinical use. *Phys Ther Rev* 1961;41:249–256.
44. Jacoby SM. Isokinetics in rehabilitation. In: Prentice WE, Voight MJ, eds. *Techniques in Musculoskeletal Rehabilitation.* New York: McGraw-Hill; 2001:153–166.
45. Jakobsson F, Borg K, Edstrom L. Fibre-type composition, structure and cytoskeletal protein location of fibres in anterior tibial muscle. *Acta Neuropathol* 1990;80:459–468.
46. Johnson BL, Nelson JK. Effect of different motivational techniques during training and in testing upon strength performance. *Res Q* 1967;38:630–636.
47. Johnson T. Age-related differences in isometric and dynamic strength and endurance. *Phys Ther* 1982;62:985–989.
48. Jordan A, Mehlsen J, Bulow M, et al. Maximal isometric strength of the cervical musculature in 100 healthy volunteers. *Spine* 1999;24:1343–1348.
49. Kanehisa H, Ilegawa S, Tsunoda N, et al. Strength and cross-sectional areas of reciprocal muscle groups in the upper arm and thigh during adolescence. *Int J Sports Med* 1995:16:54–60.
50. Kanehisa H, Yata H, Ikegawa S, et al. A cross-sectional study of the size and strength of the lower leg muscles during growth. *Eur J Appl Physiol* 1995;72:150–156.
51. Kendall FP, McCreary EK, Provance PG. *Muscles: Testing and Function*, 4th ed. Baltimore: Williams & Wilkins, 1993.
52. Kent-Braun JA, Ng AV. Specific strength and voluntary muscle activity in young and elderly women and men. *J Appl Physiol* 1999:87:22–29.
53. Kleyweg RP, Van Der Meché FGA, Schmitz PIM. Interobserver agreement in the assessment of muscle strength and functional abilities in Guillain-Barré syndrome. *Muscle Nerve* 1991;14:1103–1109.

54. Klitgaard H, Mantoni M, Schiaffino S, et al. Function, morphology and protein expression of ageing skeletal muscle: a cross-sectional study of elderly men with different training backgrounds. *Acta Physiol Scand* 1990;140:119–139.
55. Knuttgen HG, Kraemer WJ. Terminology and measurement in exercise performance. *J Appl Sport Sci Res* 1987;1:1–10.
56. Kraemer WJ, Fry AC. *Strength Testing: Development and Evaluation of Methodology. Physiological Assessment of Human Fitness*. Champaign, IL: Human Kinetics, 1995:115–138.
57. Kroemer KH. Human strength: terminology, measurement and interpretation of data. *Human Factors* 1972;12:515–522.
58. Larsson L, Sjodin B, Karlsson J. Histochemical and biochemical changes in human skeletal muscle with age in sedentary males, age 22-65 years. *Acta Physiol Scand* 1978;103:31–39.
59. Lazar RB, Yarkony GM, Ortolano D, et al. Prediction of functional outcome by motor capability after spinal cord injury. *Arch Phys Med Rehabil* 1989;70:819–822.
60. Lexell J, Taylor T. Variability in muscle fiber areas in whole human quadriceps muscle: effects of increasing age. *J Anat* 1991;174:239–249.
61. Lexell J, Taylor T, Sjostrom M. What is the cause of the ageing atrophy? Total number, size and proportion of different fiber types studied in whole vastus lateralis muscle from 15- to 83-year-old men. *J Neurol Sci* 1988;84:275–294.
62. Lilienfeld AM, Jacobs M, Willis M. A study of the reproducibility of muscle testing and certain other aspects of muscle scoring. *Phys Ther Rev* 1954;34:279–289.
63. Lindle RS, Metter EJ, Lynch NA, et al. Age and gender comparisons of muscle strength in 654 women and men aged 20-93 yr. *J Appl Physiol* 1997;83:1581–1587.
64. Lovett RW. The treatment of infantile paralysis: preliminary report. *JAMA* 1915;64:2118.
65. Lovett RW. *The treatment of Infantile Paralysis*. Philadelphia: P Blakiston, 1916.
66. Lovett RW, Martin EG. Certain aspects of infantile paralysis with a description of a method of muscle testing. *JAMA* 1916;66:729–733.
67. Lowman CL. A method of recording muscle tests. *Am J Surg* 1927;3:588–591.
68. Magee DJ. *Orthopedic Physical Assessment*, 4th ed. Philadelphia: WB Saunders, 2002.
69. Marks R. The effect of ageing and strength training on skeletal muscle. *Australian J Physiotherapy* 1992;38:9–19.
70. Martin EG, Lovett RW. A method of testing muscular strength in infantile paralysis. *JAMA* 1915;65:1512–1513.
71. Mathiowetz V, Wiemer DM, Federman SM. Grip and pinch strength: norms for 6- to 19-year-olds. *Am J Occupational Ther* 1986;40:705–711.
72. Metter EEJ, Conwit R, Tobin J, et al. Age-associated loss of power and strength in the upper extremities in women and men. *J Gerontology* 1997;52A:B267–276.
73. Michaels E: Evaluation and research in physical therapy. *Phys Ther* 1982;62:828–834.
74. Moffroid M, Whipple R, Hofkosh J, et al. A study of isokinetic exercise. *Phys Ther* 1969;49:735–747.
75. Nevill AM, Holder RL, Baxter-Jones A, et al. Modeling development changes in strength and aerobic power in children. *J Appl Physiol* 1998;84:963–970.
76. Newman LB. A new device for measuring muscle strength: the myometer. *Arch Phys Med Rehabil* 1949;30:234–237.
77. Noreau L, Vachon J. Comparison of three methods to assess muscular strength in individuals with spinal cord injury. *Spinal Cord* 1998;36:716–723.
78. Phillips BA, Lo SK, Mastaglia FL. Muscle force measured using "break" testing with a hand-held myometer in normal subjects aged 20 to 69 years. *Arch Phys Med Rehabil* 2000;81:653–661.
79. Pousson M, Lepers R, Van Hoecke J. Changes in isokinetic torque and muscular activity of elbow flexor muscles with age. *Exp Gerontology* 2001;36:1687–1698.
80. Ramos E, Frontera WR, Llopart A, et al. Muscle strength and hormonal levels in adolescence: gender related differences. *Int Sports Med* 1998;19:526–531.
81. Robertson A, Deitz J. A description of grip strength in preschool children. *Am J Occupational Ther* 1988;42:647–652.
82. Rothstein JM. Muscle biology: clinical considerations. *Phys Ther* 1982;62:1823–1830.
83. Round JM, Jones DA, Honour JW, et al. Hormonal factors in the development of differences in strength between boys and girls during adolescence: a longitudinal study. *Ann Hum Biol* 1999;26:49–62.
84. Sapega AA. Muscle performance evaluation in orthopaedic practice. *J Bone Joint Surg* 1990;72A:1562–1574.
85. Sarantini AJ, Gleim GW, Melvin M, et al. The relationship between subjective and objective measurements of strength. *J Orthop Sports Phys Ther* 1980;2:15–19.
86. Schwartz S, Cohen ME, Herbison GJ, et al. Relationship between two measures of upper extremity strength: manual muscle test compared to hand-held myometry. *Arch Phys Med Rehabil* 1992;73:1063–1068.
87. Silver M, McElroy A, Morrow L, et al. Further standardization of manual muscle testing for clinical study: applied in chronic renal disease. *Phys Ther* 1970;50:1456–1465.

88. Sinaki M, Limburg PJ, Wollan PC, et al. Correlation of trunk muscle strength with age in children 5 to 18 years old. *Mayo Clin Proc* 1996;71:1047–1054.
89. Smidt GL, Rogers MW. Factors contributing to the regulation and clinical assessment of muscular strength. *Phys Ther* 1982;62:1283–1290.
90. Stoll T, Huber E, Seifert B, et al. Maximal isometric muscle strength: normative values and gender-specific relation to age. *Clin Rheumatol* 2000;19:105–113.
91. Tabin GC, Gregg JR, Bonci T. Predictive leg strength values in immediately prepubescent and postpubescent athletes. *Am J Sports Med* 1985;13:387–389.
92. Tomlinson BE, Irving D. The number of limb motor neurons in the human lumbosacral cord throughout life. *J Neurol Sci* 1977;34:213–219.
93. Tomonaga M. Histochemical and ultrastructural changes in senile human skeletal muscle. *J Am Geriatr Soc* 1977;25:125–131.
94. Tzankoff SP, Norris AH. Effect of muscle mass decrease on age-related BMR changes. *J Appl Physiol* 1977;43:1001–1006.
95. Vandervoort AA. Effects of ageing on human neuromuscular function: implications for exercise. *Can J Spt Sci* 1992;17:178–184.
96. Wadsworth CT, Krishnan R, Sear M, et al. Intrarater reliability of manual muscle testing and hand-held dynametric muscle testing. *Phys Ther* 1987;67:1342–1347.
97. Wakim KG, Gersten JW, Martin GM. Objective recording of muscle strength. *Arch Phys Med Rehabil* 1950;31:90–99.
98. Watkins MR, Harris BA. Evaluation of isokinetic muscle performance. *Clin Sports Med* 1983;2:37–53.
99. Williams M. Manual muscle testing, development and current use. *Phys Ther Rev* 1956;36:797–805.
100. Williams M, Stutzman L. Strength variation through the range of joint motion. *Phys Ther Rev* 1959;39:145–152.
101. Wright WG. Muscle training in the treatment of infantile paralysis. *Boston Med Surg J* 1912;167:567–574.
102. Young A, Stokes M, Crowe M. Size and strength of the quadriceps muscles of old and young women. *Eur J Clin Investigation* 1984;14:282–287.

2

TECHNIQUES of MANUAL MUSCLE TESTING: UPPER EXTREMITY

■ SCAPULAR ELEVATION

UPPER TRAPEZIUS, LEVATOR SCAPULAE (Fig. 2-1)

Fig. 2-1.

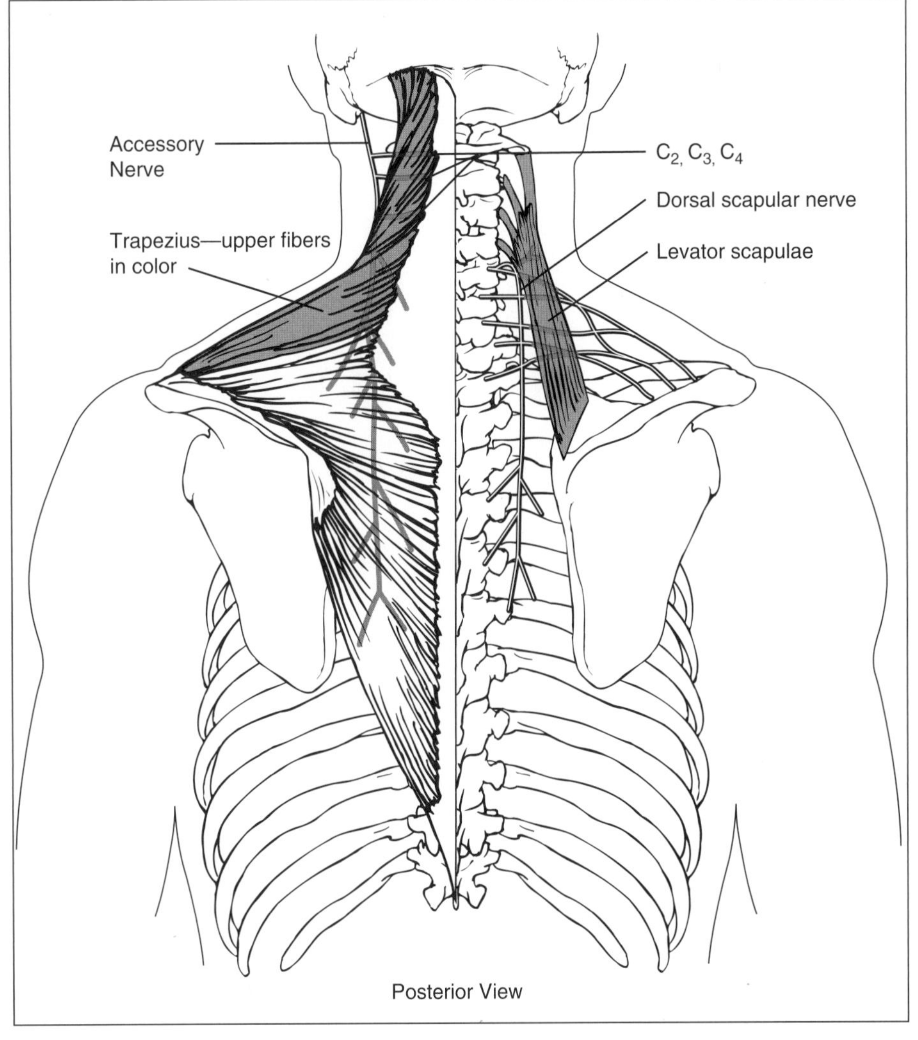

	ATTACHMENTS	NERVE SUPPLY	FUNCTION
Upper trapezius	Origin: External occipital protuberance, medial ⅓ of the superior nuchal line, ligamentum nuchae, spinous process of the seventh cervical vertebra Insertion: Lateral ⅓ of the clavicle	Peripheral nerve: Spinal portion of the accessory nerve (CN XI); ventral rami of C3, C4 Nerve root: C1–C5	Scapular elevation; upward rotation of the scapula (in conjunction with the inferior fibers)
Levator scapulae	Origin: Transverse processes of the upper four cervical vertebrae Insertion: Vertebral border of the scapula, between the superior angle and the root of the scapular spine	Peripheral nerve: Dorsal scapular nerve, C3, C4 Nerve root: C3, C4, C5	Scapular elevation, adduction, and downward rotation

Gravity-Resisted Test (Grades 5, 4, and 3)

Patient position: Seated with arms at sides, hands not in contact with supporting surface (Fig. 2-2).

Stabilization/palpation: Stabilization is unnecessary with bilateral test. Palpate upper trapezius just lateral to cervical spinous processes (Fig. 2-2).

Fig. 2-2.

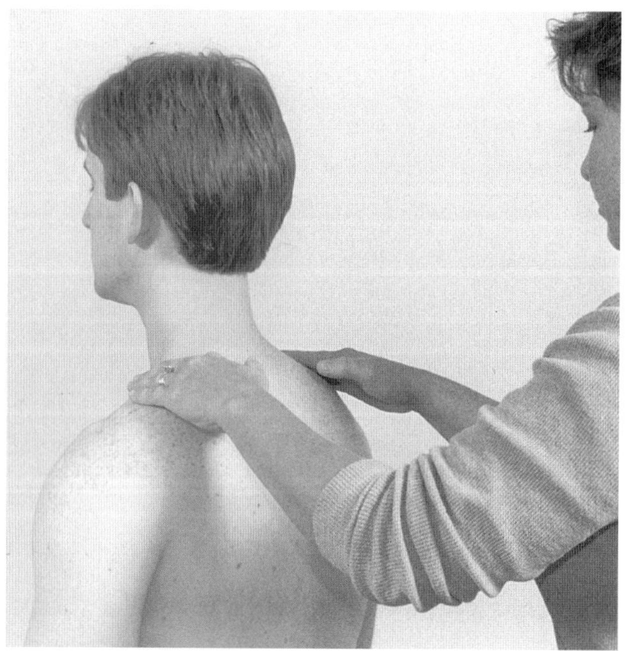

Examiner action: While instructing patient in motion desired, move patient's shoulders toward ears (scapular elevation) as far as possible. Return patient to starting position. Performing passive movement allows determination of patient's available range of motion (ROM) and shows patient exact movement desired.

Patient action: Patient performs active shoulder elevation while examiner maintains palpation of upper trapezius (Fig. 2-3).

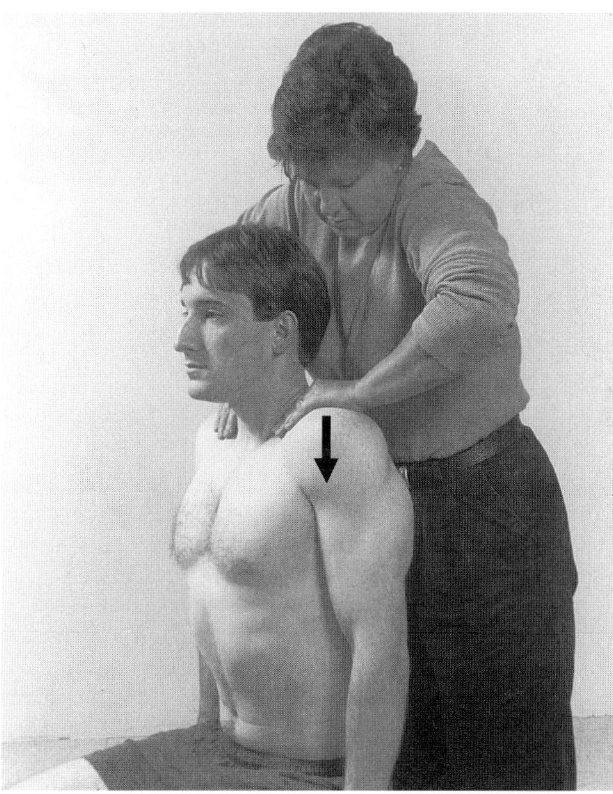

Fig. 2-3. Arrow indicates direction of resistance.

Resistance: Apply resistance over superior aspect of shoulders in an inferior direction (Fig. 2-3).

Gravity-Eliminated Test (Grades Below 3)

For patients unable to move completely through available ROM against gravity.

Patient position: Prone with arms at sides; head in neutral rotation. Shoulders may be supported anteriorly by examiner to reduce drag against supporting surface (Fig. 2-4). If support of shoulders is necessary, palpation will be impossible with bilateral test. Then, right and left muscles should be tested separately.

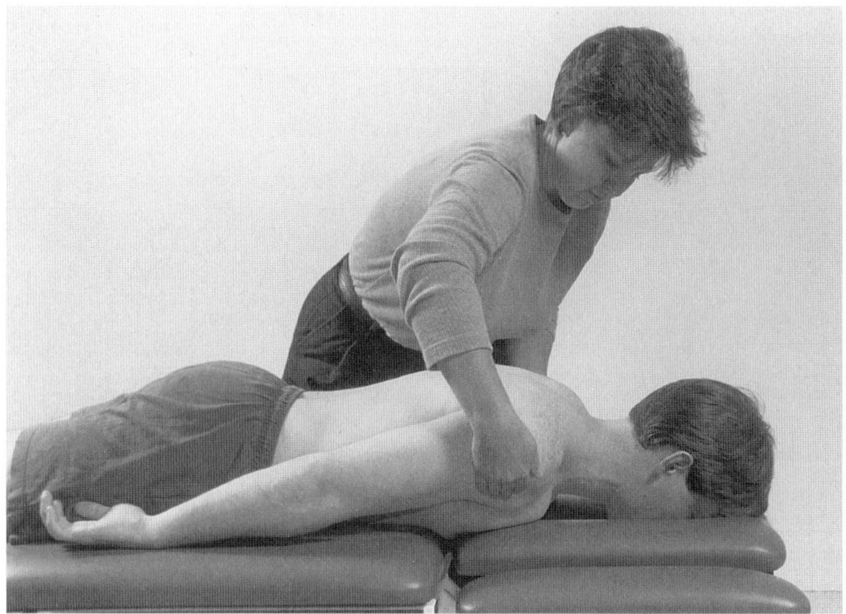

Fig. 2-4.

Stabilization/palpation: Stabilization is unnecessary with bilateral test. Palpate upper trapezius just lateral to cervical spinous processes (Fig. 2-5).

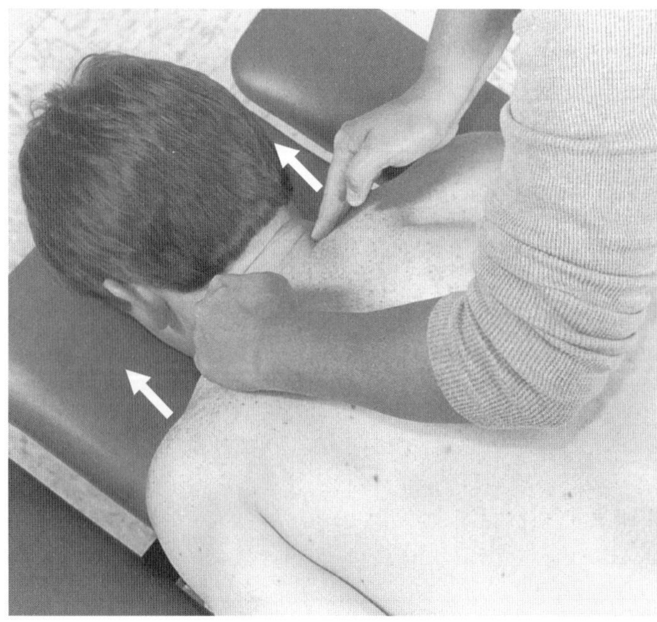

Fig. 2-5. Arrows indicate direction of movement.

Examiner action: As in gravity-resisted test.

Patient action: As in gravity-resisted test (Fig. 2-5).

■ SCAPULAR ADDUCTION

MIDDLE TRAPEZIUS (Fig. 2-6)

Fig. 2-6.

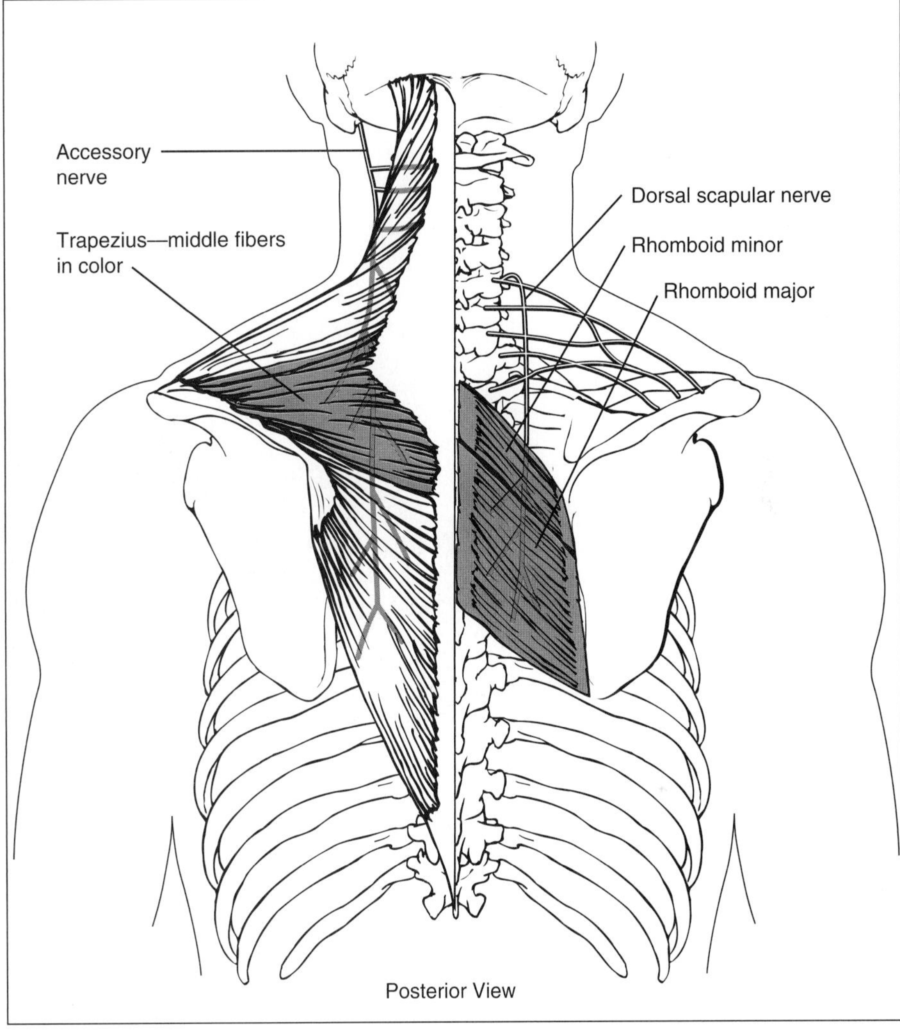

	ATTACHMENTS	NERVE SUPPLY	FUNCTION
Middle trapezius	Origin: Spinous processes of the 1st through 5th thoracic vertebrae and intervening supraspinal ligament Insertion: Medial border of the acromion process of the scapula; the spine of the scapula	Peripheral nerve: Spinal portion of the accessory nerve (CN XI); ventral rami of C3, C4 Nerve root: C1–C5	Scapular adduction

Gravity-Resisted Test (Grades 5, 4, and 3)

Patient position: Prone with upper extremity in 90° shoulder abduction and full lateral rotation, 90° elbow flexion. Patient's head is turned to contralateral side (Fig. 2-7).

Fig. 2-7.

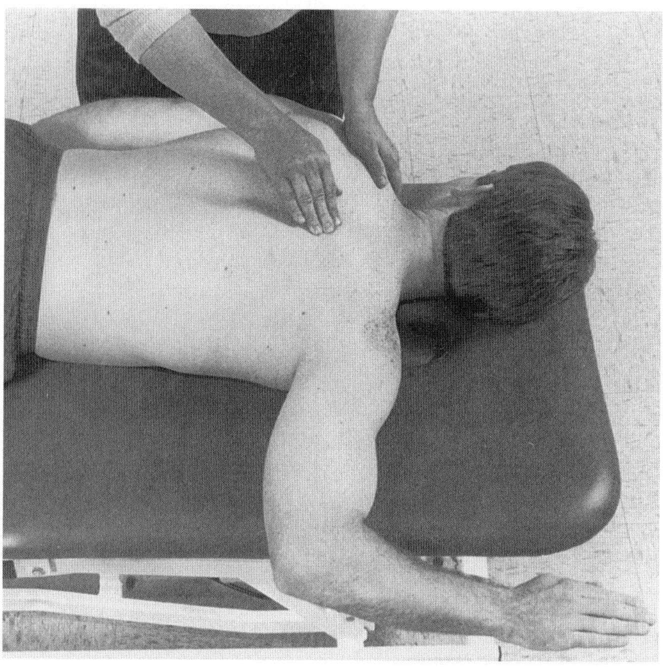

Stabilization/palpation: Stabilize with one hand over opposite thorax to prevent trunk rotation. Palpate middle trapezius between vertebral border of scapula and spinous processes of lower cervical and upper thoracic vertebrae ipsilaterally (Fig. 2-7).

Examiner action: While instructing patient in motion desired, move patient's scapula through full range of adduction while keeping upper extremity positioned as described earlier. Return patient to starting position. Performing passive movement allows determination of patient's available ROM and shows patient exact movement desired.

Patient action:

Patient performs active scapular adduction (accompanied by horizontal abduction of arm) while examiner maintains stabilization of thorax and palpation of middle trapezius (Fig. 2-8).

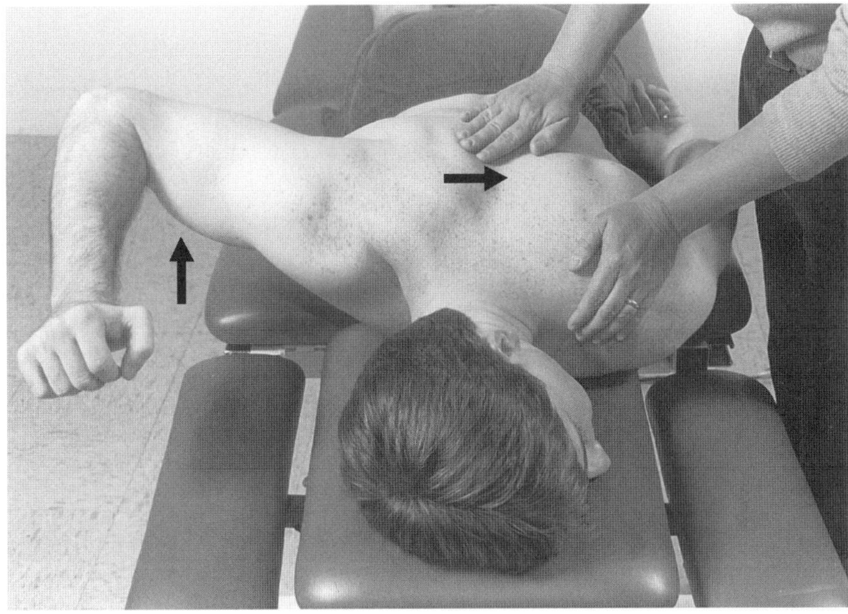

Fig. 2-8. Arrows indicate direction of movement.

Resistance:

Apply resistance over lateral aspect of scapula in direction of scapular abduction. Palpating hand is moved to lateral aspect of scapula to apply resistance (Fig. 2-9).

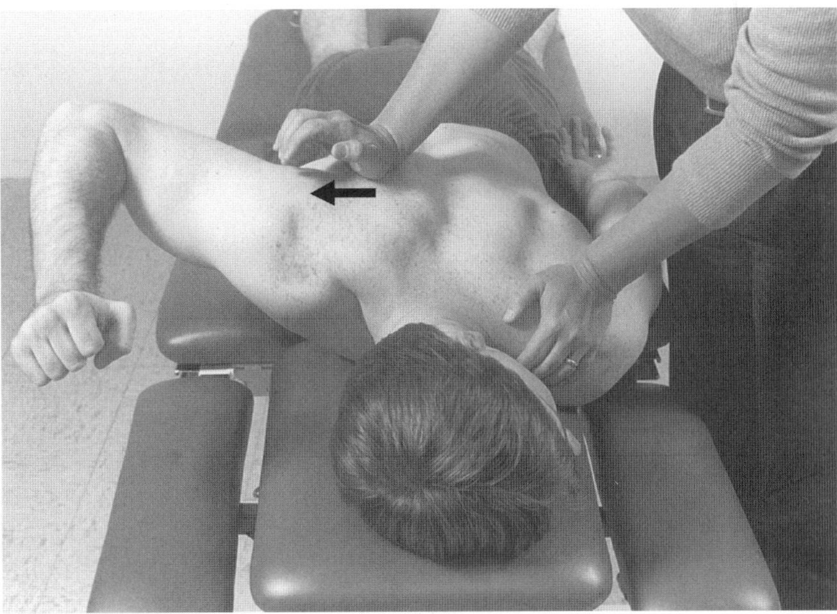

Fig. 2-9. Arrow indicates direction of resistance.

Gravity-Eliminated Test (Grades Below 3)

For patients unable to move completely through available ROM against gravity.

Patient position: Seated with shoulder abducted to 90° and in full lateral rotation, elbow slightly flexed. Upper extremity should be supported on a firm, smooth surface. Talcum powder and a cloth may be placed between limb and supporting surface to reduce friction (Fig. 2-10; starting position of upper extremity not shown).

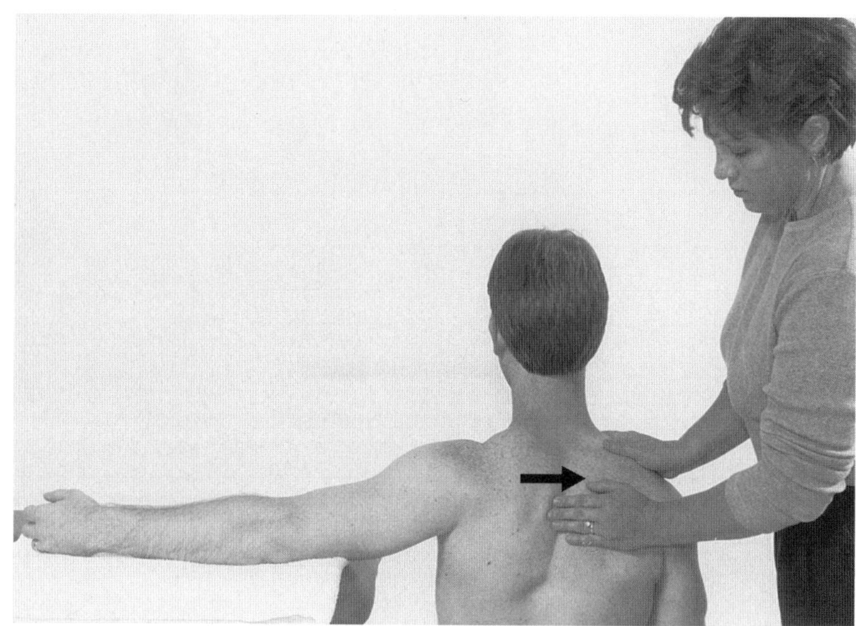

Fig. 2-10. Arrow indicates direction of movement.

Stabilization/palpation: Stabilize over superior aspect of opposite shoulder to prevent trunk rotation. Palpation occurs as in gravity-resisted test (Fig. 2-10).

Examiner action: As in gravity-resisted test.

Patient action: As in gravity-resisted test (Fig. 2-10).

COMMON SUBSTITUTIONS

1. Patient may rotate trunk toward ipsilateral side; can be prevented through stabilization of thorax.
2. In presence of middle trapezius weakness, contraction of posterior deltoid will still allow horizontal abduction of humerus. Care should be taken to observe scapula for movement so that horizontal abduction of humerus is not mistaken for scapular adduction.

■ SCAPULAR ADDUCTION—ALTERNATIVE TEST

MIDDLE TRAPEZIUS

Lever arm in this alternative test is increased by applying resistance on forearm rather than scapula. Application of resistance on forearm requires strong posterior deltoid and triceps muscles. This test is advocated by Kendall et al. (1993).

Gravity-Resisted Test (Grades 5, 4, and 3)

Patient position: Prone with upper extremity in 90° shoulder abduction and complete external rotation, 0° elbow extension. Patient's head is turned to contralateral side (Fig. 2-11).

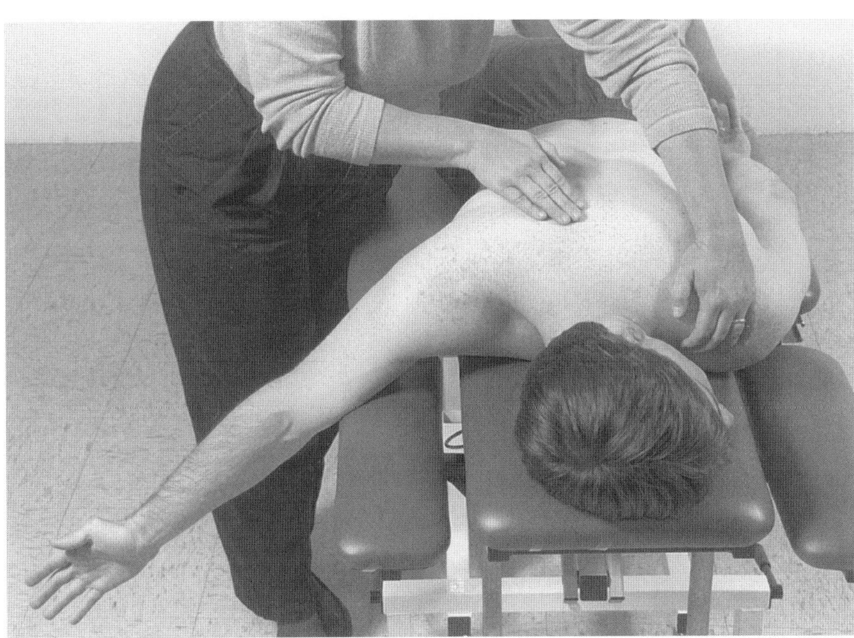

Fig. 2-11.

Stabilization/palpation: Stabilize with one hand over opposite thorax to prevent trunk rotation. Palpate middle trapezius between vertebral border of scapula and spinous processes of lower cervical and upper thoracic vertebrae ipsilaterally (Fig. 2-11).

Examiner action: While instructing patient in motion desired, move patient's scapula through full range of adduction, keeping upper extremity positioned as described earlier. Return patient to starting position. Performing passive movement allows determination of patient's available ROM and shows patient exact movement desired.

Patient action: Patient performs active scapular adduction (accompanied by horizontal abduction of arm) while examiner maintains stabilization of thorax and palpation of middle trapezius (Fig. 2-12).

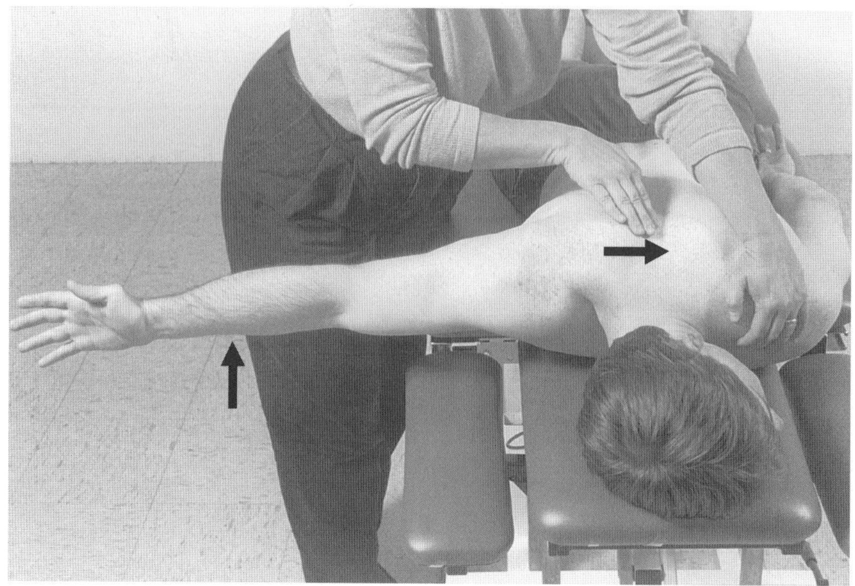

Fig. 2-12. Arrows indicate direction of movement.

Resistance:

Apply resistance over dorsum of distal forearm in direction of horizontal adduction of arm. Palpating hand is moved to distal forearm to apply resistance. Patient is graded on ability to keep *scapula,* not humerus, fixed during resistance (Fig. 2-13).

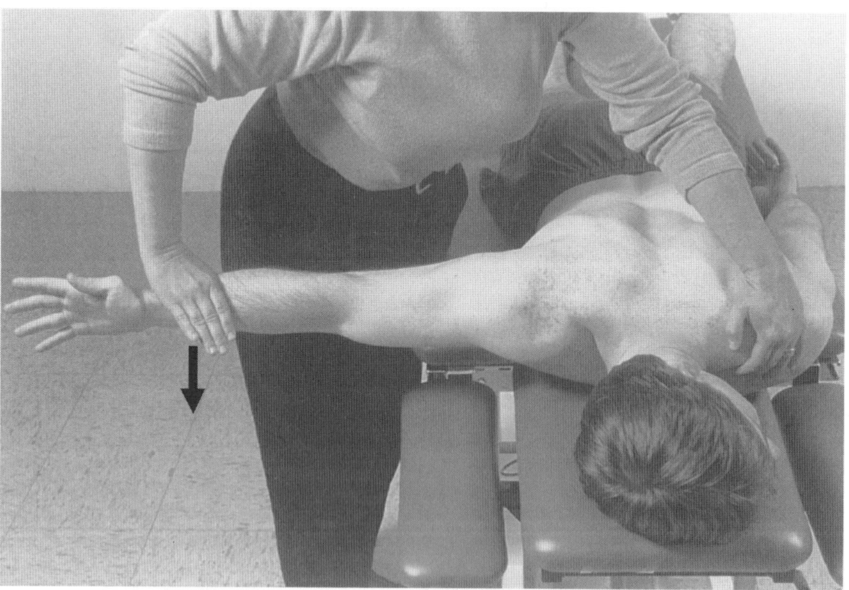

Fig. 2-13. Arrow indicates direction of resistance.

Gravity-Eliminated Test (Grades Below 3)

For patients unable to move completely through available ROM against gravity.

Patient position: Seated with shoulder abducted to 90° and in full lateral rotation, elbow slightly flexed. Upper extremity should be supported on a firm, smooth surface. Talcum powder and a cloth may be placed between limb and supporting surface to reduce friction (Fig. 2-14; starting position of upper extremity not shown).

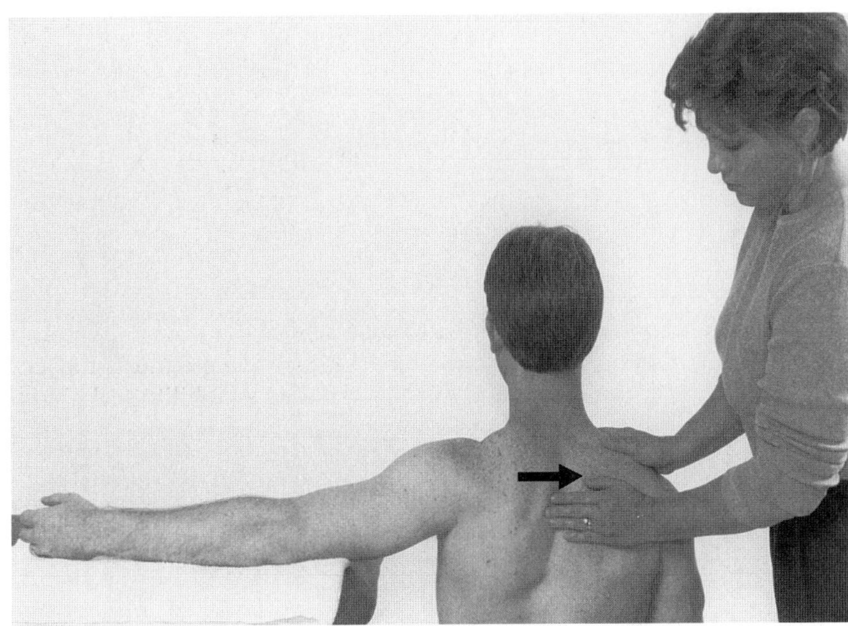

Fig. 2-14. Arrow indicates direction of movement.

Stabilization/palpation: Stabilize over superior aspect of opposite shoulder to prevent trunk rotation. Palpation occurs as in gravity-resisted test (Fig. 2-14).

Examiner action: As in gravity-resisted test (see p. 28).

Patient action: As in gravity-resisted test (see Fig. 2-14).

COMMON SUBSTITUTIONS

1. Patient may rotate trunk toward ipsilateral side; can be prevented through stabilization of thorax.
2. In presence of middle trapezius weakness, contraction of posterior deltoid will still allow horizontal abduction of humerus. Care should be taken to observe scapula for movement so that horizontal abduction of humerus is not mistaken for scapular adduction.

■ SCAPULAR ADDUCTION AND DEPRESSION

LOWER TRAPEZIUS (Fig. 2-15)

Fig. 2-15.

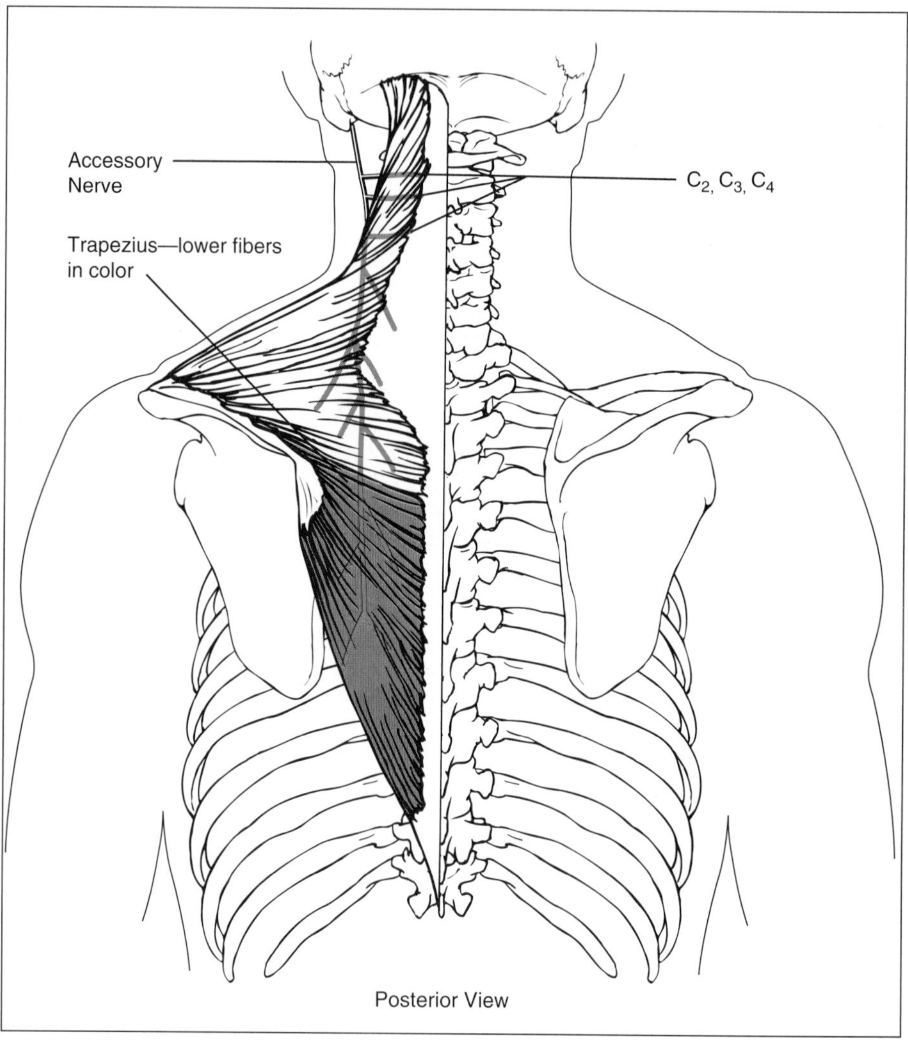

	ATTACHMENTS	NERVE SUPPLY	FUNCTION
Lower trapezius	Origin: Spinous processes of the 6th through 12th thoracic vertebrae and intervening supraspinal ligaments Insertion: Tubercle on the medial end of the scapular spine	Peripheral nerve: Spinal portion of the accessory nerve (CN XI); ventral rami of C3, C4 Nerve root: C1–C5	Scapular depression, upward rotation of the scapula (in conjunction with the superior fibers)

Gravity-Resisted Test (Grades 5 and 4)

Patient position: Prone with upper extremity in approximately 130° shoulder abduction, 0° elbow extension. Patient's head is turned to contralateral side (Fig. 2-16).

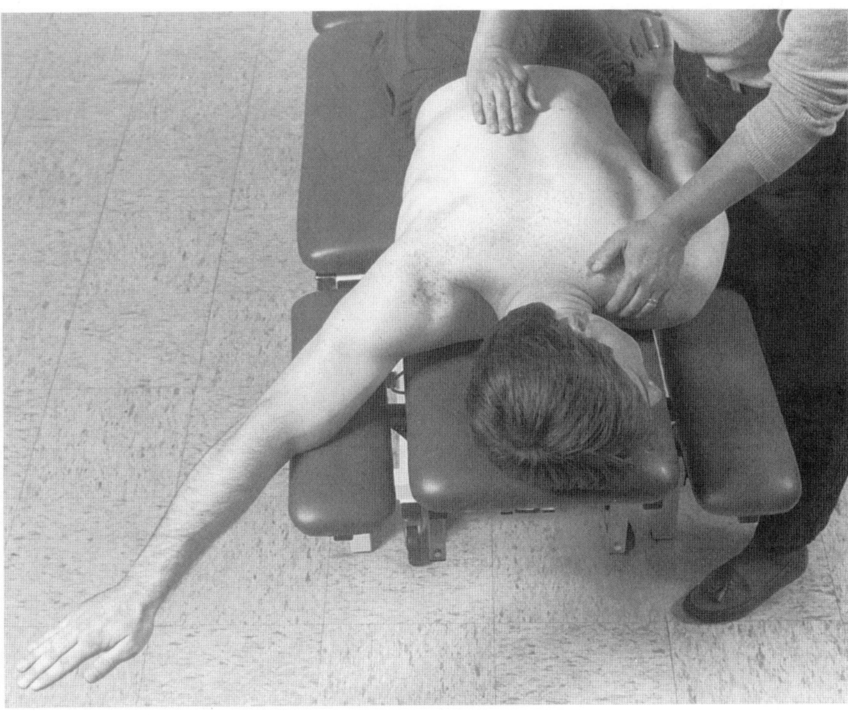

Fig. 2-16.

Stabilization/palpation: Stabilize with one hand over posterior aspect of opposite thorax. Palpate lower trapezius between root of scapular spine and spinous processes of lower thoracic vertebrae (Fig. 2-16).

Examiner action: While instructing patient in motion desired, move patient's scapula through full range of adduction and depression by elevating arm off table, keeping patient's shoulder and elbow in position described earlier. Return patient to starting position. Performing passive movement allows determination of patient's available ROM and shows patient exact movement desired.

Patient action:

Patient performs adduction and depression of scapula by elevating arm, while examiner maintains stabilization of thorax and palpation of lower trapezius (Fig. 2-17).

Fig. 2-17. Arrows indicate direction of movement.

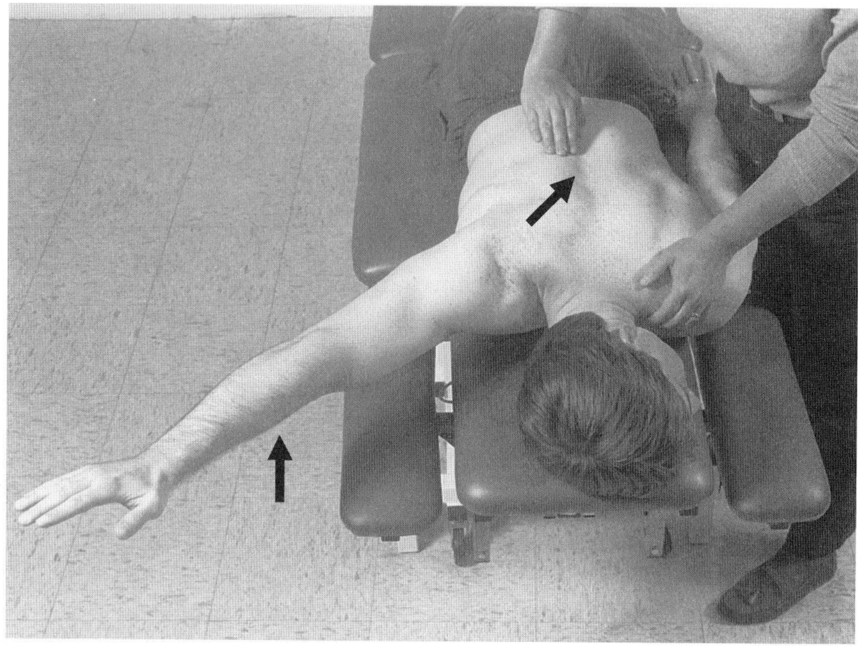

Resistance:

Apply resistance over lateral aspect of scapula in direction of scapular abduction and elevation. Palpating hand is moved to lateral aspect of scapula to apply resistance (Fig. 2-18).

Fig. 2-18. Arrow indicates direction of resistance.

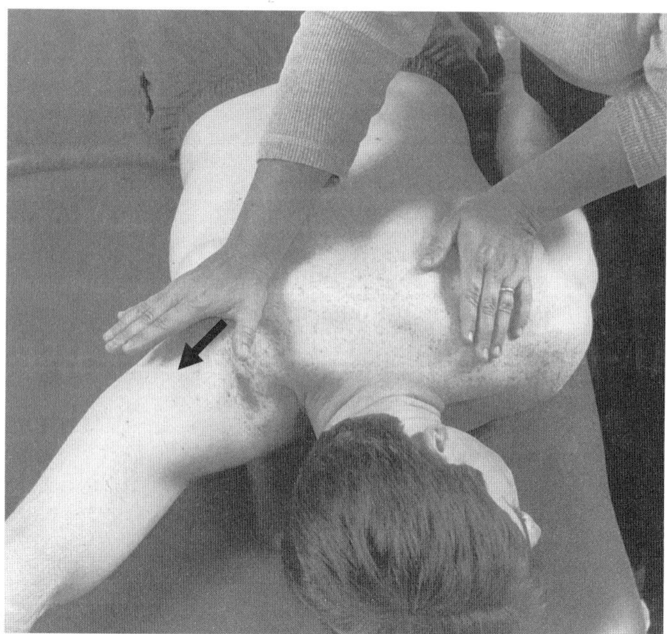

Grades 3 and Below

There is no separate test of this muscle for grades below 3. Grading is altered as follows to accommodate lack of a gravity-eliminated position:

For grade 3: Patient elevates arm through full available ROM with accompanying scapular adduction and downward rotation but against no resistance.

For grade 2: Patient elevates arm through partial ROM against no resistance.

For grade 1: No motion, but a palpable contraction is present. Palpation occurs as described earlier (see Fig. 2-16).

For grade 0: No motion or contraction is present.

■ SCAPULAR ADDUCTION AND DOWNWARD ROTATION

RHOMBOID MAJOR AND MINOR (Fig. 2-19)

Fig. 2-19.

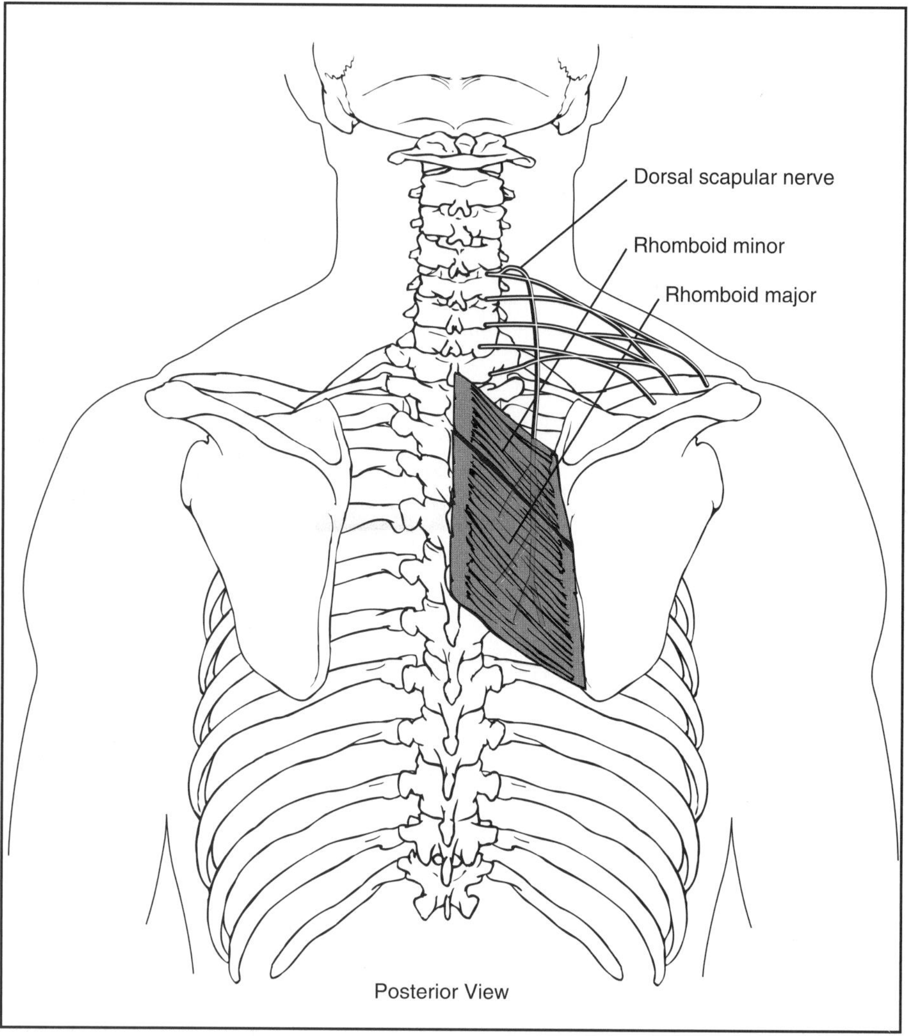

	ATTACHMENTS	NERVE SUPPLY	FUNCTION
Rhomboid major	Origin: Spinous processes of T2–T5 and intervening supraspinous ligament Insertion: Vertebral border of the scapula between the spine and the inferior angle	Peripheral nerve: Dorsal scapular nerve Nerve root: C5	Adduction, downward rotation, and elevation of the scapula
Rhomboid minor	Origin: Spinous processes of C7 and T1 and the inferior aspect of the ligamentum nuchae Insertion: Base of the spine of the scapula	Peripheral nerve: Dorsal scapular nerve Nerve root: C5	Adduction and elevation of the scapula

Gravity-Resisted Test (Grades 5, 4, and 3)

Patient position: Prone with upper extremity behind back. Shoulder in medial rotation and adduction so dorsum of hand is in contact with ipsilateral gluteal region. Patient's head is turned to contralateral side (Fig. 2-20).

Fig. 2-20.

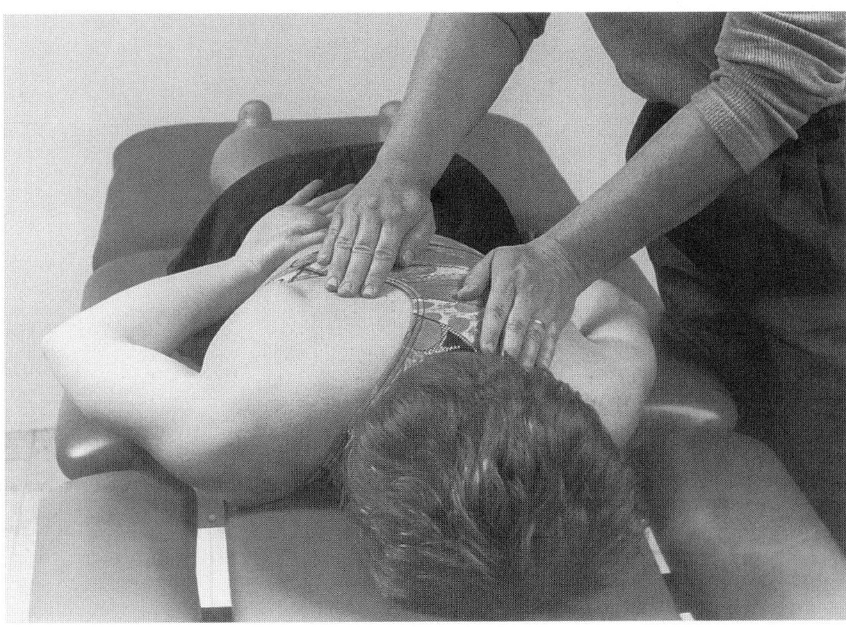

Stabilization/palpation: Stabilize with one hand over contralateral thorax. Palpate over ipsilateral rhomboids between vertebral border of scapula and spinous processes of C7 to T5 (Fig. 2-20).

Examiner action: While instructing patient in motion desired, move patient's scapula through full range of adduction and downward rotation while raising dorsum of patient's hand away from back. Return patient to starting position. Performing passive movement allows determination of patient's available ROM and shows patient exact movement desired.

Patient action: Patient performs scapular adduction and downward rotation (dorsum of patient's hand should not be allowed to remain in contact with body). Examiner maintains palpation and stabilization during patient's movement (Fig. 2-21).

Resistance: Apply resistance on vertebral border of scapula in direction of scapular abduction and upward rotation. Palpating hand is moved to vertebral border of scapula to apply resistance (Fig. 2-22).

Fig. 2-21. Arrows indicate direction of movement.

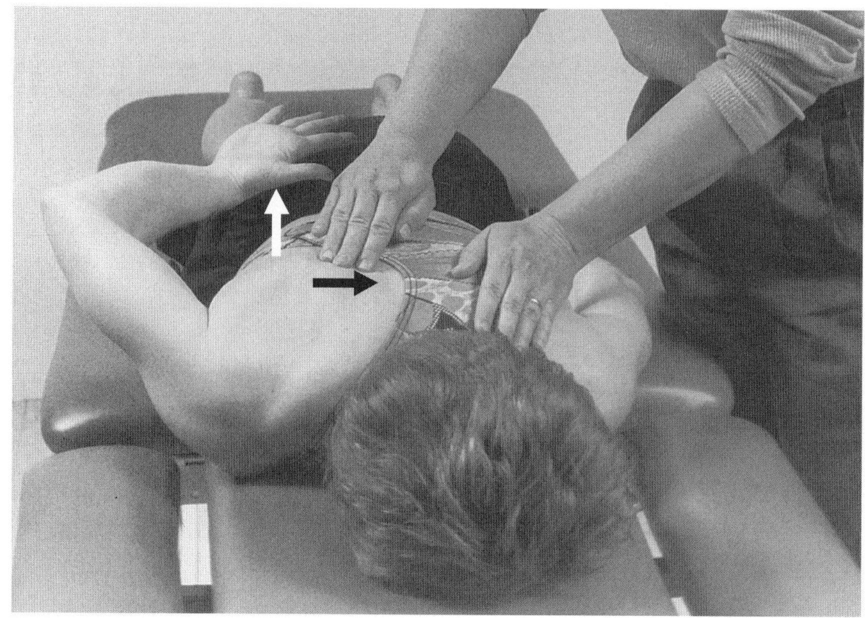

Fig. 2-22. Arrow indicates direction of resistance.

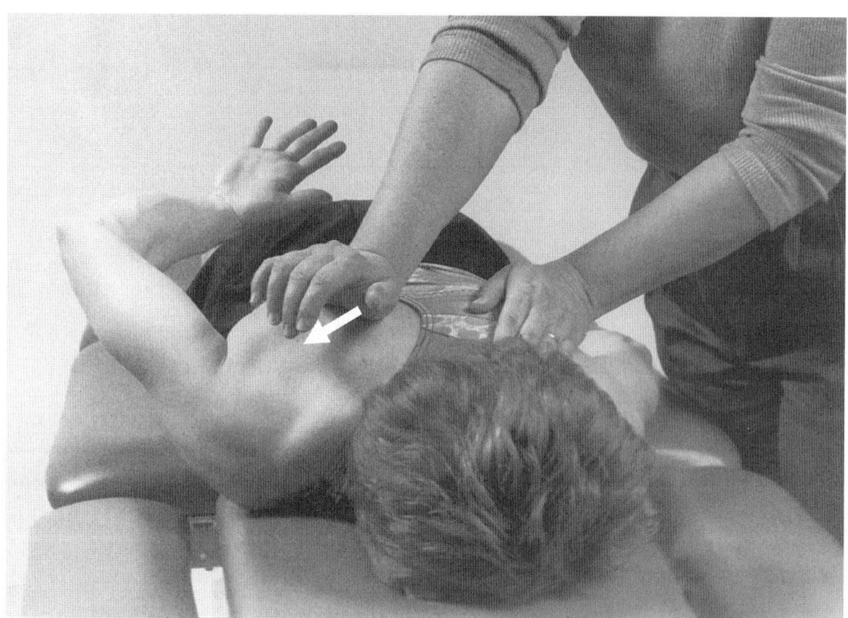

Gravity-Eliminated Test (Grades Below 3)

For patients unable to move completely through available ROM against gravity.

Patient position: Seated with arm to be tested behind back. Shoulder in medial rotation and adduction so dorsum of hand is in contact with ipsilateral gluteal region.

Stabilization/palpation: Stabilize over ipsilateral shoulder girdle to prevent trunk rotation. Palpation occurs as in gravity-resisted test (Fig. 2-23).

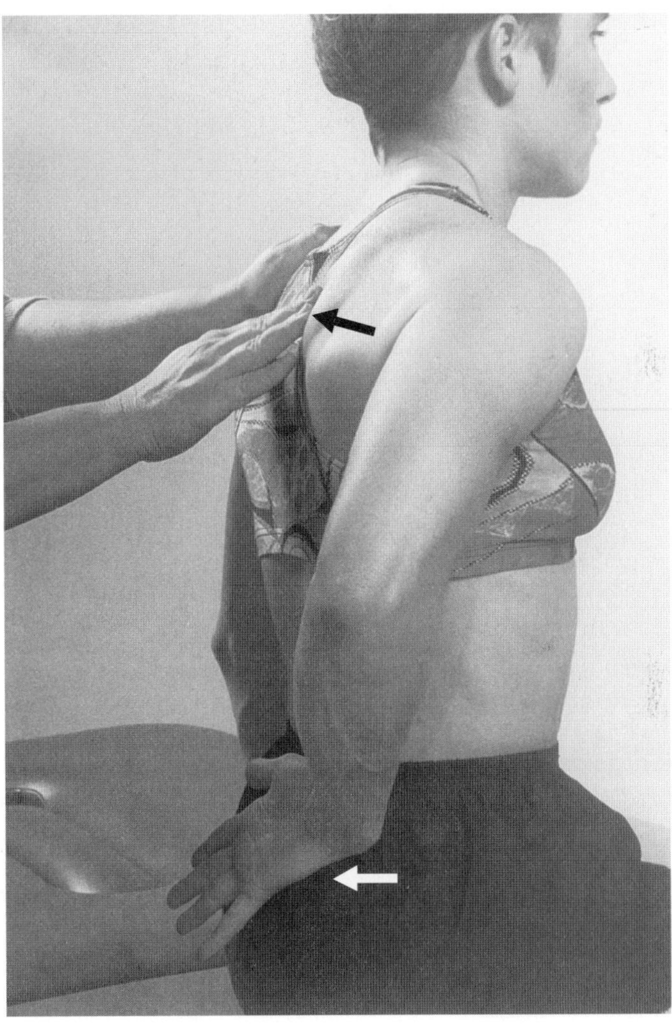

Fig. 2-23. Arrows indicate direction of movement.

Examiner action: As in gravity-resisted test.

Patient action: As in gravity-resisted test (Fig. 2-23).

COMMON SUBSTITUTIONS

1. Tipping of scapula anteriorly; occurs via contraction of pectoralis minor muscle and can be detected by movement of humeral head toward examining table.
2. Rotation of trunk toward side being tested; can be controlled by careful stabilization of thorax.

▪ SCAPULAR ADDUCTION AND DOWNWARD ROTATION–ALTERNATIVE TEST

RHOMBOID MAJOR AND MINOR

Gravity-Resisted Test (Grades 5 and 4)

Patient position: Prone with upper extremity in 0° shoulder adduction, full elbow flexion, full forearm pronation. Patient's head is turned to contralateral side (Fig. 2-24).

Fig. 2-24.

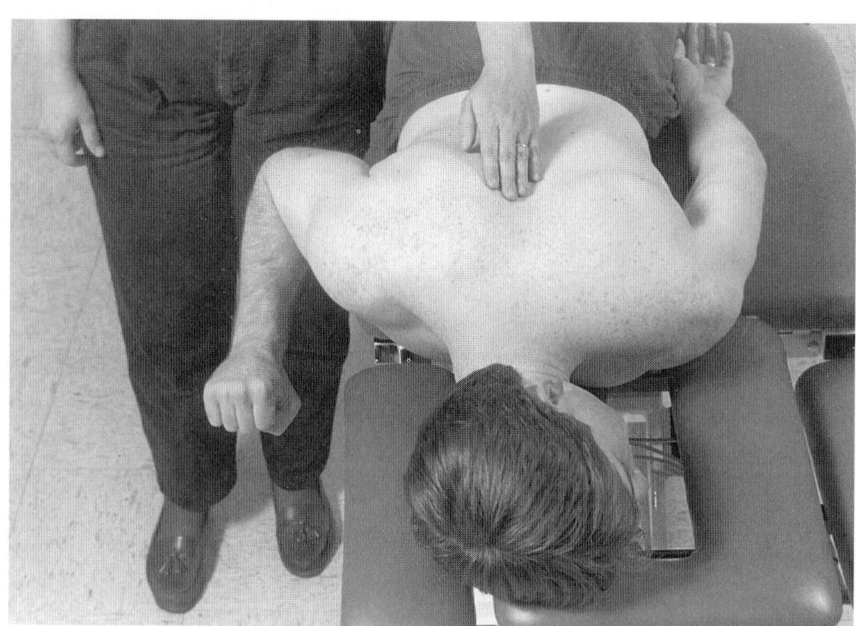

Stabilization/palpation: No stabilization necessary; palpate ipsilateral rhomboids between vertebral border of scapula and spinous processes of C7–T5 (Fig. 2-24).

Examiner action: While instructing patient in motion desired, move patient's scapula through full range of adduction and downward rotation while keeping patient's elbow flexed and forearm pronated. Return patient to starting position. Performing passive movement allows determination of patient's available ROM and shows patient exact movement desired.

Patient action: Patient performs active scapular adduction and downward rotation by extending and adducting humerus. Elbow and forearm are maintained in original positions. Examiner maintains palpation during patient movement (Fig. 2-25).

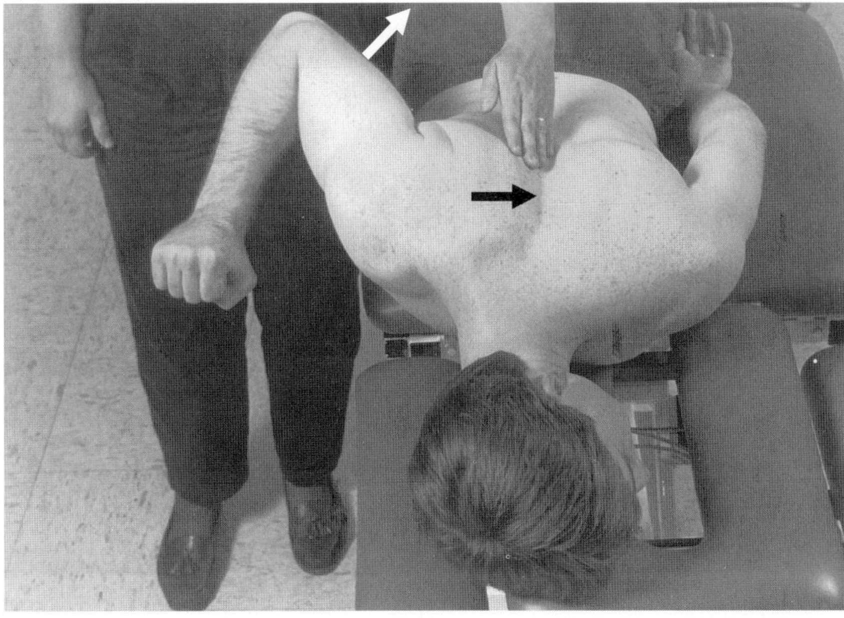

Fig. 2-25. Arrows indicate direction of movement.

Resistance: Apply resistance against distal end of humerus in direction of abduction and flexion (Fig. 2-26). Examiner grades muscle on basis of *scapular,* not humeral, movement. Note: If shoulder extensors are weak, resistance should be applied on scapula.

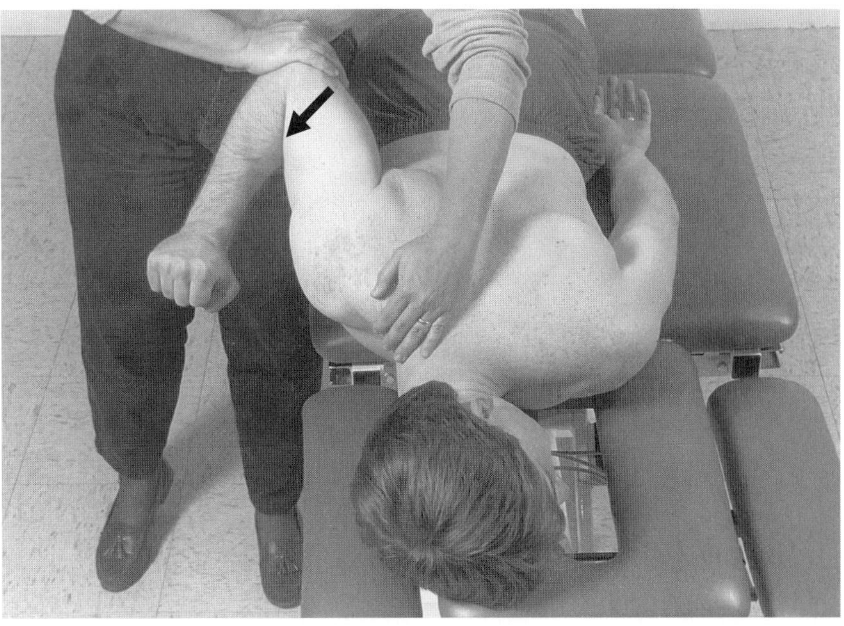

Fig. 2-26. Arrow indicates direction of resistance.

Grades 3 and Below

There is no separate test of this muscle for grades below 3. Grading is altered as follows to accommodate lack of a gravity-eliminated position.

For grade 3: Patient extends and adducts humerus through full ROM with accompanying scapular adduction and downward rotation but against no resistance.

For grade 2: Patient moves arm and scapula through partial ROM against no resistance.

For grade 1: No motion, but a palpable contraction is present. Palpation occurs as described earlier (see Fig. 2-24).

For grade 0: No motion or contraction is present.

■ SCAPULAR ABDUCTION AND UPWARD ROTATION

SERRATUS ANTERIOR: OPTION I (Fig. 2-27)

Option I test is gravity-resisted for that portion of serratus anterior that abducts scapula, but positioning prevents examiner from visualizing scapula during movement. As a result, winging of scapula may be missed. Option II allows visualization of scapula but is not a true gravity-resisted test.

Fig. 2-27.

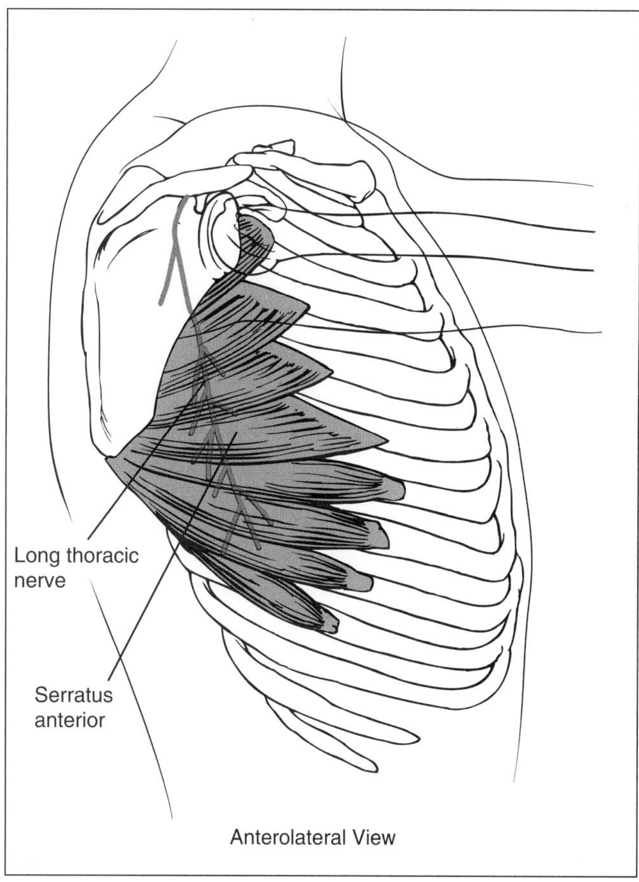

	ATTACHMENTS	NERVE SUPPLY	FUNCTION
Serratus anterior	Origin: Anterosuperior aspect of the upper eight or nine ribs Insertion: Anterior surface of the vertebral border of the scapula	Peripheral nerve: Long thoracic nerve Nerve root: C5–C7	Scapular abduction, upward rotation of the scapula (inferior fibers)

Gravity-Resisted Test (Grades 5, 4, and 3)

Patient position: Supine with upper extremity in 90° shoulder flexion, 0° elbow extension (Fig. 2-28).

Fig. 2-28.

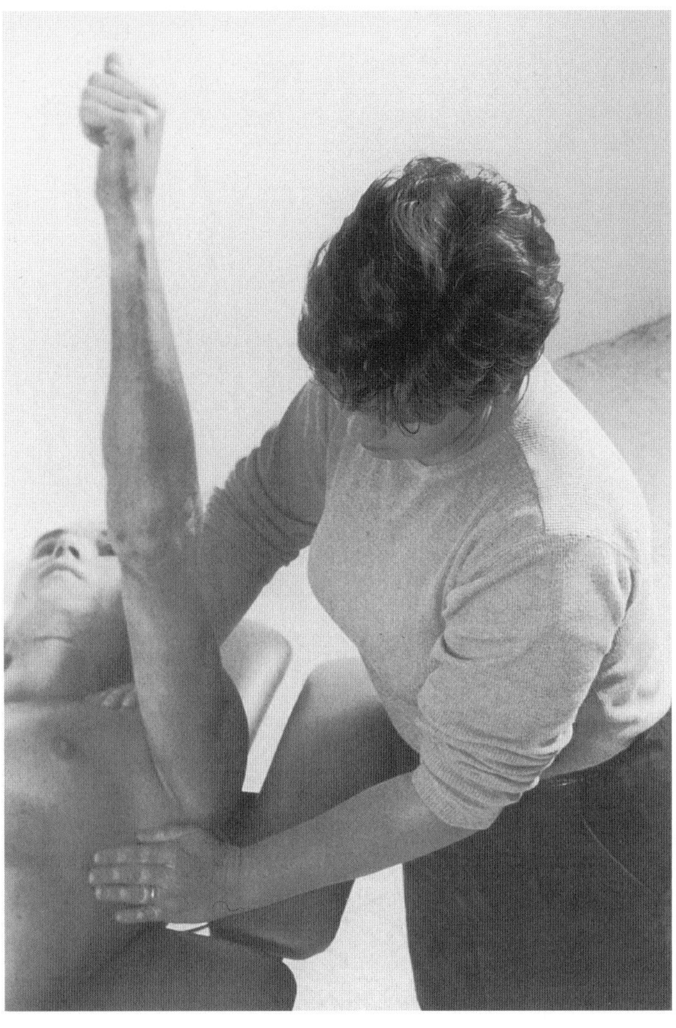

Stabilization/palpation: Stabilize with one hand over ipsilateral thorax to prevent trunk rotation. Palpate serratus anterior over lateral aspect of upper eight or nine ribs, just anterior to lateral border of scapula (Fig. 2-28).

Examiner action: While instructing patient in motion desired, move patient's scapula through full range of abduction by moving patient's hand vertically toward ceiling. Patient's elbow should remain extended. Return patient to starting position. Performing passive movement allows determination of patient's available ROM and shows patient exact movement desired.

Patient action:

Patient performs active scapular abduction by moving hand vertically toward ceiling. Examiner maintains stabilization of thorax and palpation of serratus during patient's movement (Fig. 2-29). Palpation of scapula for "winging" of vertebral border also should occur (not shown).

Fig. 2-29. Arrow indicates direction of movement.

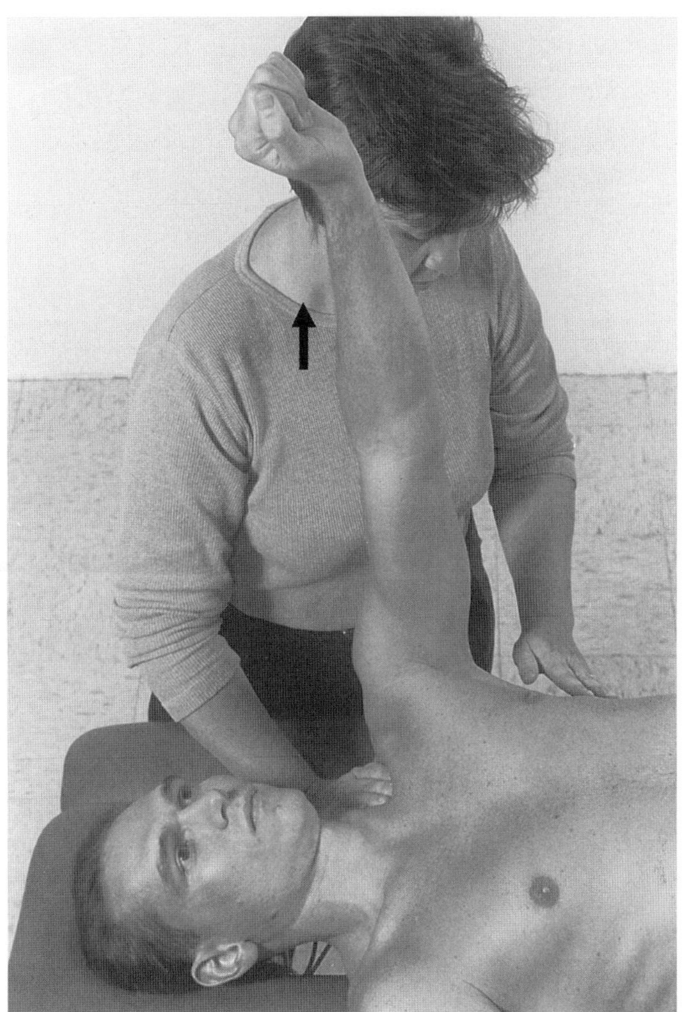

Resistance: Apply resistance by grasping patient's wrist and elbow and pushing downward toward table in direction of scapular adduction. Palpating and stabilizing hands are moved to patient's wrist and elbow to apply resistance (Fig. 2-30).

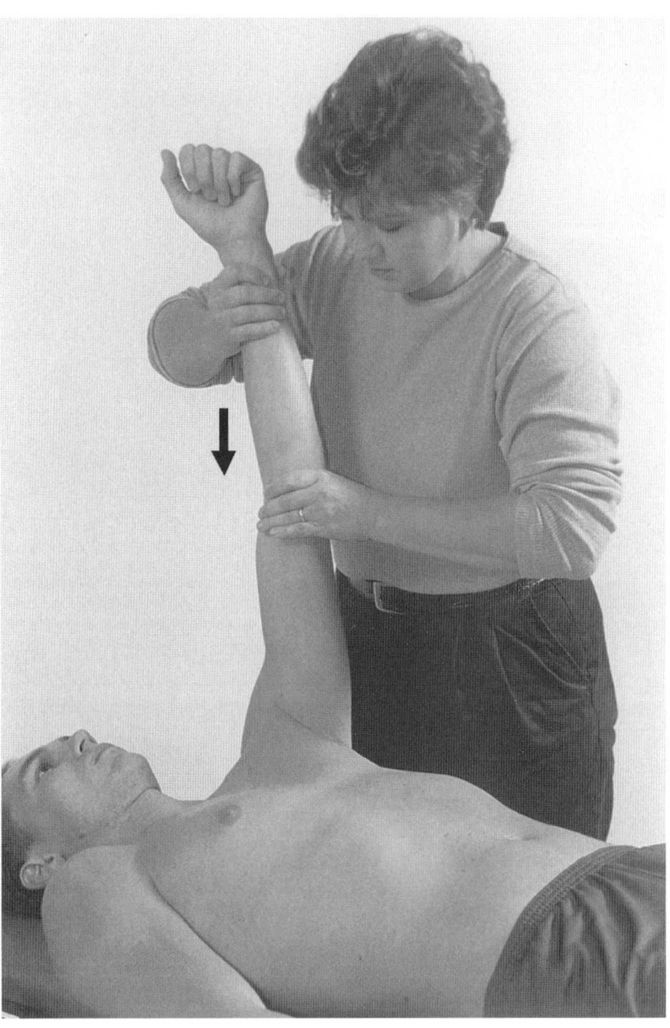

Fig. 2-30. Arrow indicates direction of resistance.

Gravity-Eliminated Test (Grades Below 3)

For patients unable to move completely through available ROM against gravity.

Patient position:

Seated with upper extremity to be tested in scapular adduction and 90° shoulder flexion, 0° elbow extension, arm supported on flat surface. Talcum powder and a cloth may be placed between limb and supporting surface to reduce friction (Fig. 2-31; starting position of upper extremity not shown).

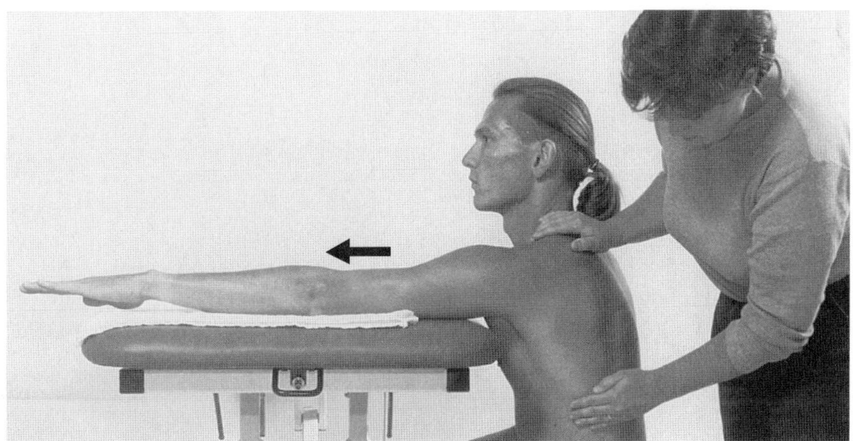

Fig. 2-31. Arrow indicates direction of movement.

Stabilization/palpation:

Stabilize over superior aspect of ipsilateral shoulder girdle. Palpation occurs as in gravity-resisted test (Fig. 2-31).

Examiner action:

While instructing patient in motion desired, move patient's scapula through full range of abduction by sliding patient's arm directly forward on table. Patient's elbow should remain extended. Return patient to starting position.

Patient action:

Patient slides upper extremity directly forward along table by abducting scapula. Palpation and stabilization are maintained during patient's movement (Fig. 2-31).

COMMON SUBSTITUTION

Rotation of trunk away from side being tested; can be controlled via stabilization of thorax.

SERRATUS ANTERIOR: OPTION II

Option II allows visualization of scapula, providing opportunity for examiner to check for scapular winging, denoting serratus anterior weakness. However, because serratus anterior does not act completely against gravity in this position, Option II is not a true gravity-resisted test.

Gravity-Resisted Test (Grades 5 and 4)

Patient position: Seated with upper extremity in approximately 120° shoulder flexion 0° elbow extension (Fig. 2-32).

Fig. 2-32.

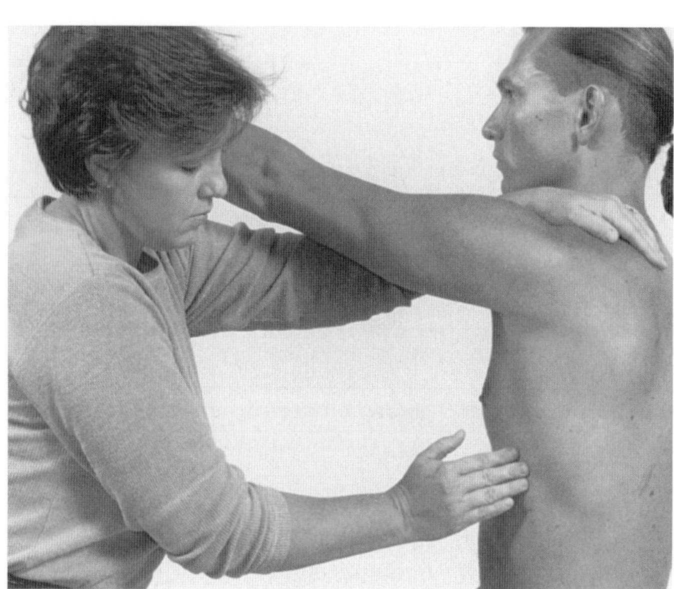

Stabilization/palpation: Stabilize with one hand over superior aspect of ipsilateral thorax to prevent trunk rotation. Palpate serratus anterior over lateral aspect of upper eight or nine ribs, just anterior to lateral border of scapula (Fig. 2-32).

Examiner action: While instructing patient in motion desired, move patient's scapula through full range of abduction by moving arm directly forward while keeping elbow extended and shoulder flexed to 120°. Return patient to starting position. Performing passive movement allows determination of patient's available ROM and shows patient exact movement desired.

Patient action: Patient abducts scapula by moving hand directly forward while maintaining elbow in 0° extension and shoulder in 120° flexion. Examiner maintains stabilization of thorax and palpation of serratus during patient's movement (Fig. 2-33).

Resistance: Apply resistance in direction of scapular adduction by grasping patient's wrist and elbow and applying pressure through long axis of upper extremity. Palpating and stabilizing hands are moved to patient's wrist and elbow to apply resistance (Fig. 2-34).

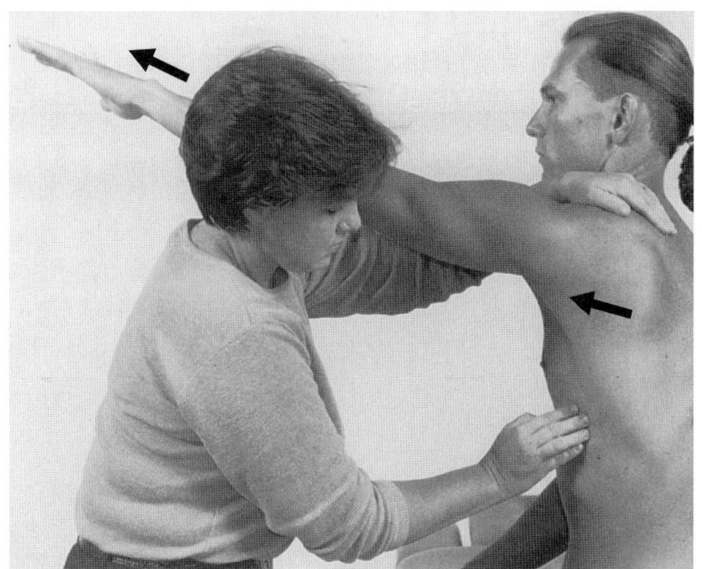

Fig. 2-33. Arrows indicate direction of movement.

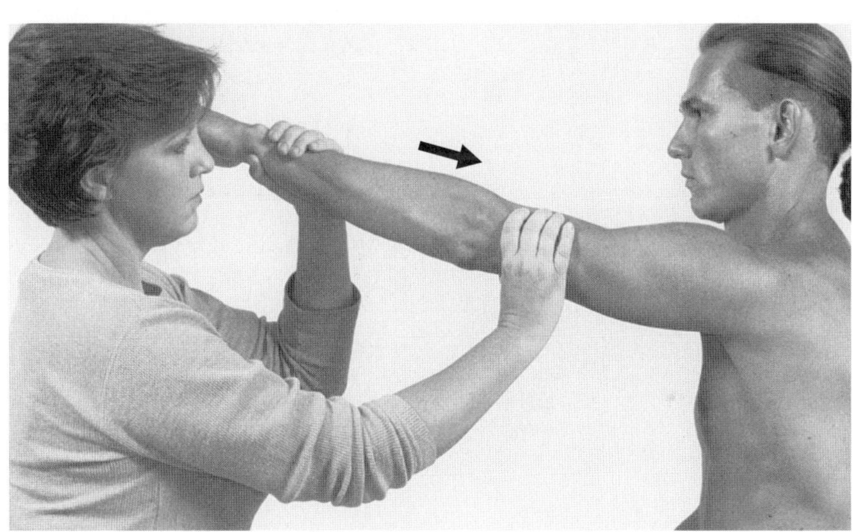

Fig. 2-34. Arrow indicates direction of resistance.

Grades 3 and Below

There is no separate test of this muscle for grades below 3. Grading is altered as follows to accommodate lack of a gravity-eliminated position.

For grade 3: Patient moves scapula through full range of abduction against no resistance.

For grade 2: Patient moves scapula through partial range of abduction against no resistance.

For grade 1: No motion, but a palpable contraction is present. Palpation occurs as described earlier (see Fig. 2-32).

For grade 0: No motion or contraction is present.

COMMON SUBSTITUTION

See option I test for serratus anterior.

■ SHOULDER FLEXION

ANTERIOR DELTOID, CORACOBRACHIALIS (Fig. 2-35)

Fig. 2-35.

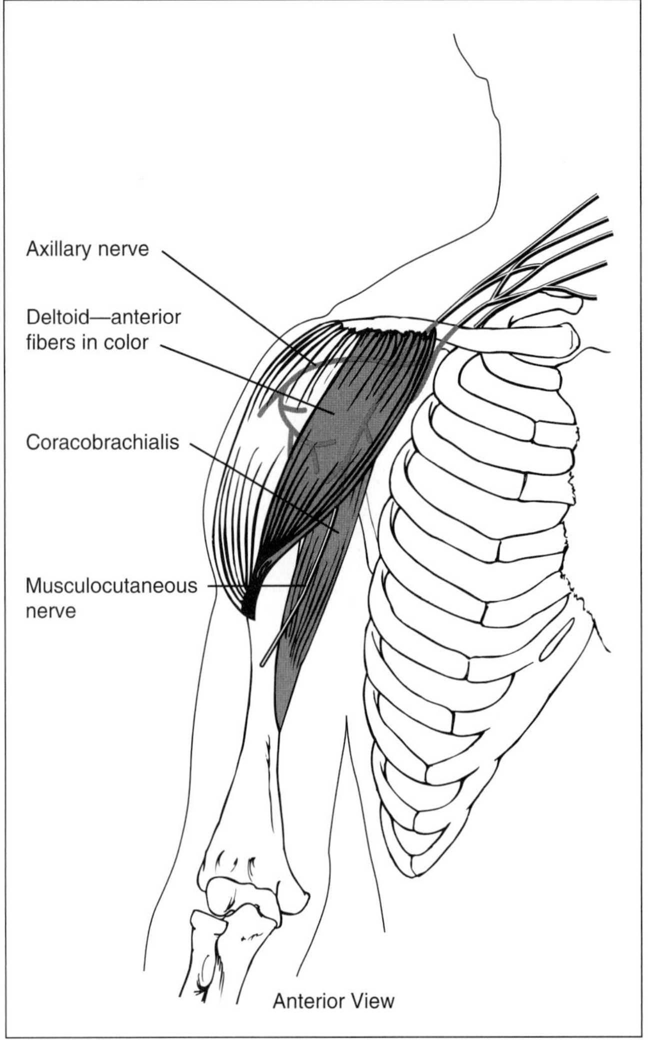

	ATTACHMENTS	NERVE SUPPLY	FUNCTION
Anterior deltoid	Origin: Anterosuperior aspect of the lateral ⅓ of the clavicle Insertion: Deltoid tuberosity of the humerus	Peripheral nerve: Axillary nerve Nerve root: C5, C6	Flexion of the shoulder joint
Coracobrachialis	Origin: Coracoid process of the scapula Insertion: Medial aspect of the middle ⅓ of the shaft of the humerus	Peripheral nerve: Musculocutaneous nerve Nerve root: C6, C7	Flexion and adduction of the shoulder joint

Gravity-Resisted Test (Grades 5, 4, and 3)

Patient position: Seated with upper extremity in 0° shoulder flexion and adduction, 0° elbow extension, palm facing trunk (Fig. 2-36).

Fig. 2-36.

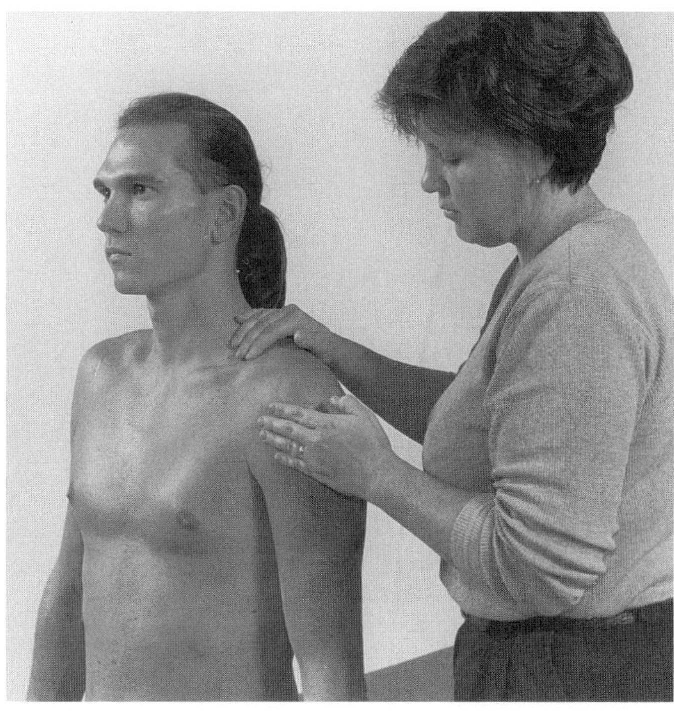

Stabilization/palpation: Stabilize over superior aspect of ipsilateral shoulder, taking care to avoid pressure over fibers of anterior deltoid. Palpate anterior deltoid over proximal, anterior aspect of humerus (Fig. 2-36).

Examiner action: While instructing patient in motion desired, move patient's arm into 90° of shoulder flexion. Return patient to starting position. Performing passive movement allows determination of patient's available ROM and shows patient exact movement desired.

Patient action:

Patient flexes shoulder to 90°, keeping forearm in neutral position, while examiner stabilizes ipsilateral shoulder and palpates anterior deltoid (Fig. 2-37).

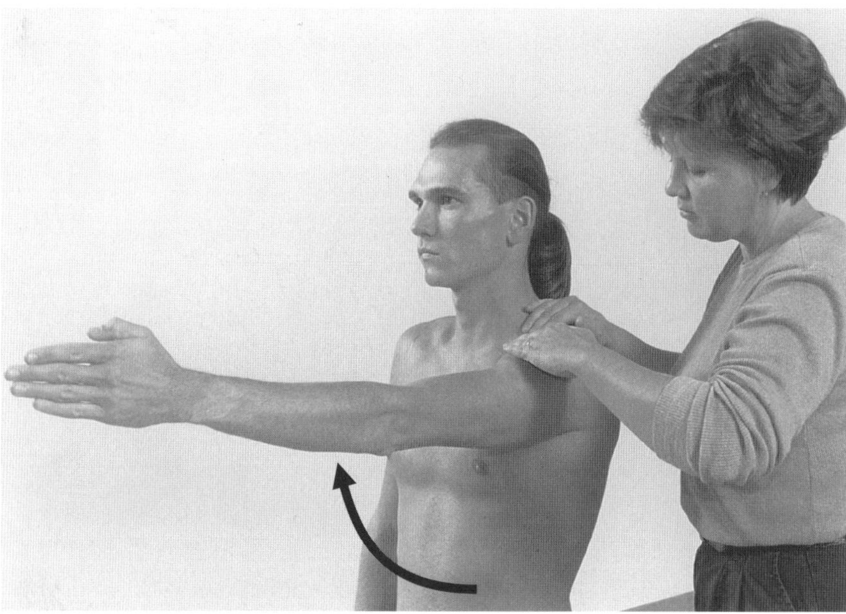

Fig. 2-37. Arrow indicates direction of movement.

Resistance:

Apply resistance just proximal to elbow in direction of shoulder extension. Palpating hand is moved to distal humerus to apply resistance (Fig. 2-38).

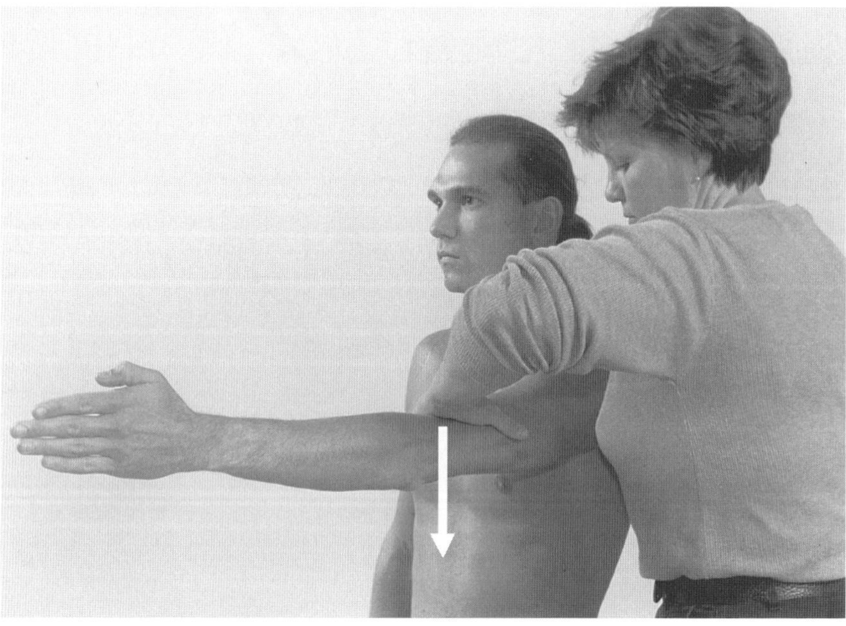

Fig. 2-38. Arrow indicates direction of resistance.

Gravity-Eliminated Test (Grades Below 3)

For patients unable to move completely through available ROM against gravity.

Patient position: Side-lying with arm to be tested uppermost and supported on a powder board. Talcum powder and a cloth may be placed between limb and supporting surface to reduce friction (Fig. 2-39). Patient begins motion in 0° shoulder flexion, with palm facing trunk (not shown).

Fig. 2-39. Arrow indicates direction of movement.

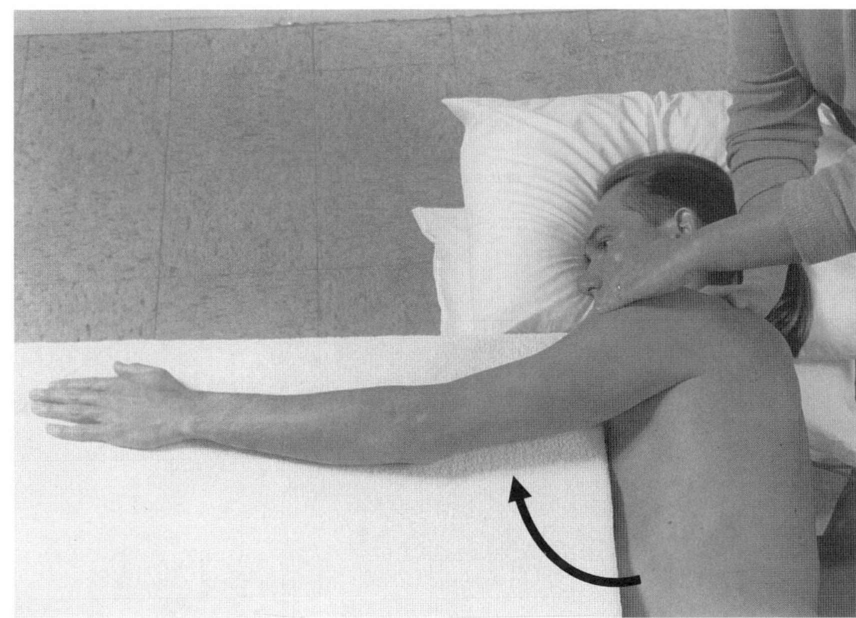

Stabilization/palpation: As in gravity-resisted test (Fig. 2-39).

Examiner action: As in gravity-resisted test.

Patient action: As in gravity-resisted test (Fig. 2-39).

COMMON SUBSTITUTION

Biceps brachii long head; patient will rotate humerus laterally during shoulder flexion. May be controlled by maintaining neutral position of humerus during test.

SHOULDER FLEXION—ALTERNATIVE TEST

ANTERIOR DELTOID

This test is designed to minimize activity of biceps brachii (accomplished by flexing elbow) and pectoralis major (accomplished by maintaining shoulder in partial abduction) during shoulder flexion. Thus relative activity of anterior deltoid is theoretically greater in this testing position (similar to test recommended by Kendall et al. [1993]).

Gravity-Resisted Test (Grades 5 and 4)

Patient position: Seated with upper extremity in 0° shoulder adduction and slight lateral rotation, 90° elbow flexion (Fig. 2-40).

Fig. 2-40.

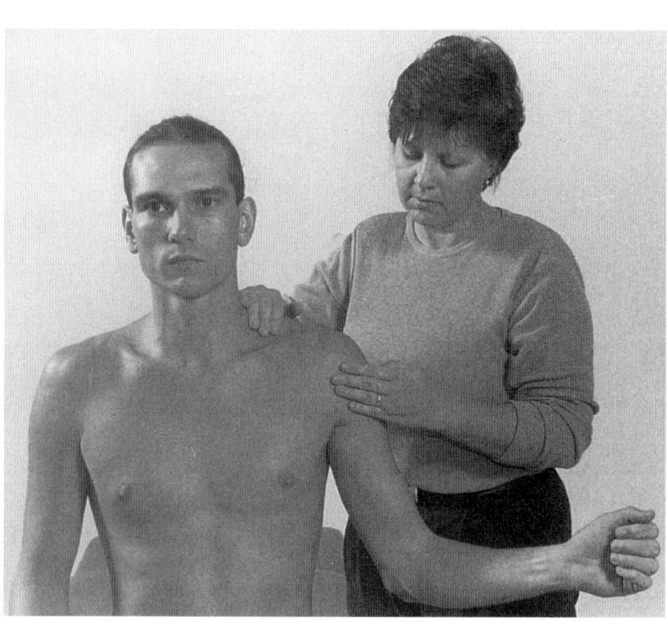

Stabilization/palpation: Stabilize with one hand over superior aspect of ipsilateral shoulder, taking care to avoid pressure over fibers of anterior deltoid. Palpate anterior deltoid just distal to anterior aspect of acromion (Fig. 2-40).

Examiner action: While instructing patient in motion desired, elevate patient's arm 90° in a plane halfway between flexion and abduction, maintaining elbow in flexion and shoulder in slight lateral rotation. Return patient to starting position. Performing passive movement allows determination of patient's available ROM and shows patient exact movement desired.

Patient action: Patient elevates arm in oblique plane, halfway between flexion and abduction, while maintaining elbow in flexion and shoulder in slight lateral rotation. Examiner maintains palpation and stabilization during patient's movement (Fig. 2-41).

Resistance: Apply resistance just proximal to elbow in direction of shoulder extension and adduction. Palpating hand is moved to distal humerus to apply resistance (Fig. 2-42).

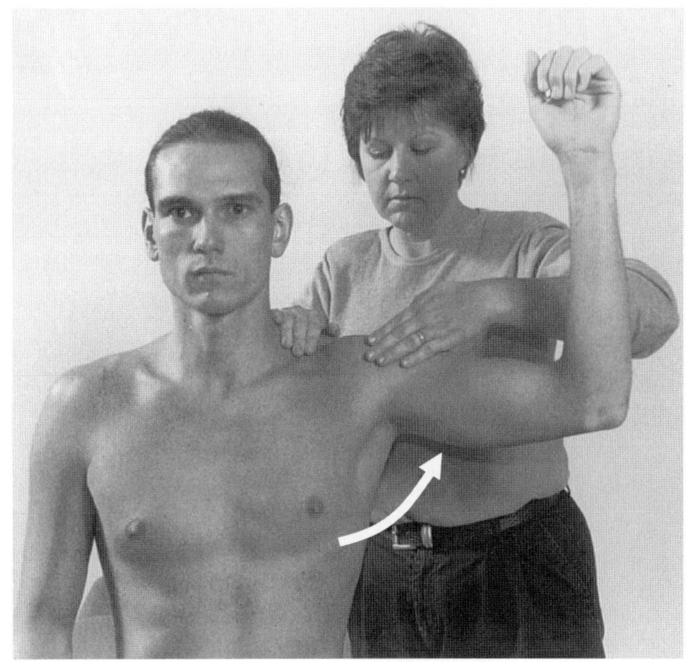

Fig. 2-41. Arrow indicates direction of movement.

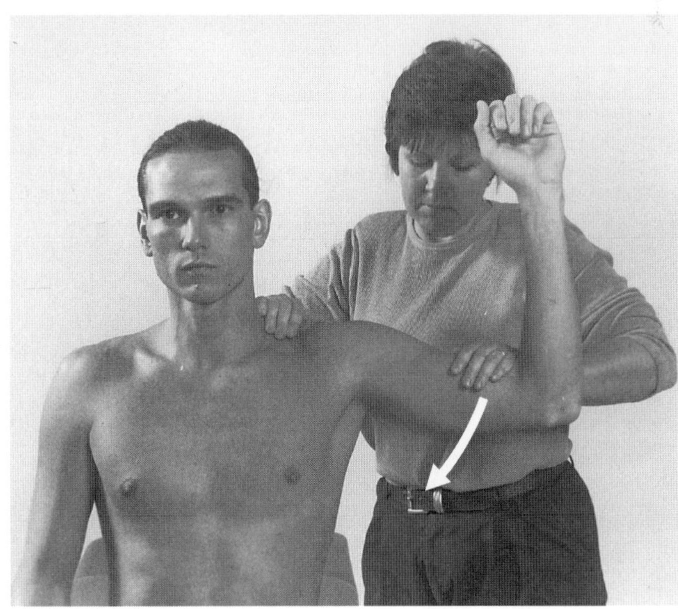

Fig. 2-42. Arrow indicates direction of resistance.

Grades 3 and Below

There is no separate test of this muscle for grades below 3. Grading is altered as follows to accommodate lack of a gravity-eliminated position.

For grade 3: Patient elevates arm through full ROM against no resistance.

For grade 2: Patient elevates arm through partial ROM against no resistance.

For grade 1: No motion, but a palpable contraction is present. Palpation occurs as described earlier (see Fig. 2-40).

For grade 0: No motion or contraction is present.

■ SHOULDER FLEXION AND ADDUCTION

CORACOBRACHIALIS

Gravity-Resisted Test (Grades 5 and 4)

Patient position: Seated with upper extremity in 0° shoulder adduction and full external rotation, 90° elbow flexion, full forearm supination (Fig. 2-43).

Fig. 2-43.

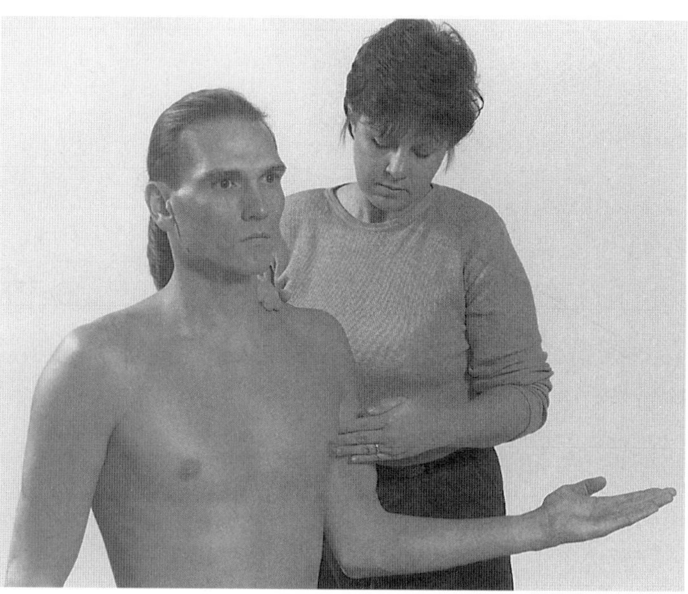

Stabilization/palpation: Stabilize over superior aspect of shoulder. Palpate coracobrachialis along anteromedial aspect of arm in its upper third (Fig. 2-43).

Examiner action: While instructing patient in motion desired, move patient's arm into shoulder flexion (90°) and adduction, taking care to maintain external rotation of shoulder, flexion of elbow, and supination of forearm. Return patient to starting position. Performing passive movement allows determination of patient's available ROM and shows patient exact movement desired.

Patient action: Patient flexes and adducts humerus while maintaining external rotation of shoulder, flexion of elbow, and supination of forearm. Examiner maintains palpation and stabilization during patient's movement (Fig. 2-44).

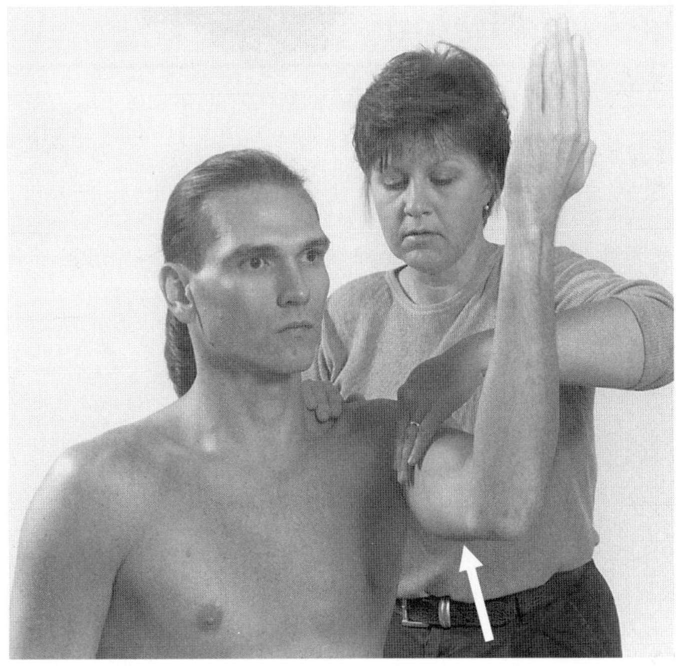

Fig. 2-44. Arrow indicates direction of movement.

Resistance: Apply resistance over anterior aspect of distal humerus in direction of shoulder extension. Palpating hand is moved to distal humerus to apply resistance (Fig. 2-45).

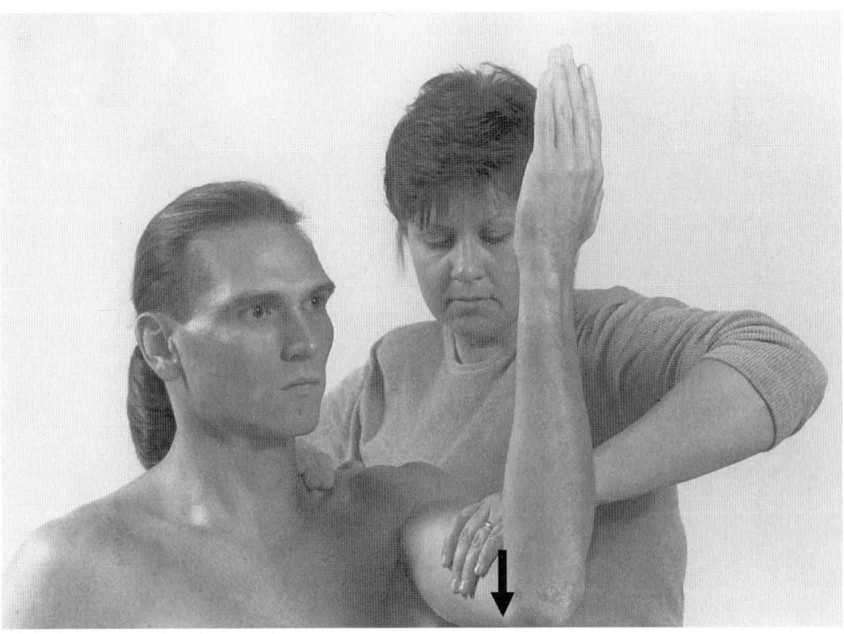

Fig. 2-45. Arrow indicates direction of resistance.

Grades 3 and Below

There is no separate test of this muscle for grades below 3. Grading is altered as follows to accommodate lack of a gravity-eliminated position.

For grade 3: Patient flexes and adducts humerus through full ROM against no resistance.

For grade 2: Patient flexes and adducts humerus through partial ROM against no resistance.

For grade 1: No motion, but a palpable contraction is present. Palpation occurs as described earlier (see Fig. 2-43).

For grade 0: No motion or contraction is present.

■ SHOULDER EXTENSION

LATISSIMUS DORSI, TERES MAJOR, POSTERIOR DELTOID (Fig. 2-46)

Fig. 2-46.

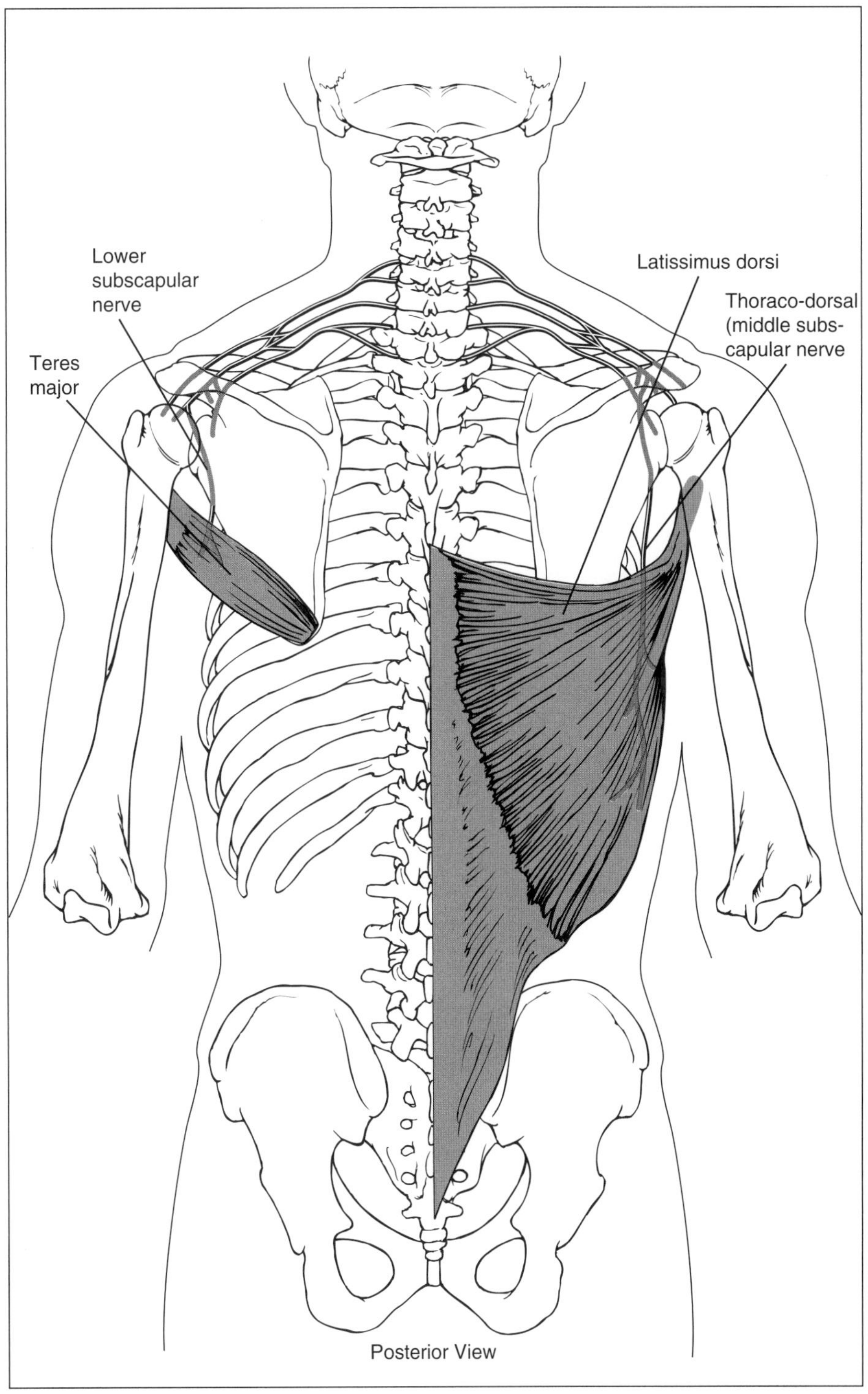

	ATTACHMENTS	NERVE SUPPLY	FUNCTION
Latissimus dorsi	Origin: Spinous processes of sacral, lumbar, and lower six thoracic vertebrae and the supraspinal ligament via the thoracolumbar fascia, iliac crest, and lower three to four ribs Insertion: Floor of the intertubercular groove of the humerus	Peripheral nerve: Thoracodorsal nerve Nerve root: C6–C8	Extension, adduction, and medial rotation of the shoulder
Teres major	Origin: Posterior surface of the inferior angle of the scapula Insertion: Medial lip of the intertubercular groove of the humerus	Peripheral nerve: Lower subscapular nerve Nerve root: C5, C6	Adduction, extension, and medial rotation of the shoulder
Posterior deltoid	Origin: Inferior aspect of the spine of the scapula Insertion: Deltoid tuberosity of the humerus	Peripheral nerve: Axillary nerve Nerve root: C5, C6	Extension of the shoulder

Gravity-Resisted Test (Grades 5, 4, and 3)

Patient position: Prone with upper extremity in 0° shoulder adduction and full medial rotation (palm facing ceiling), 0° elbow extension (Fig. 2-47).

Stabilization/palpation: Stabilize with one hand over ipsilateral thorax (or scapula if scapular stabilizers are weak). Palpate latissimus dorsi along lateral side of rib cage (Fig. 2-47).

Fig. 2-47.

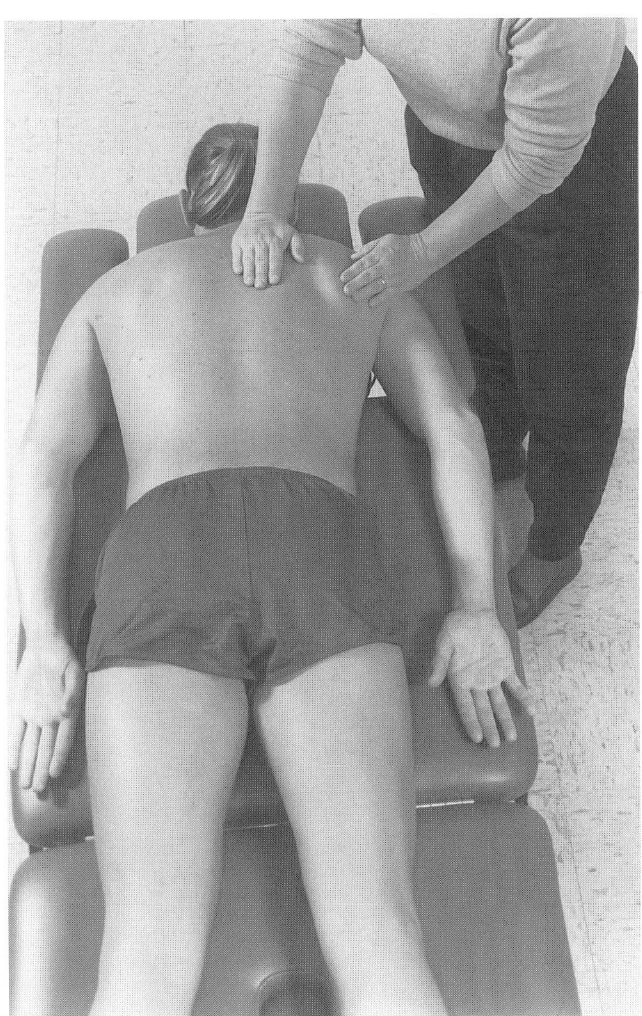

Examiner action: While instructing patient in motion desired, move patient's arm into shoulder extension while keeping shoulder medially rotated and adducted. Return patient to starting position. Performing passive movement allows determination of patient's available ROM and shows patient exact movement desired.

Patient action: Patient raises arm through full range of shoulder extension while keeping shoulder adducted and medially rotated. Examiner maintains palpation and stabilization during patient's movement (Fig. 2-48).

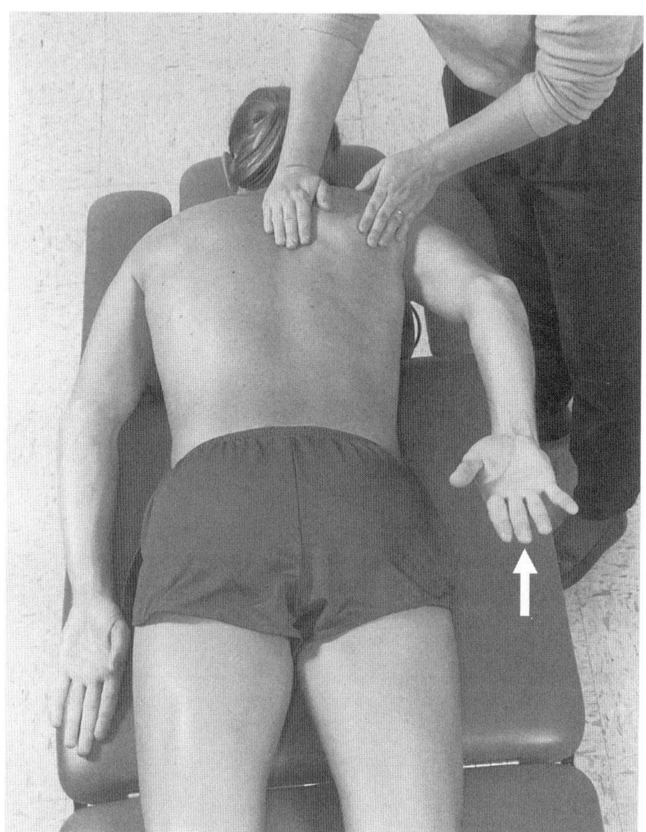

Fig. 2-48. Arrow indicates direction of movement.

Resistance: Apply resistance just proximal to elbow in direction of shoulder flexion. Palpating hand is moved to distal humerus to apply resistance (Fig. 2-49).

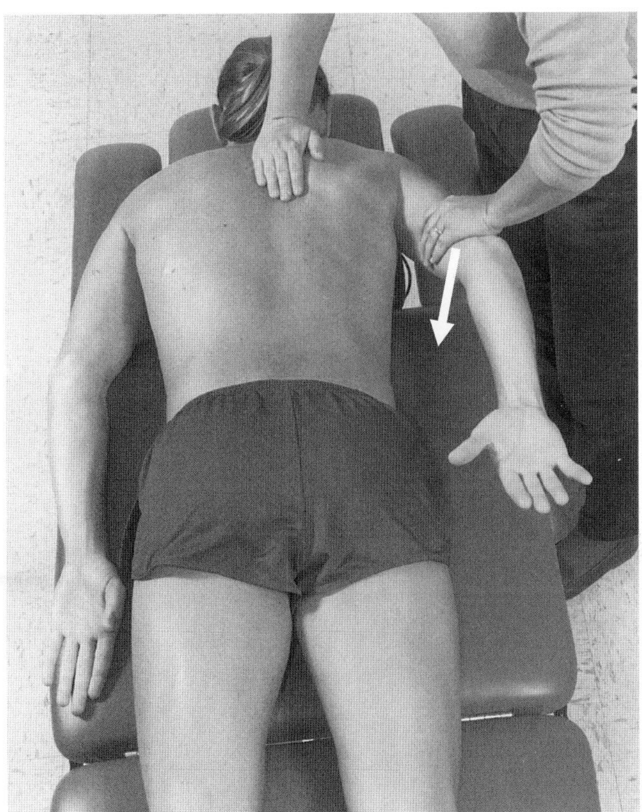

Fig. 2-49. Arrow indicates direction of resistance.

Gravity-Eliminated Test (Grades Below 3)

For patients unable to move completely through available ROM against gravity.

Patient position: Side-lying with arm to be tested uppermost and on a powder board. Talcum powder and a cloth may be placed between limb and supporting surface to reduce friction (Fig. 2-50). Patient begins motion positioned in 0° shoulder extension and adduction, full shoulder medial rotation, and 0° elbow extension (initial arm position not shown).

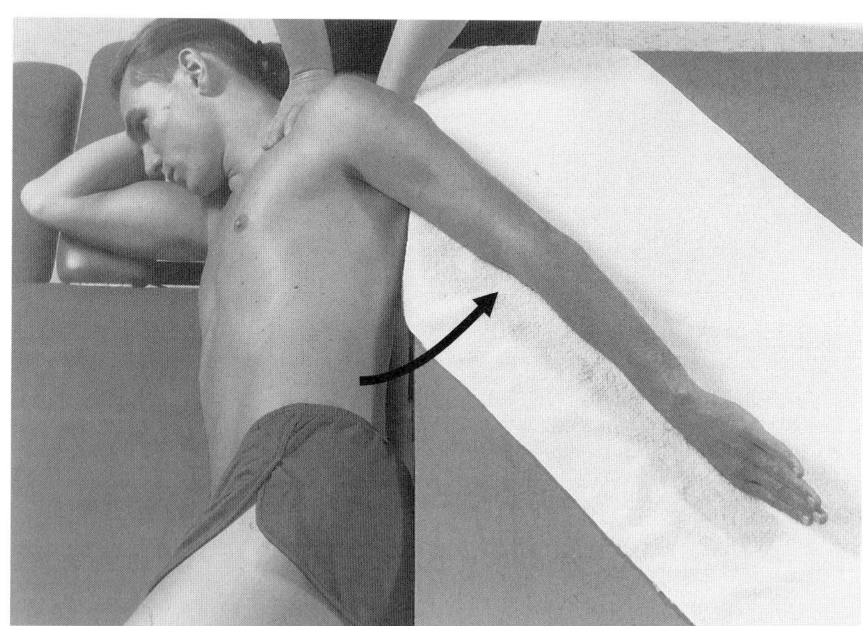

Fig. 2-50. Arrow indicates direction of movement.

Stabilization/palpation: Stabilize over ipsilateral thorax (or scapula if scapular stabilizers are weak) with one hand while palpating muscles tested with other hand (Fig. 2-50).

Examiner action: As in gravity-resisted test.

Patient action: Patient slides arm along surface through full range of shoulder extension while keeping shoulder medially rotated and adducted. Palpation and stabilization are maintained during active movement by patient (Fig. 2-50).

COMMON SUBSTITUTION

Long head of triceps brachii may substitute for primary shoulder extensors. In this case, patient will position humerus in lateral rotation. Substitution by triceps may be prevented by maintaining humerus in medial rotation.

■ SHOULDER ABDUCTION

MIDDLE DELTOID: SUPRASPINATUS (Figs. 2-51 and 2-52)

Fig. 2-51.

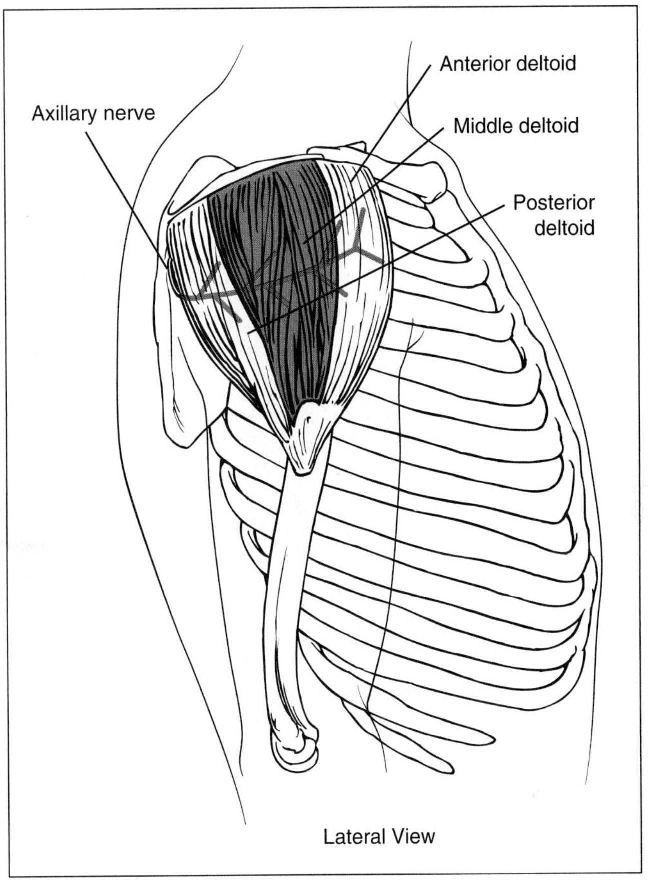

Fig. 2-52.

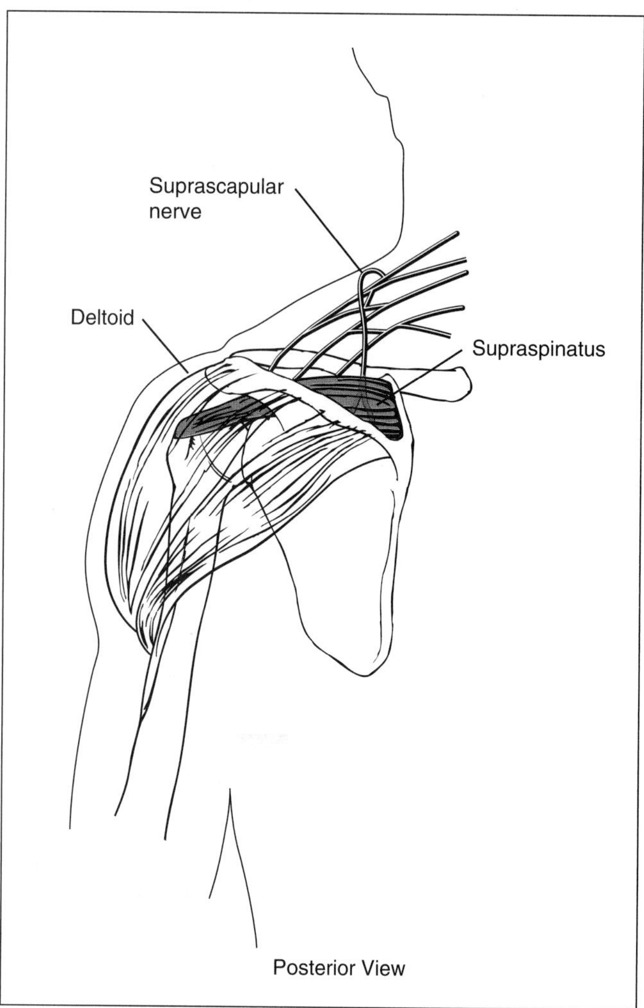

	ATTACHMENTS	NERVE SUPPLY	FUNCTION
Middle deltoid	Origin: Acromion process of the scapula Insertion: Deltoid tuberosity of the humerus	Peripheral nerve: Axillary nerve Nerve root: C5, C6	Abduction of the shoulder
Supraspinatus	Origin: Supraspinatus fossa of the scapula Insertion: Greater tubercle of the humerus	Peripheral nerve: Suprascapular nerve Nerve root: C5	Abduction and lateral rotation of the shoulder

Gravity-Resisted Test (Grades 5, 4, and 3)

Patient position: Seated with upper extremity to be tested in 0° shoulder abduction, 0° elbow extension, and forearm neutral (Fig. 2-53).

Fig. 2-53.

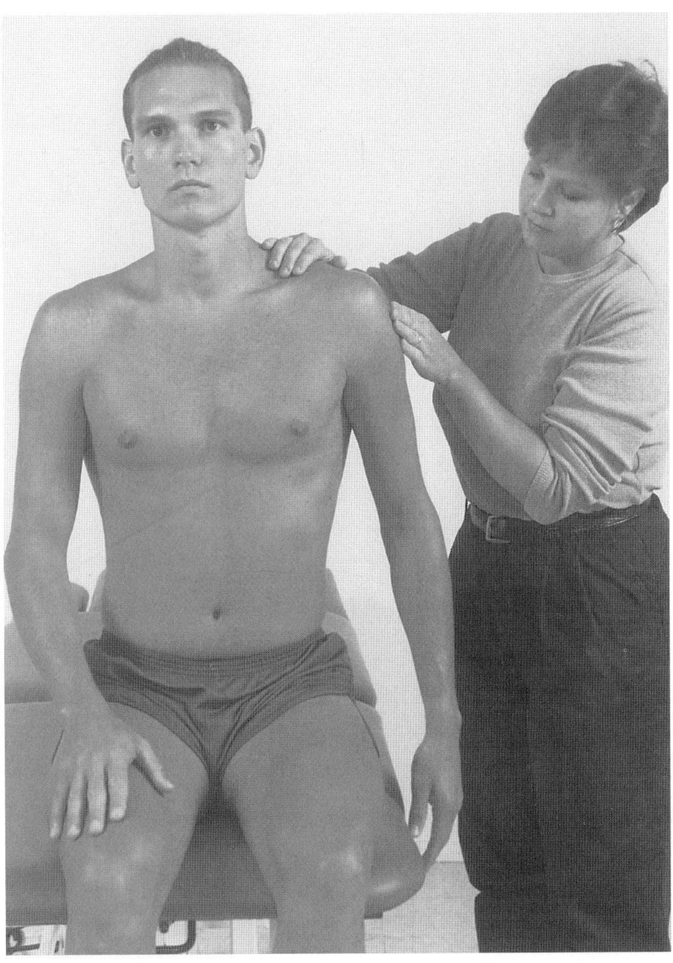

Stabilization/palpation: Stabilize over superior aspect of shoulder (avoiding pressure on deltoid). Palpate middle deltoid over superior lateral aspect of humerus (Fig. 2-53).

Examiner action: While instructing patient in motion desired, move patient's arm into 90° of shoulder abduction. Return patient to starting position. Performing passive movement allows determination of patient's available ROM and shows patient exact movement desired.

Patient action: Patient raises arm to 90° shoulder abduction. Examiner maintains palpation and stabilization during patient's movement (Fig. 2-54).

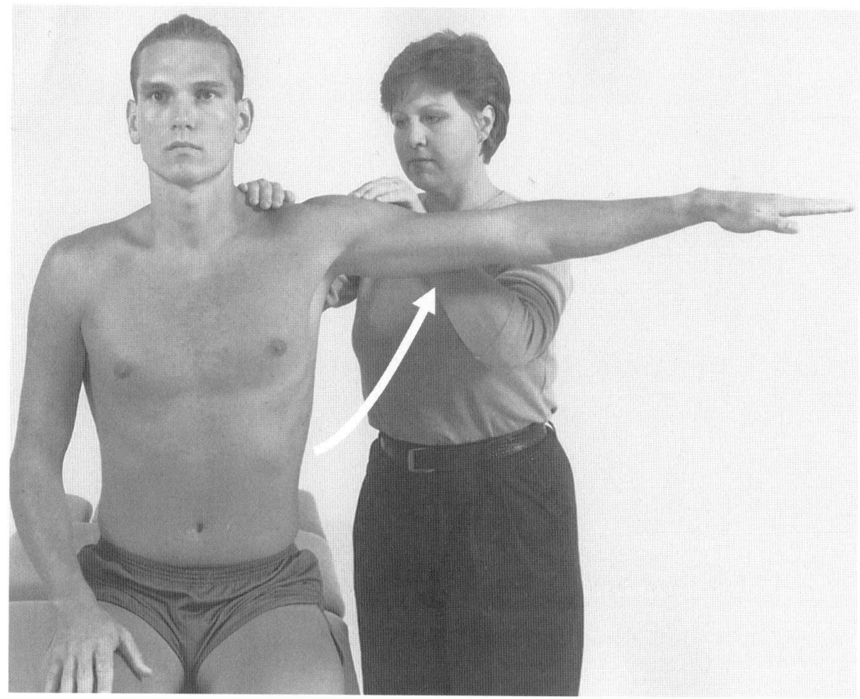

Fig. 2-54. Arrow indicates direction of movement.

Resistance: Apply resistance just proximal to elbow in direction of shoulder adduction. Palpating hand is moved to distal humerus to apply resistance (Fig. 2-55).

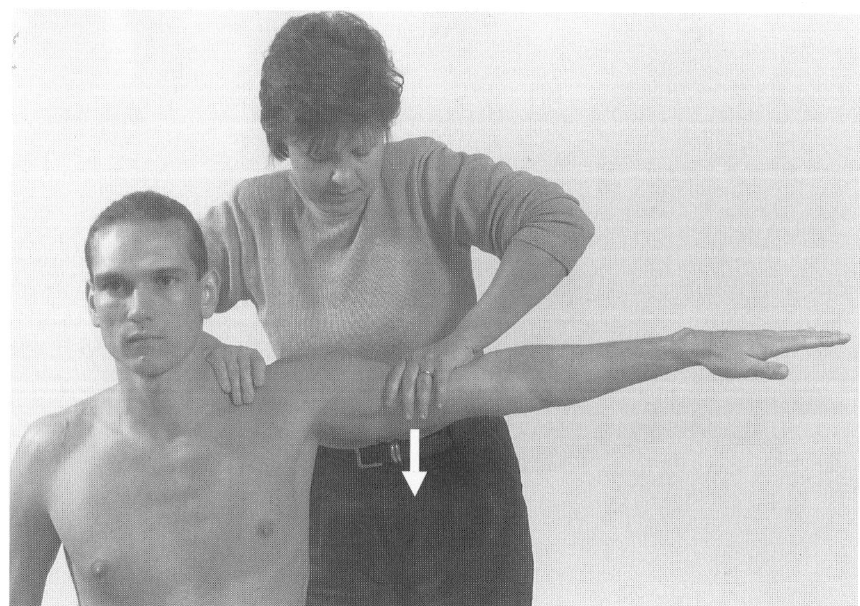

Fig. 2-55. Arrow indicates direction of resistance.

Gravity-Eliminated Test (Grades Below 3)

For patients unable to move completely through available ROM against gravity.

Patient position: Supine on firm surface with arm to be tested in 0° shoulder abduction, 0° elbow extension, forearm neutral.

Stabilization/palpation: As in gravity-resisted test (Fig. 2-56).

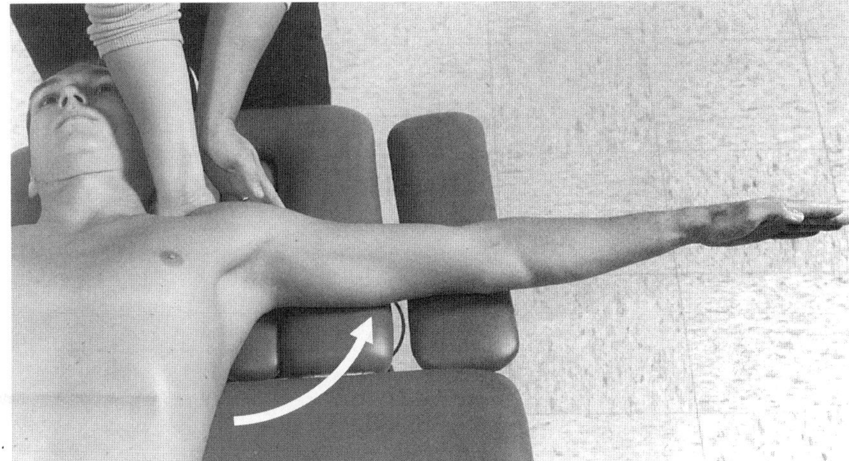

Fig. 2-56. Arrow indicates direction of movement.

Examiner action: As in gravity-resisted test.

Patient action: Patient slides arm along surface to 90° shoulder abduction. Examiner maintains palpation and stabilization during patient's movement (Fig. 2-56).

COMMON SUBSTITUTIONS

1. Long head of biceps brachii: Patient may substitute with biceps by rotating humerus laterally during abduction. Control of this substitution may be achieved by maintaining humerus in neutral rotation during test.
2. In presence of a weak supraspinatus, patient may lean trunk toward ipsilateral side, thus initiating abduction passively.
3. Elevation of ipsilateral shoulder may give appearance of abduction. This can be controlled by stabilization over superior aspect of ipsilateral shoulder during test.

CLINICAL COMMENT: DELTOID MUSCLE AND C5 NEUROLOGIC ASSESSMENT

The deltoid muscle is a key muscle for examining the integrity of the C5 spinal nerve or neurologic segment of the spinal cord. Complete assessment of the C5 neurologic level includes:

Strength assessment of:
Deltoid (pp. 69–71)
Biceps brachii (C5 and C6; 99–102)
Reflex testing of:
Biceps reflex (C5 and C6; p. 547)
Sensory testing of:
Skin over middle deltoid (C5 dermatome; pp. 528–532)

■ SHOULDER HORIZONTAL ABDUCTION

POSTERIOR DELTOID (Fig. 2-57)

Fig. 2-57.

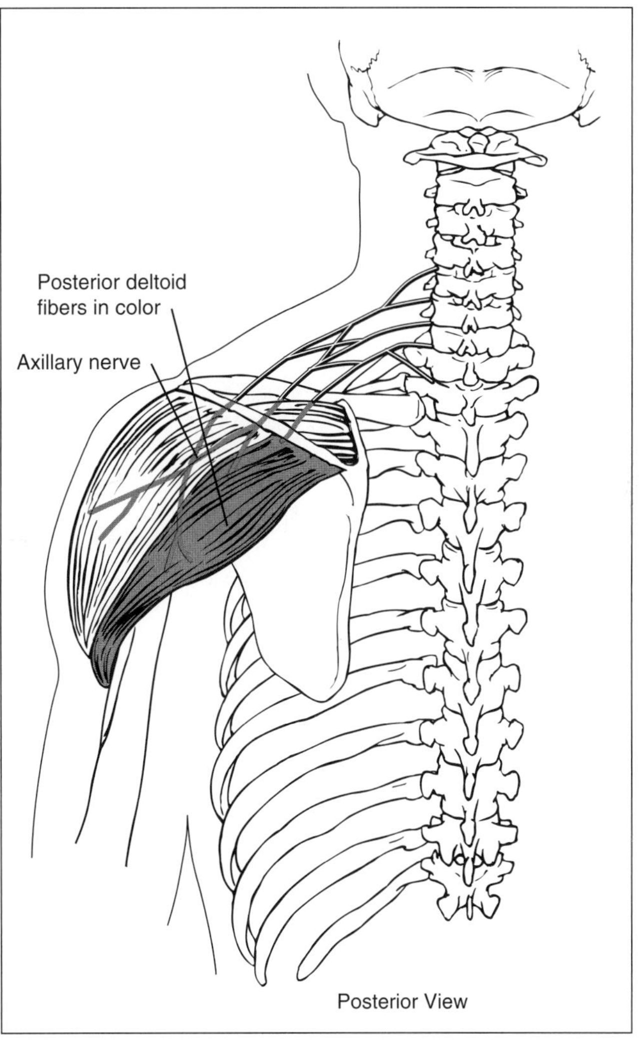

	ATTACHMENTS	NERVE SUPPLY	FUNCTION
Posterior deltoid	Origin: Inferior aspect of the spine of the scapula Insertion: Deltoid tuberosity of the humerus	Peripheral nerve: Axillary nerve Nerve root: C5, C6	Extension of the shoulder

Gravity-Resisted Test (Grades 5, 4, and 3)

Patient position: Prone with upper extremity in 90° shoulder abduction, 90° elbow flexion; forearm hanging vertically off side of table. Patient's head is turned to contralateral side (Fig. 2-58).

Fig. 2-58.

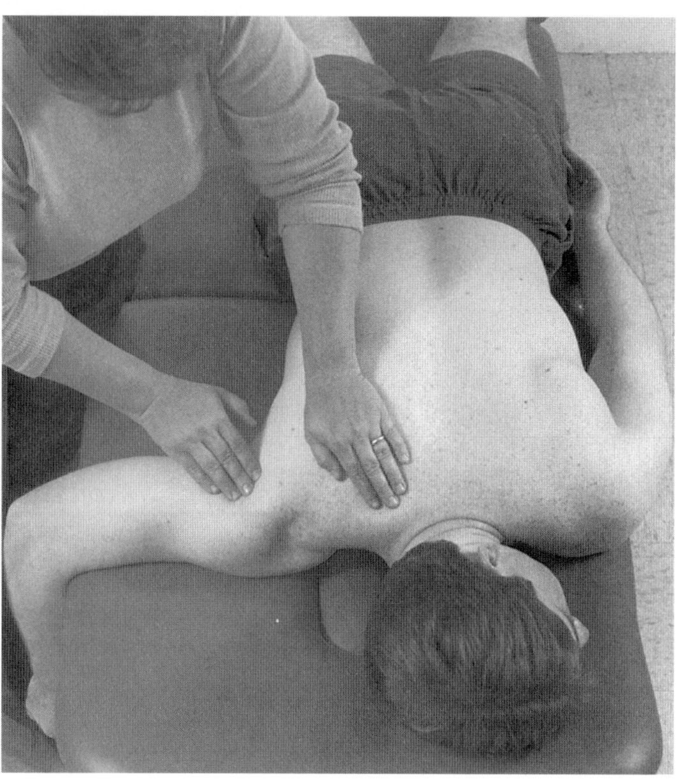

Stabilization/palpation: Stabilize with one hand over ipsilateral scapula. Palpate fibers of posterior deltoid over posterior, superior aspect of humerus (Fig. 2-58).

Examiner action: While instructing patient in motion desired, move patient's humerus into horizontal abduction, keeping elbow flexed. Return patient to starting position. Performing passive movement allows determination of patient's available ROM and shows patient exact movement desired.

Patient action: Have patient perform active horizontal shoulder abduction while examiner maintains stabilization of scapula and palpation of posterior deltoid (Fig. 2-59).

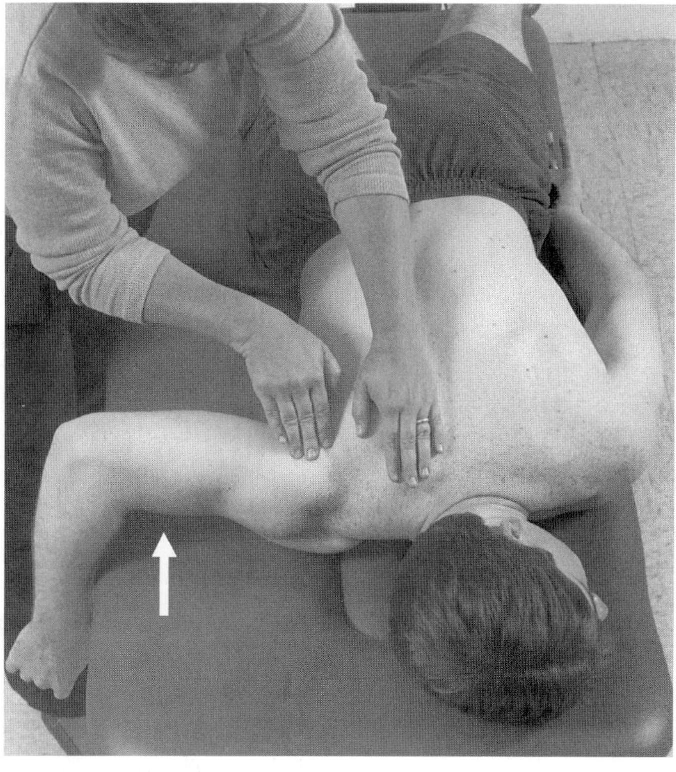

Fig. 2-59. Arrow indicates direction of movement.

Resistance: Apply resistance over distal humerus in direction of horizontal adduction. Palpating hand is moved to distal end of humerus to apply resistance (Fig. 2-60).

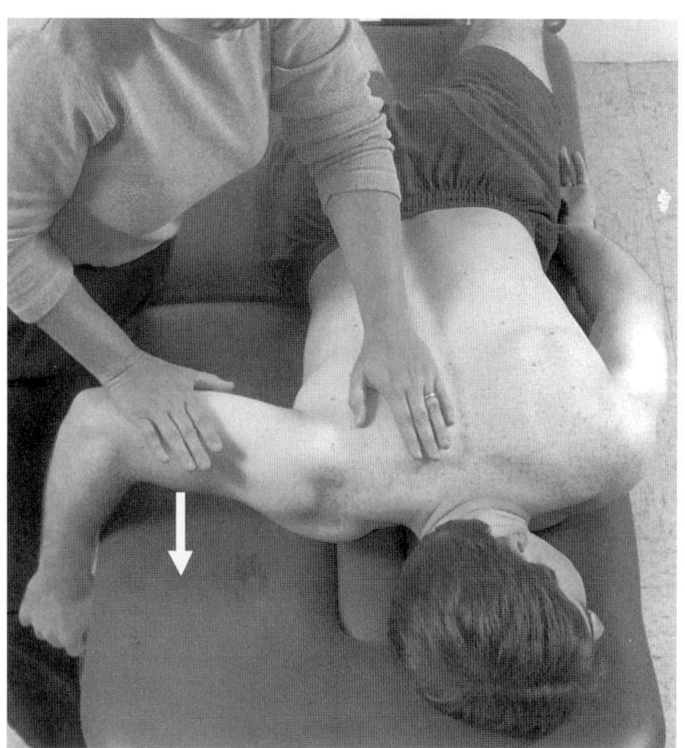

Fig. 2-60. Arrow indicates direction of resistance.

Gravity-Eliminated Test (Grades Below 3)

For patients unable to move completely through available ROM against gravity.

Patient position: Seated with shoulder abducted to 90°, humerus in neutral rotation, elbow flexed to 90°. Upper extremity should be supported on a smooth, firm surface. Talcum powder and a cloth may be placed between limb and supporting surface to reduce friction (Fig. 2-61; starting position of upper extremity not shown).

Stabilization/palpation: Stabilize over superior aspect of ipsilateral shoulder to prevent trunk rotation. Palpation occurs as in gravity-resisted test (Fig. 2-61).

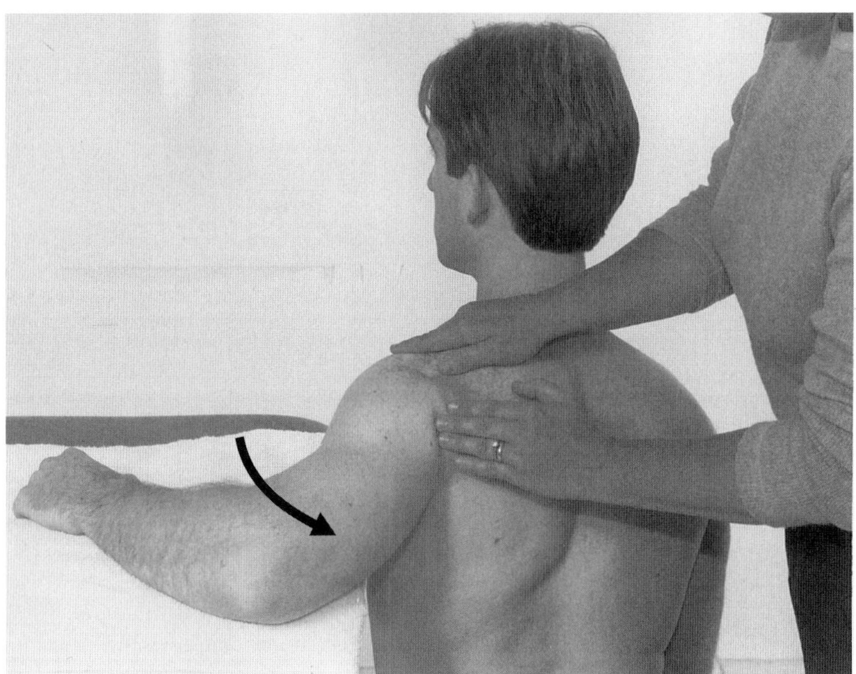

Fig. 2-61. Arrow indicates direction of movement.

Examiner action: As in gravity-resisted test.

Patient action: Patient abducts shoulder horizontally through ROM. Examiner maintains palpation and stabilization during patient's movement (Fig. 2-61).

COMMON SUBSTITUTION

Long head of triceps brachii: Elbow should remain flexed during test to prevent substitution by triceps.

■ SHOULDER HORIZONTAL ADDUCTION

PECTORALIS MAJOR (Fig. 2-62)

Fig. 2-62.

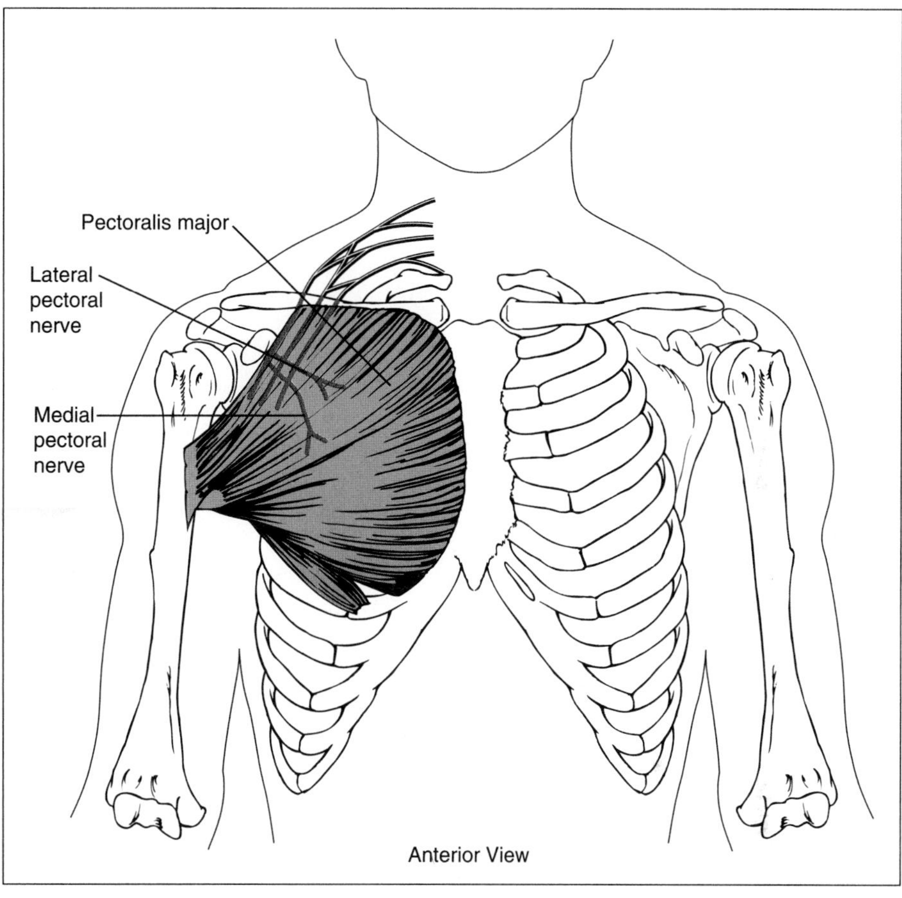

	ATTACHMENTS	NERVE SUPPLY	FUNCTION
Pectoralis major	Origin: Clavicular portion: Anterior surface of the medial ½ of the clavicle Sternocostal portion: Anterior surface of the sternum, cartilage of ribs 1–7, aponeurosis of the external abdominal oblique Insertion: Lateral lip of the intertubercular groove of the humerus	Peripheral nerve: Medial and lateral pectoral nerves Nerve root: C5–8, T1	Adduction and medial rotation of the shoulder Other functions: Clavicular portion: Flexion and horizontal adduction of the shoulder Sternocostal portion: Extension of the shoulder from a flexed position

Gravity-Resisted Test (Grades 5, 4, and 3)

Patient position: Supine with upper extremity in 90° shoulder abduction, 90° elbow flexion, forearm vertical (Fig. 2-63).

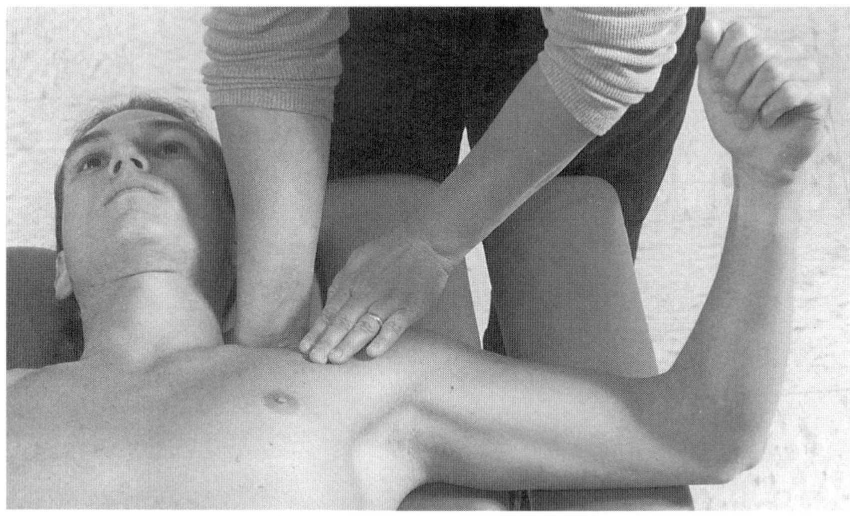

Fig. 2-63.

Stabilization/palpation: Stabilize over ipsilateral shoulder/upper thorax to prevent trunk rotation. Palpate ipsilateral pectoralis major inferior to lateral third of clavicle on anterior border of axilla (Fig. 2-63).

Examiner action: While instructing patient in motion desired, horizontally adduct patient's shoulder by bringing patient's arm across chest and keeping elbow flexed. Return patient to starting position. Performing passive movement allows determination of patient's available ROM and shows patient exact movement desired.

Patient action: Have patient horizontally adduct shoulder, bringing arm across chest. Examiner maintains palpation and stabilization during patient's movement (Fig. 2-64).

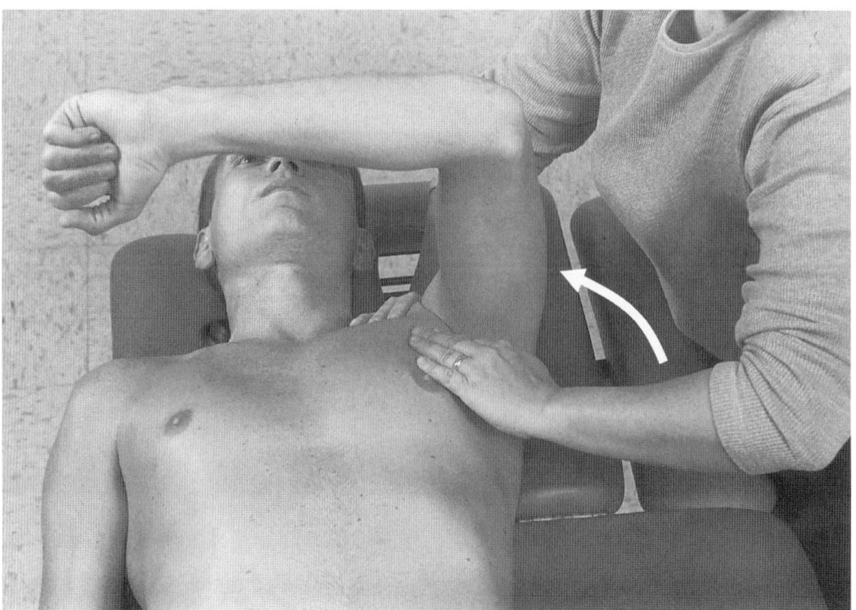

Fig. 2-64. Arrow indicates direction of movement.

Resistance: Apply resistance just proximal to elbow in direction of horizontal abduction. Palpating hand is moved to distal humerus to apply resistance (Fig. 2-65).

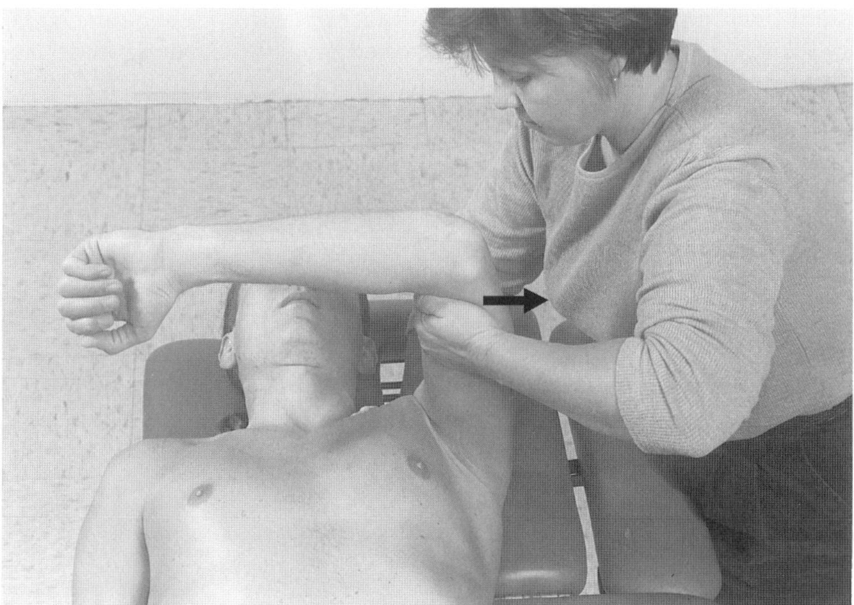

Fig. 2-65. Arrow indicates direction of resistance.

Gravity-Eliminated Test (Grades Below 3)

For patients unable to move completely through available ROM against gravity.

Patient position:

Seated half-facing table with shoulder in 90° abduction, elbow flexed to 90°, arm supported on table. Talcum powder and a cloth may be placed between limb and supporting surface to reduce friction (Fig. 2-66; initial upper extremity position not shown).

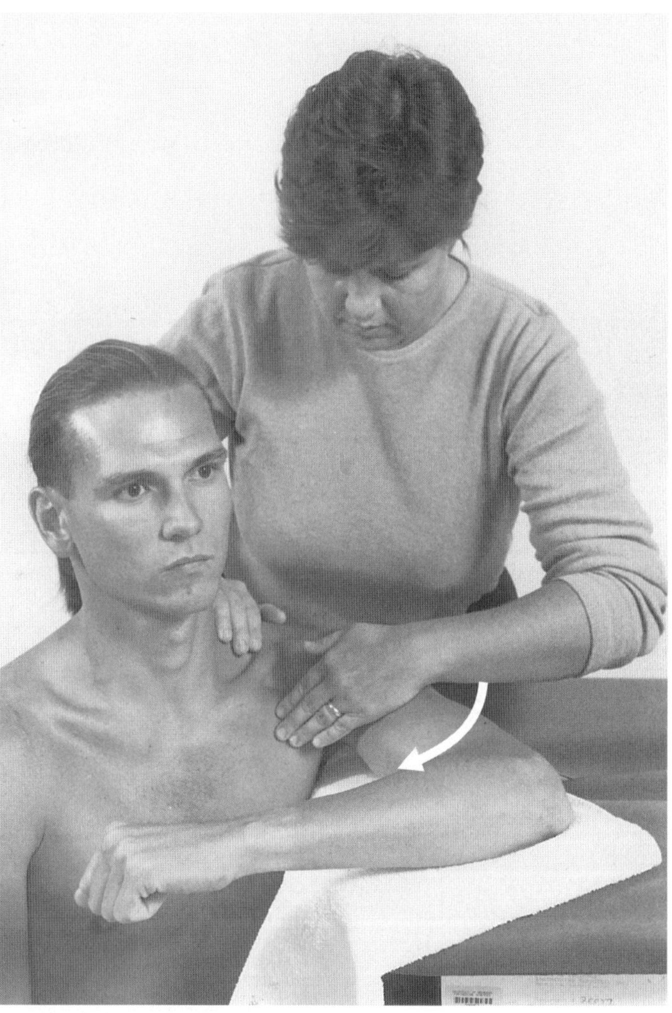

Fig. 2-66. Arrow indicates direction of movement.

Stabilization/palpation:

Stabilize over superior aspect of ipsilateral shoulder. Palpation occurs as in gravity-resisted test (Fig. 2-66).

Examiner action:

As in gravity-resisted test.

Patient action:

Patient adducts shoulder horizontally by sliding arm along table across chest. Examiner maintains palpation and stabilization during patient's movement (Fig. 2-66).

COMMON SUBSTITUTION

Rotation of trunk toward opposite side; can be prevented through stabilization of ipsilateral thorax.

■ SHOULDER HORIZONTAL ADDUCTION—ALTERNATIVE TEST I

PECTORALIS MAJOR, CLAVICULAR HEAD

This test (adapted from Kendall et al. [1993]) is used to differentiate between two heads of pectoralis major.

Gravity-Resisted Test (Grades 5 and 4)

Patient position: Supine with upper extremity in 90° shoulder flexion and slight medial rotation; 0° elbow extension (if triceps strength is sufficient) (Fig. 2-67).

Fig. 2-67.

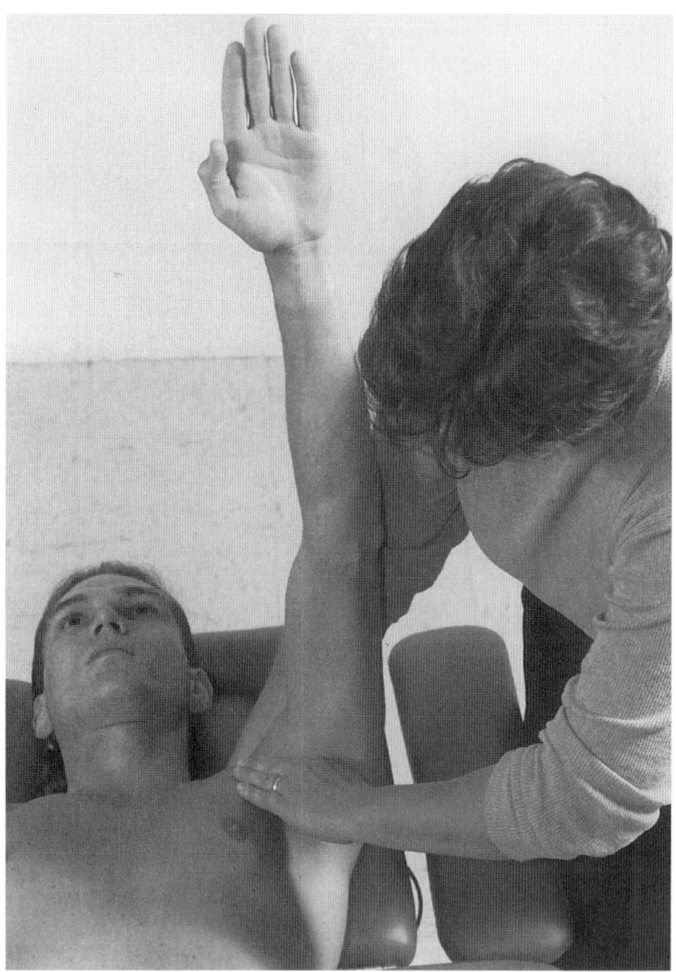

Stabilization/palpation: Stabilize over ipsilateral shoulder/upper thorax to prevent trunk rotation. Palpate pectoralis major inferior to lateral third of clavicle on anterior border of axilla (Fig. 2-67).

Examiner action: While instructing patient in motion desired, adduct patient's shoulder horizontally by bringing patient's arm across chest while keeping elbow extended. Return patient to starting position. Performing passive movement allows determination of patient's available ROM and shows patient exact movement desired.

Patient action: Have patient horizontally adduct shoulder, bringing arm across chest while examiner maintains stabilization of thorax and palpation of pectoralis major (Fig. 2-68).

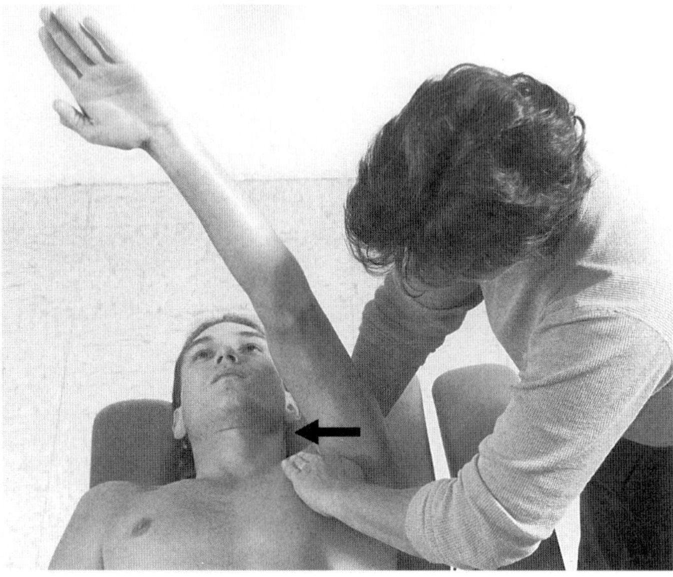

Fig. 2-68. Arrow indicates direction of movement.

Resistance: Apply resistance just proximal to elbow in direction of horizontal abduction. Palpating hand is moved to distal humerus to apply resistance (Fig. 2-69).

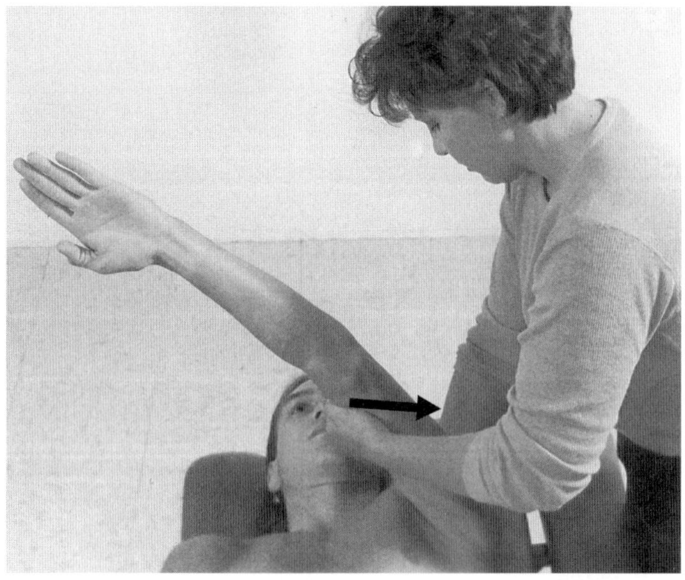

Fig. 2-69. Arrow indicates direction of resistance.

Grades 3 and Below

There is no separate test of this muscle for grades below 3. Grading is altered as follows to accommodate a lack of gravity-eliminated position.

For grade 3: Patient moves joint through full ROM without resistance.

For grade 2: Patient moves joint through partial ROM.

For grade 1: No motion, but a palpable contraction is present. Palpation occurs as described earlier (see Fig. 2-67).

For grade 0: No motion or contraction is present.

COMMON SUBSTITUTION

Rotation of trunk toward opposite side; can be prevented through stabilization of ipsilateral thorax.

■ *SHOULDER HORIZONTAL ADDUCTION— ALTERNATIVE TEST II*

PECTORALIS MAJOR: STERNOCOSTAL HEAD

This test (adapted from Kendall et al. [1993]) is used to differentiate between two heads of pectoralis major.

Gravity-Resisted Test (Grades 5 and 4)

Patient position: Supine with upper extremity in 90° shoulder flexion and slight medial rotation, 0° elbow extension (if triceps strength is sufficient) (Fig. 2-70).

Fig. 2-70.

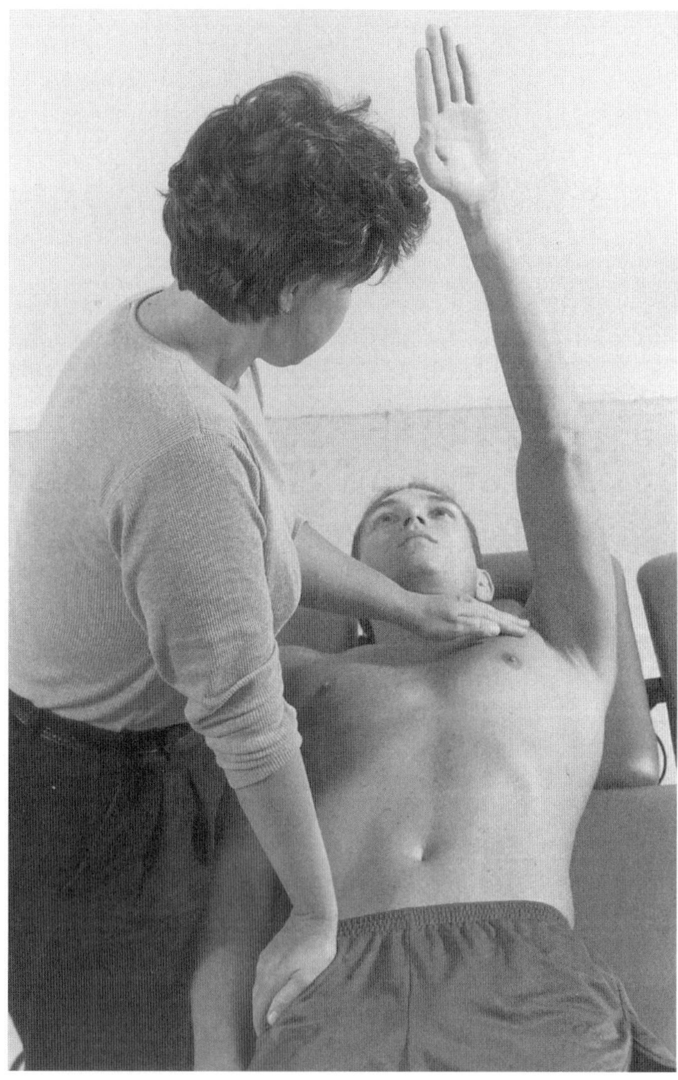

Stabilization/palpation: Stabilize over contralateral iliac crest to prevent trunk rotation. Palpate pectoralis major inferior to lateral third of clavicle on anterior border of axilla (Fig. 2-70).

Examiner action: While instructing patient in motion desired, horizontally adduct and extend patient's shoulder so that patient's hand approaches opposite iliac crest. Return patient to starting position. Performing passive movement allows determination of patient's available ROM and shows patient exact motion desired.

Patient action: Patient adducts upper extremity across body toward opposite hip while examiner maintains stabilization of pelvis and palpation of pectoralis major (Fig. 2-71).

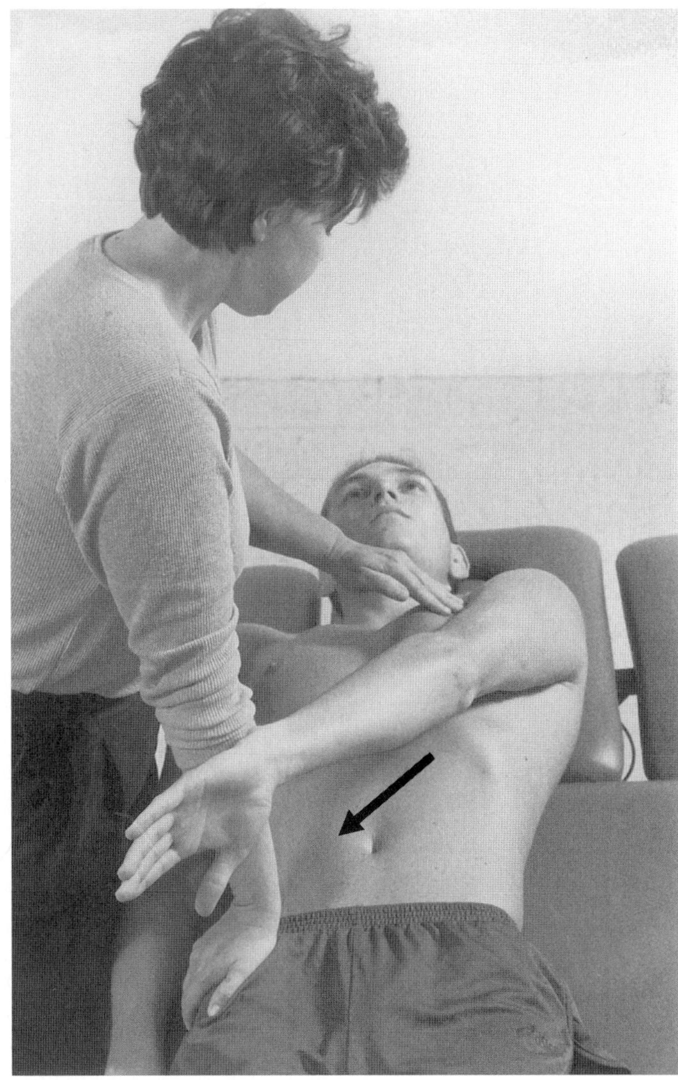

Fig. 2-71. Arrow indicates direction of movement.

Resistance: Apply resistance just proximal to wrist in direction of shoulder abduction and flexion. Palpating hand is moved to distal forearm to apply resistance (Fig. 2-72).

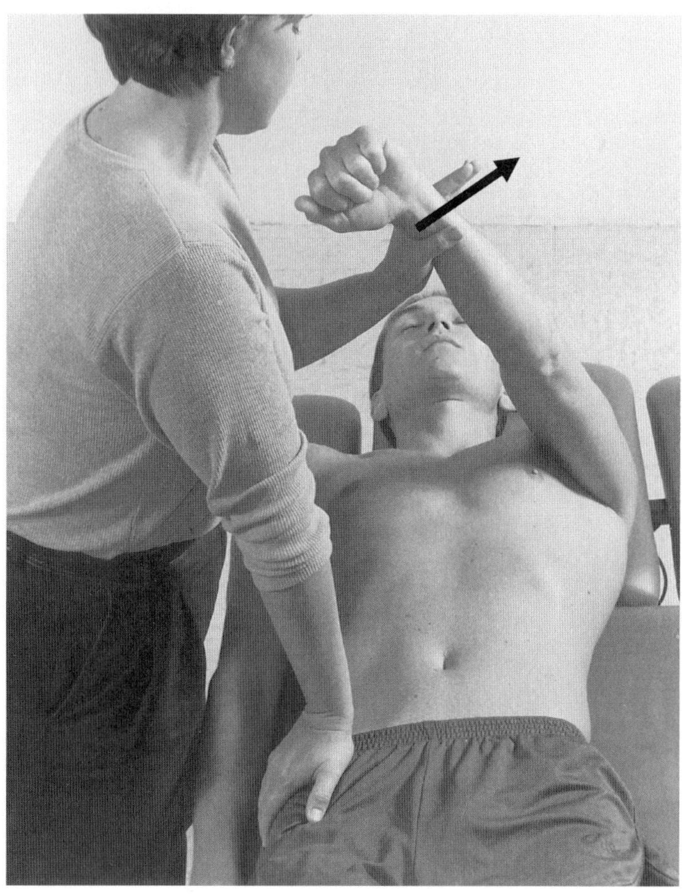

Fig. 2-72. Arrow indicates direction of resistance.

Grades 3 and Below

There is no separate test of this muscle for grades below 3. Grading is altered as follows to accommodate lack of a gravity-eliminated position.

For grade 3: Patient moves joint through full ROM without resistance.

For grade 2: Patient moves joint through partial ROM.

For grade 1: No motion, but a palpable contraction is present. Palpation occurs as described previously (Fig. 2-70).

For grade 0: No motion or contraction is present.

■ SHOULDER MEDIAL ROTATION

SUBSCAPULARIS, PECTORALIS MAJOR, LATISSIMUS DORSI, TERES MAJOR (Fig. 2-73)

Fig. 2-73.

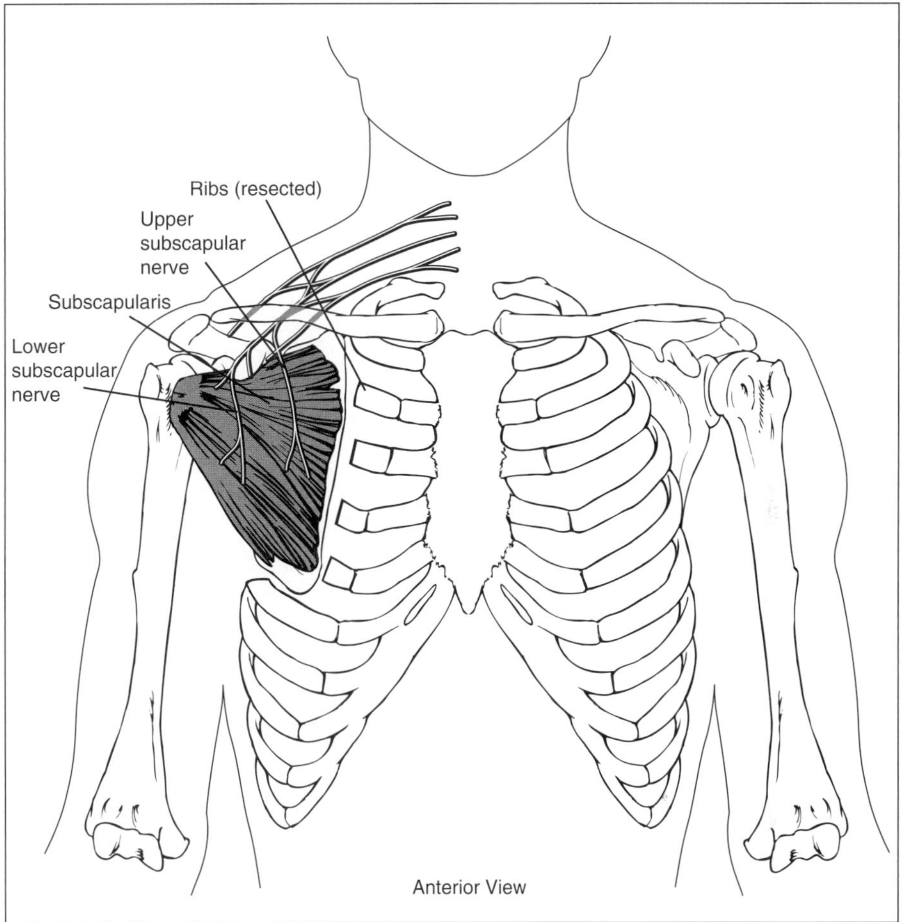

	ATTACHMENTS	NERVE SUPPLY	FUNCTION
Subscapularis	Origin: Subscapular fossa of the scapula Insertion: Lesser tubercle of the humerus	Peripheral nerve: Upper and lower subscapular nerves Nerve root: C5, C6	Medial rotation of the shoulder
Pectoralis major	Origin: Clavicular portion: Anterior surface of the medial ½ of the clavicle Sternocostal portion: Anterior surface of the sternum, cartilage of ribs 1–7, aponeurosis of the external abdominal oblique Insertion: Lateral lip of the intertubercular groove of the humerus	Peripheral nerve: Medial and lateral pectoral nerves Nerve root: C5–8, T1	Adduction and medial rotation of the shoulder Other functions: Clavicular portion: Flexion and horizontal adduction of the shoulder Sternocostal portion: Extension of the shoulder from a flexed position
Latissimus dorsi	Origin: Spinous processes of the sacral, lumbar, and lower six thoracic vertebrae and supraspinal ligament via the thoracolumbar fascia, iliac crest, and lower three to four ribs Insertion: Floor of the intertubercular groove of the humerus	Peripheral nerve: Thoracodorsal nerve Nerve root: C6–C8	Extension, adduction, and medial rotation of the shoulder
Teres major	Origin: Posterior surface of the inferior angle of the scapula Insertion: Medial lip of the intertubercular groove of the humerus	Peripheral nerve: Lower subscapular nerve Nerve root: C5, C6	Adduction, extension, and medial rotation of the shoulder

Gravity-Resisted Test (Grades 5, 4, and 3)

Patient position: Prone with upper extremity in 90° shoulder abduction, 90° elbow flexion, forearm hanging vertically off side of table. Horizontal position of humerus is maintained by folded towel placed between table and patient's humerus (Fig. 2-74).

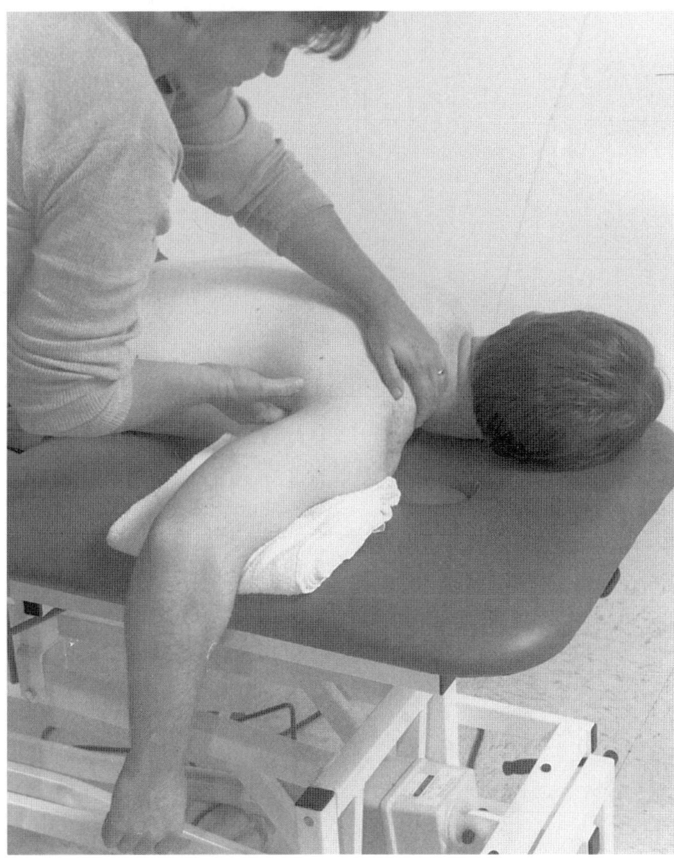

Fig. 2-74.

Stabilization/palpation: Stabilize over ipsilateral thorax (or scapula if scapular stabilizers are weak; avoid pressure on tested muscles). Palpate subscapularis deep in axilla along anterior surface of scapula with patient in a prone position (Fig. 2-74).

Examiner action: While instructing patient in motion desired, rotate patient's humerus medially, maintaining elbow in flexed position. Return patient to starting position. Performing passive movement allows determination of patient's available ROM and shows patient exact movement desired.

Patient action:

Patient moves through full range of shoulder medial rotation while examiner maintains stabilization of thorax and palpation of subscapularis (Fig. 2-75).

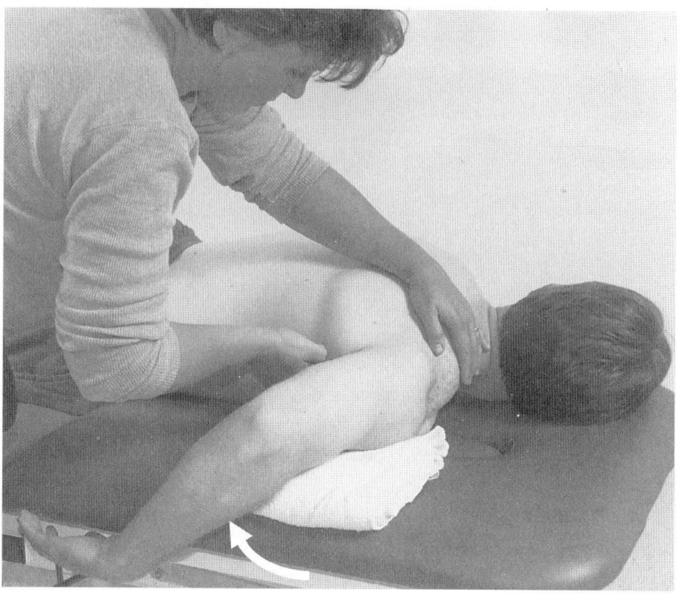

Fig. 2-75. Arrow indicates direction of movement.

Resistance:

Apply resistance just proximal to wrist in direction of lateral rotation of shoulder. Palpating hand is moved to distal forearm to apply resistance (Fig. 2-76).

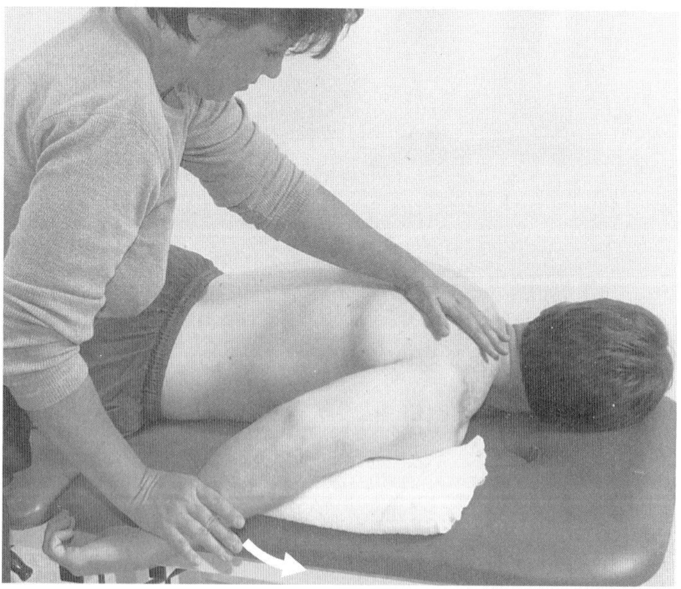

Fig. 2-76. Arrow indicates direction of resistance.

Gravity-Eliminated Test (Grades Below 3)

For patients unable to move completely through available ROM against gravity.

Patient position: Prone with upper extremity in 90° shoulder flexion, full lateral shoulder rotation, 0° elbow extension, arm hanging vertically off side of table (Fig. 2-77).

Fig. 2-77.

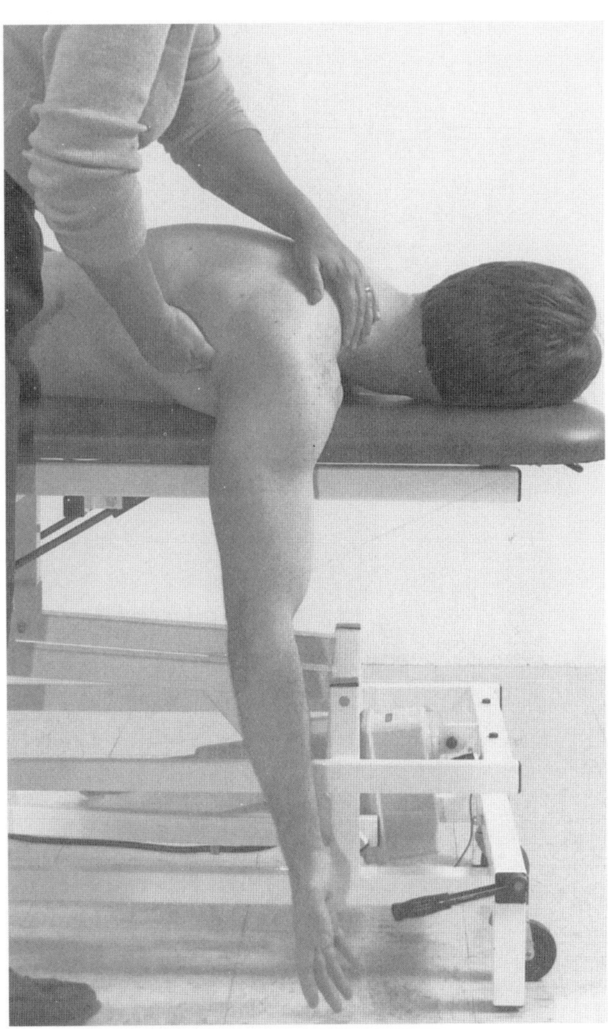

Stabilization/palpation: As in gravity-eliminated test (Fig. 2-77).

Examiner action: While instructing patient in motion desired, rotate humerus medially along its long axis, maintaining elbow in extension. Return patient to starting position.

Patient action: Patient moves through full range of medial rotation while examiner maintains stabilization of thorax and palpation of subscapularis (Fig. 2-78).

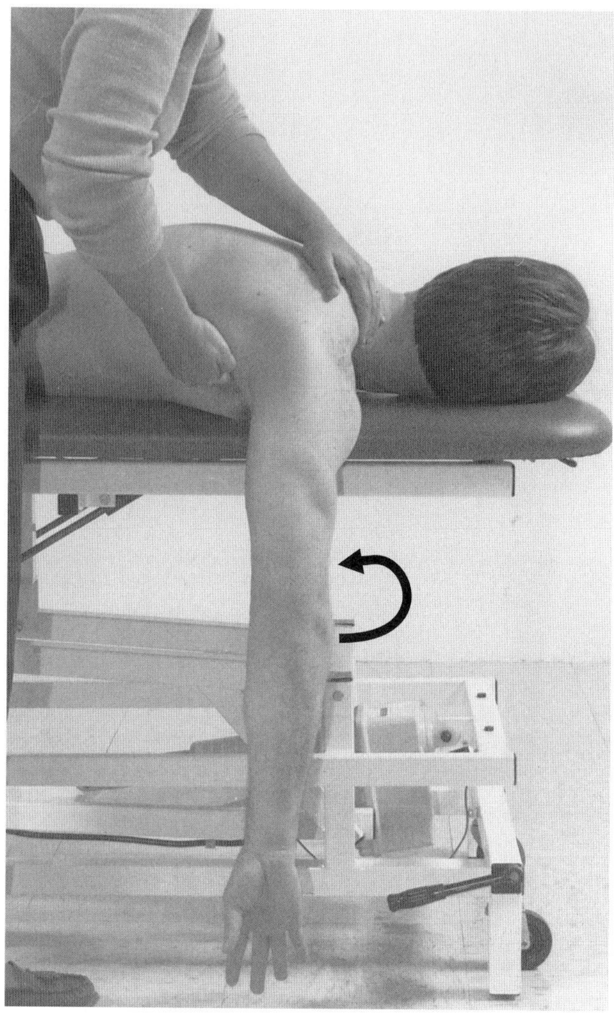

Fig. 2-78. Arrow indicates direction of movement.

COMMON SUBSTITUTION

During gravity-eliminated test, patient may appear to be rotating humerus medially by pronating forearm. Care should be taken to ensure that motion is occurring at glenohumeral joint.

SHOULDER LATERAL ROTATION

INFRASPINATUS: TERES MINOR (Fig. 2-79)

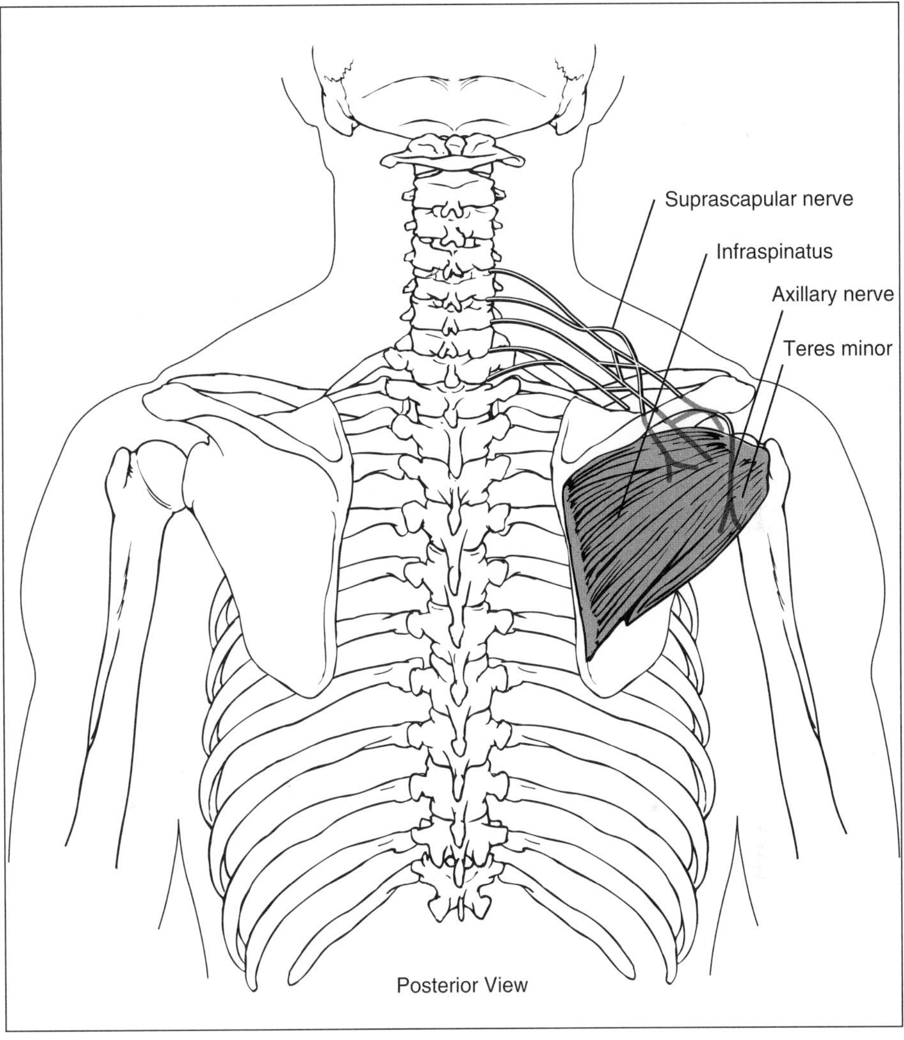

Fig. 2-79.

	ATTACHMENTS	NERVE SUPPLY	FUNCTION
Infraspinatus	Origin: Infraspinatus fossa of the scapula Insertion: Greater tubercle of the humerus	Peripheral nerve: Suprascapular nerve Nerve root: C5, C6	Lateral rotation of the shoulder
Teres minor	Origin: Superior ⅔ of the posterior surface of the axillary border of the scapula Insertion: Greater tubercle of the humerus	Peripheral nerve: Axillary nerve Nerve root: C5	Lateral rotation of the shoulder

Gravity-Resisted Test (Grades 5, 4, and 3)

Patient position: Prone with upper extremity in 90° abduction, 90° elbow flexion, forearm hanging vertically off side of table. Horizontal position of humerus is maintained by folded towel placed between table and patient's humerus (Fig. 2-80).

Fig. 2-80.

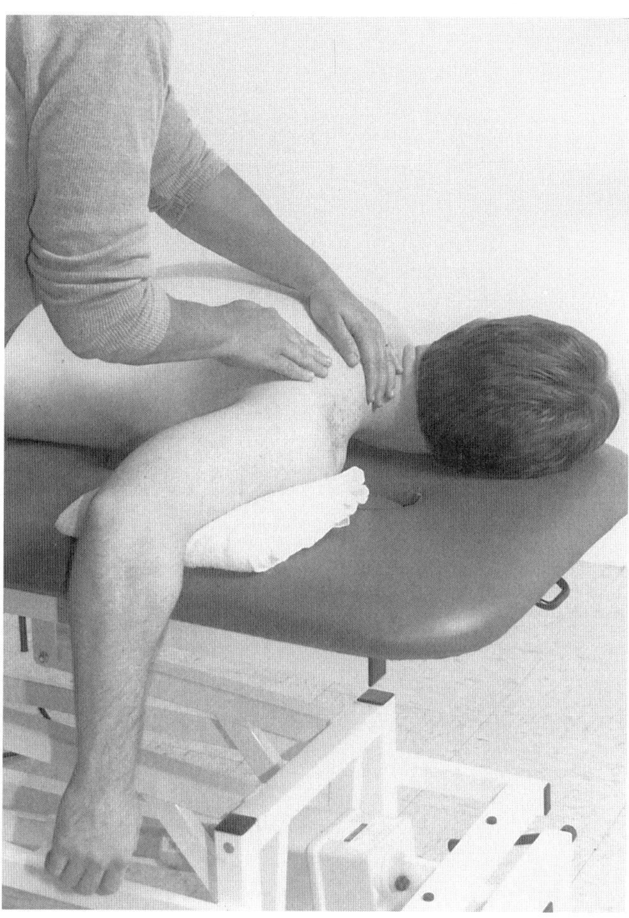

Stabilization/palpation: Stabilize over ipsilateral thorax (or scapula if scapular stabilizers are weak; avoid pressure on tested muscles). Palpate infraspinatus and teres minor below spine of scapula over posterior surface of body (infraspinatus) and axillary border (teres minor) of scapula (Fig. 2-80).

Examiner action: While instructing patient in motion desired, rotate patient's humerus laterally, maintaining elbow in a flexed position. Return patient to starting position. Performing passive movement allows determination of patient's available ROM and shows patient exact movement desired.

Patient action:

Patient moves through full range of lateral rotation while examiner maintains stabilization of thorax and palpation of infraspinatus and teres minor (Fig. 2-81).

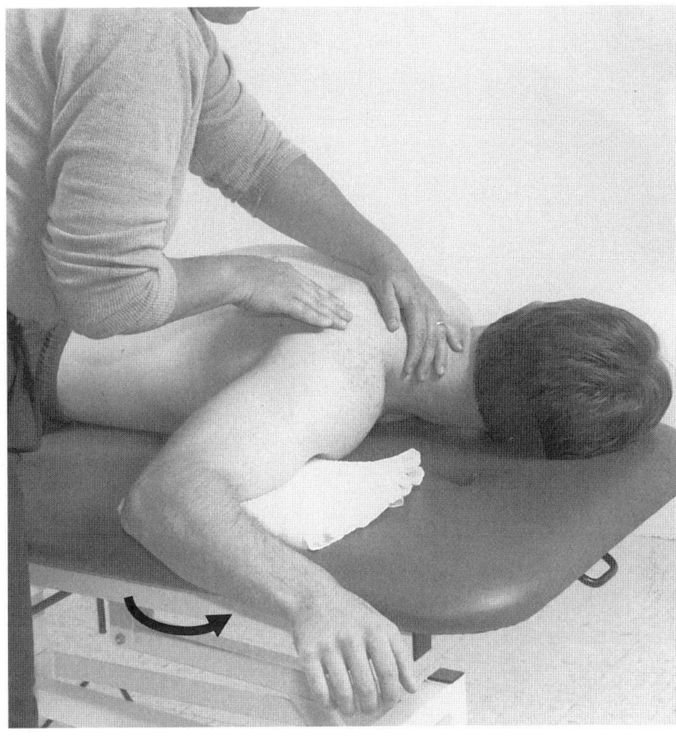

Fig. 2-81. Arrow indicates direction of movement.

Resistance:

Apply resistance just proximal to wrist in direction of medial rotation of shoulder. Palpating hand is moved to distal forearm to apply resistance (Fig. 2-82).

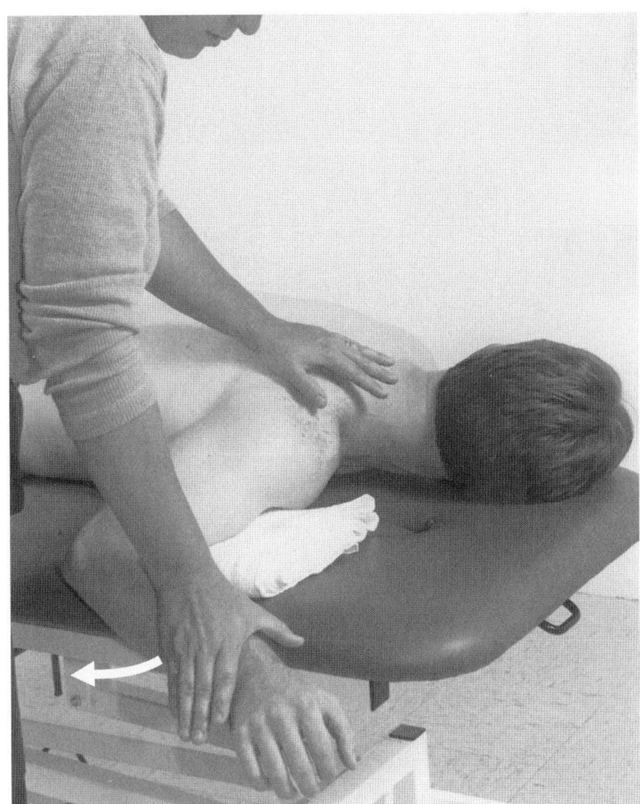

Fig. 2-82. Arrow indicates direction of resistance.

Gravity-Eliminated Test (Grades Below 3)

For patients unable to move completely through available ROM against gravity.

Patient position: Prone with shoulder flexed to 90° and in full medial rotation, elbow extended, arm hanging vertically off side of table (Fig. 2-83).

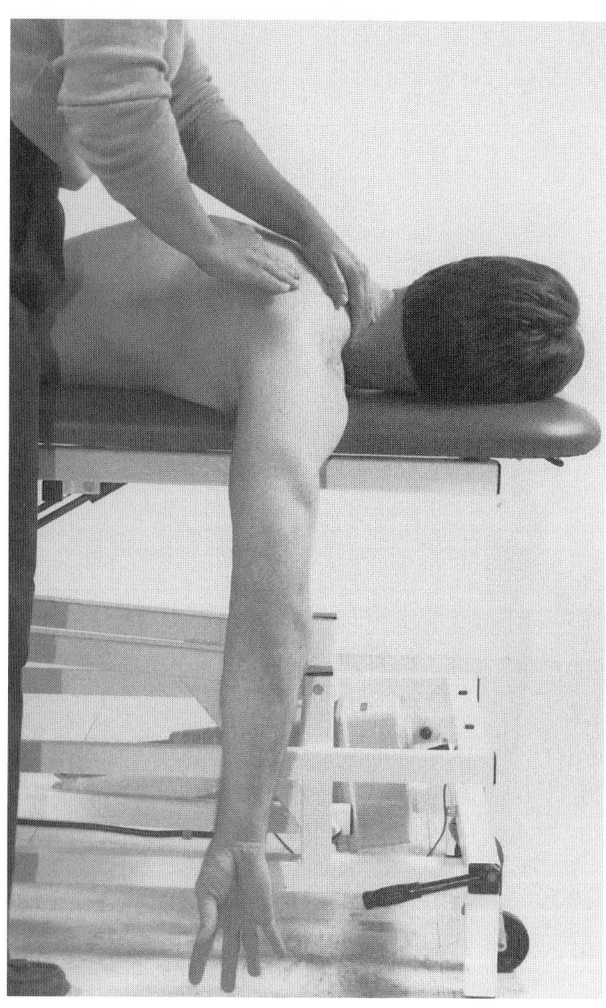

Fig. 2-83.

Stabilization/palpation: As in gravity-resisted test (Fig. 2-83).

Examiner action: While instructing patient in motion desired, rotate humerus laterally along its long axis, maintaining elbow in extension. Return patient to starting position.

Patient action: Patient moves through full range of lateral rotation while examiner maintains stabilization of thorax and palpation of infraspinatus and teres minor (Fig. 2-84).

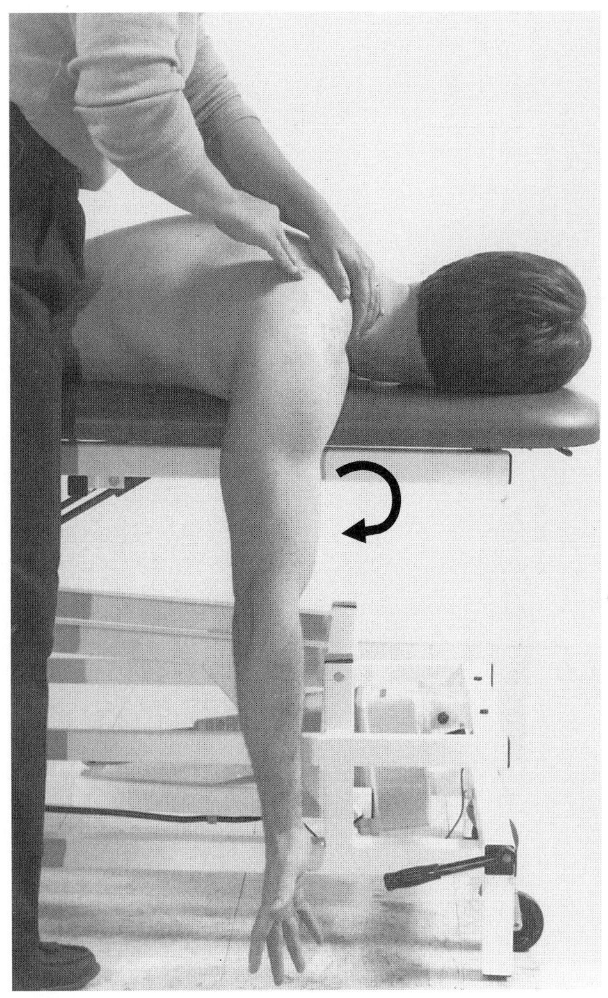

Fig. 2-84. Arrow indicates direction of movement.

COMMON SUBSTITUTION

During gravity-eliminated test, patient may appear to be rotating humerus laterally by supinating forearm. Care should be taken to ensure that motion is occurring at glenohumeral joint.

ELBOW FLEXION

BICEPS BRACHII (Fig. 2-85)

Fig. 2-85.

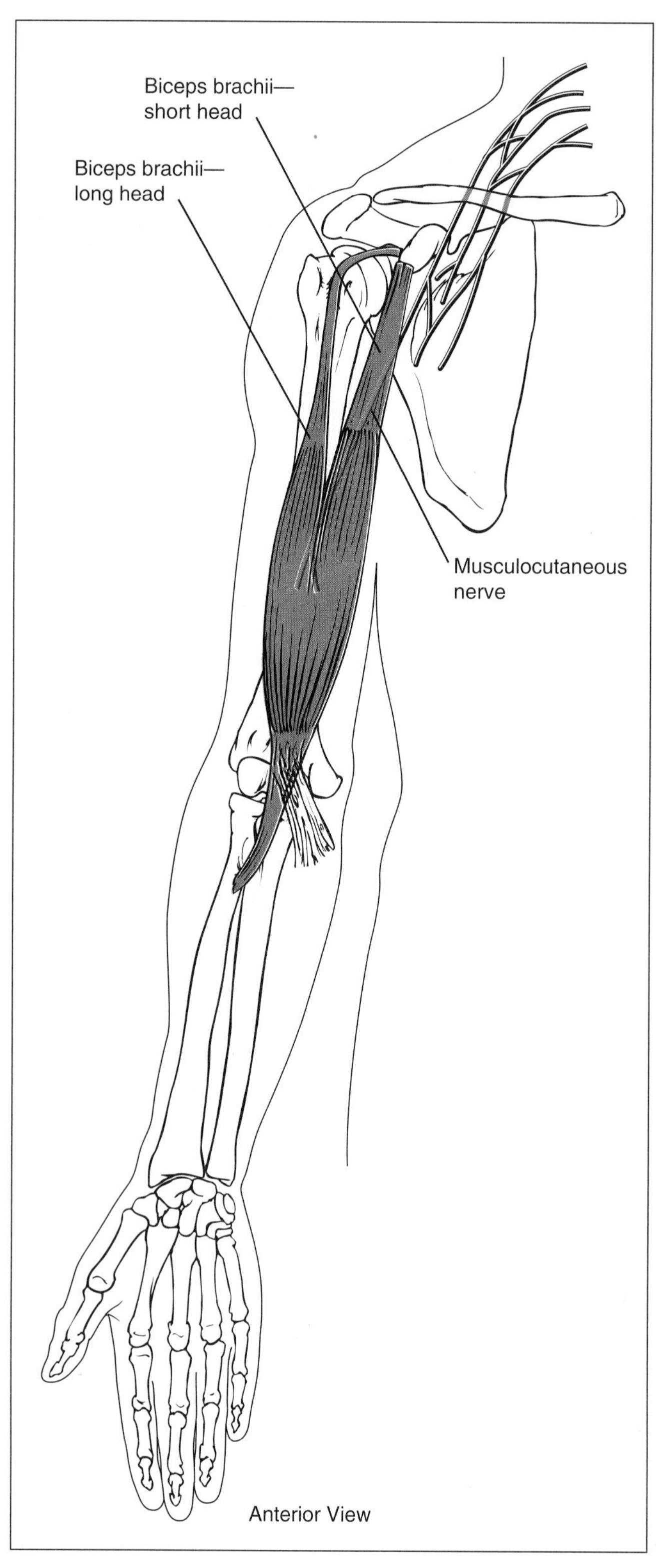

	ATTACHMENTS	NERVE SUPPLY	FUNCTION
Biceps brachii	Origin: Short head: Coracoid process of the scapula Long head: Supraglenoid tuberosity of the scapula Insertion: Tuberosity of the radius	Peripheral nerve: Musculocutaneous nerve Nerve root: C5, C6	Flexion of the elbow; supination of the forearm; assists in flexion of the shoulder

Gravity-Resisted Test (Grades 5, 4, and 3)

Patient position: Seated with upper extremity in 0° shoulder adduction, 0° elbow extension, forearm supination (Fig. 2-86).

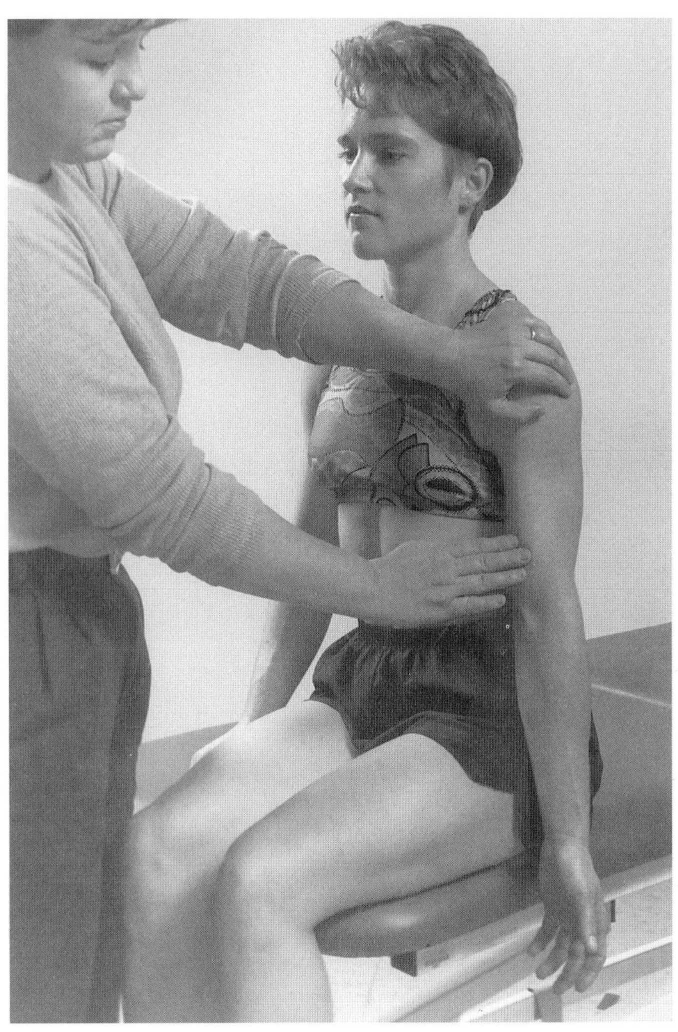

Fig. 2-86.

Stabilization/palpation: Stabilize over anterosuperior aspect of ipsilateral humerus. Palpate biceps brachii over middle third of anterior arm (Fig. 2-86).

Examiner action: While instructing patient in motion desired, flex patient's elbow, maintaining forearm in full supination. Return patient to starting position. Performing passive movement allows determination of patient's available ROM and shows patient exact movement desired.

Patient action: Patient flexes elbow through full ROM while examiner maintains stabilization of humerus and palpation of biceps (Fig. 2-87).

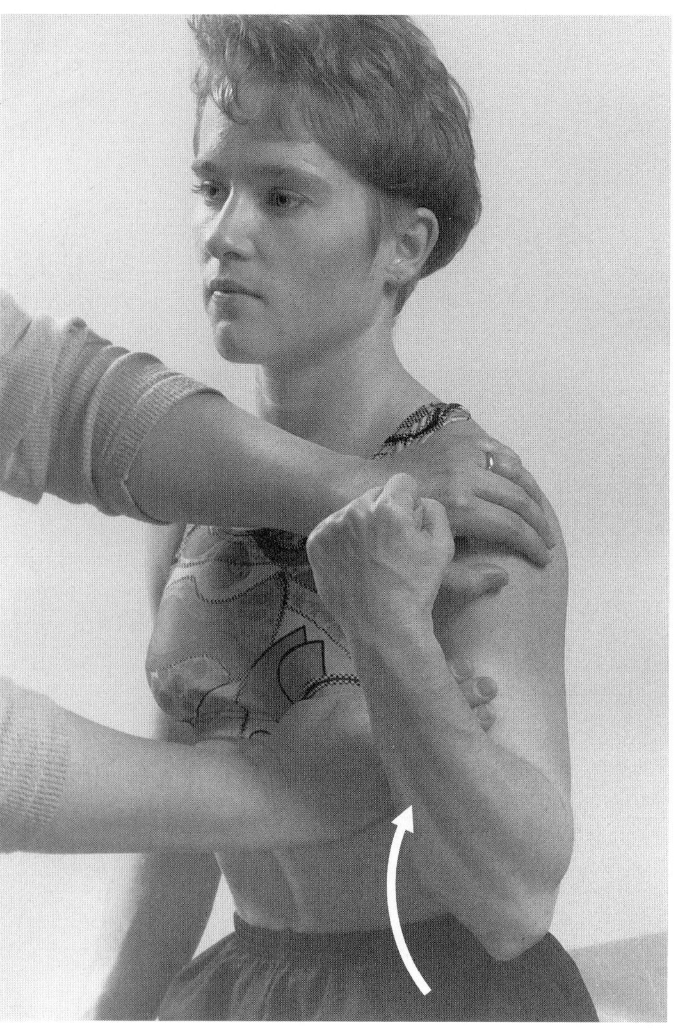

Fig. 2-87. Arrow indicates direction of movement.

Resistance: Apply resistance just proximal to wrist in direction of elbow extension. Palpating hand is moved to distal forearm to apply resistance (Fig. 2-88).

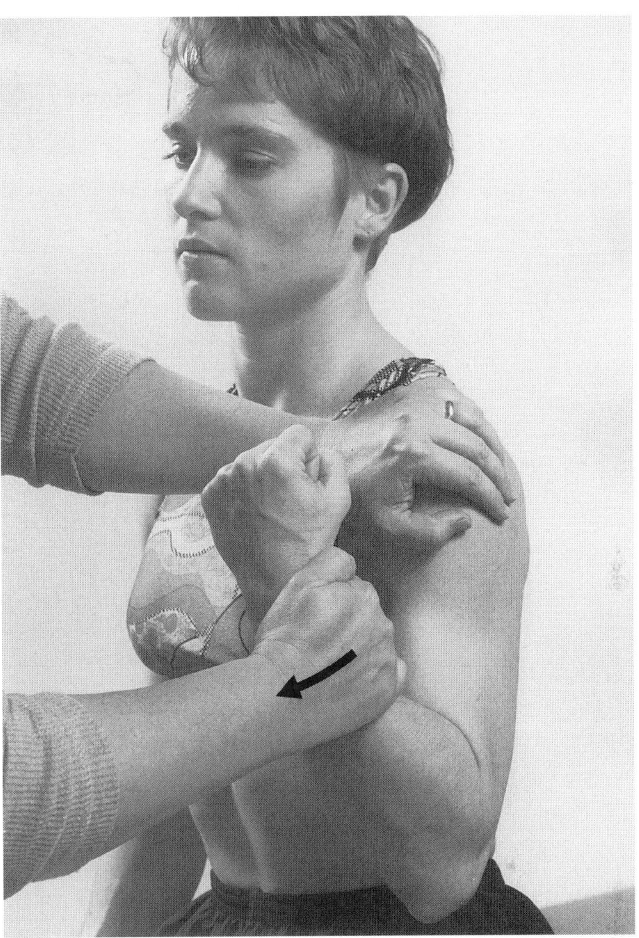

Fig. 2-88. Arrow indicates direction of resistance.

Gravity-Eliminated Test (Grades Below 3)

For patients unable to move completely through available ROM against gravity.

Patient position: Seated with arm supported on table; shoulder abducted to 90°, elbow extended, forearm fully supinated. Talcum powder and a cloth may be placed between limb and supporting surface to reduce friction (Fig. 2-89; initial elbow position not shown).

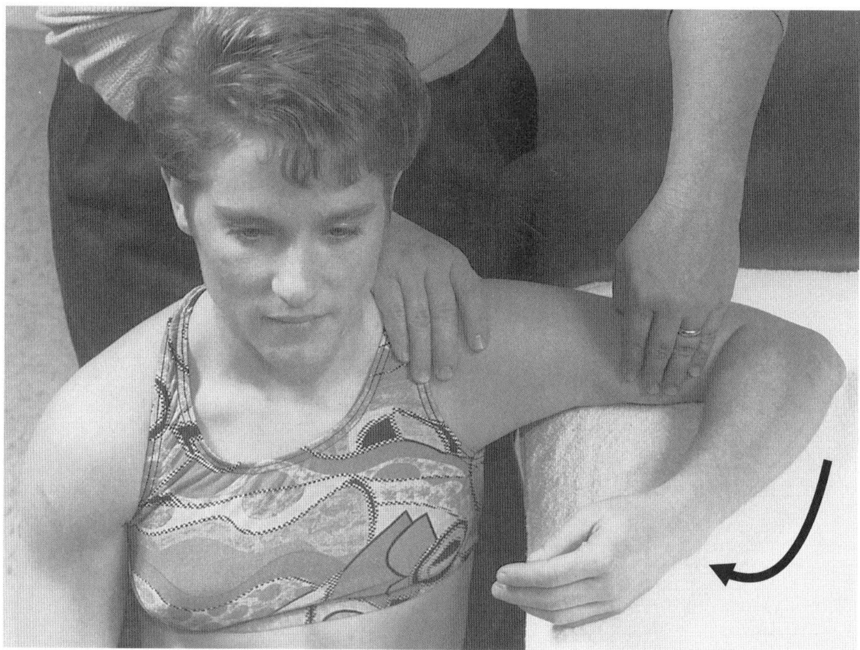

Fig. 2-89. Arrow indicates direction of movement.

Stabilization/palpation: Stabilize over anterosuperior aspect of ipsilateral humerus. Palpate muscle as in gravity-resisted test (Fig. 2-89).

Examiner action: As in gravity-resisted test.

Patient action: Patient flexes elbow through full ROM by sliding forearm along table while examiner maintains stabilization of humerus and palpation of biceps (Fig. 2-89).

CLINICAL COMMENT: BICEPS BRACHII MUSCLE AND C6 NEUROLOGIC ASSESSMENT

The biceps brachii muscle is a key muscle for examining the integrity of the C6 spinal nerve or neurologic segment of the spinal cord. Complete assessment of the C6 neurologic level includes:

Strength assessment of:
Biceps brachii (pp. 99–102)
Wrist extensors (pp. 134-142)

Reflex testing of:
Brachioradialis reflex (p. 548)
Biceps reflex (C5 and C6; p. 547)

Sensory testing of:
Skin over thumb and lateral forearm (C6 dermatome; pp. 528-532)

▪ ELBOW FLEXION

BRACHIALIS (Fig. 2-90)

Fig. 2-90.

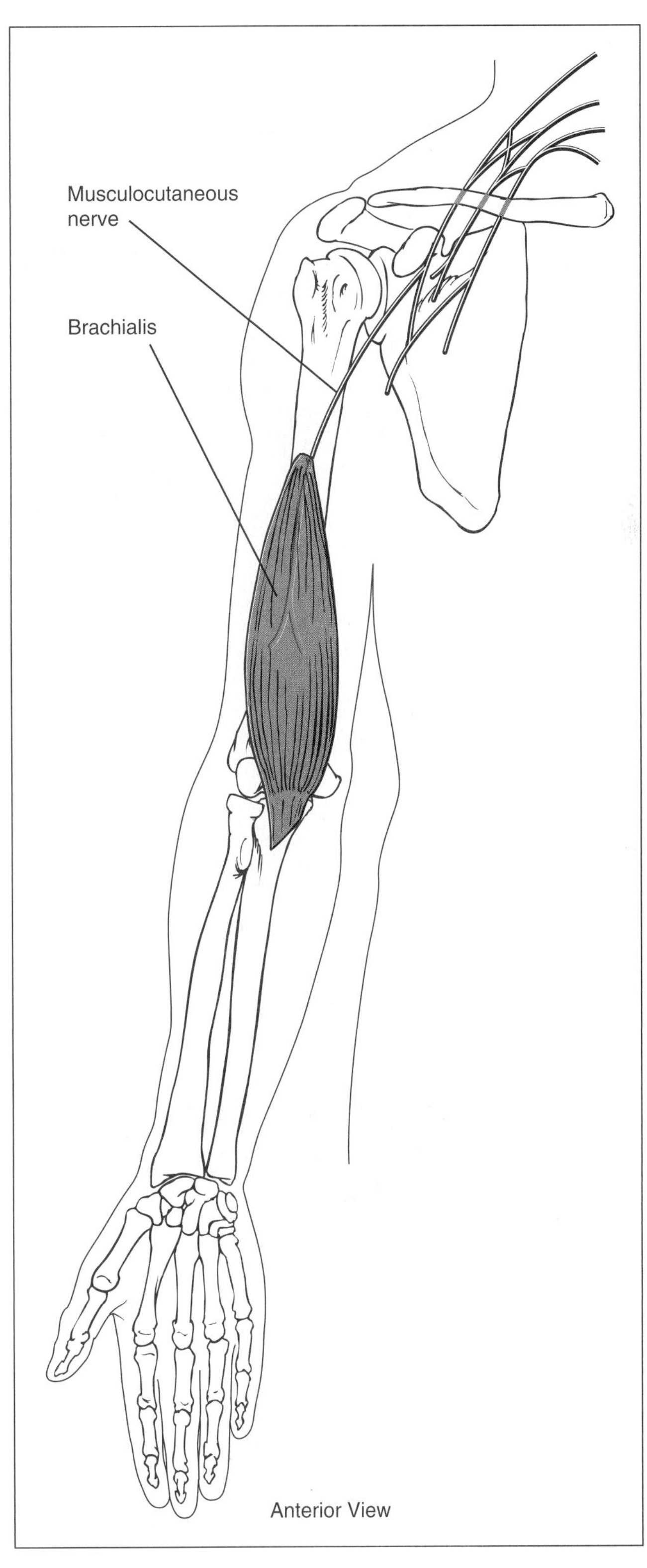

	ATTACHMENTS	NERVE SUPPLY	FUNCTION
Brachialis	Origin: Distal ½ of the anterior aspect of the humeral shaft; medial and lateral intermuscular septa Insertion: Tuberosity and coronoid process of the ulna	Peripheral nerve: Musculocutaneous nerve Nerve root: C5, C6	Flexion of the elbow

Gravity-Resisted Test (Grades 5, 4, and 3)

Patient position: Seated with upper extremity in 0° shoulder adduction, 0° elbow extension, forearm pronation (Fig. 2-91).

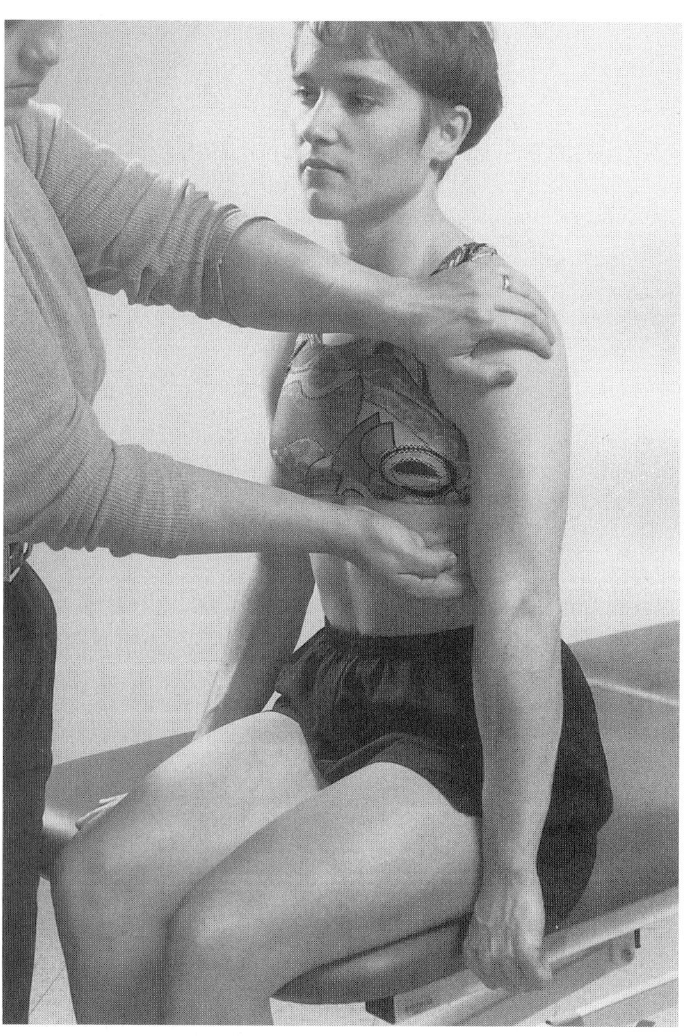

Fig. 2-91.

Stabilization/palpation: Stabilize over anterosuperior aspect of ipsilateral humerus. Palpate brachialis medial to distal attachment of biceps brachii (Fig. 2-91).

Examiner action:

While instructing patient in motion desired, flex patient's elbow, maintaining forearm in full pronation. Return patient to starting position. Performing passive movement allows determination of patient's available ROM and shows patient exact movement desired.

Patient action:

Patient flexes elbow through full ROM while examiner maintains stabilization of humerus and palpation of brachialis (Fig. 2-92).

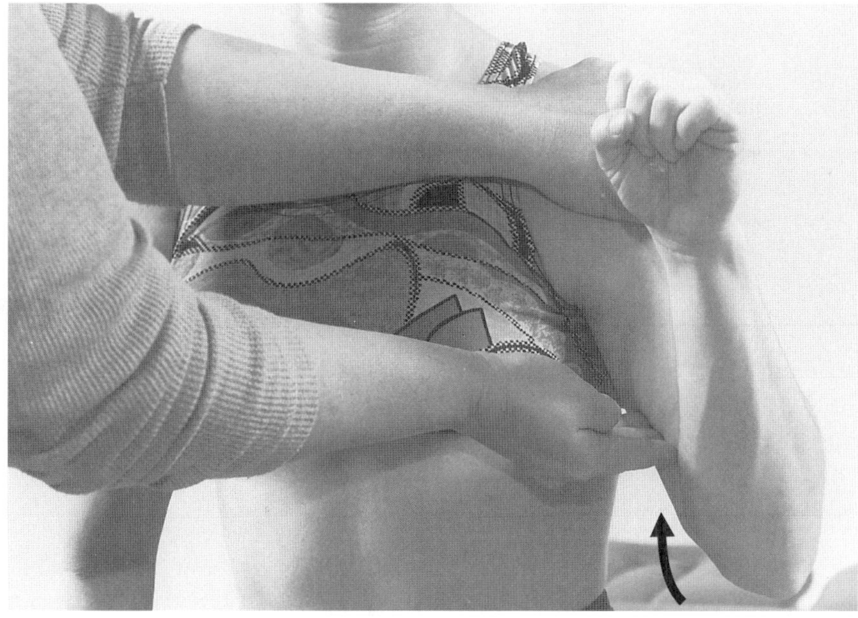

Fig. 2-92. Arrow indicates direction of movement.

Resistance:

Apply resistance just proximal to wrist in direction of elbow extension. Palpating hand is moved to distal forearm to apply resistance (Fig. 2-93).

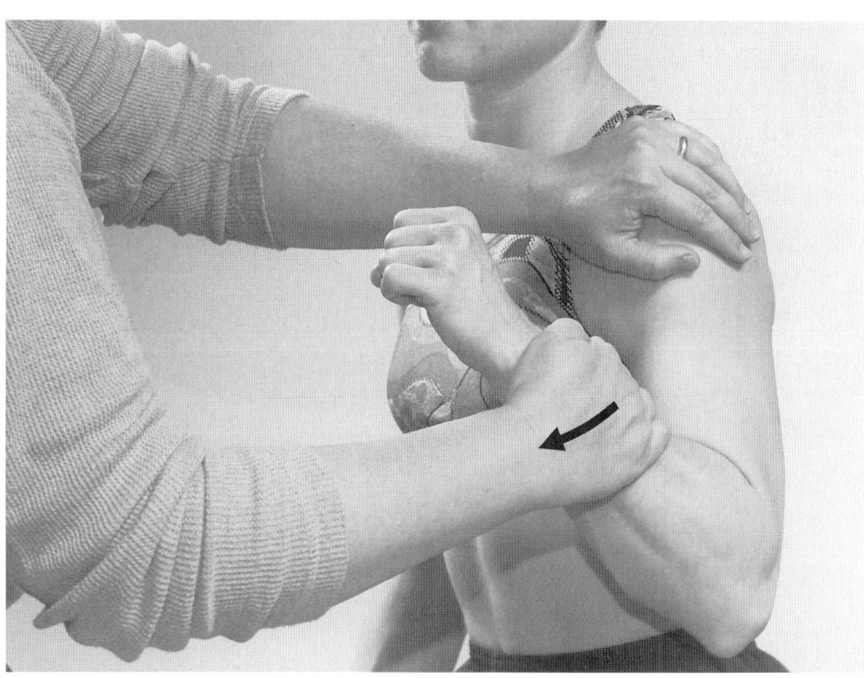

Fig. 2-93. Arrow indicates direction of resistance.

Gravity-Eliminated Test (Grades Below 3)

For patients unable to move completely through available ROM against gravity.

Patient position:

Seated with arm supported on table. Shoulder is abducted to 90°, elbow extended, forearm pronated. Talcum powder and a cloth may be placed between limb and supporting surface to reduce friction (Fig. 2-94; initial elbow position not shown).

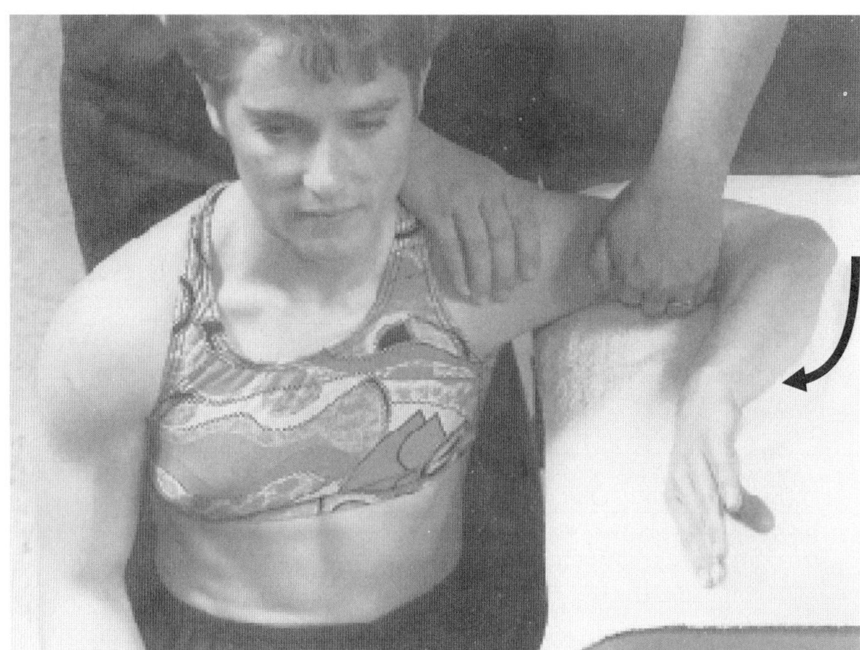

Fig. 2-94. Arrow indicates direction of movement.

Stabilization/palpation:

Stabilize over anterosuperior aspect of ipsilateral humerus. Palpate muscle as in gravity-resisted test (Fig. 2-94).

Examiner action:

As in gravity-resisted test.

Patient action:

Patient flexes elbow through full ROM by sliding forearm along table while examiner maintains stabilization of humerus and palpation of brachialis (Fig. 2-94).

■ ELBOW FLEXION

BRACHIORADIALIS (Fig. 2-95)

Fig. 2-95.

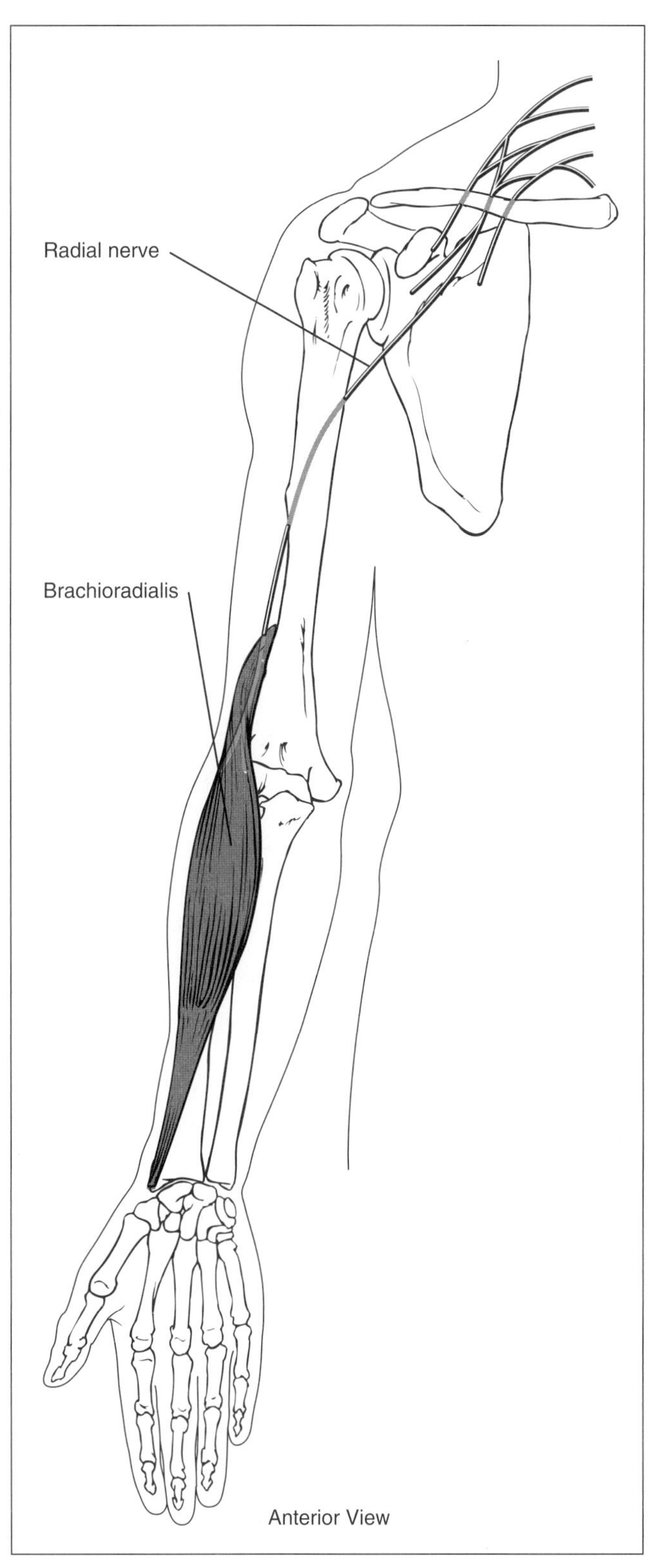

	ATTACHMENTS	NERVE SUPPLY	FUNCTION
Brachioradialis	Origin: Upper ⅔ of the lateral supracondylar ridge of the humerus; lateral intermuscular septum Insertion: Styloid process of the radius	Peripheral nerve: Radial nerve Nerve root: C5, C6	Flexion of the elbow

Gravity-Resisted Test (Grades 5, 4, and 3)

Patient position: Seated with upper extremity in 0° shoulder adduction, 0° elbow extension, neutral forearm rotation (halfway between pronation and supination) (Fig. 2-96).

Fig. 2-96.

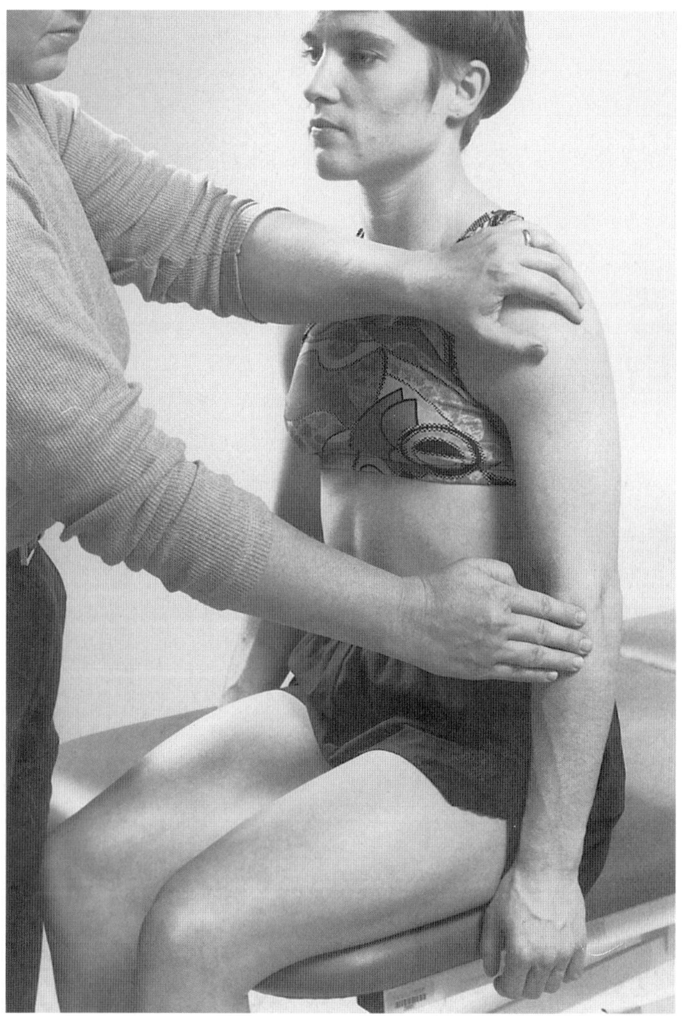

Stabilization/palpation: Stabilize over anterosuperior aspect of ipsilateral humerus. Palpate brachioradialis over anterolateral aspect of forearm just distal to lateral epicondyle of humerus (Fig. 2-96).

Examiner action:

While instructing patient in motion desired, flex patient's elbow, maintaining forearm in neutral position. Return patient to starting position. Performing passive movement allows determination of patient's available ROM and shows patient exact motion desired.

Patient action:

Patient flexes elbow through full ROM while examiner maintains stabilization of humerus and palpation of brachioradialis (Fig. 2-97).

Fig. 2-97. Arrow indicates direction of movement.

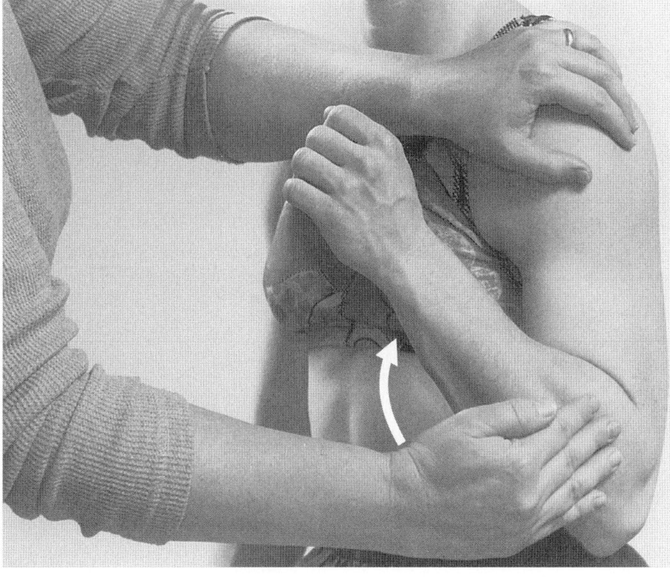

Resistance:

Apply resistance just proximal to wrist in direction of elbow extension. Palpating hand is moved to distal forearm to apply resistance (Fig. 2-98).

Fig. 2-98. Arrow indicates direction of resistance.

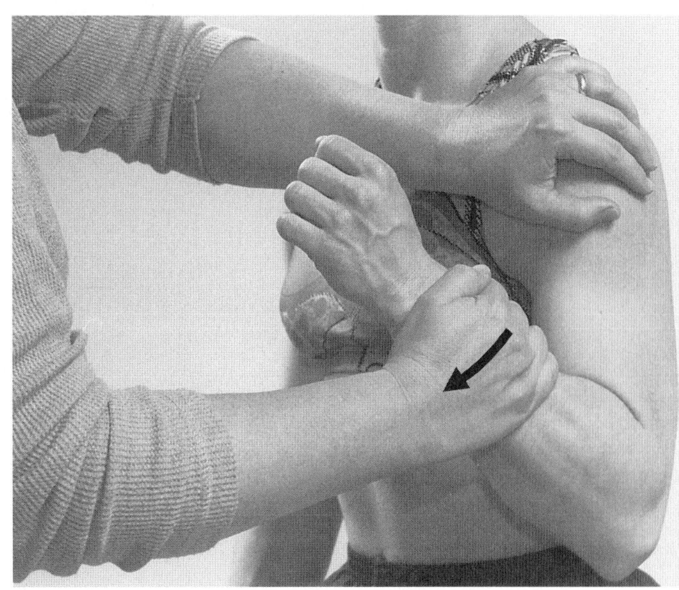

Gravity-Eliminated Test (Grades Below 3)

For patients unable to move completely through available ROM against gravity.

Patient position: Seated with arm supported on table, shoulder abducted to 90°, elbow extended, forearm in neutral rotation (halfway between pronation and supination). Talcum powder and a cloth may be placed between limb and supporting surface to reduce friction (Fig. 2-99; initial elbow position not shown).

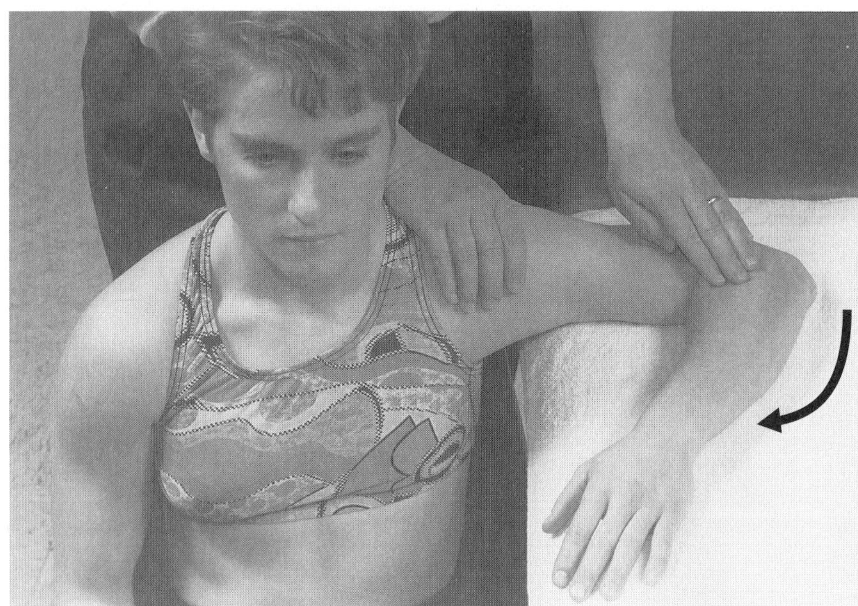

Fig. 2-99. Arrow indicates direction of movement.

Stabilization/palpation: As in gravity-resisted test (Fig. 2-99).

Examiner action: As in gravity-resisted test.

Patient action: Patient flexes elbow through full ROM by sliding forearm along table. Examiner maintains stabilization of humerus and palpation of brachioradialis during patient movement (Fig. 2-99).

■ ELBOW EXTENSION

TRICEPS BRACHII: ANCONEUS (Fig. 2-100)

Fig. 2-100.

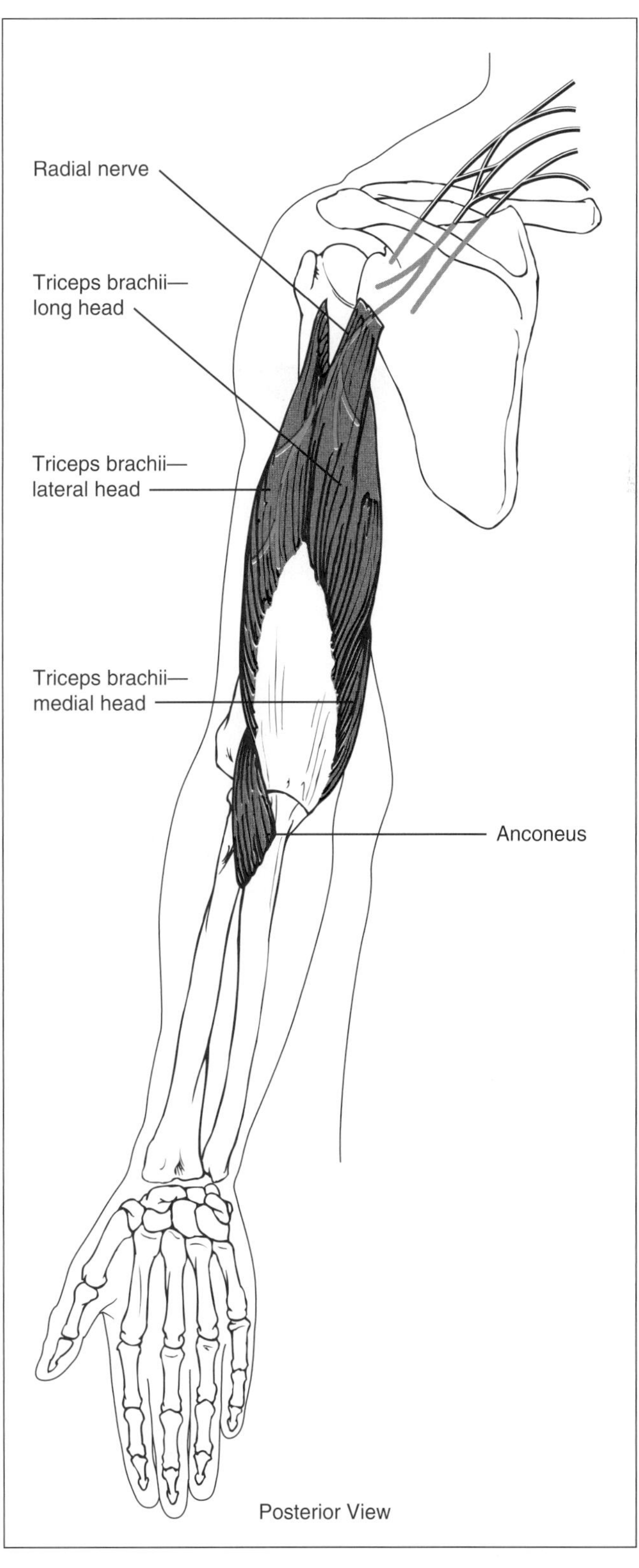

	ATTACHMENTS	NERVE SUPPLY	FUNCTION
Triceps brachii	Origin: Long head: Infraglenoid tuberosity of the scapula; Lateral head: Posterior and lateral surfaces of the humeral shaft; Medial head: Posterior and medial surfaces of the humeral shaft. Insertion: Olecranon process of the ulna	Peripheral nerve: Radial nerve Nerve root: C7, C8	Extension of the elbow; the long head assists in extending the shoulder
Anconeus	Origin: Lateral epicondyle of the humerus Insertion: Lateral surface of the olecranon; superior ¼ of the posterior aspect of the ulna	Peripheral nerve: Radial nerve Nerve root: C7, C8	Assists in extending the elbow

Gravity-Resisted Test (Grades 5, 4, and 3)

Patient position: Supine with upper extremity in 90° shoulder flexion, full elbow flexion, full forearm supination (Fig. 2-101).

Fig. 2-101.

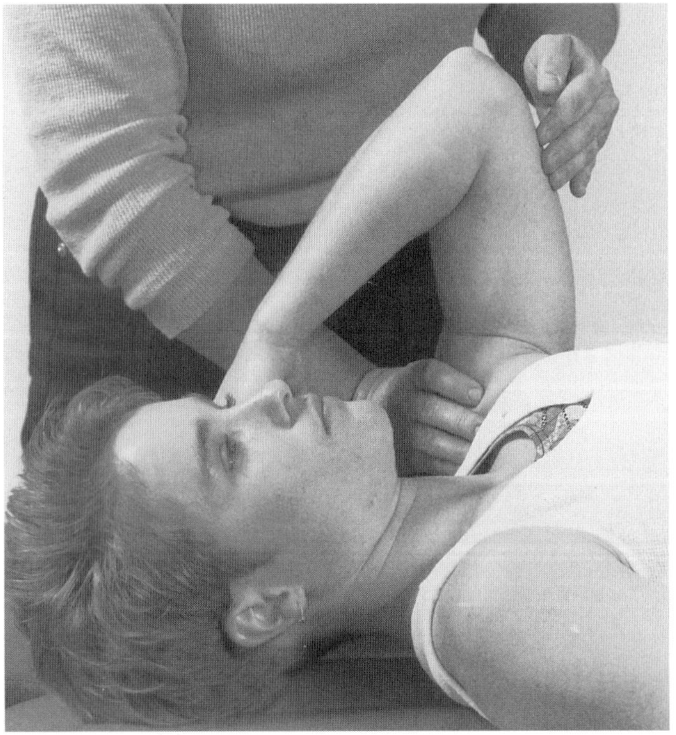

Stabilization/palpation: Stabilize over anterior aspect of ipsilateral shoulder. Palpate triceps over posterior surface of humerus (Fig. 2-101).

Examiner action:

While instructing patient in motion desired, extend patient's elbow, maintaining shoulder in 90° flexion. Return patient to starting position. Performing passive movement allows determination of patient's available ROM and shows patient exact motion desired.

Patient action:

Patient extends elbow through full ROM while examiner maintains stabilization of shoulder and palpation of triceps (Fig. 2-102).

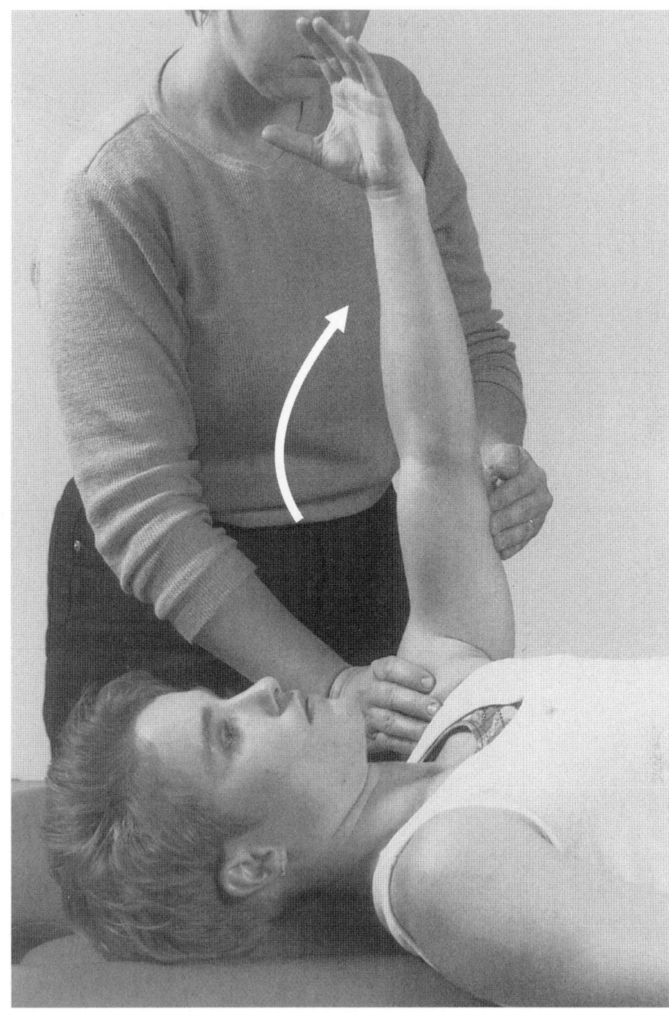

Fig. 2-102. Arrow indicates direction of movement.

Resistance: Flex patient's elbow slightly, then apply resistance just proximal to wrist in direction of elbow flexion. Care should be taken to avoid applying resistance to fully extended elbow. Palpating hand is moved to distal forearm to apply resistance (Fig. 2-103).

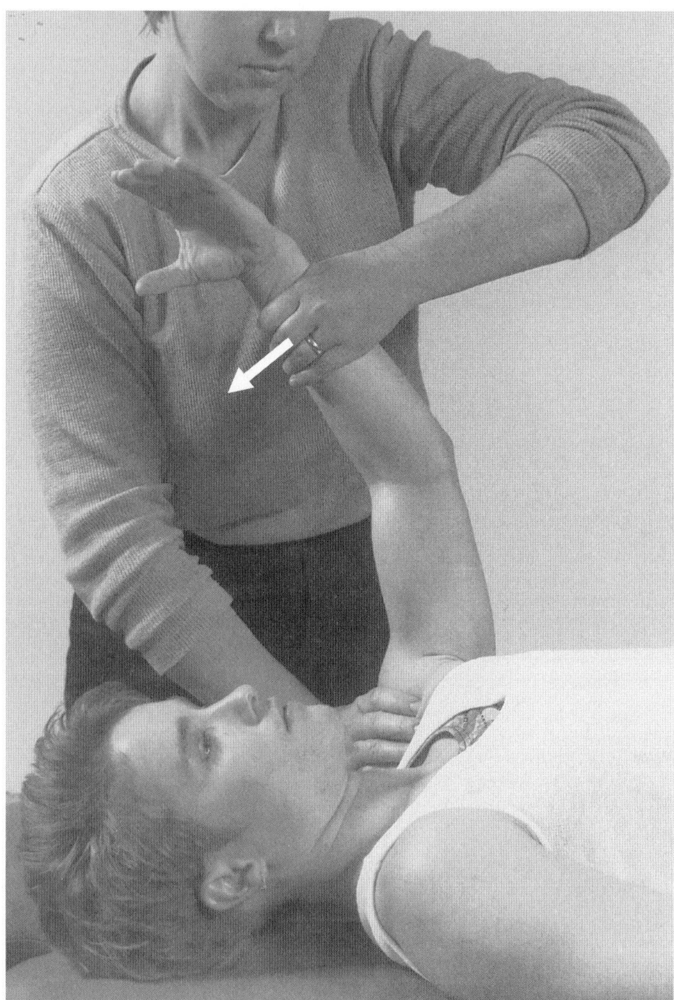

Fig. 2-103. Arrow indicates direction of resistance.

Gravity-Eliminated Test (Grades Below 3)

For patients unable to move completely through available ROM against gravity.

Patient position: Seated with arm supported on table, shoulder abducted to 90°, elbow fully flexed, forearm supinated. Talcum powder and a cloth may be placed between limb and supporting surface to reduce friction (Fig. 2-104; initial elbow position not shown).

Stabilization/palpation: As in gravity-resisted test (Fig. 2-104).

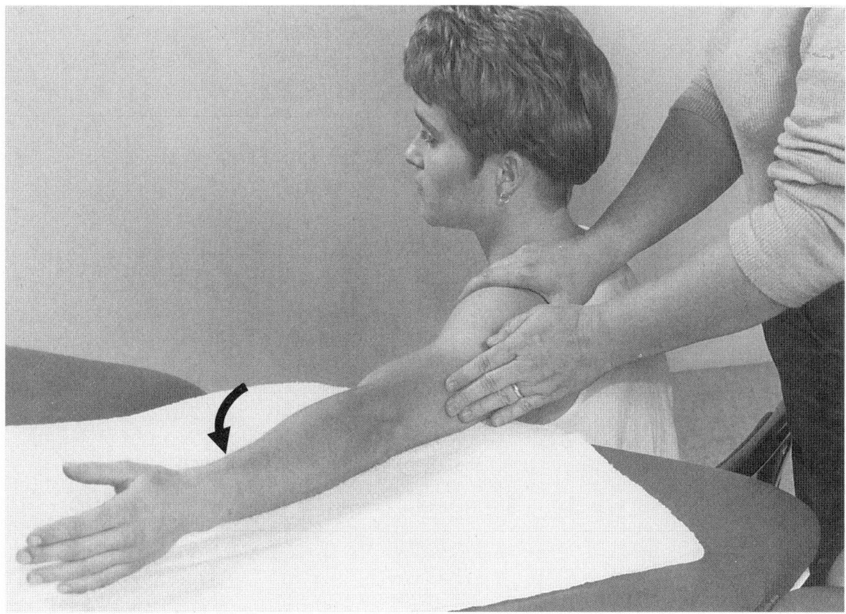

Fig. 2-104. Arrow indicates direction of movement.

Examiner action: As in gravity-resisted test, but shoulder should be maintained in 90° *abduction.*

Patient action: Patient extends elbow through full ROM. Examiner maintains stabilization of shoulder and palpation of triceps during patient movement (Fig. 2-104).

COMMON SUBSTITUTION

During gravity-eliminated test, patient may use lateral rotation of shoulder to substitute for elbow extension. Care should be taken to prevent lateral rotation of shoulder during gravity-eliminated test.

CLINICAL COMMENT: TRICEPS BRACHII MUSCLE AND C7 NEUROLOGIC ASSESSMENT

The triceps brachii muscle is a key muscle for examining the integrity of the C7 spinal nerve or neurologic segment of the spinal cord. Complete assessment of the C7 neurologic level includes:

Strength assessment of:
Triceps brachii (pp. 112–115)
Wrist flexors (pp. 126–129)
Finger extensors (pp. 158–160)

Reflex testing of:
Triceps reflex (p. 549)

Sensory testing of:
Skin over middle finger (C7 dermatome; pp. 528-532)

■ FOREARM SUPINATION

SUPINATOR: BICEPS BRACHII (Fig. 2-105)

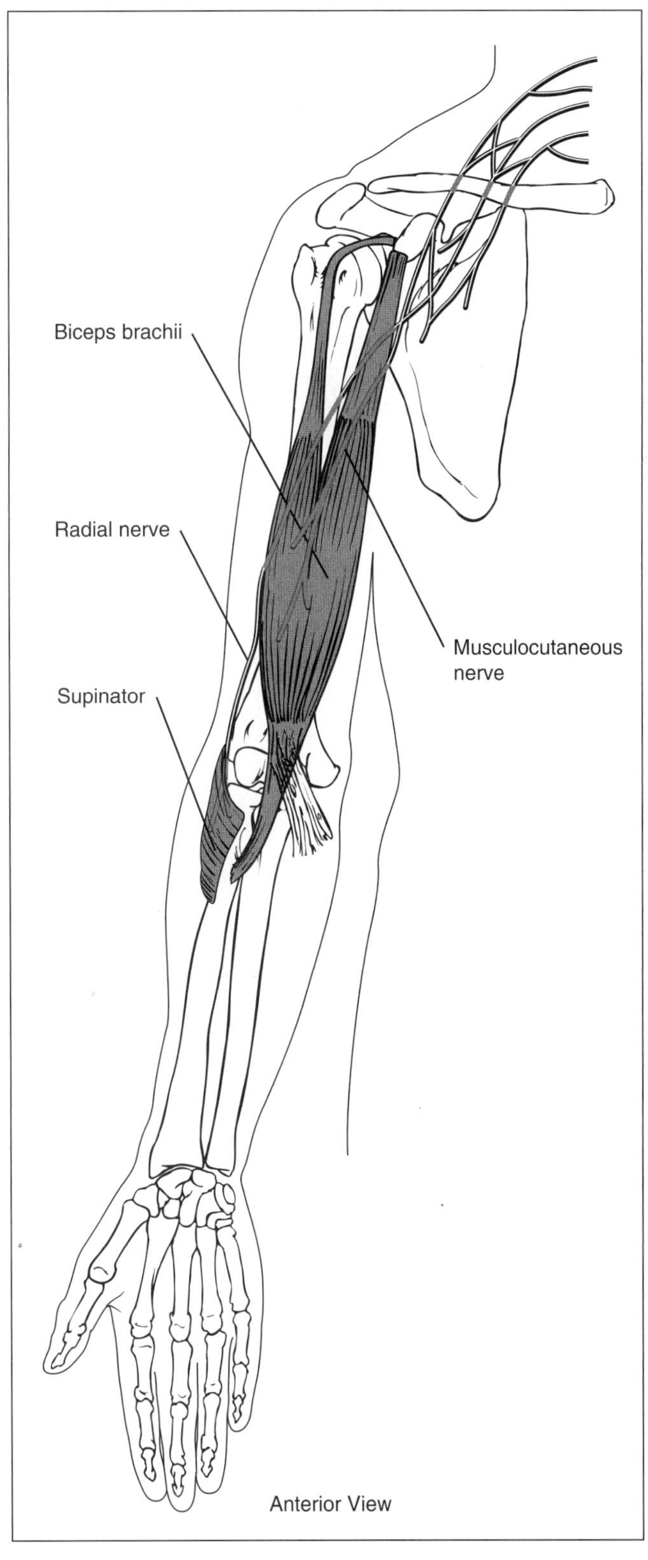

Fig. 2-105.

	ATTACHMENTS	NERVE SUPPLY	FUNCTION
Supinator	Origin: Lateral epicondyle of the humerus, supinator crest of the ulna, radial collateral ligament of the elbow, annular ligament of the radius Insertion: Tuberosity and oblique line of the radius, dorsolateral surface of the upper ⅓ of the radial shaft	Peripheral nerve: Deep branch of the radial nerve Nerve root: C6	Supination of the forearm
Biceps brachii	Origin: Short head: Coracoid process of the scapula Long head: Supraglenoid tuberosity of the scapula Insertion: Tuberosity of the radius	Peripheral nerve: Musculocutaneous nerve Nerve root: C5, C6	Flexion of the elbow; supination of the forearm; assists in flexion of the shoulder

Gravity-Resisted Test (Grades 5, 4, and 3)

Patient position: Seated with upper extremity in 0° shoulder abduction, 90° elbow flexion, full forearm pronation (Fig. 2-106).

Fig. 2-106.

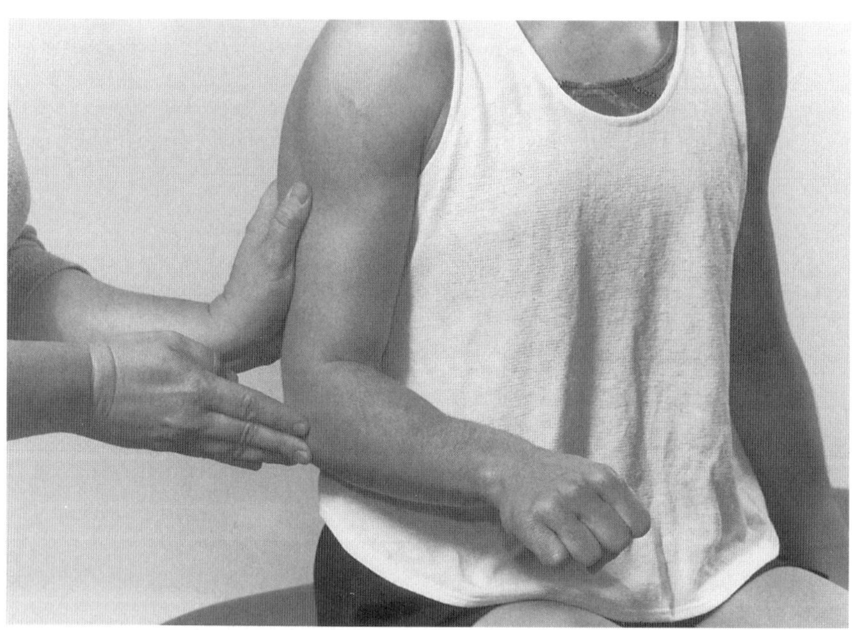

Stabilization/palpation: Stabilize on inferolateral aspect of humerus, to prevent shoulder abduction. Palpate biceps on anterior aspect of humerus and supinator on posterosuperior aspect of radius, just distal to radial head. Palpation of supinator is shown (Fig. 2-106).

Examiner action: While instructing patient in motion desired, supinate patient's forearm, maintaining elbow in 90° flexion. Return patient to starting position. Performing passive movement allows determination of patient's available ROM and shows patient exact motion desired.

Patient action: Patient supinates forearm through full ROM while examiner maintains stabilization of humerus and palpation of biceps/supinator (Fig. 2-107).

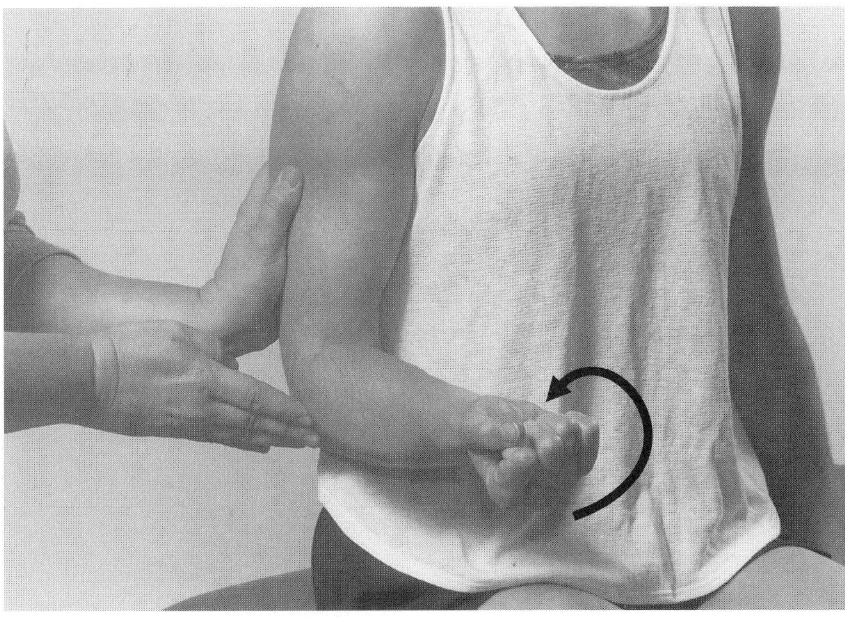

Fig. 2-107. Arrow indicates direction of movement.

Resistance: Apply resistance along volar surface of ulna and dorsal surface of radius in direction of pronation. Palpating hand is moved to distal forearm to apply resistance (Fig. 2-108).

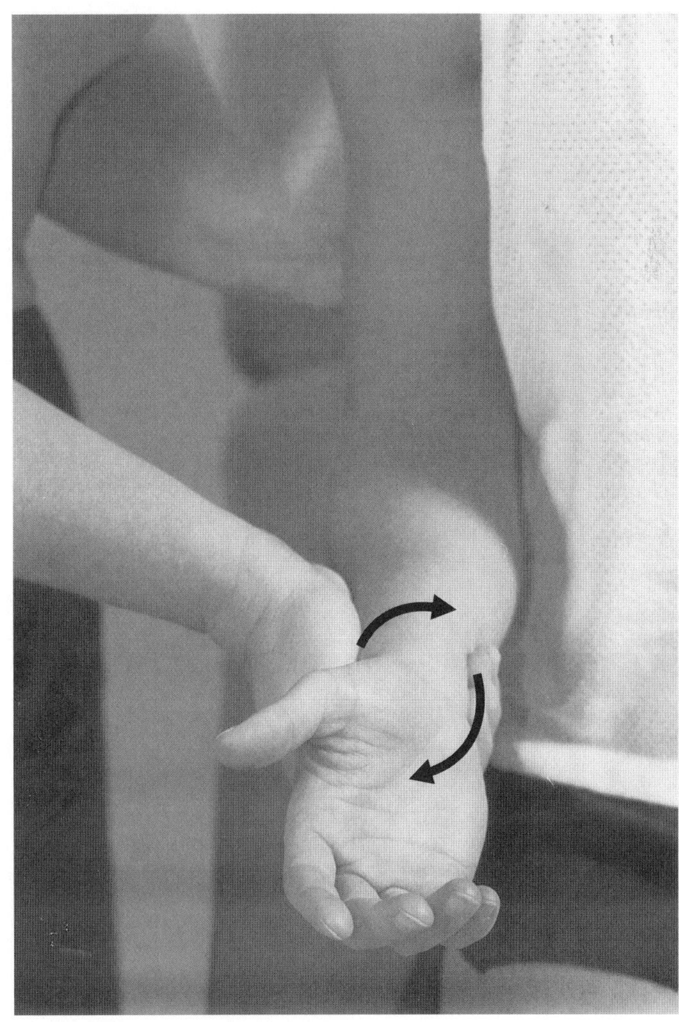

Fig. 2-108. Arrows indicate direction of resistance.

Gravity-Eliminated Test (Grades Below 3)

For patients unable to move completely through available ROM against gravity.

Patient position: Seated with upper extremity in 90° shoulder flexion, 90° elbow flexion, full forearm pronation. Arm should be supported on a flat surface (Fig. 2-109; initial forearm position not shown).

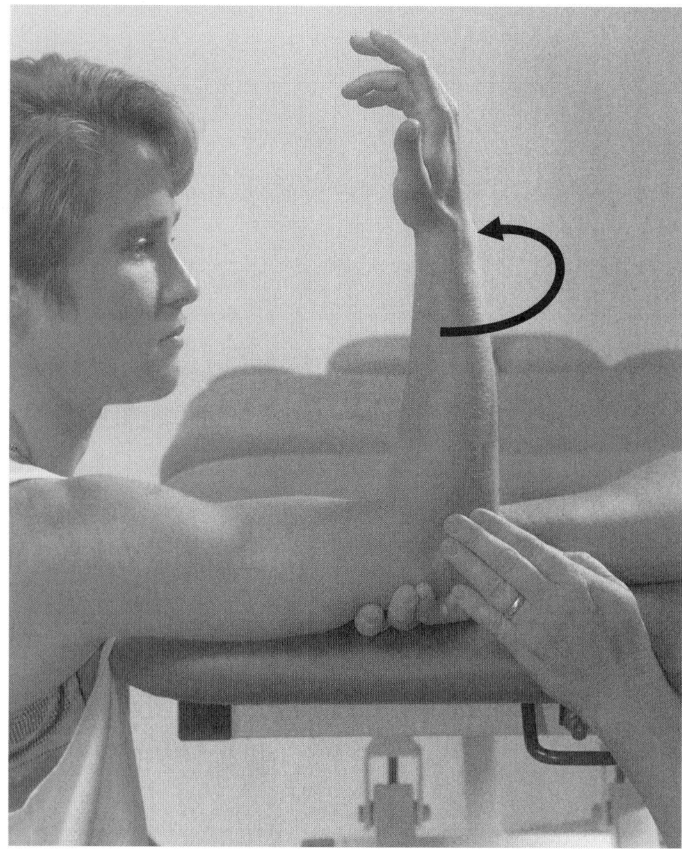

Fig. 2-109. Arrow indicates direction of movement.

Stabilization/palpation: Examiner stabilizes along posterior aspect of elbow. Palpation occurs as in gravity-resisted test (Fig. 2-109).

Examiner action: As in gravity-resisted test.

Patient action: Patient supinates forearm through full ROM while examiner maintains stabilization of distal forearm and palpation of biceps/supinator (Fig. 2-109).

COMMON SUBSTITUTION

Adduction and lateral rotation of shoulder may mimic forearm supination during gravity-resisted test. Care should be taken to maintain patient's humerus in adduction during gravity-resisted test.

■ FOREARM PRONATION

PRONATOR QUADRATUS: PRONATOR TERES (Fig. 2-110)

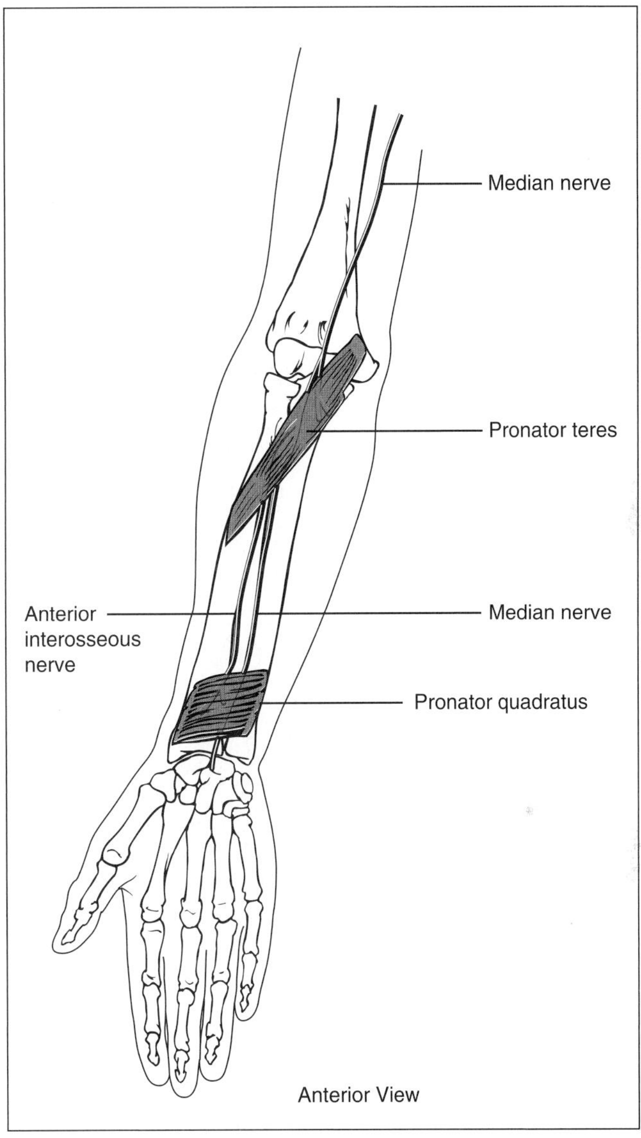

Fig. 2-110.

	ATTACHMENTS	NERVE SUPPLY	FUNCTION
Pronator quadratus	Origin: Anterior aspect of the distal ¼ of the ulna Insertion: Anterior aspect of the distal ¼ of the radius	Peripheral nerve: Median nerve Nerve root: C8, T1	Pronation of the forearm
Pronator teres	Origin: Humeral head: Medial epicondylar ridge of the humerus, common forearm flexor tendon Ulnar head: Coronoid process of the ulna Insertion: Lateral surface of the midshaft of the radius	Peripheral nerve: Median nerve Nerve root: C6, C7	Pronation of the forearm; assists in flexion of the elbow

Gravity-Resisted Test (Grades 5, 4, and 3)

Patient position:

Seated with upper extremity in 0° shoulder abduction, 90° elbow flexion, full forearm supination (Fig. 2-111).

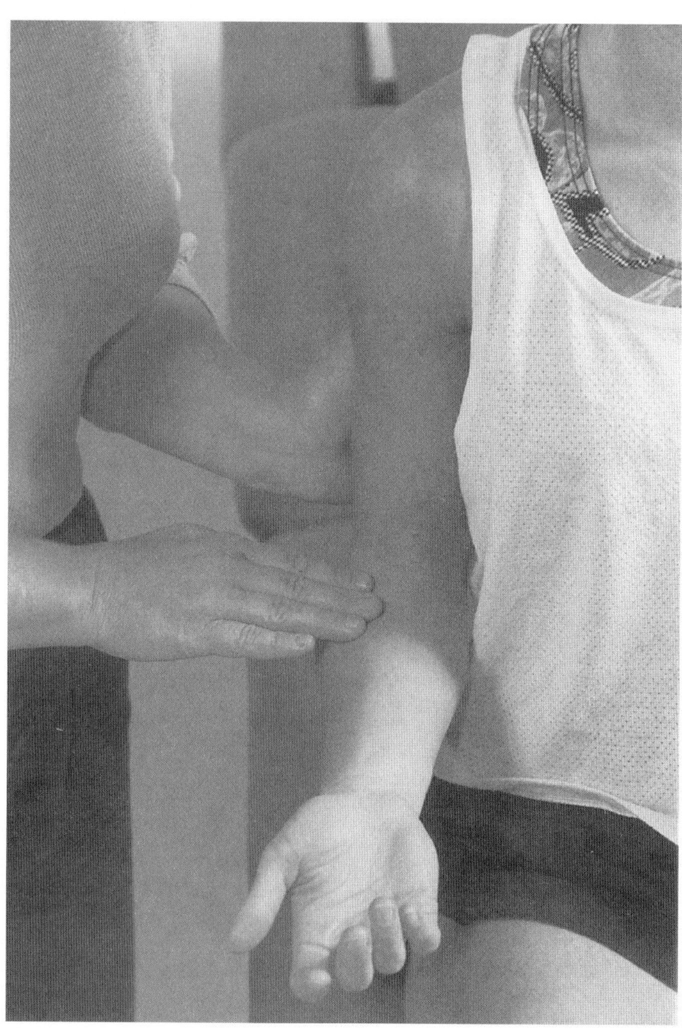

Fig. 2-111.

Stabilization/palpation:

Stabilize over inferolateral aspect of humerus, preventing shoulder abduction. Palpate pronator teres along anterior surface of proximal third of forearm. Pronator quadratus is deep and not accessible to palpation (Fig. 2-111).

Examiner action:

While instructing patient in motion desired, pronate patient's forearm, maintaining elbow in 90° flexion. Return patient to starting position. Performing passive movement allows determination of patient's available ROM and shows patient exact motion desired.

Patient action:

Patient pronates forearm through full ROM while examiner maintains stabilization of humerus and palpation of pronator teres (Fig. 2-112).

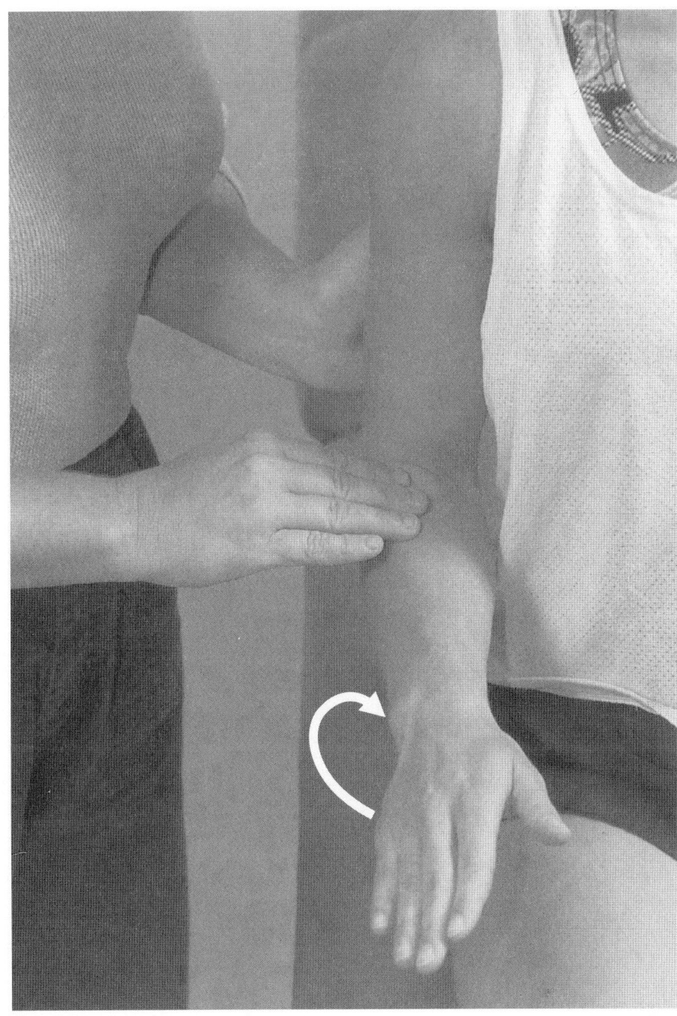

Fig. 2-112. Arrow indicates direction of movement.

Resistance: Apply resistance along volar surface of radius and dorsal surface of ulna in direction of supination. Palpating hand is moved to distal forearm to apply resistance (Fig. 2-113).

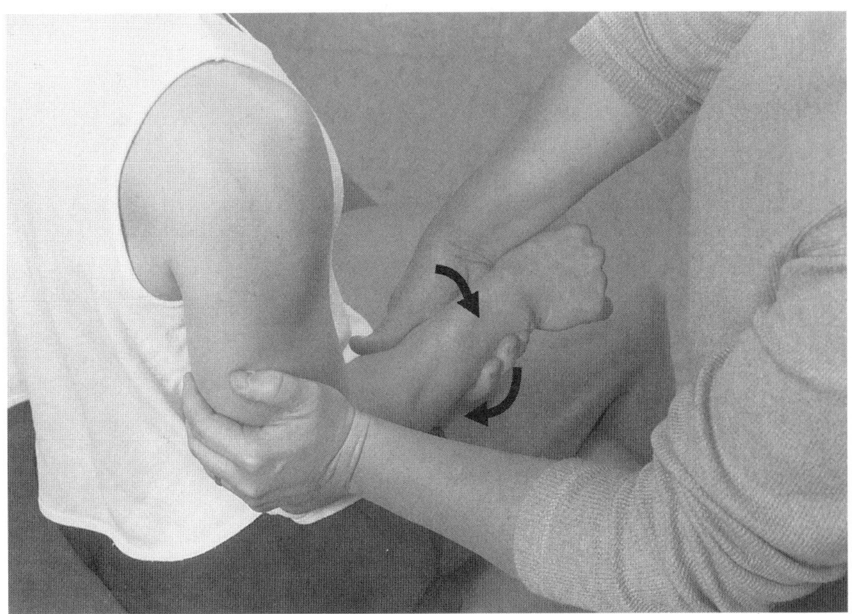

Fig. 2-113. Arrows indicate direction of resistance.

Gravity-Eliminated Test (Grades Below 3)

For patients unable to move completely through available ROM against gravity.

Patient position: Seated with upper extremity to be tested in 90° shoulder flexion, 90° elbow flexion, full forearm supination. Arm should be supported on a flat surface (Fig. 2-114; initial forearm position is not shown).

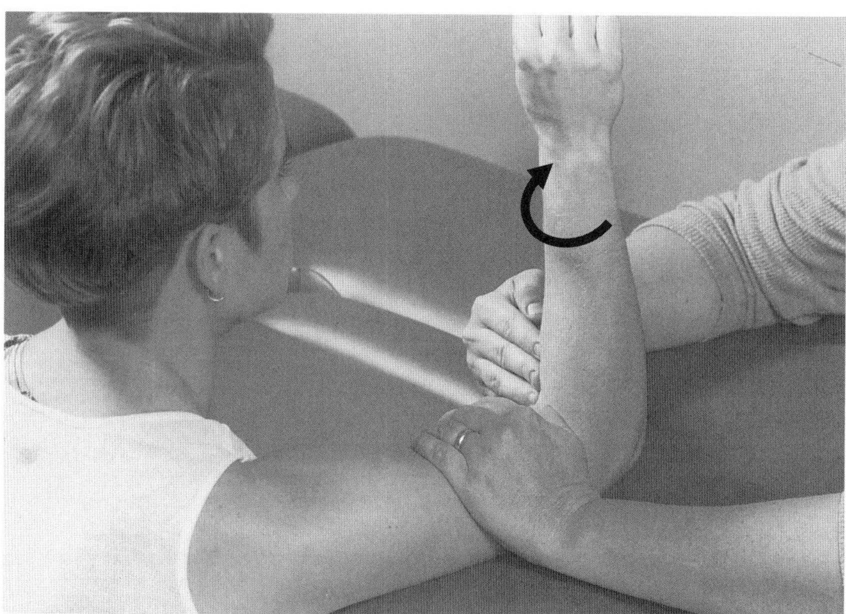

Fig. 2-114. Arrow indicates direction of movement.

Stabilization/palpation: Stabilize on anterior surface of arm, just proximal to elbow. Palpate as in gravity-resisted test (Fig. 2-114).

Examiner action: As in gravity-resisted test.

Patient action: Patient pronates forearm through full ROM while examiner maintains stabilization of humerus and palpation of pronator teres (Fig. 2-114).

COMMON SUBSTITUTION

Abduction and medial rotation of shoulder may mimic forearm pronation during gravity-resisted test. Care should be taken to maintain patient's humerus in adduction during gravity-resisted test.

■ WRIST FLEXION AND RADIAL DEVIATION

FLEXOR CARPI RADIALIS (Fig. 2-115)

Fig. 2-115.

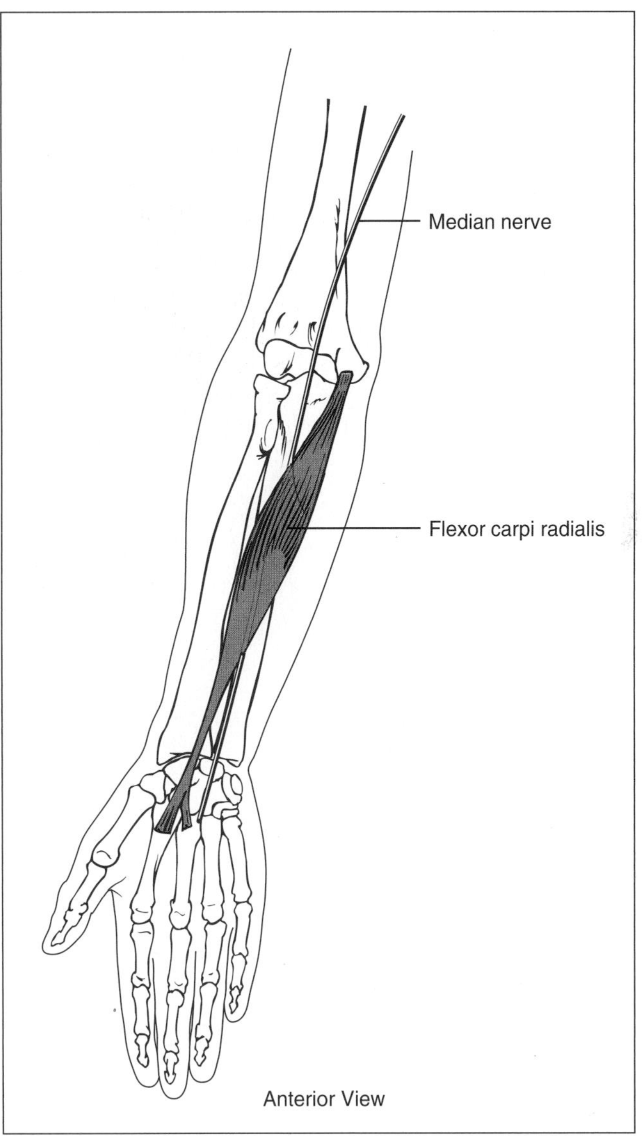

	ATTACHMENTS	NERVE SUPPLY	FUNCTION
Flexor carpi radialis	Origin: Medial epicondyle of the humerus via the common forearm flexor tendon; antebrachial fascia Insertion: Base of 2nd and 3rd metacarpals	Peripheral nerve: Median nerve Nerve root: C6, C7	Flexion and abduction (radial deviation) of the wrist

Gravity-Resisted Test (Grades 5, 4, and 3)

Patient position: Seated with forearm supinated and supported on a flat surface, wrist in neutral position (Fig. 2-116).

Fig. 2-116.

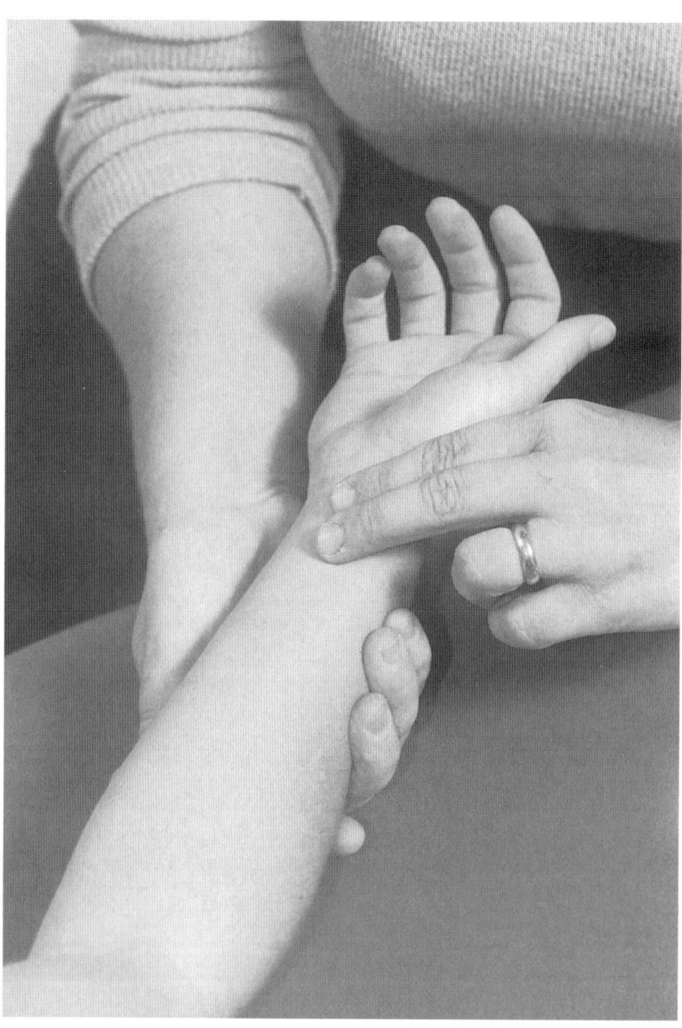

Stabilization/palpation: Stabilize on posterior aspect of distal forearm. Palpate tendon of flexor carpi radialis at base of second metacarpal, just lateral to midline of forearm (Fig. 2-116).

Examiner action: While instructing patient in motion desired, flex patient's wrist and deviate it to radial side. Return patient to starting position. Performing passive movement allows determination of patient's available ROM and shows patient exact motion desired.

Patient action: Patient flexes and deviates wrist to radial side while examiner maintains stabilization of forearm and palpation of flexor carpi radialis (Fig. 2-117).

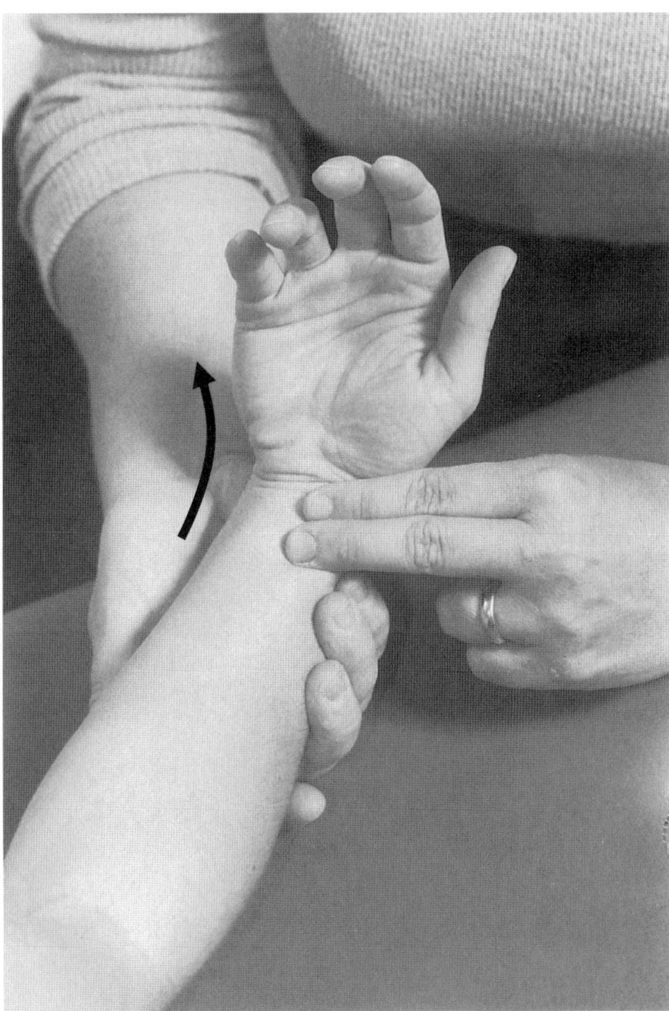

Fig. 2-117. Arrow indicates direction of movement.

Resistance: Apply resistance along volar aspect of bases of first and second metacarpals in direction of wrist extension and ulnar deviation. Palpating hand is moved to metacarpals to apply resistance (Fig. 2-118).

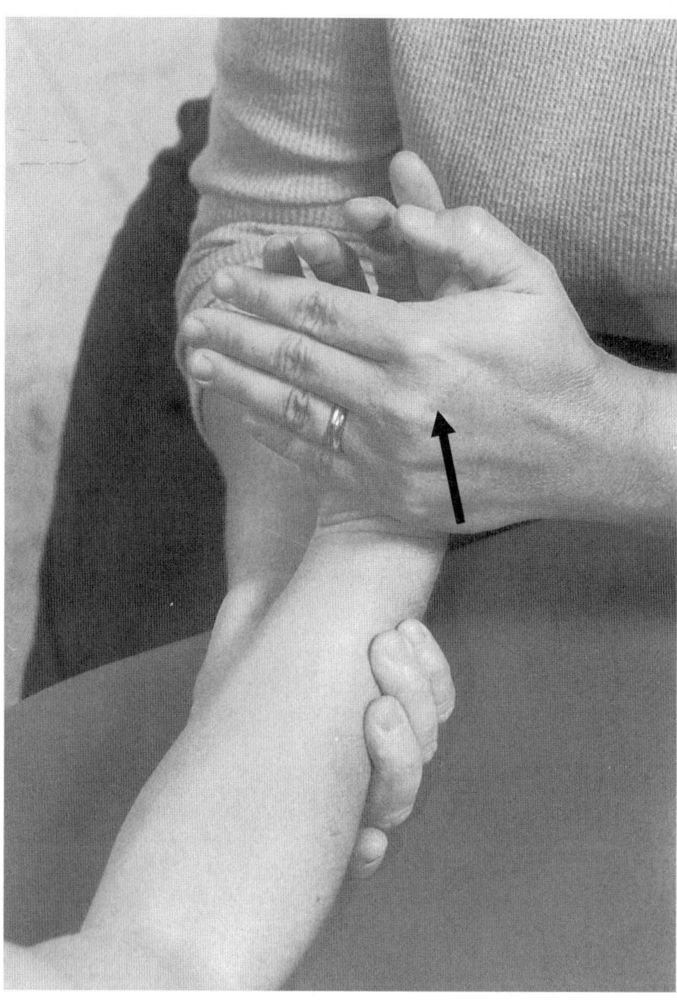

Fig. 2-118. Arrow indicates direction of resistance.

Gravity-Eliminated Test (Grades Below 3)

For patients unable to move through available ROM against gravity.

Patient position: Seated with forearm in neutral rotation (halfway between supination and pronation), wrist in neutral position, forearm supported on a flat surface (Fig. 2-119; initial position of wrist not shown).

Stabilization/palpation: Stabilize along radial side of forearm. Palpate as in gravity-resisted test (Fig. 2-119).

Examiner action: While instructing patient in motion desired, flex patient's wrist. Return patient to starting position.

Patient action: Patient flexes wrist through full ROM while examiner maintains stabilization of forearm and palpation of flexor carpi radialis (Fig. 2-119).

COMMON SUBSTITUTION

Long-finger flexors: Care should be taken to prevent fingers from flexing during test to eliminate substitution by flexor digitorum superficialis or profundus.

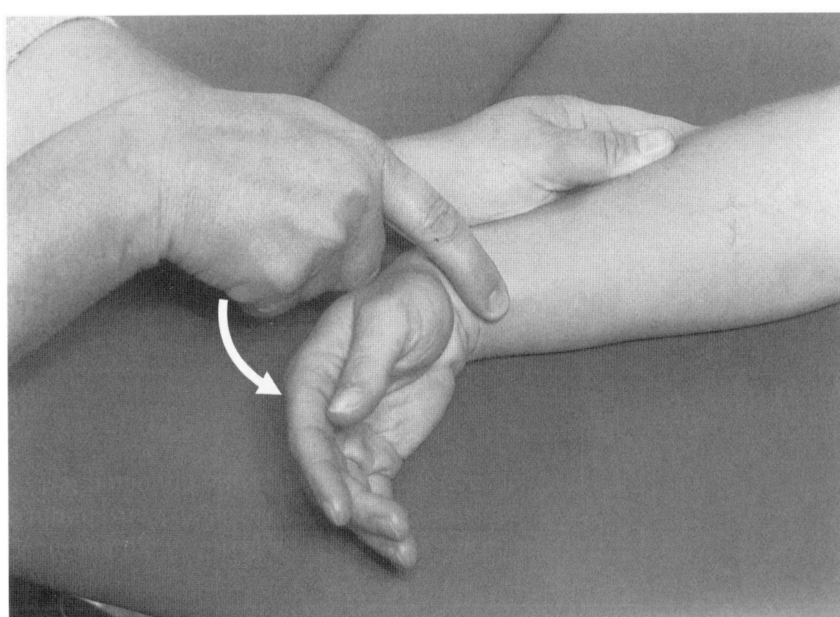

Fig. 2-119. Arrow indicates direction of movement.

■ WRIST FLEXION AND ULNAR DEVIATION

FLEXOR CARPI ULNARIS (Fig. 2-120)

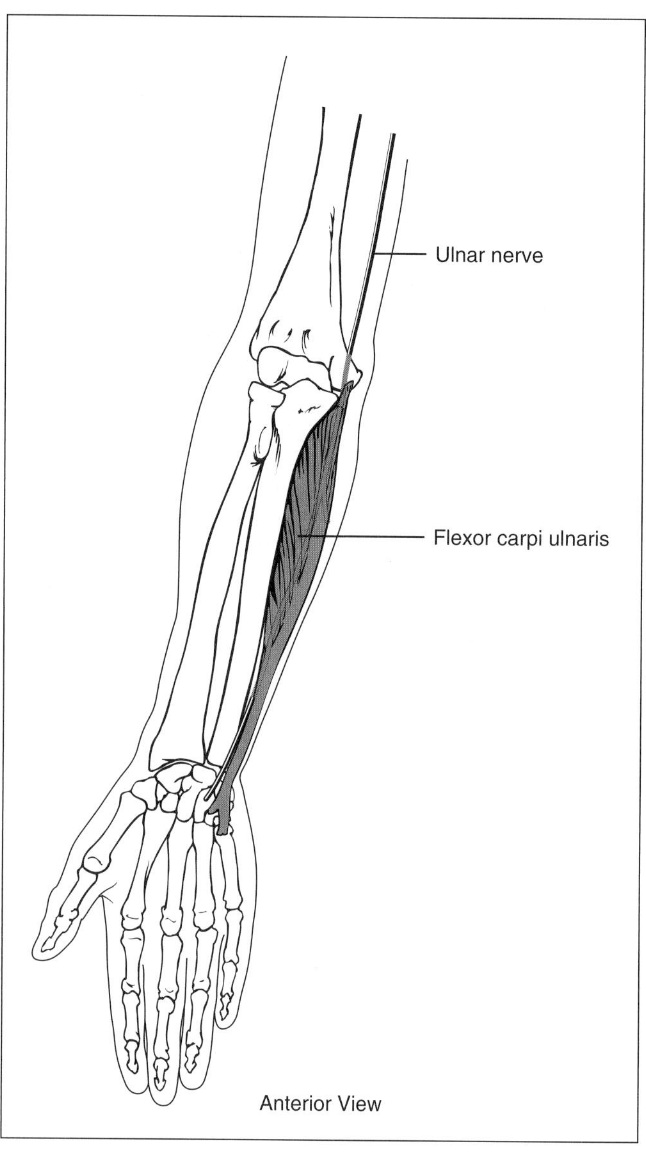

Fig. 2-120.

	ATTACHMENTS	NERVE SUPPLY	FUNCTION
Flexor carpi ulnaris	Origin: Humeral head: Medial epicondyle of the humerus via the common forearm flexor tendon Ulnar head: Upper ⅔ of the posterior border of the ulna Insertion: Pisiform bone	Peripheral nerve: Ulnar nerve Nerve root: C8, T1	Flexion and adduction (ulnar deviation) of the wrist

Gravity-Resisted Test (Grades 5, 4, and 3)

Patient position: Seated with forearm supinated and supported on a flat surface, wrist in neutral position (Fig. 2-121).

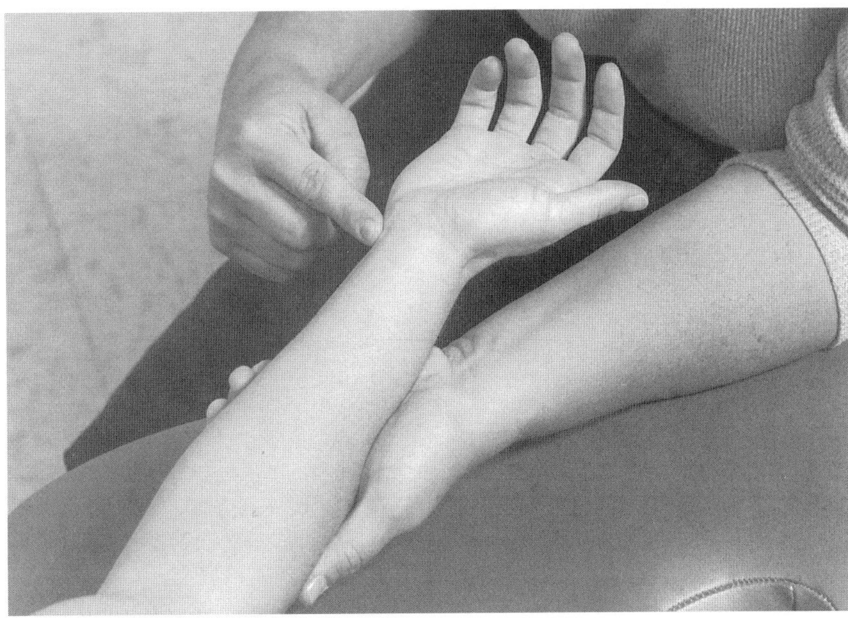

Fig. 2-121.

Stabilization/palpation: Stabilize on posterior aspect of distal forearm. Palpate tendon of flexor carpi ulnaris just proximal to pisiform bone (Fig. 2-121).

Examiner action: While instructing patient in motion desired, flex patient's wrist and deviate it to ulnar side. Return patient to starting position. Performing passive movement allows determination of patient's available ROM and shows patient exact motion desired.

Patient action: Patient flexes and deviates wrist to ulnar side while examiner maintains stabilization of forearm and palpation of flexor carpi ulnaris (Fig. 2-122).

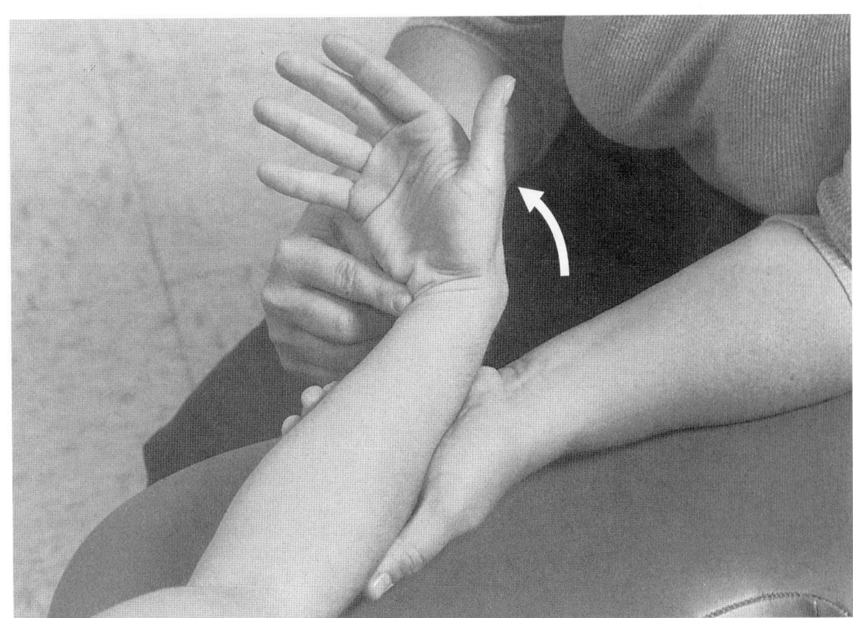

Fig. 2-122. Arrow indicates direction of movement.

Resistance: Apply resistance along volar aspect of fifth metacarpal bone in direction of wrist extension and radial deviation. Palpating hand is moved to metacarpal to apply resistance (Fig. 2-123).

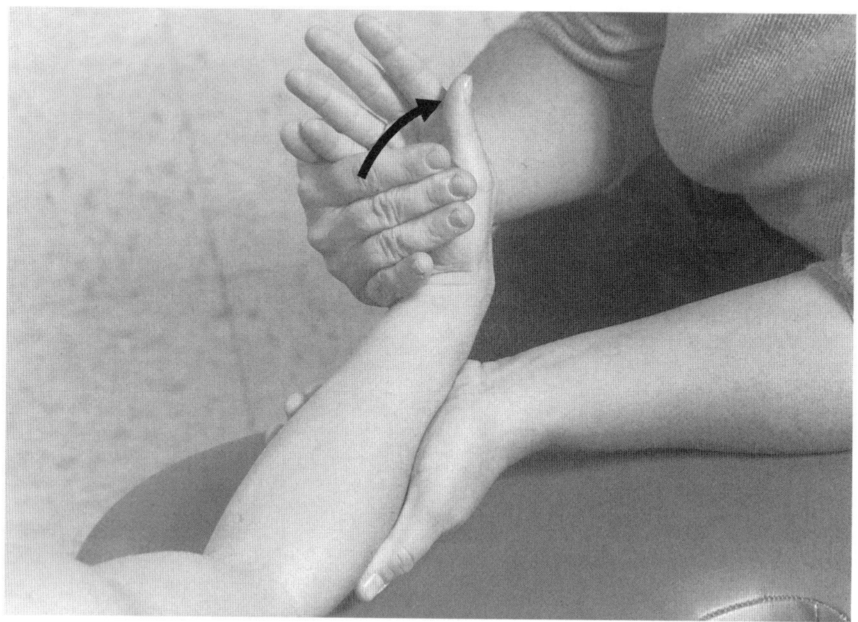

Fig. 2-123. Arrow indicates direction of resistance.

Gravity-Eliminated Test (Grades Below 3)

For patients unable to move completely through available ROM against gravity.

Patient position: Seated with forearm in neutral rotation (halfway between supination and pronation) and supported on a flat surface, wrist in neutral position (Fig. 2-124; initial position of wrist not shown).

Stabilization/palpation: Stabilize along radial side of forearm. Palpate as described in gravity-resisted test (Fig. 2-124).

Examiner action: While instructing patient in motion desired, flex patient's wrist. Return patient to starting position.

Patient action: Patient flexes wrist through full ROM for both flexor carpi radialis and ulnaris. Examiner maintains stabilization and palpation during active movement by patient (Fig. 2-124).

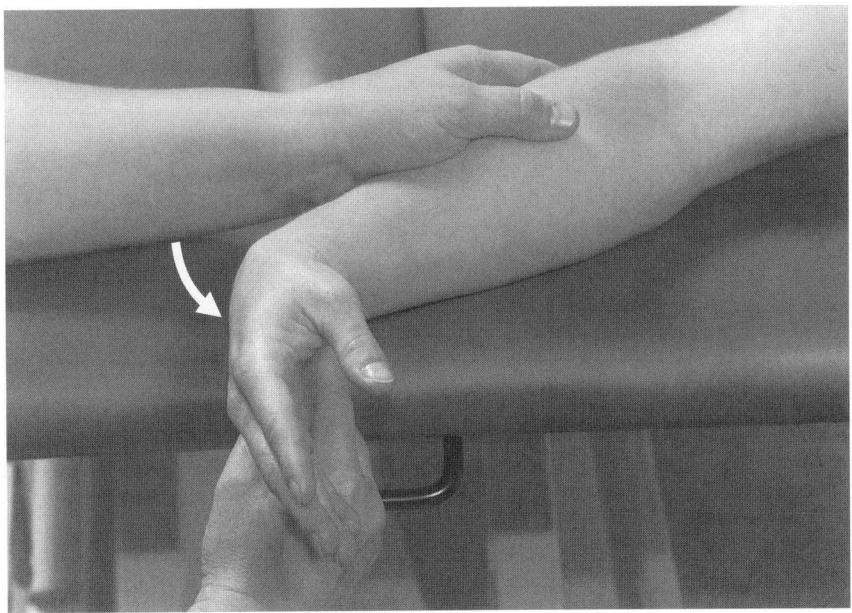

Fig. 2-124. Arrow indicates direction of movement.

COMMON SUBSTITUTION

See test for flexor carpi radialis.

CLINICAL COMMENT: WRIST FLEXOR MUSCLES AND C7 NEUROLOGICAL ASSESSMENT

The wrist flexor muscles (flexor carpi radialis and flexor carpi ulnaris) are key muscles for examining the integrity of the C7 spinal nerve or neurological segment of the spinal cord. Complete assessment of the C7 neurological level includes:

Strength assessment of:
Triceps brachii (pp. 112-115)
Wrist flexors (pp. 126-129)
Finger extensors (pp. 158-160)
Reflex testing of:
Triceps reflex (p. 549)
Sensory testing of:
Skin over middle finger (C7 dermatome; pp. 528-532)

WRIST EXTENSION AND RADIAL DEVIATION

EXTENSOR CARPI RADIALIS LONGUS AND BREVIS (Fig. 2-125)

Fig. 2-125.

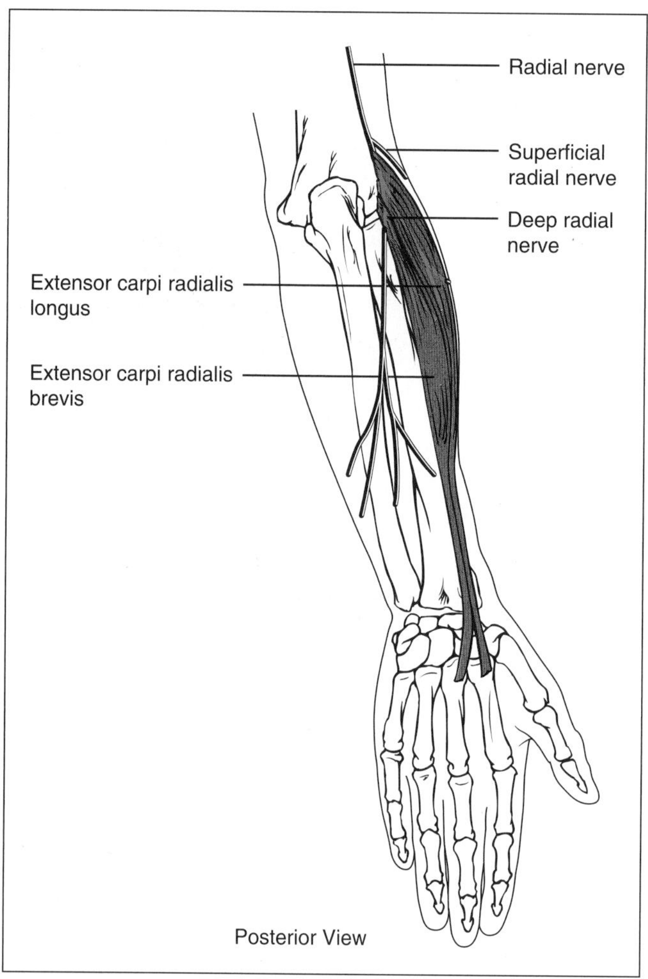

	ATTACHMENTS	NERVE SUPPLY	FUNCTION
Extensor carpi radialis longus	Origin: Lateral supra-condylar ridge of the humerus; the common extensor tendon Insertion: Base of the 2nd metacarpal bone	Peripheral nerve: Radial nerve Nerve root: C6, C7	Extension and abduction (radial deviation) of the wrist; assists in extension of the elbow
Extensor carpi radialis brevis	Origin: Lateral epicondyle of the humerus; the common extensor tendon; radial collateral ligament of the elbow Insertion: Base of the 3rd metacarpal bone	Peripheral nerve: Radial nerve Nerve root: C6, C7	Extension and abduction (radial deviation) of the wrist

Gravity-Resisted Test (Grades 5, 4, and 3)

Patient position: Seated with forearm pronated and supported on a flat surface, wrist in neutral position (Fig. 2-126).

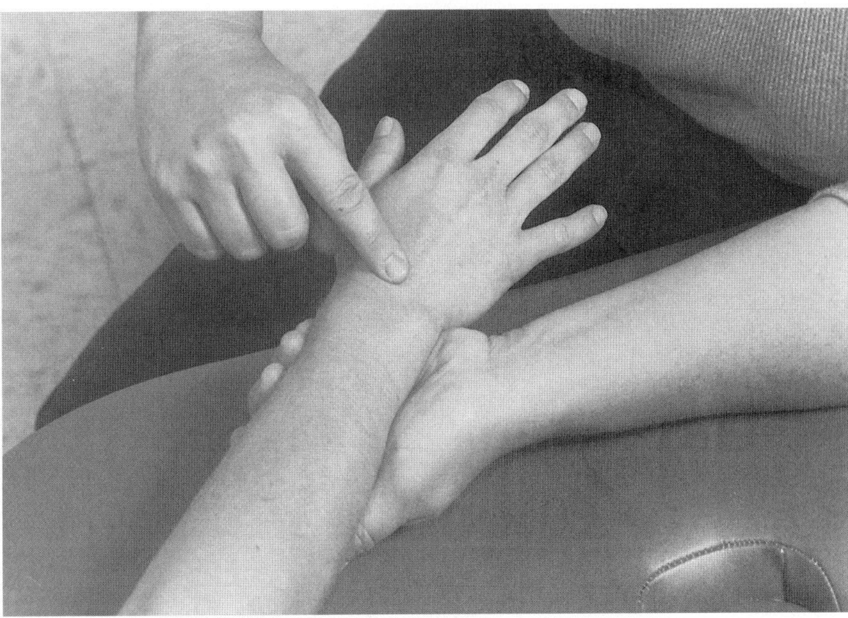

Fig. 2-126.

Stabilization/palpation: Stabilize anterior aspect of distal forearm. Palpate tendons of extensor carpi radialis longus and brevis just proximal to bases of second and third metacarpals (Fig. 2-126).

Examiner action: While instructing patient in movement desired, extend patient's wrist and deviate it to radial side. Return patient to starting position. Performing passive movement allows determination of patient's available ROM and shows patient exact motion desired.

Patient action:

Patient extends and deviates wrist to radial side while examiner maintains stabilization of forearm and palpation of extensor carpi radialis muscles (Fig. 2-127).

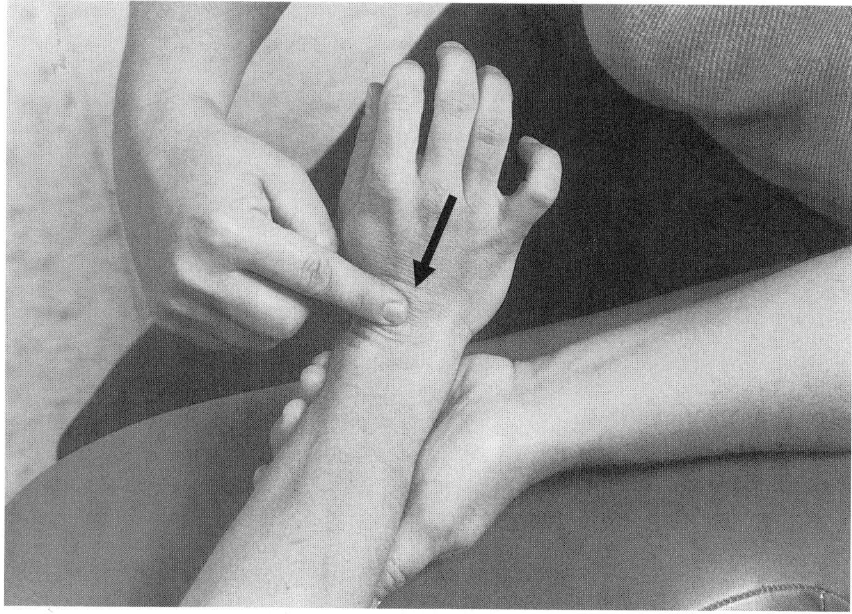

Fig. 2-127. Arrow indicates direction of movement.

Resistance:

Apply resistance along dorsal aspect of first and second metacarpals in direction of wrist flexion and ulnar deviation (Fig. 2-128).

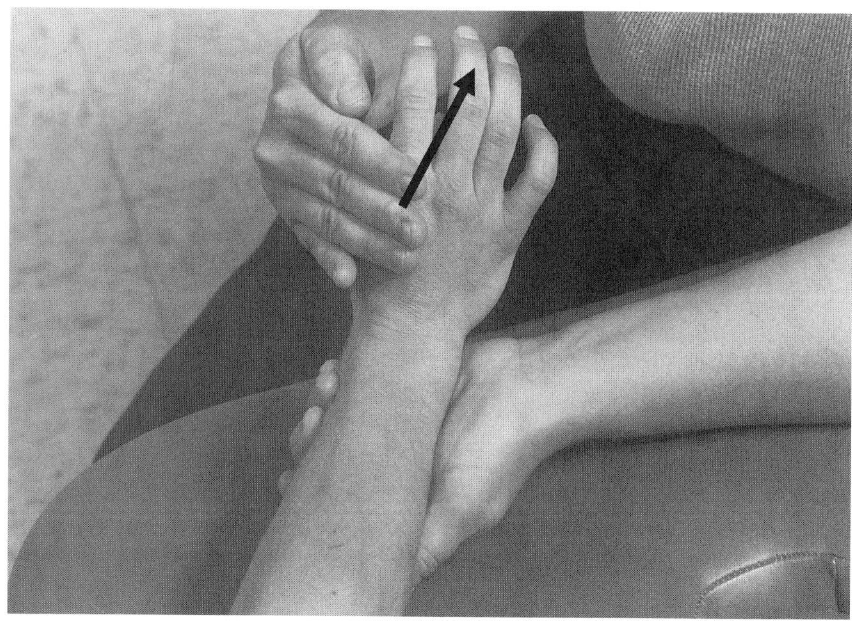

Fig. 2-128. Arrow indicates direction of resistance.

Gravity-Eliminated Test (Grades Below 3)

For patients unable to move completely through available ROM against gravity.

Patient position: Seated with forearm in neutral rotation (halfway between supination and pronation), wrist in neutral position, forearm supported on a flat surface (Fig. 2-129; initial position of wrist not shown).

Fig. 2-129. Arrow indicates direction of movement.

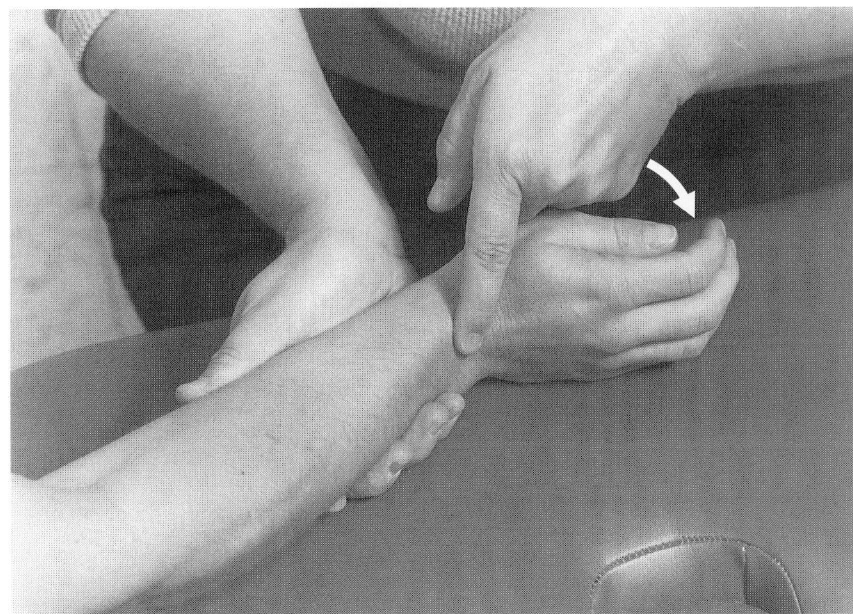

Stabilization/palpation: Stabilize along volar surface of distal forearm. Palpate tendons of extensor carpi radialis longus and brevis as in gravity-resisted test (Fig. 2-129).

Examiner action: While instructing patient in movement desired, extend patient's wrist. Return patient to starting position.

Patient action: Patient extends wrist through full ROM while examiner maintains stabilization of forearm and palpation of extensor carpi radialis muscles (Fig. 2-129).

COMMON SUBSTITUTION

Finger extensors: Care should be taken to prevent fingers from extending during test to eliminate substitution by finger extensors.

CLINICAL COMMENT: WRIST EXTENSOR MUSCLES AND C6 NEUROLOGIC ASSESSMENT

The wrist extensor muscles (extensor carpi radialis longus and brevis, extensor carpi ulnaris) are key muscles for examining the integrity of the C6 spinal nerve or neurological segment of the spinal cord. Complete assessment of the C6 neurologic level includes:

Strength assessment of:
Biceps brachii (pp. 99-102)
Wrist extensors (pp. 134-142)

Reflex testing of:
Brachioradialis reflex (p. 548)
Biceps reflex (C5 and C6; p. 547)

Sensory testing of:
Skin over thumb and lateral forearm (C6 dermatome; pp. 528-532)

■ WRIST EXTENSION AND ULNAR DEVIATION

EXTENSOR CARPI ULNARIS (Fig. 2-130)

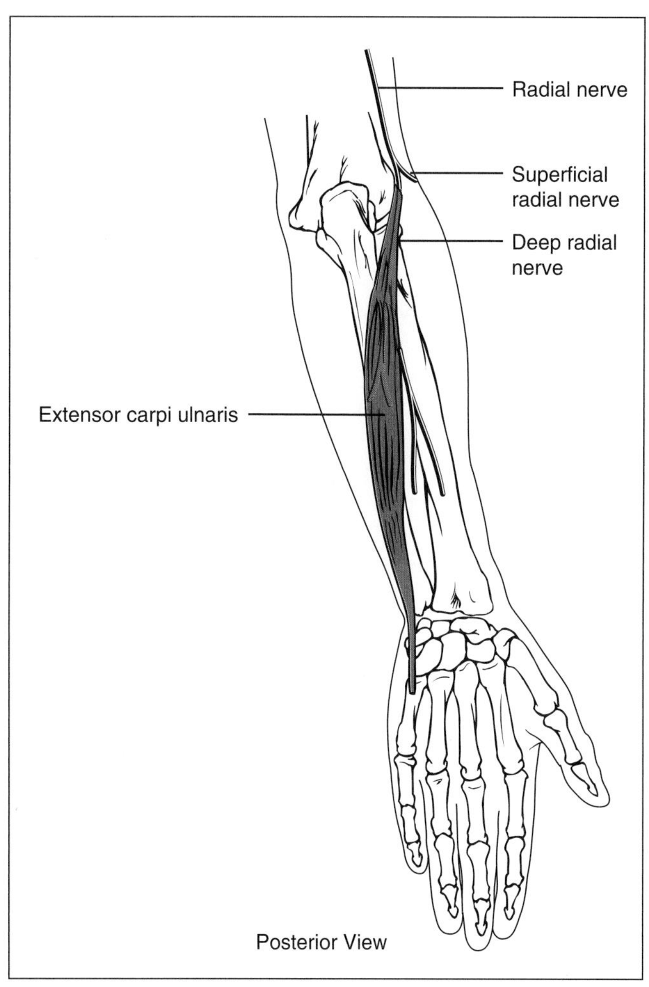

Fig. 2-130.

	ATTACHMENTS	NERVE SUPPLY	FUNCTION
Extensor carpi ulnaris	Origin: Lateral epicondyle of the humerus via the common extensor tendon; dorsal border of the ulna Insertion: Base of 5th metacarpal bone	Peripheral nerve: Deep radial nerve Nerve root: C6–C8	Extension and adduction (ulnar deviation) of the wrist

Gravity-Resisted Test (Grades 5, 4, and 3)

Patient position: Seated with forearm pronated and supported on a flat surface, wrist in neutral position (Fig. 2-131).

Fig. 2-131.

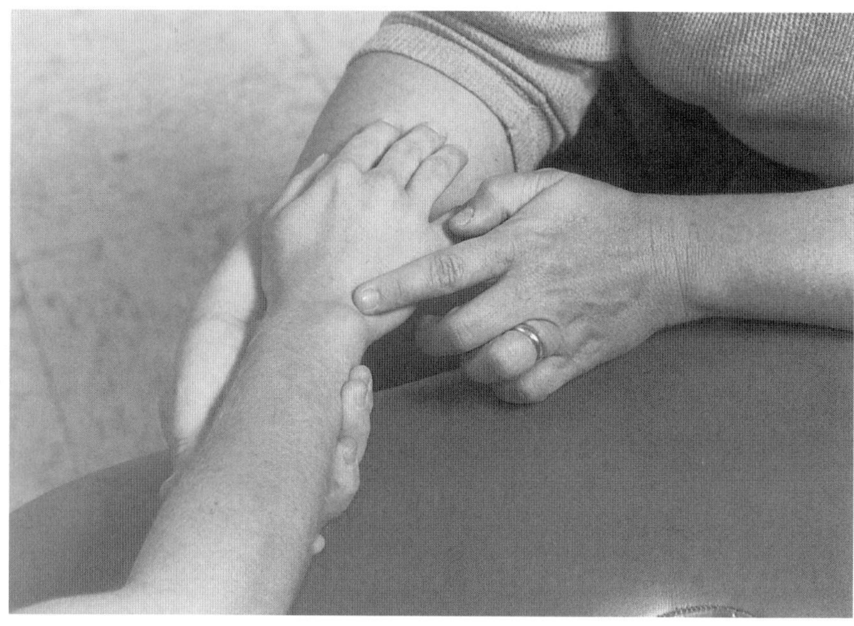

Stabilization/palpation: Stabilize anterior aspect of distal forearm. Palpate tendon of extensor carpi ulnaris on ulnar side of wrist, just distal to ulnar styloid process (Fig. 2-131).

Examiner action: While instructing patient in movement desired, extend patient's wrist and deviate it to ulnar side. Return patient to starting position. Performing passive movement allows determination of patient's available ROM and shows patient exact motion desired.

Patient action:

Patient extends and deviates wrist to ulnar side while examiner maintains stabilization of forearm and palpation of extensor carpi ulnaris (Fig. 2-132).

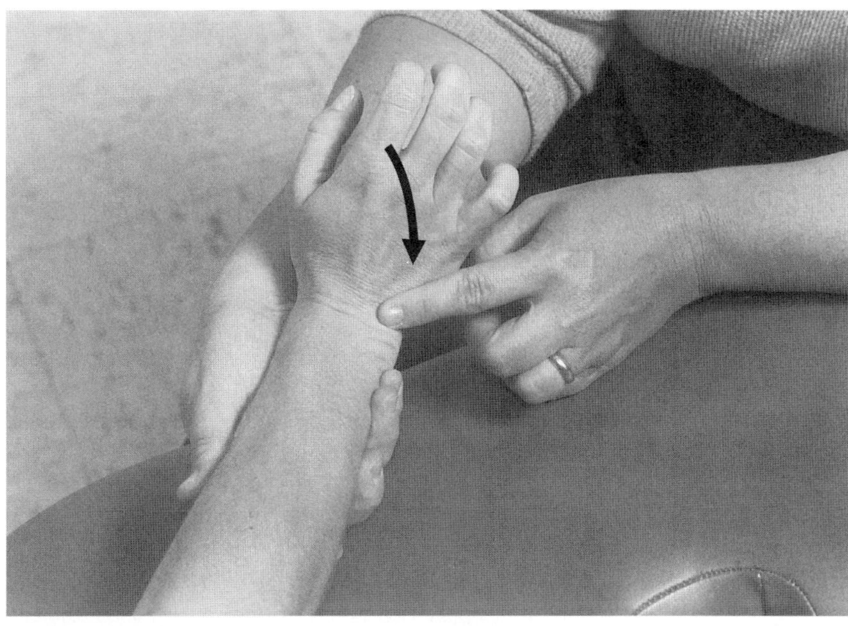

Fig. 2-132. Arrow indicates direction of movement.

Resistance:

Apply resistance along dorsal aspect of fifth metacarpal in direction of wrist flexion and radial deviation (Fig. 2-133).

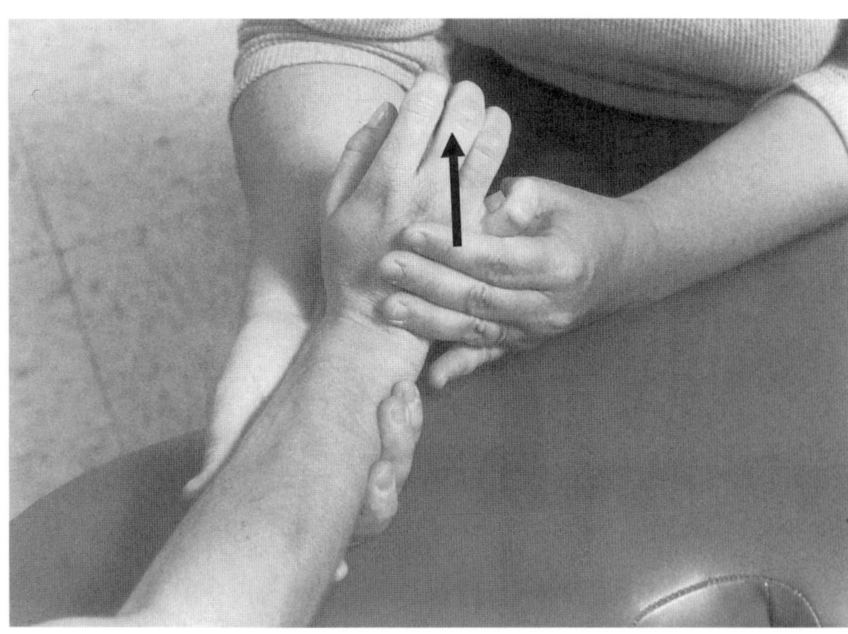

Fig. 2-133. Arrow indicates direction of resistance.

Gravity-Eliminated Test (Grades Below 3)

For patients unable to move completely through available ROM against gravity.

Patient position: Seated with forearm in neutral rotation (halfway between supination and pronation) and supported on a flat surface, wrist in neutral position (Fig. 2-134; initial wrist position not shown).

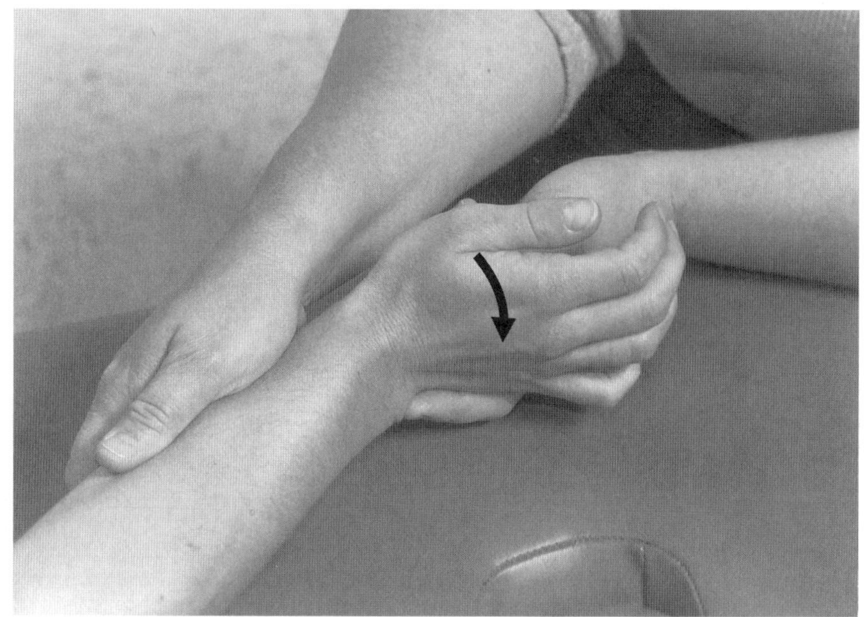

Fig. 2-134. Arrow indicates direction of movement.

Stabilization/palpation: Stabilize along radial side of distal forearm. Palpate extensor carpi ulnaris as in gravity-resisted test (Fig. 2-134).

Examiner action: While instructing patient in movement desired, extend patient's wrist. Return patient to starting position.

Patient action: Patient extends wrist through full ROM while examiner maintains stabilization of forearm and palpation of extensor carpi ulnaris (Fig. 2-134).

COMMON SUBSTITUTION

See test for extensor carpi radialis longus and brevis.

■ FINGER FLEXION (METACARPOPHALANGEAL)

LUMBRICALS, PALMAR AND DORSAL INTEROSSEI (Fig. 2-135)

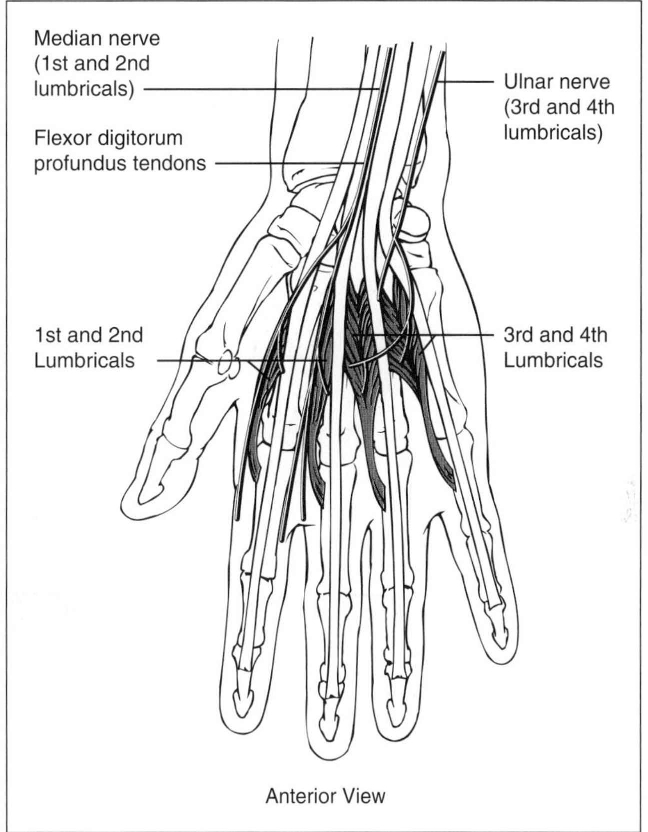

Fig. 2-135.

	ATTACHMENTS	NERVE SUPPLY	FUNCTION
Lumbricals	Origin: Tendons of the flexor digitorum profundus. 1st: Radial side of the tendon of the index finger; 2nd: radial side of the tendon of the middle finger; 3rd: tendons of the middle and ring fingers; 4th: tendons of the ring and little fingers Insertion: Radial side of the extensor hood of the corresponding finger	Peripheral nerve: 1st and 2nd Lumbricals: median nerve; 3rd and 4th Lumbricals: ulnar nerve Nerve root: C8, T1	Flexion of MCP joints 2–5; extension of the PIP and DIP joints of digits 2–5
Palmar interossei	Origin: Palmar surface of metacarpal bones 2, 4 and 5. 1st: Ulnar side of the 2nd metacarpal bone; 2nd: radial side of the 4th metacarpal bone; 3rd: radial side of the 5th metacarpal bone Insertion: 1st: Ulnar side of the base of the proximal phalanx and the extensor hood of the 2nd digit; 2nd: radial side of the base of the proximal phalanx and the extensor hood of the 4th digit; 3rd: radial side of the base of the proximal phalanx and the extensor hood of the 5th digit	Peripheral nerve: Ulnar nerve Nerve root: C8, T1	Adduction and flexion of the 2nd, 4th, and 5th MCP joints; extension of the PIP and DIP joints of digits 2, 4, and 5
Dorsal interossei	Origin: By two heads from adjacent metacarpal bones Insertion: 1st: Radial side of the proximal phalanx and the extensor hood of the 2nd digit; 2nd: radial side of the proximal phalanx and the extensor hood of the 3rd digit; 3rd: ulnar side of the proximal phalanx and the extensor hood of the 3rd digit; 4th: ulnar side of the proximal phalanx and the extensor hood of the 4th digit	Peripheral nerve: Ulnar nerve Nerve root: C8, T1	Abduction and flexion of the 2nd, 3rd, and 4th MCP joints; extension of the PIP and DIP joints of digits 2, 3, and 4

Gravity-Resisted Test (Grades 5, 4, and 3)

Patient position: Seated with forearm fully supinated and supported on a flat surface, wrist in neutral position, fingers extended (Fig. 2-136).

Fig. 2-136.

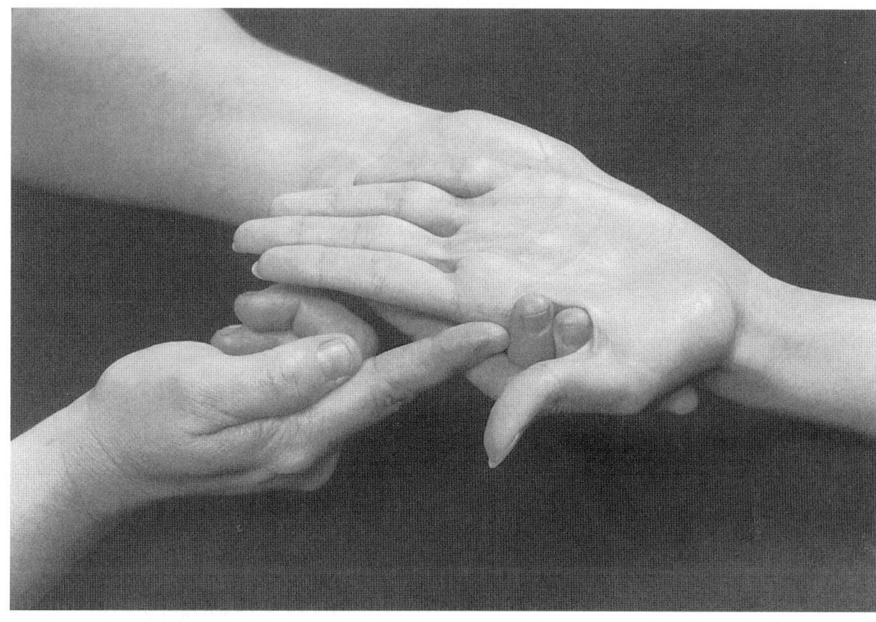

Stabilization/palpation: Stabilize over distal dorsal surface of second through fifth metacarpals. Palpation of lumbricals is difficult, but contraction may be detectable in palm, along radial aspect of second through fifth metacarpals (Fig. 2-136).

Examiner action: While instructing patient in movement desired, flex patient's fingers at metacarpophalangeal (MCP) joints while keeping interphalangeal (IP) joints extended. Return patient to starting position. Performing passive movement allows determination of patient's available ROM and shows patient exact motion desired.

Patient action:

Patient flexes MCP joints while extending IP joints. Examiner maintains stabilization of metacarpals and palpation of lumbricals during active movement by patient (Fig. 2-137).

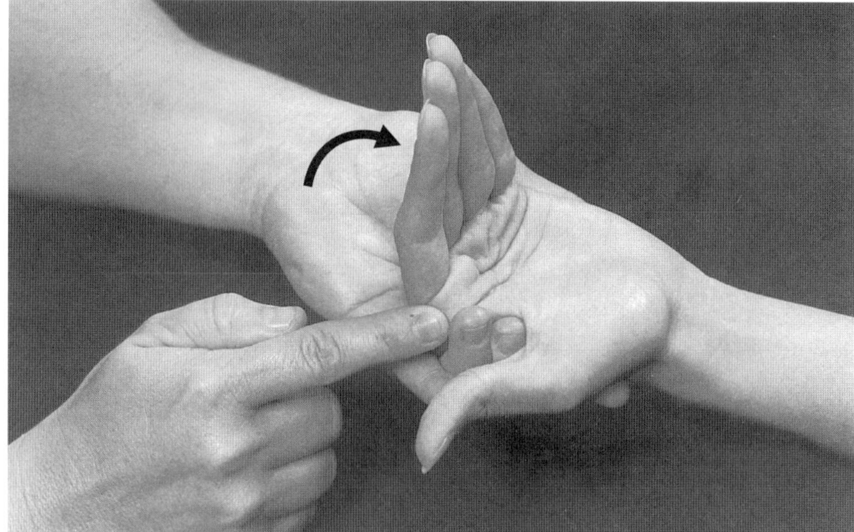

Fig. 2-137. Arrow indicates direction of movement.

Resistance:

Apply resistance with one finger along volar surface of proximal phalanx of second through fifth digits individually in direction of MCP extension (Fig. 2-138; resistance on second digit is shown). Resistance also may be applied separately on dorsal surface of middle and distal phalanges of second through fifth digits in direction of IP flexion (not shown). Palpating hand is moved to proximal phalanges to apply resistance.

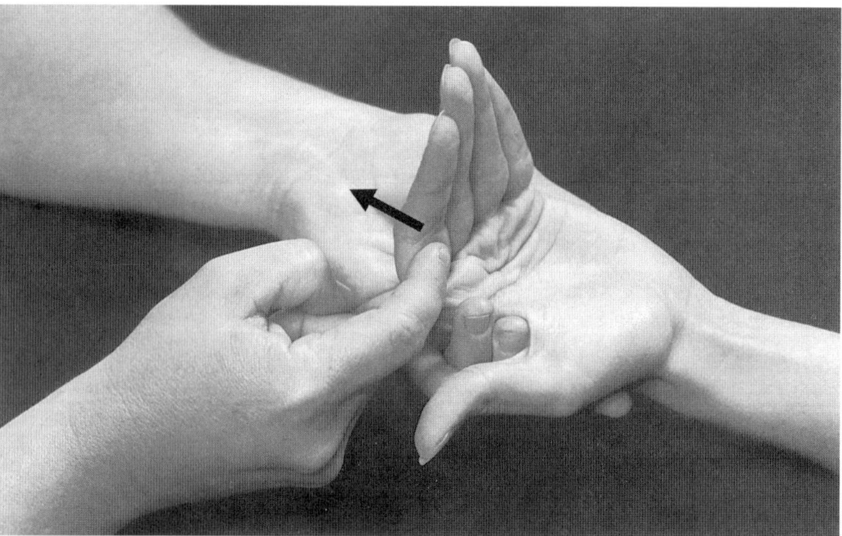

Fig. 2-138. Arrow indicates direction of resistance.

Gravity-Eliminated Test (Grades Below 3)

For patients unable to move completely through available ROM against gravity.

Patient position: Seated with forearm in neutral rotation and supported on a flat surface, wrist in neutral position, fingers extended (Fig. 2-139; initial finger position not shown).

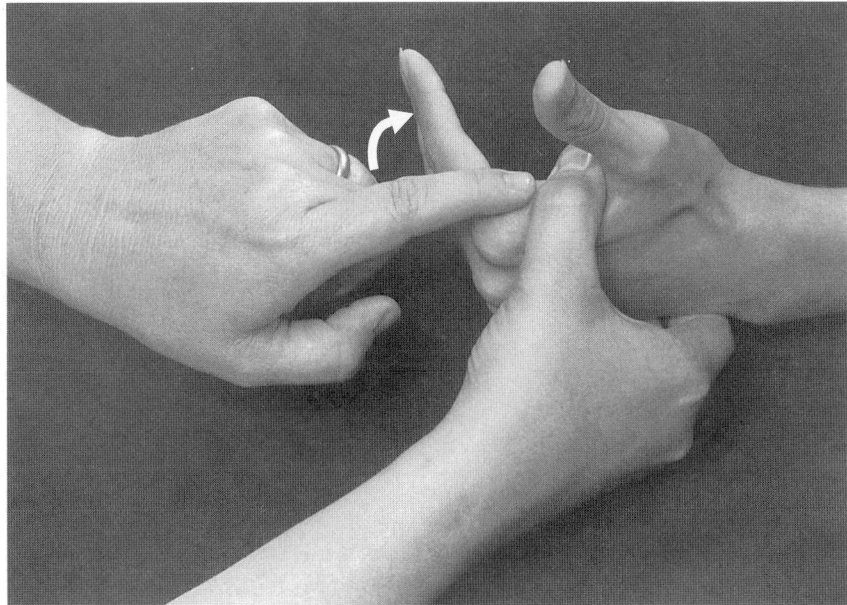

Fig. 2-139. Arrow indicates direction of movement.

Stabilization/palpation: Stabilize over dorsal surface of second through fifth metacarpals. Palpate lumbricals as in gravity-resisted test (Fig. 2-139).

Examiner action: As in gravity-resisted test.

Patient action: Patient flexes at MCP joints while extending IP joints. Examiner maintains stabilization of metacarpals and palpation of lumbricals during active movement by patient (Fig. 2-139).

■ FINGER FLEXION (PROXIMAL INTERPHALANGEAL)

FLEXOR DIGITORUM SUPERFICIALIS (Fig. 2-140)

Fig. 2-140.

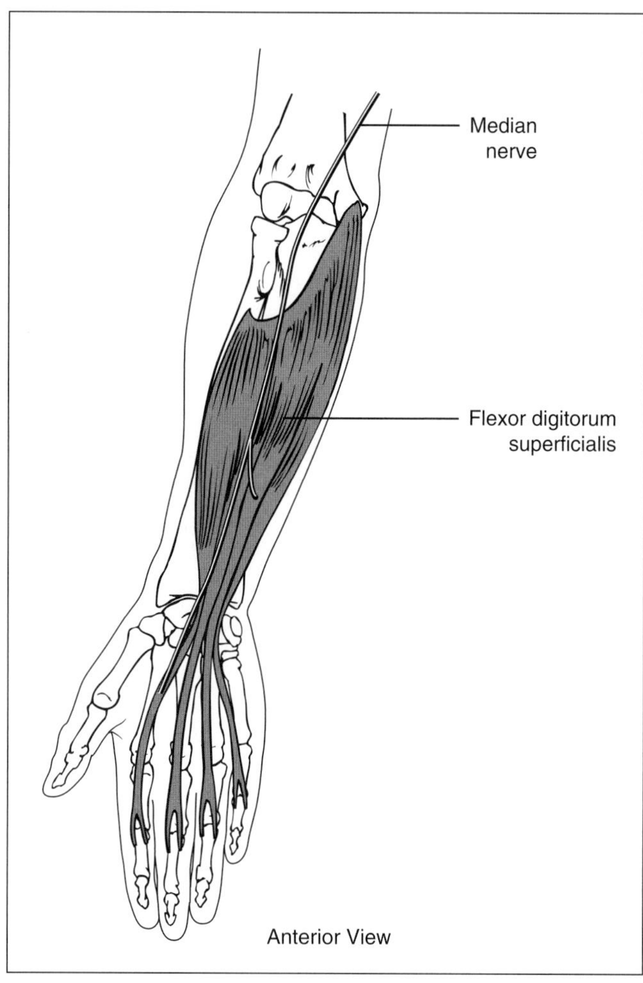

	ATTACHMENTS	NERVE SUPPLY	FUNCTION
Flexor digitorum superficialis	Origin: Humeroulnar head: Medial epicondyle of the humerus via the common flexor tendon, the ulnar collateral ligament of the elbow; the coronoid process of the ulna Radial head: Anterior surface of the radius Insertion: Via two slips into the sides of the middle phalanx of digits 2–5	Peripheral nerve: Median nerve Nerve root: C7, C8, T1	Flexion of the PIP joints of digits 2–5; assists in flexion of the MCP joints of digits 2–5 and of the wrist

Grades 5 and 4

Patient position: Seated with forearm supinated and supported on a flat surface, wrist in neutral position, fingers extended (Fig. 2-141).

Fig. 2-141.

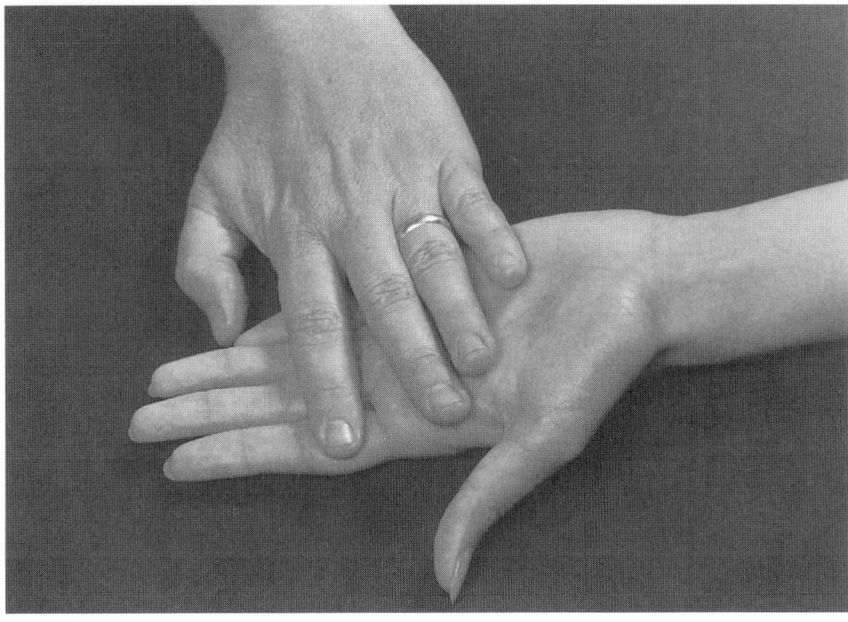

Stabilization/palpation: Stabilize over palmar surface of proximal phalanges of second through fifth digits. With same hand, palpate tendons of flexor digitorum superficialis over palmar surface of proximal phalanges of second through fifth digits (Fig. 2-141).

Examiner action: While instructing patient in motion desired, flex patient's fingers at proximal interphalangeal (PIP) joints, while keeping distal interphalangeal (DIP) joints extended. Return patient to starting position. Performing passive movement allows determination of patient's available ROM and shows patient exact motion desired.

Patient action:

Patient flexes PIP joints of second through fifth digits without accompanying flexion of DIP joints. Examiner maintains stabilization of proximal phalanges and palpation of flexor tendons during active movement by patient (Fig. 2-142).

Fig. 2-142. Arrow indicates direction of movement.

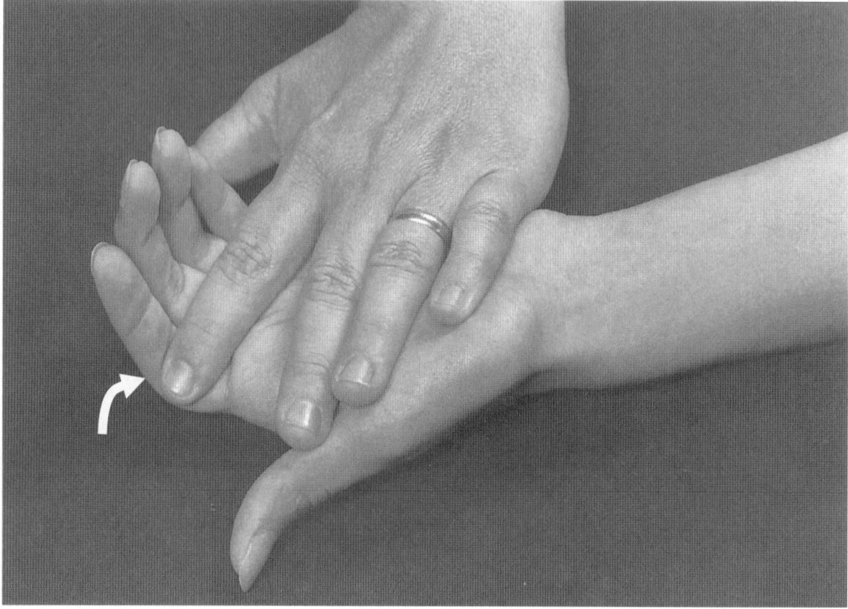

Resistance:

Use one finger to apply resistance on palmar surface of middle phalanges of second through fifth digits individually (Fig. 2-143).

Fig. 2-143. Arrow indicates direction of resistance.

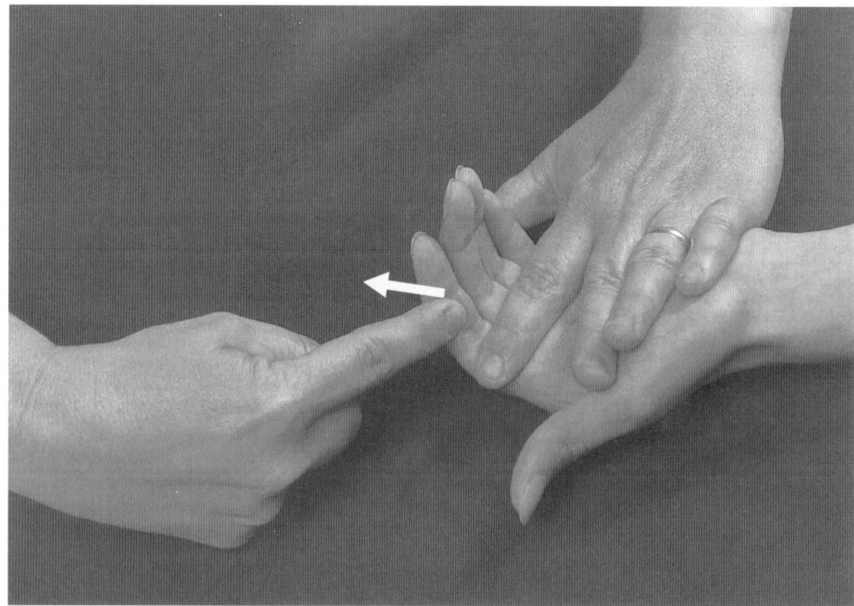

Grades 3 and Below

There is no separate test of these muscles for grades below 3. Grading is altered as follows to accommodate lack of a gravity-eliminated position.

For grade 3: Patient flexes joint through full ROM without resistance.

For grade 2: Patient flexes joint through partial ROM.

For grade 1: No motion, but a palpable contraction is present. Palpation occurs as described earlier (see Fig. 2-141).

For grade 0: No motion or contraction is present.

COMMON SUBSTITUTION

Flexor digitorum profundus; patient should flex at proximal joint without flexing distal joint to avoid substitution by flexor digitorum profundus.

■ FINGER FLEXION (DISTAL INTERPHALANGEAL)

FLEXOR DIGITORUM PROFUNDUS (Fig. 2-144)

Fig. 2-144.

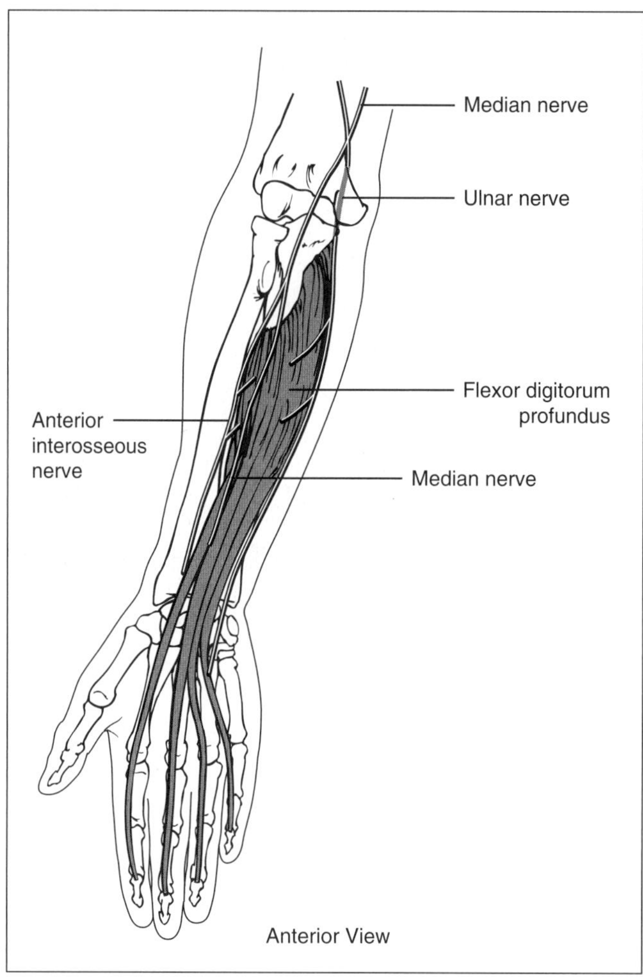

	ATTACHMENTS	NERVE SUPPLY	FUNCTION
Flexor digitorum profundus	Origin: Upper ¾ of the ulna, the coronoid process of the ulna, and the interosseus membrane Insertion: Base of the distal phalanges of digits 2–5	Peripheral nerve: Median and ulnar nerves Nerve root: C8, T1	Flexion of the DIP joints of digits 2–5; assists in flexing the PIP and MCP joints of digits

Grades 5 and 4

Patient position: Seated with forearm supinated and supported on a flat surface, wrist in neutral position, fingers extended (Fig. 2-145).

Fig. 2-145.

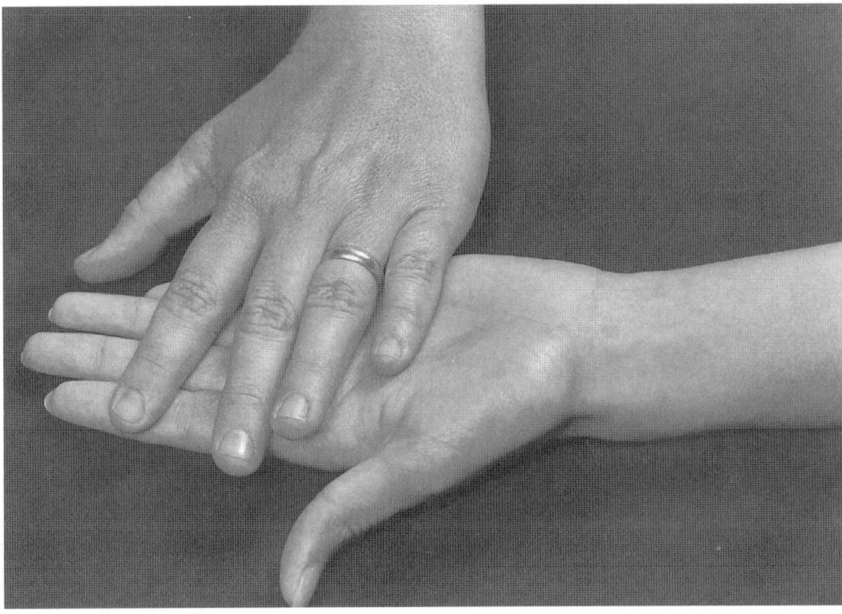

Stabilization/palpation: Stabilize over palmar surface of middle phalanges of second through fifth digits. With same hand, palpate tendons of flexor digitorum profundus over palmar surface of middle phalanges of second through fifth digits (Fig. 2-145).

Examiner action: While instructing patient in movement desired, flex patient's fingers at DIP joints. Return patient to starting position. Performing passive movement allows determination of patient's available ROM and shows patient exact motion desired.

Patient action:

Patient flexes DIP joints of second through fifth digits individually. (Note: Patient will be unable to flex DIP without accompanying flexion of PIP unless firm stabilization is used.) Examiner maintains stabilization of middle phalanges and palpation of flexor tendons during active movement by patient (Fig. 2-146).

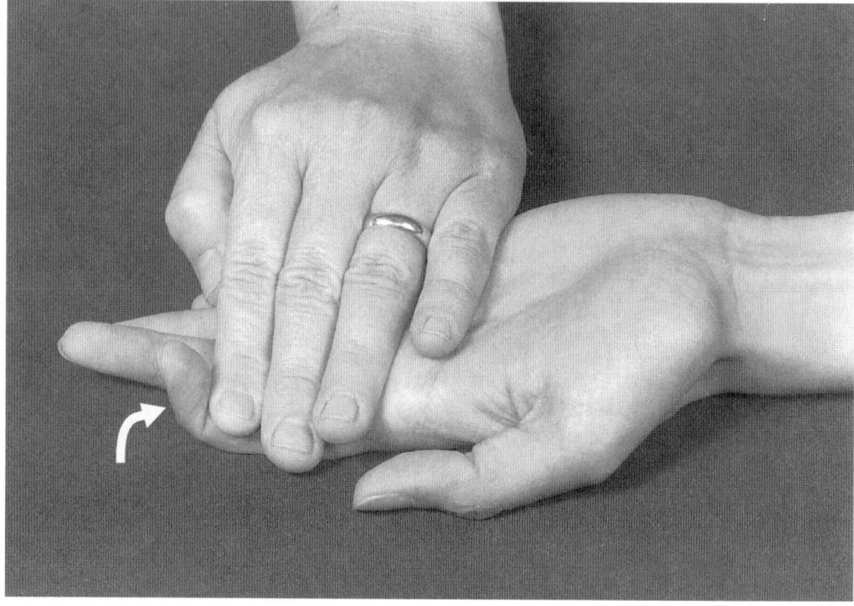

Fig. 2-146. Arrow indicates direction of movement.

Resistance:

Use one finger to apply resistance on palmar surface of distal phalanges of second through fifth digits individually (Fig. 2-147).

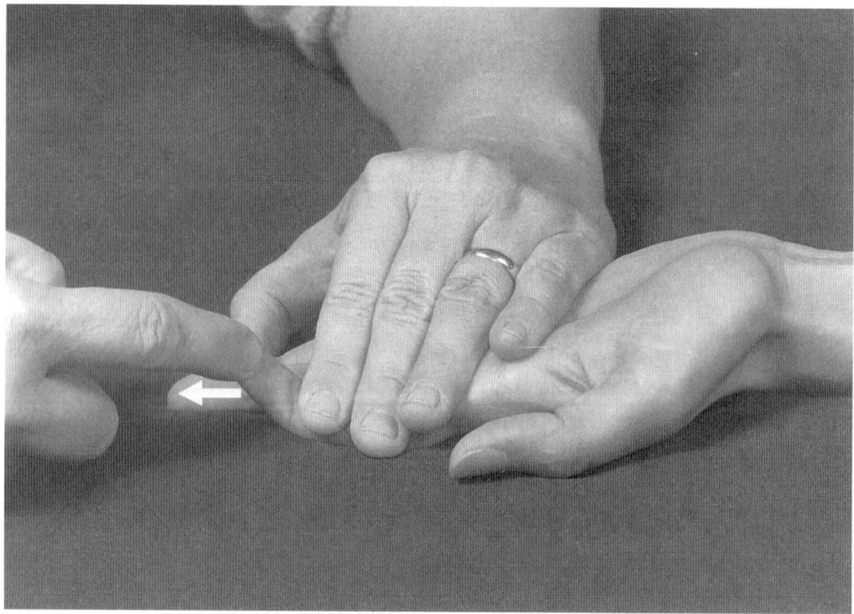

Fig. 2-147. Arrow indicates direction of resistance.

Grades 3 and Below

There is no separate test of these muscles for grades below 3. Grading is altered as follows to accommodate lack of a gravity-eliminated position.

For grade 3: Patient flexes joint through full ROM without resistance.

For grade 2: Patient flexes joint through partial ROM.

For grade 1: No motion, but a palpable contraction is present. Palpation occurs as described earlier (see Fig. 2-145).

For grade 0: No motion or contraction is present.

CLINICAL COMMENT: FLEXOR DIGITORUM PROFUNDUS AND C8 NEUROLOGIC ASSESSMENT

The flexor digitorum profundus muscle is a key muscle for examining the integrity of the C8 spinal nerve or neurologic segment of the spinal cord. Complete assessment of the C8 neurologic level includes:

Strength assessment of:
Flexor digitorum profundus (pp. 153–155)
Sensory testing of:
Skin over ulnar side of hand, particularly little finger (C8 dermatome; pp. 528-532)
No reflex for C8

■ FINGER EXTENSION

EXTENSOR DIGITORUM, EXTENSOR INDICIS, AND EXTENSOR DIGITI MINIMI (Figs. 2-148 and 2-149)

Fig. 2-148.

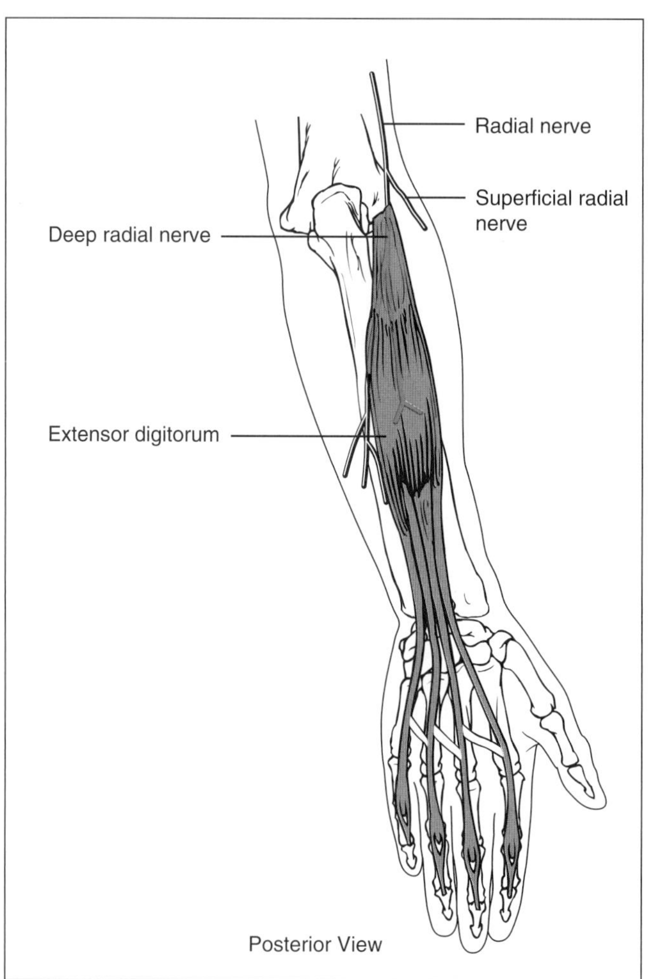

Fig. 2-149.

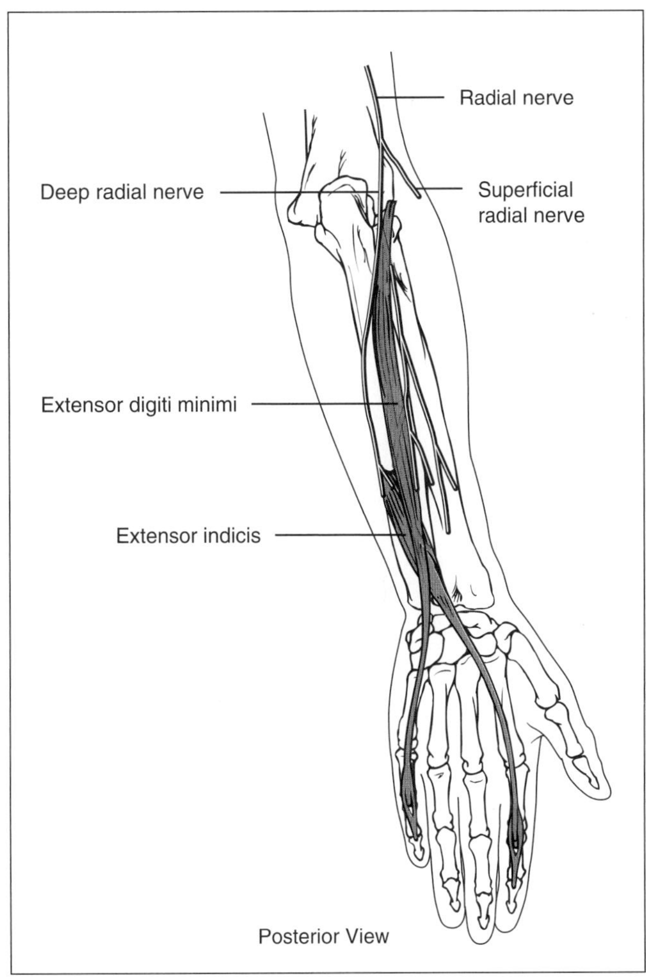

	ATTACHMENTS	NERVE SUPPLY	FUNCTION
Extensor digitorum	Origin: Lateral epicondyle of the humerus via the common extensor tendon; antebrachial fascia Insertion: Middle and distal phalanges of digits 2–5 via the extensor hood or expansion	Peripheral nerve: Deep radial nerve Nerve root: C6–C8	Extension of digits 2–5; assists in wrist extension
Extensor indicis	Origin: Posterior surface of the ulna; interosseous membrane Insertion: Extensor hood of the index finger	Peripheral nerve: Deep radial nerve Nerve root: C6–C8	Extension of the index finger; assists in wrist extension
Extensor digiti minimi	Origin: Lateral epicondyle of the humerus via the common extensor tendon; intermuscular septa Insertion: Extensor hood on the dorsum of the proximal phalanx of digit 5	Peripheral nerve: Deep radial nerve Nerve root: C6–C8	Extension of digit 5; assists in wrist extension

Gravity-Resisted Test (Grades 5, 4, and 3)

Patient position: Seated with forearm pronated and supported on a flat surface, wrist in neutral position, fingers are allowed to extend past edge of surface in a position of flexion (Fig. 2-150).

Fig. 2-150.

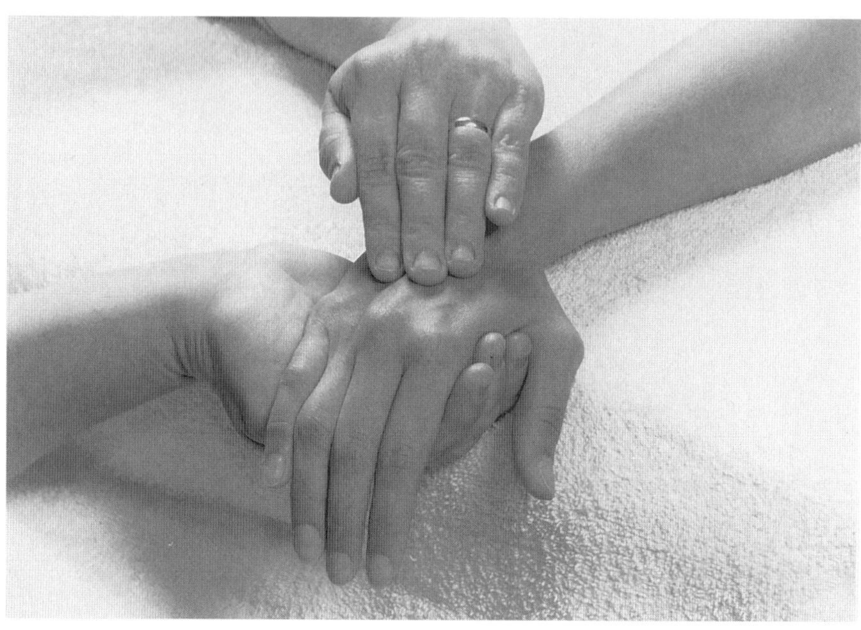

Stabilization/palpation: Stabilize over palmar aspect of second through fifth metacarpals. Palpate tendons of extensor digitorum along dorsal surface of corresponding metacarpal bone. Palpate tendon of extensor indicis just to ulnar side of extensor digitorum tendon for second digit; palpate tendon of extensor digiti minimi just to ulnar side of extensor digitorum tendon for fifth digit (Fig. 2-150).

Examiner action: While instructing patient in movement desired, extend patient's fingers at MCP joints while allowing IP joints to remain flexed. Return patient to starting position. Performing passive movement allows determination of patient's available ROM and shows patient exact motion desired.

Patient action: Patient extends second through fifth digits at MCP joints through full ROM. Examiner maintains stabilization of metacarpals and palpation of extensor tendons during active movement by patient (Fig. 2-151).

Resistance: Use one finger to apply resistance individually along dorsal surface of proximal phalanx of second through fifth digits in direction of flexion. Index finger of palpating hand is moved to proximal phalanx to apply resistance (Fig. 2-152).

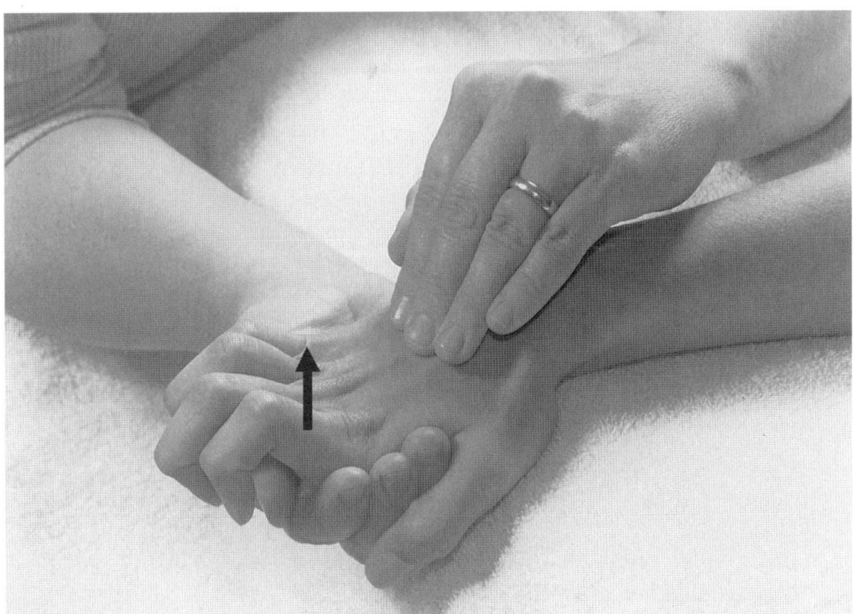

Fig. 2-151. Arrow indicates direction of movement.

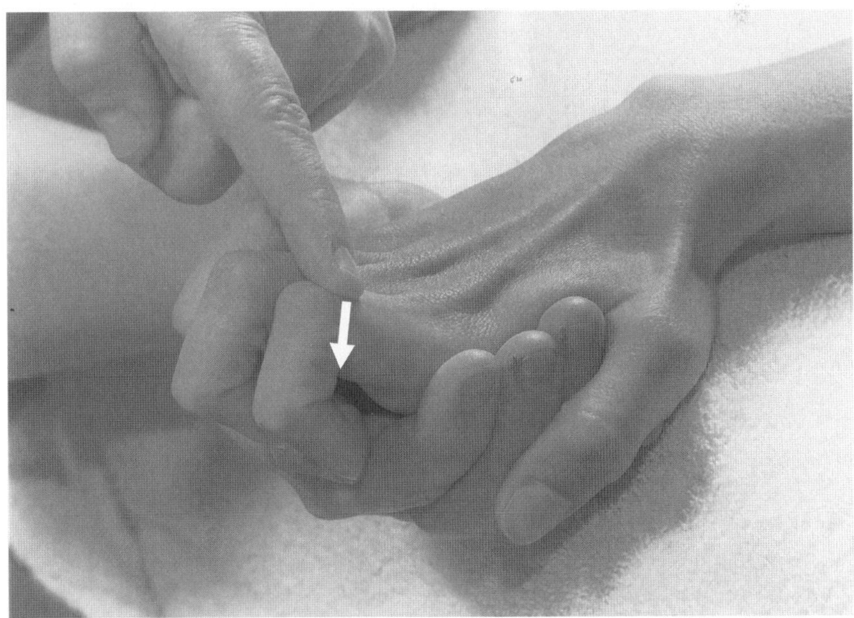

Fig. 2-152. Arrow indicates direction of resistance.

Gravity-Eliminated Test (Grades Below 3)

For patients unable to move completely through available ROM against gravity.

Patient position: Seated with forearm in neutral rotation (halfway between pronation and supination) and supported on a flat surface, wrist in neutral position, fingers flexed at MCP joints (Fig. 2-153; initial finger position not shown).

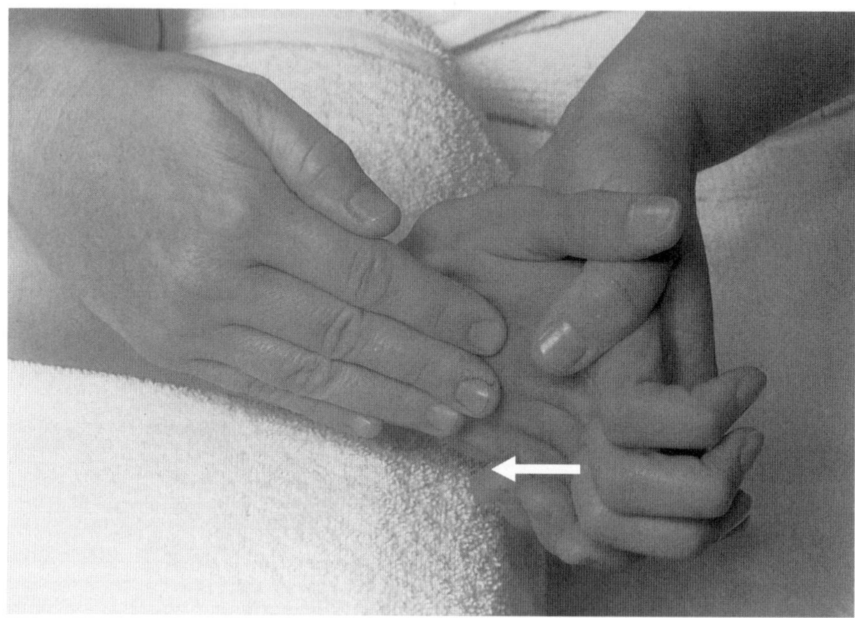

Fig. 2-153. Arrow indicates direction of movement.

Stabilization/palpation: Stabilize over palmar aspect of second through fifth metacarpals. Palpate extensor tendons as described in gravity-resisted test (Fig. 2-153).

Examiner action: As in gravity-resisted test.

Patient action: Patient extends second through fifth digits at MCP joints through full ROM. Examiner maintains stabilization of metacarpals and palpation of extensor tendons during active movement by patient (Fig. 2-153).

CLINICAL COMMENT: FINGER EXTENSOR MUSCLES AND C7 NEUROLOGIC ASSESSMENT

The finger extensor muscles (extensor digitorum, extensor indicis, extensor digiti minimi) are key muscles for examining the integrity of the C7 spinal nerve or neurologic segment of the spinal cord. Complete assessment of the C7 neurologic level includes:

Strength assessment of:
Triceps brachii (pp. 112–115)
Wrist flexors (pp. 126–129)
Finger extensors (pp. 158–160)
Reflex testing of:
Triceps reflex (p. 549)
Sensory testing of:
Skin over the middle finger (C7 dermatome; pp. 528-532)

FINGER ABDUCTION

DORSAL INTEROSSEI, ABDUCTOR DIGITI MINIMI (Fig. 2-154)

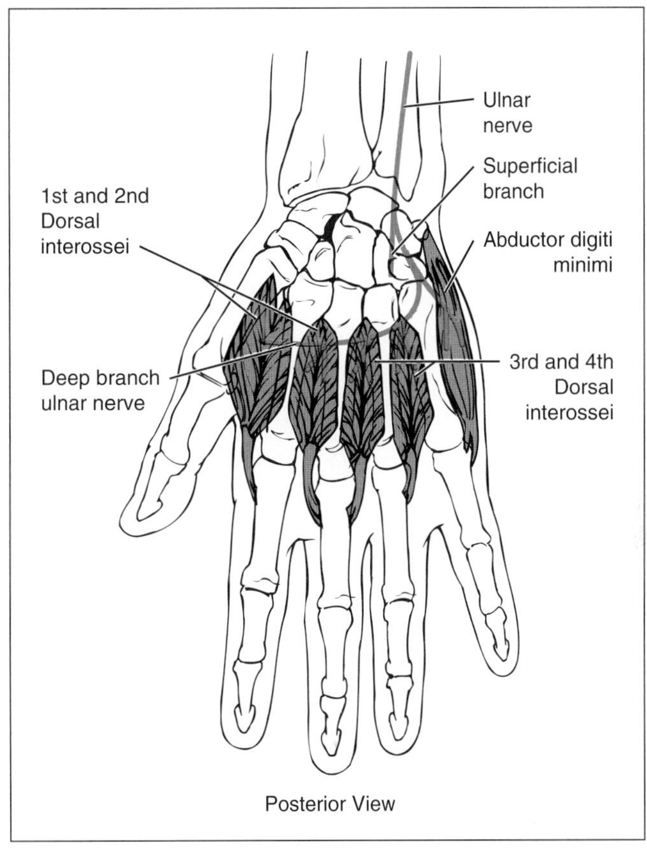

Fig. 2-154.

	ATTACHMENTS	NERVE SUPPLY	FUNCTION
Dorsal interossei	Origin: By two heads from adjacent metacarpal bones Insertion: 1st: Radial side of the proximal phalanx and the extensor hood of the 2nd digit; 2nd: radial side of the proximal phalanx and the extensor hood of the 3rd digit; 3rd: ulnar side of the proximal phalanx and the extensor hood of the 3rd digit; 4th: ulnar side of the proximal phalanx and the extensor hood of the 4th digit	Peripheral nerve: Ulnar nerve Nerve root: C8, T1	Abduction and flexion of the 2nd, 3rd, and 4th MCP joints; extension of the PIP and DIP joints of digits 2–4
Abductor digiti minimi	Origin: Pisiform bone and the tendon of flexor carpi ulnaris Insertion: Ulnar side of the base of the proximal phalanx of the 5th digit; aponeurosis of the extensor digiti minimi	Peripheral nerve: Ulnar nerve Nerve root: C8, T1	Abduction and flexion of the 5th MCP joint

Grades 5 and 4

Patient position: Seated with forearm pronated and supported on a flat surface, wrist in neutral position, fingers adducted and allowed to extend beyond supporting surface (Fig. 2-155).

Fig. 2-155.

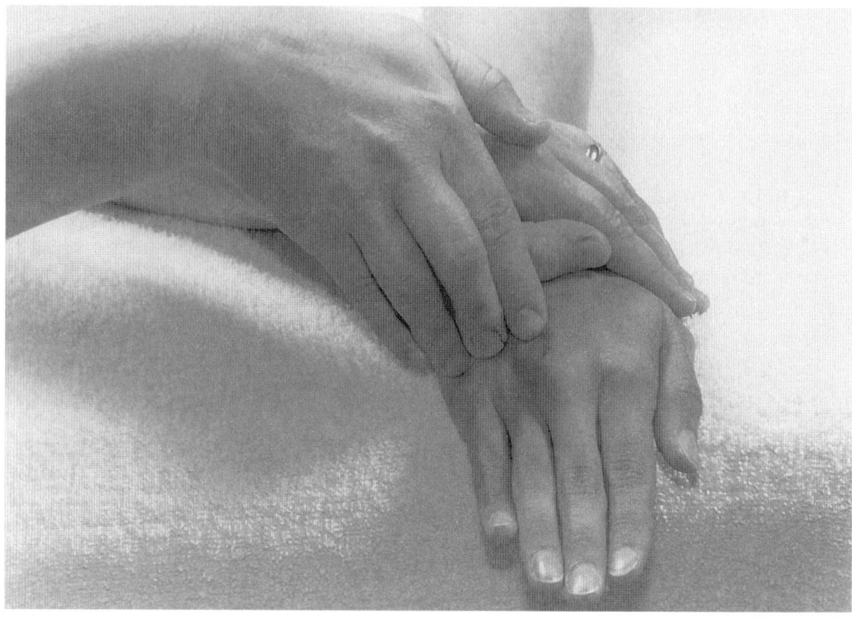

Stabilization/palpation: Stabilize over dorsal surface of second through fifth metacarpals. Dorsal interossei are difficult to palpate, but contraction may be detected along dorsoradial aspect of second and third metacarpals and along dorsoulnar aspect of third and fourth metacarpals. Palpate abductor digiti minimi along ulnar aspect of fifth metacarpal (Fig. 2-155).

Examiner action: While instructing patient in movement desired, abduct patient's fingers. Return patient to starting position. Performing passive movement allows determination of patient's available ROM and shows patient exact motion desired.

Patient action:

Patient abducts fingers through full ROM (third digit should be abducted toward both second and fourth digits). Examiner maintains stabilization of metacarpals and palpation of MCP abductors during patient motion (Fig. 2-156).

Fig. 2-156. Arrows indicate direction of movement.

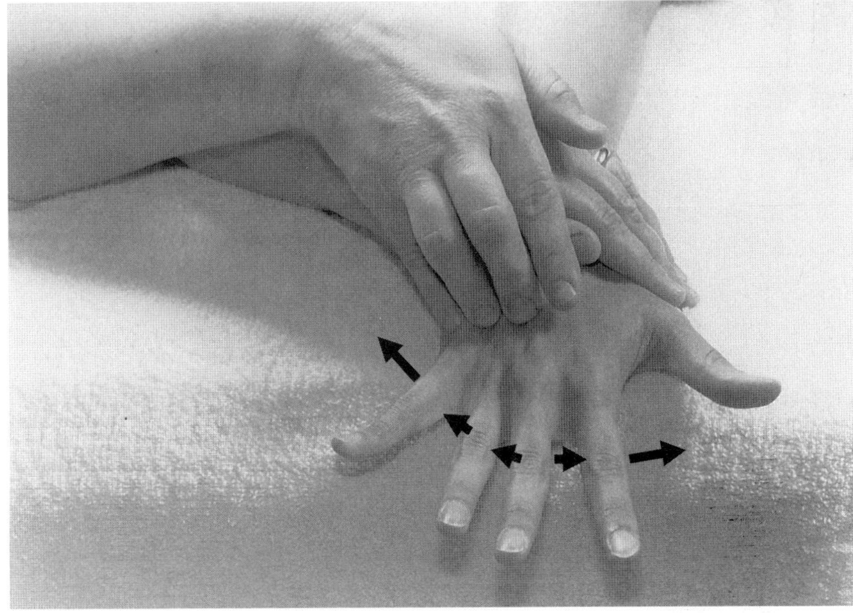

Resistance:

Use one finger to apply resistance along proximal phalanx of each finger individually as follows: on radial side of second digit in direction of adduction; on radial side of third digit in direction of adduction; on ulnar side of third digit in direction of adduction; on ulnar side of fourth digit in direction of adduction; and on ulnar side of fifth digit (abductor digiti minimi) in direction of adduction (Fig. 2-157; resistance for abductor digiti minimi shown).

Fig. 2-157. Arrow indicates direction of resistance.

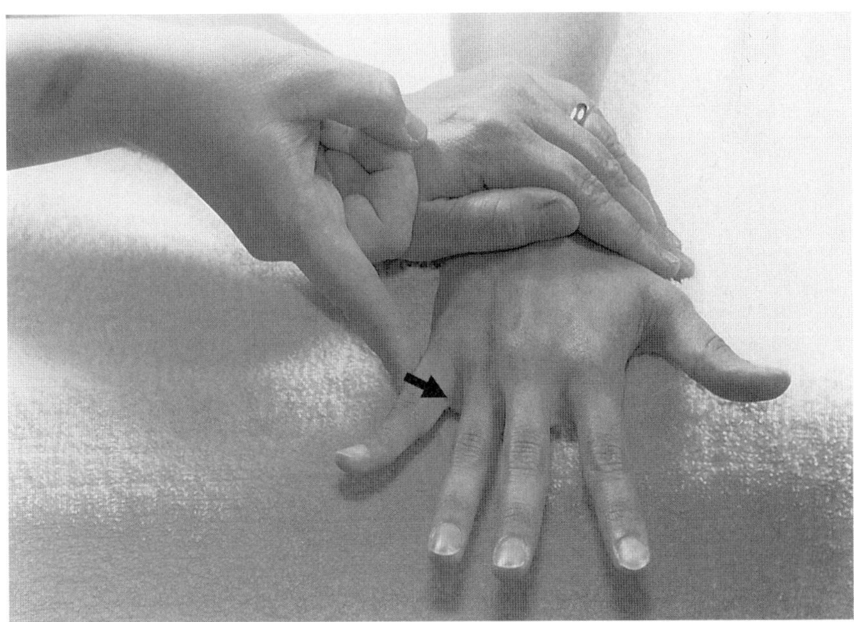

Grades 3 and Below

There is no separate test of these muscles for grades below 3. Grading is altered as follows to accommodate lack of a gravity-eliminated position.

For grade 3: Patient abducts fingers through full ROM without resistance.

For grade 2: Patient abducts fingers through partial ROM.

For grade 1: No motion, but a palpable contraction is present. Palpation occurs as described earlier (Fig. 2-155).

For grade 0: No motion or contraction is present.

CLINICAL COMMENT: FINGER ABDUCTORS AND ADDUCTORS AND T1 NEUROLOGIC ASSESSMENT

The abductors (dorsal interossei and abductor digiti minimi) and adductors (palmar interossei) of the MCP joints of digits 2-5 are key muscles for examining the integrity of the T1 spinal nerve or neurologic segment of the spinal cord. Complete assessment of the T1 neurologic level includes:

Strength assessment of:

MCP abductors (pp. 162–164)

MCP adductors (pp. 166–167)

Sensory testing of:

Skin over the medial aspect of the elbow (T1 dermatome; pp. 528-532)

■ FINGER ADDUCTION

PALMAR INTEROSSEI (Fig. 2-158)

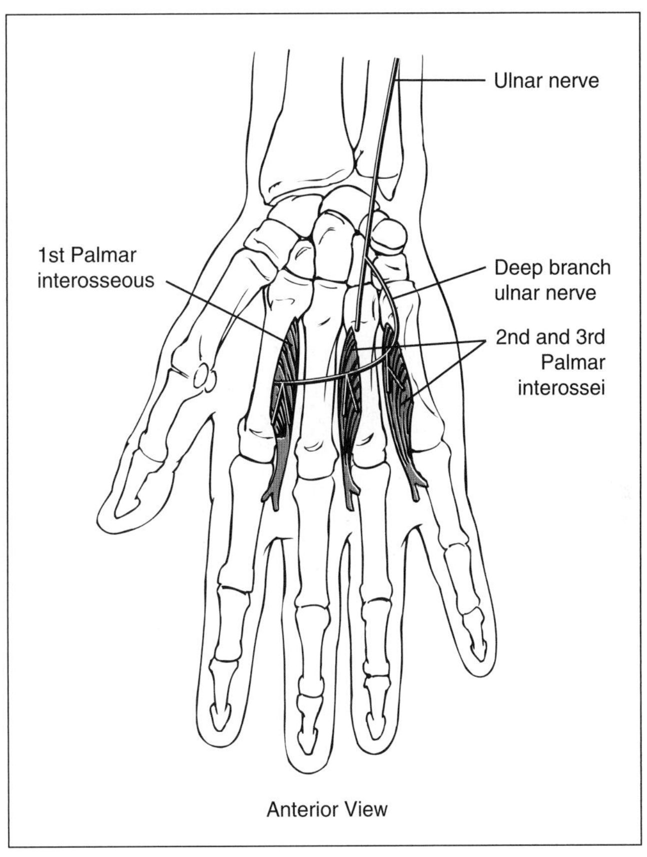

Fig. 2-158.

	ATTACHMENTS	NERVE SUPPLY	FUNCTION
Palmar interossei	Origin: Palmar surface of metacarpal bones 2, 4, and 5. 1st: Ulnar side of the 2nd metacarpal bone; 2nd: radial side of the 4th metacarpal bone; 3rd: radial side of the 5th metacarpal bone Insertion: 1st: Ulnar side of the base of the proximal phalanx and the extensor hood of the 2nd digit; 2nd: radial side of the base of the proximal phalanx and the extensor hood of the 4th digit; 3rd: radial side of the base of the proximal phalanx and the extensor hood of the 5th digit	Peripheral nerve: Ulnar nerve Nerve root: C8, T1	Adduction and flexion of the 2nd, 4th, and 5th MCP joints; extension of the proximal and distal IP joints of digits 2, 4, and 5

Grades 5 and 4

Patient position: Seated with forearm pronated and supported on a flat surface, wrist in neutral position, fingers fully abducted and allowed to extend beyond supporting surface (Fig. 2-159).

Fig. 2-159.

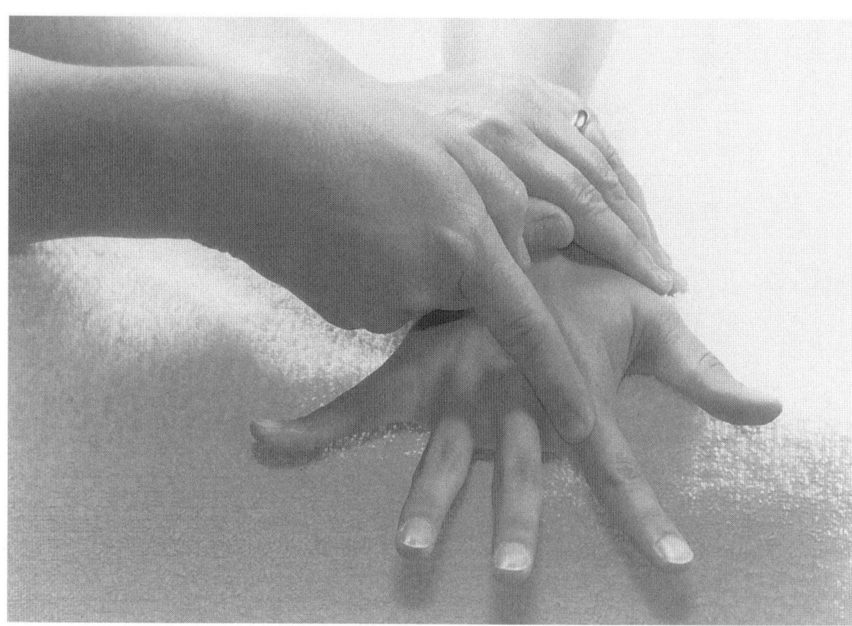

Stabilization/palpation: Stabilize over dorsal surface of second through fifth metacarpals. Palmar interossei are difficult to palpate, but contraction may be detected at base of proximal phalanges of second digit (ulnar side) and fourth and fifth digits (radial side) (Fig. 2-159).

Examiner action: While instructing patient in desired movement, adduct patient's fingers. Return patient to starting position. Performing passive movement allows determination of patient's available ROM and shows patient exact motion desired.

Patient action: Patient adducts fingers through full ROM while examiner maintains stabilization of metacarpals and palpation of palmar interossei (Fig. 2-160).

Resistance: Use one finger to apply resistance along proximal phalanx of each finger individually as follows: on ulnar side of second digit in direction of abduction; on radial side of fourth digit in direction of abduction; on radial side of fifth digit in direction of abduction (Fig. 2-161; resistance for first palmar interosseous muscle shown).

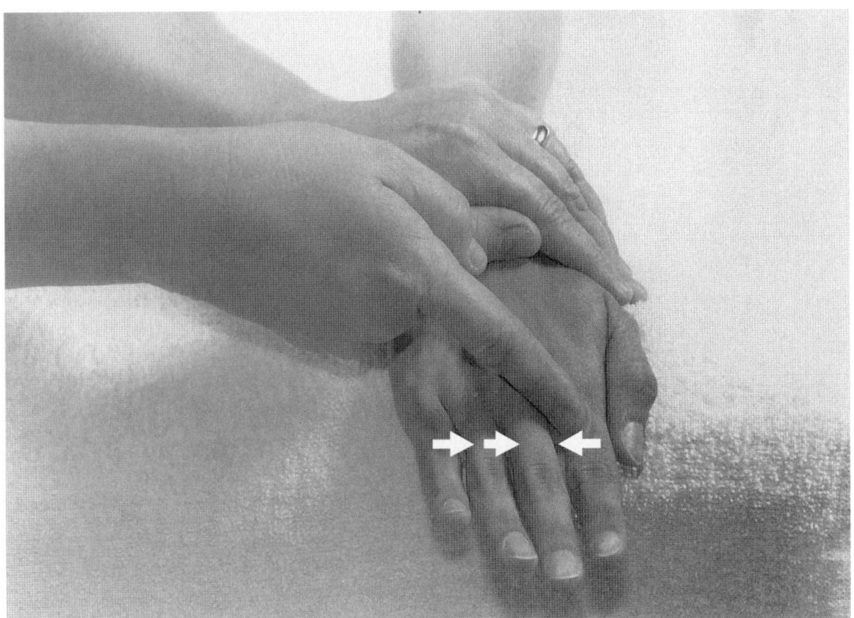

Fig. 2-160. Arrows indicate direction of movement.

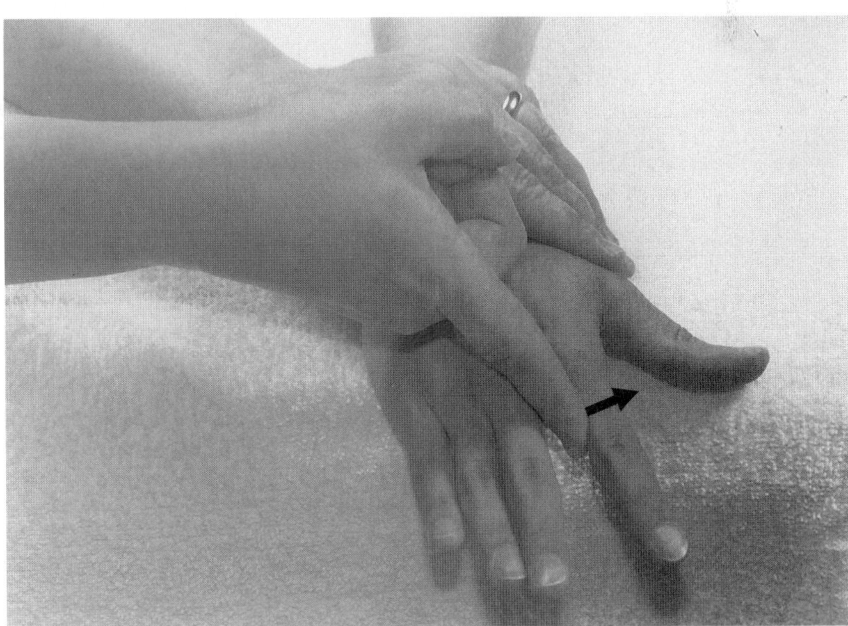

Fig. 2-161. Arrow indicates direction of resistance.

Grades 3 and Below

There is no separate test of these muscles for grades below 3. Grading is altered as follows to accommodate lack of a gravity-eliminated position.

For grade 3: Patient adducts fingers through full ROM without resistance.

For grade 2: Patient adducts fingers through partial ROM.

For grade 1: No motion, but a palpable contraction is present. Palpation occurs as described earlier (see Fig. 2-159).

For grade 0: No motion or contraction is present.

■ THUMB FLEXION (METACARPOPHALANGEAL)

FLEXOR POLLICIS BREVIS (Fig. 2-162)

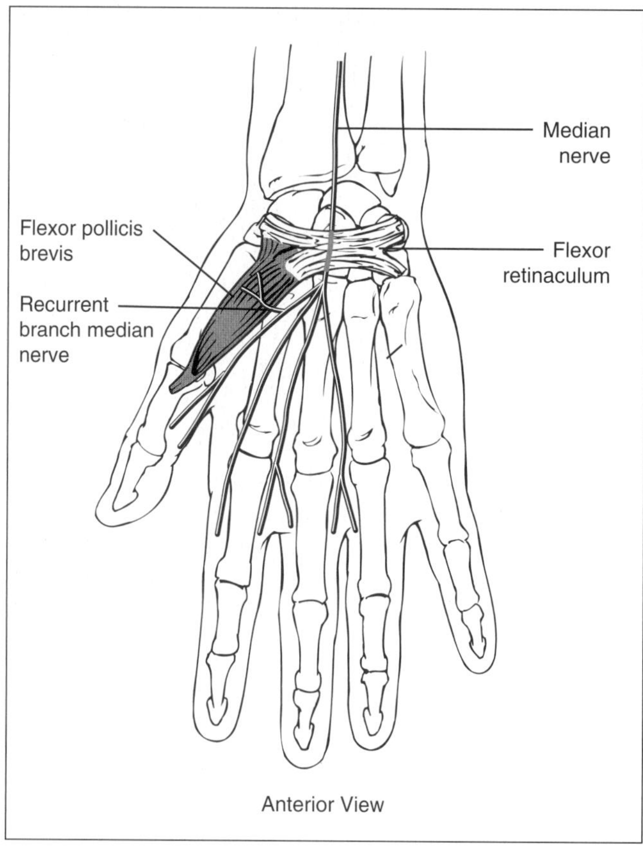

Fig. 2-162.

	ATTACHMENTS	NERVE SUPPLY	FUNCTION
Flexor pollicis brevis	Origin: Flexor retinaculum, trapezium, trapezoid, and capitate bones Insertion: Radial side of the base of the proximal phalanx of the thumb	Peripheral nerve: Median and ulnar nerves Nerve root: C8, T1	Flexion of the MCP joint of the thumb

Grades 5 and 4

Patient position: Seated with forearm supinated and supported on a flat surface, wrist in neutral position, MCP and IP joints of thumb are extended (Fig. 2-163).

Fig. 2-163.

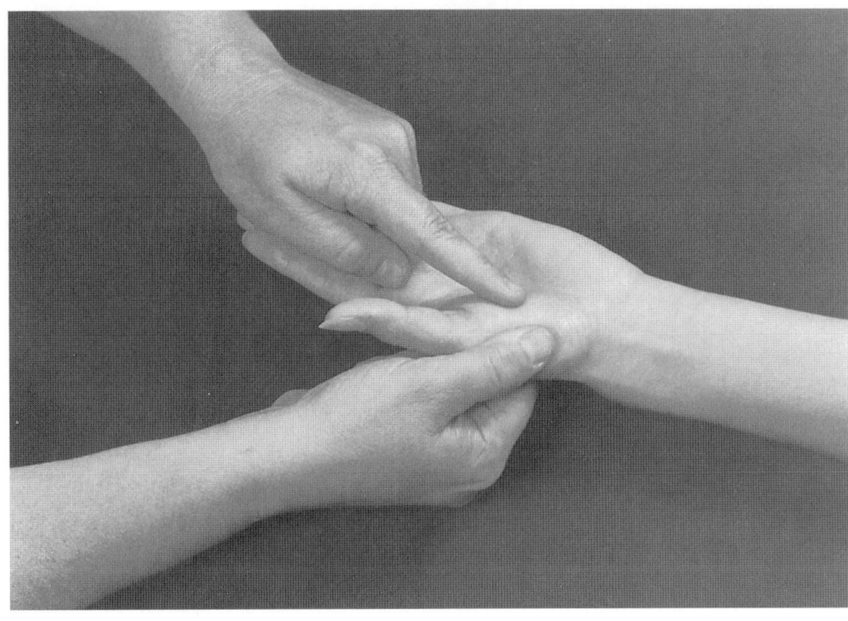

Stabilization/palpation: Stabilize sides of first metacarpal. Palpate flexor pollicis brevis over volar aspect of first metacarpal bone (Fig. 2-163).

Examiner action: While instructing patient in movement desired, flex MCP joint of patient's thumb while keeping IP joint of thumb extended. Return patient to starting position. Performing passive movement allows determination of patient's available ROM and shows patient exact motion desired.

Patient action:

Patient flexes MCP joint of thumb without flexing IP joint. Examiner maintains stabilization of metacarpal and palpation of flexor pollicis brevis during patient's active movement (Fig. 2-164).

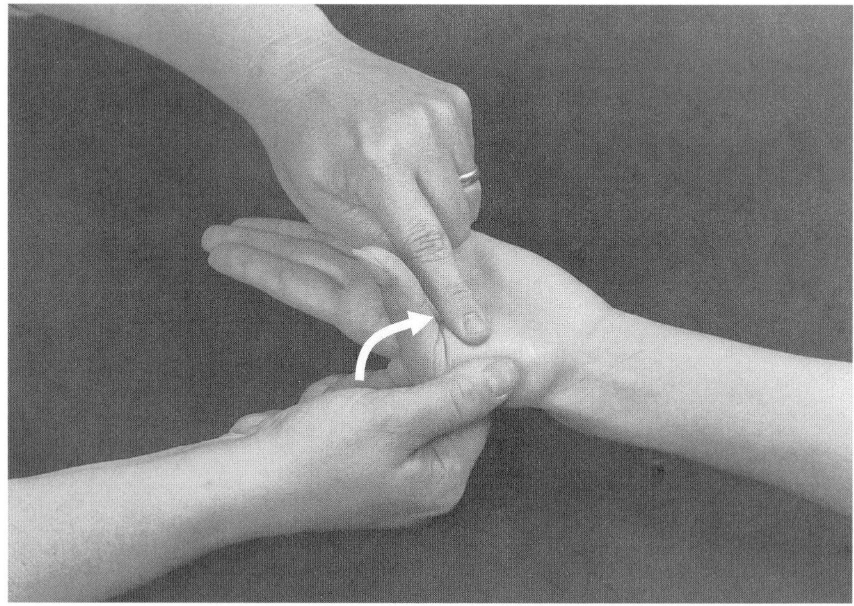

Fig. 2-164. Arrow indicates direction of movement.

Resistance:

Use one finger to apply resistance along volar aspect of proximal phalanx of thumb in direction of MCP extension. Palpating hand is moved to proximal phalanx to apply resistance (Fig. 2-165).

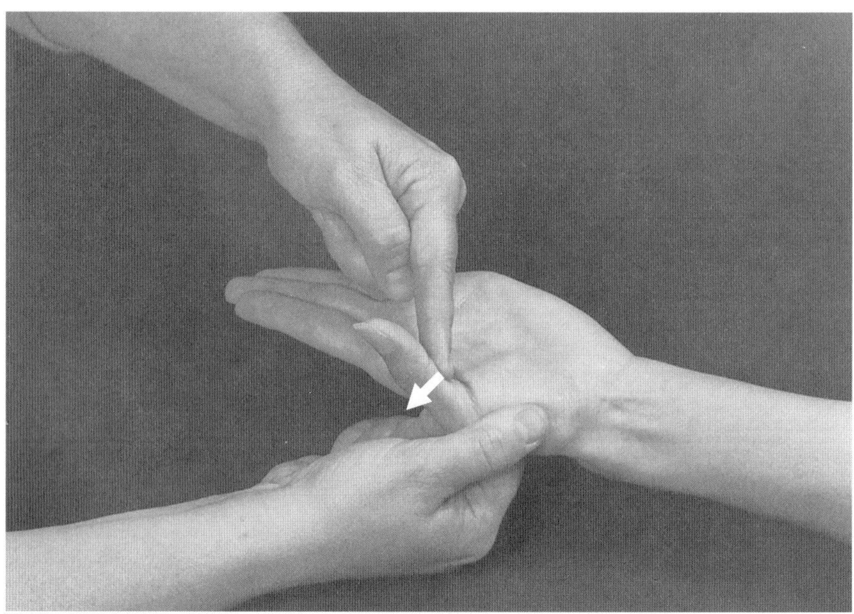

Fig. 2-165. Arrow indicates direction of resistance.

Grades 3 and Below

There is no separate test of this muscle for grades below 3. Grading is altered as follows to accommodate lack of a gravity-eliminated position.

For grade 3: Patient flexes joint through full ROM without resistance.

For grade 2: Patient flexes joint through partial ROM.

For grade 1: No motion, but a palpable contraction is present. Palpation occurs as described earlier (see Fig. 2-163).

For grade 0: No motion or contraction is present.

COMMON SUBSTITUTION

Flexor pollicis longus; patient should flex MCP joint without flexing IP joint to avoid substitution by flexor pollicis longus.

■ THUMB FLEXION (INTERPHALANGEAL)

FLEXOR POLLICIS LONGUS (Fig. 2-166)

Fig. 2-166.

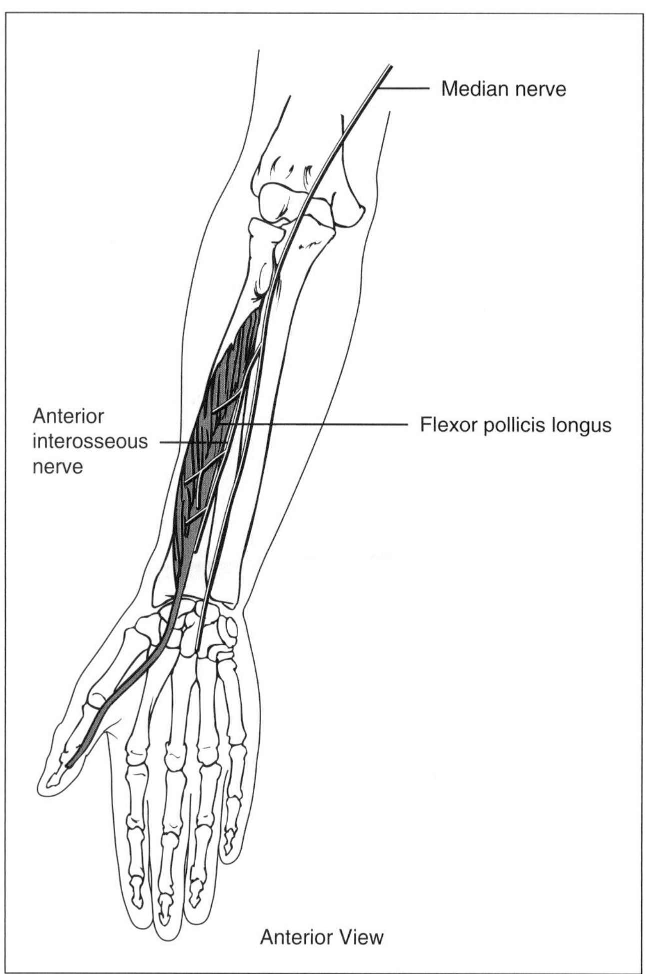

	ATTACHMENTS	NERVE SUPPLY	FUNCTION
Flexor pollicis longus	Origin: Anterior aspect of the radius, the coronoid process of the ulna, and the interosseous membrane Insertion: Base of the distal phalanx of the thumb	Peripheral nerve: Anterior interosseous (median) nerve Nerve root: C8, T1	Flexion of the IP joint of the thumb; assists in flexion of the MCP joint of the thumb

Grades 5 and 4

Patient position: Seated with forearm supinated and supported on a flat surface, wrist in neutral position, MCP and IP joints of thumb are extended (Fig. 2-167).

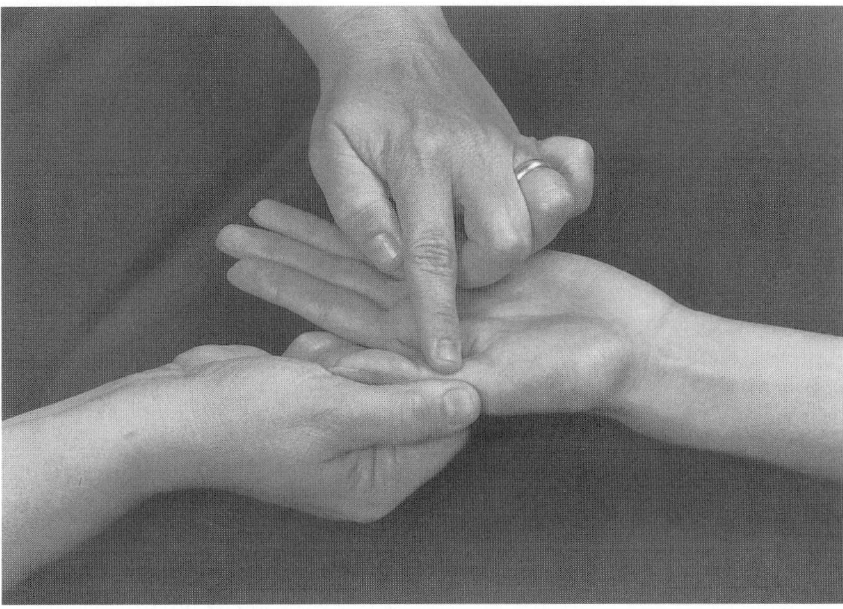

Fig. 2-167.

Stabilization/palpation: Stabilize sides of proximal phalanx of thumb. Palpate tendon of flexor pollicis longus on volar aspect of proximal phalanx of thumb (Fig. 2-167).

Examiner action: While instructing patient in motion desired, flex IP joint of patient's thumb. Return patient to starting position. Performing passive movement allows determination of patient's available ROM and shows patient exact motion desired.

Patient action: Patient flexes IP joint of thumb. (Note: Patient will be unable to flex IP joint without also flexing MCP joint unless firm stabilization is used.) Examiner maintains stabilization of proximal phalanx and palpation of flexor pollicis longus tendon during active movement by patient (Fig. 2-168).

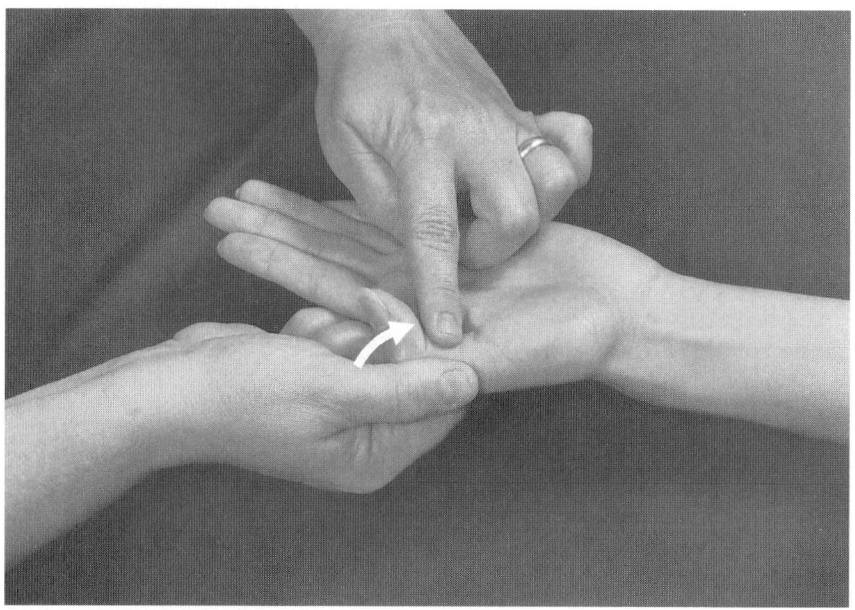

Fig. 2-168. Arrow indicates direction of movement.

Resistance: Use one finger to apply resistance along volar aspect of distal phalanx of thumb in direction of IP extension. Palpating hand is moved to distal phalanx to apply resistance (Fig. 2-169).

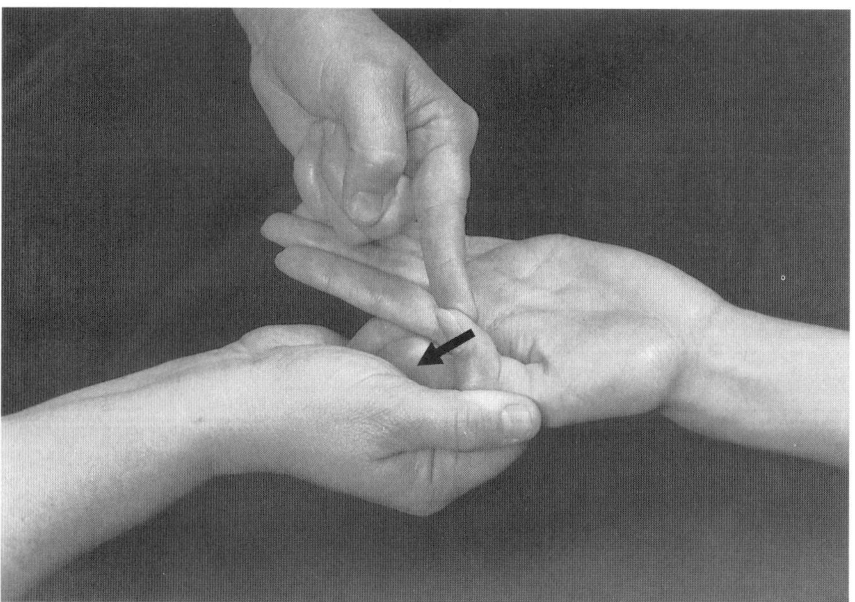

Fig. 2-169. Arrow indicates direction of resistance.

Grades 3 and Below

There is no separate test of this muscle for grades below 3. Grading is altered as follows to accommodate lack of a gravity-eliminated position.

For grade 3: Patient flexes joint through full ROM without resistance.

For grade 2: Patient flexes joint through partial ROM.

For grade 1: No motion, but a palpable contraction is present. Palpation occurs as described earlier (see Fig. 2-167).

For grade 0: No motion or contraction is present.

■ THUMB EXTENSION (METACARPOPHALANGEAL)

EXTENSOR POLLICIS BREVIS (Fig. 2-170)

Fig. 2-170.

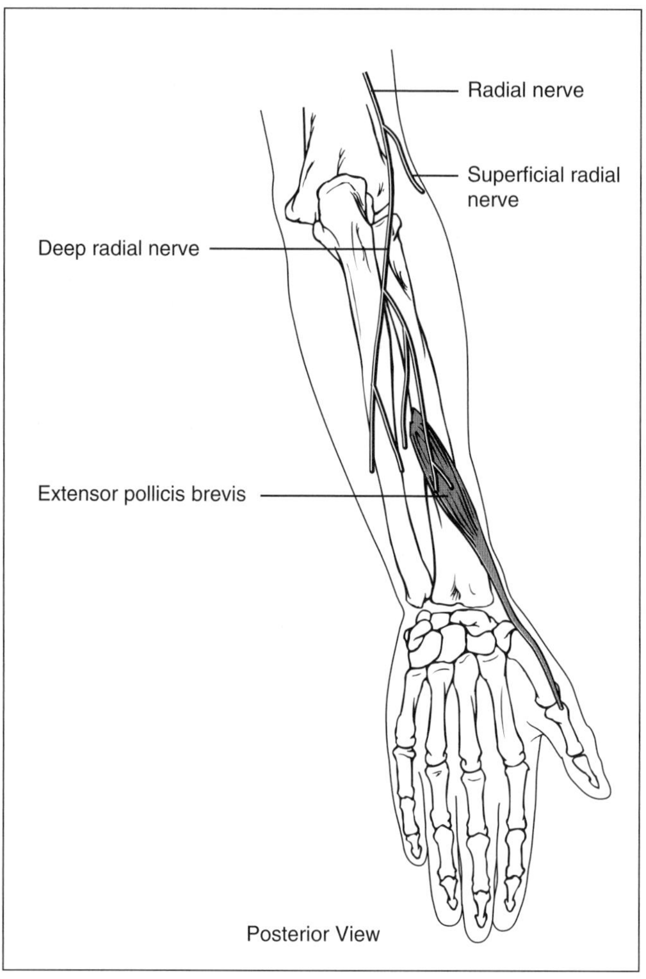

	ATTACHMENTS	NERVE SUPPLY	FUNCTION
Extensor pollicis brevis	Origin: Posterior aspect of the radius; the interosseous membrane Insertion: Base of the proximal phalanx of the thumb	Peripheral nerve: Deep radial nerve Nerve root: C6, C7	Extension of the MCP and carpornatacerpal (CMC) joints of the thumb

Grades 5 and 4

Patient position:

Seated with forearm in neutral rotation (halfway between pronation and supination) and supported on a flat surface, wrist in neutral position, MCP and IP joints of thumb slightly flexed (Fig. 2-171).

Fig. 2-171.

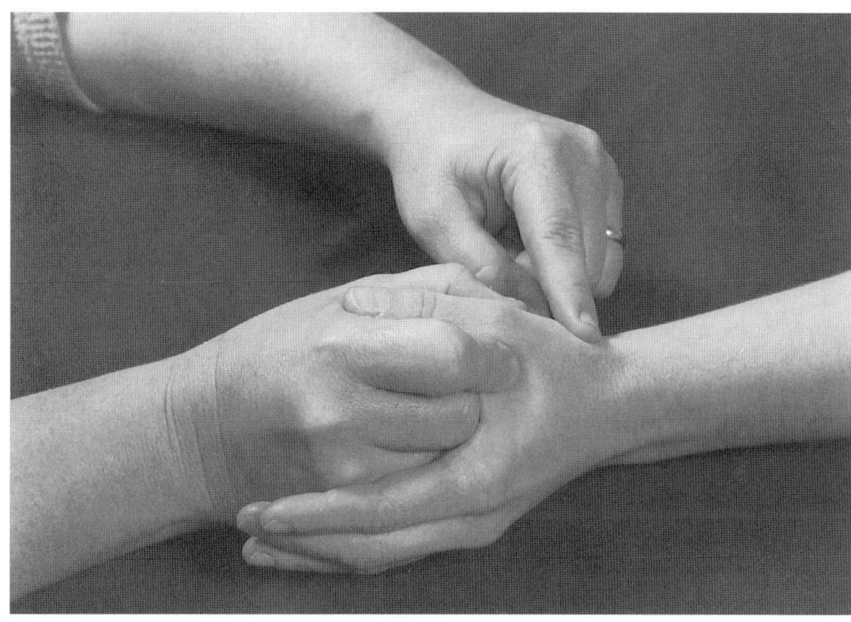

Stabilization/palpation:

Stabilize sides of first metacarpal bone. Palpate tendon of extensor pollicis brevis on dorsal surface of first metacarpal bone, just radial to tendon of extensor pollicis longus (Fig. 2-171).

Examiner action:

While instructing patient in motion desired, extend MCP joint of patient's thumb while maintaining IP joint of thumb in flexion. Return patient to starting position. Performing passive movement allows determination of patient's available ROM and shows patient exact motion desired.

Patient action:

Patient extends MCP joint of thumb without extending IP joint. Examiner maintains stabilization of first metacarpal and palpation of extensor pollicis brevis tendon during active movement by patient (Fig. 2-172).

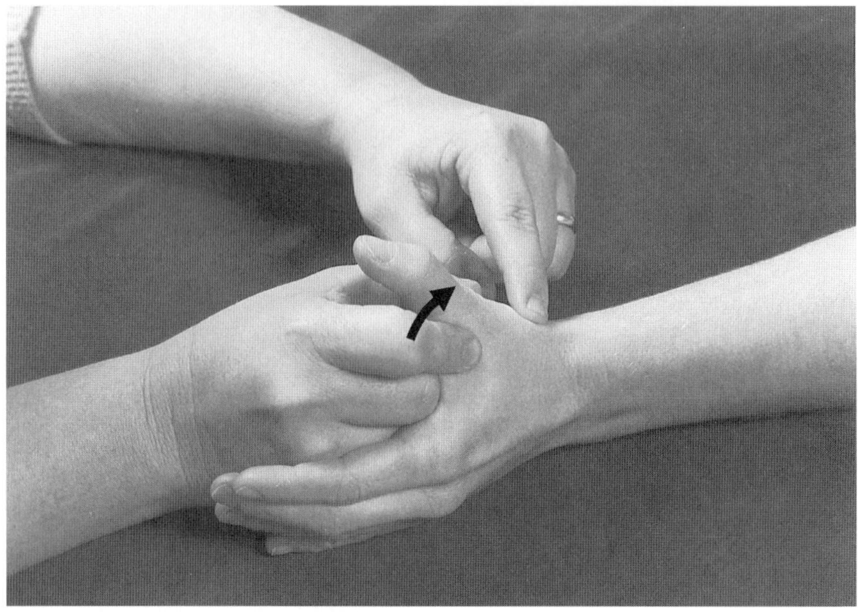

Fig. 2-172. Arrow indicates direction of movement.

Resistance:

Use one finger to apply resistance along dorsal surface of proximal phalanx of thumb in direction of MCP flexion. Palpating hand is moved to proximal phalanx to apply resistance (Fig. 2-173).

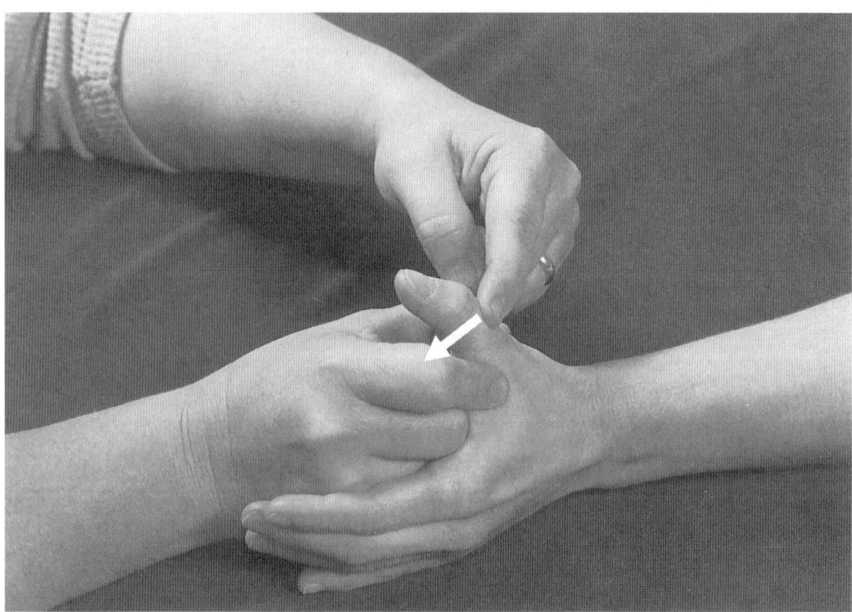

Fig. 2-173. Arrow indicates direction of resistance.

Grades 3 and Below

There is no separate test of this muscle for grades below 3. Grading is altered as follows to accommodate lack of a gravity-eliminated position.

For grade 3: Patient extends joint through full ROM without resistance.

For grade 2: Patient extends joint through partial ROM.

For grade 1: No motion, but a palpable contraction is present. Palpation occurs as described earlier (see Fig. 2-171).

For grade 0: No motion or contraction is present.

COMMON SUBSTITUTION

Extensor pollicis longus: Patient should extend MCP joint while keeping IP joint slightly flexed to avoid substitution by extensor pollicis longus.

■ THUMB EXTENSION (INTERPHALANGEAL)

EXTENSOR POLLICIS LONGUS (Fig. 2-174)

Fig. 2-174.

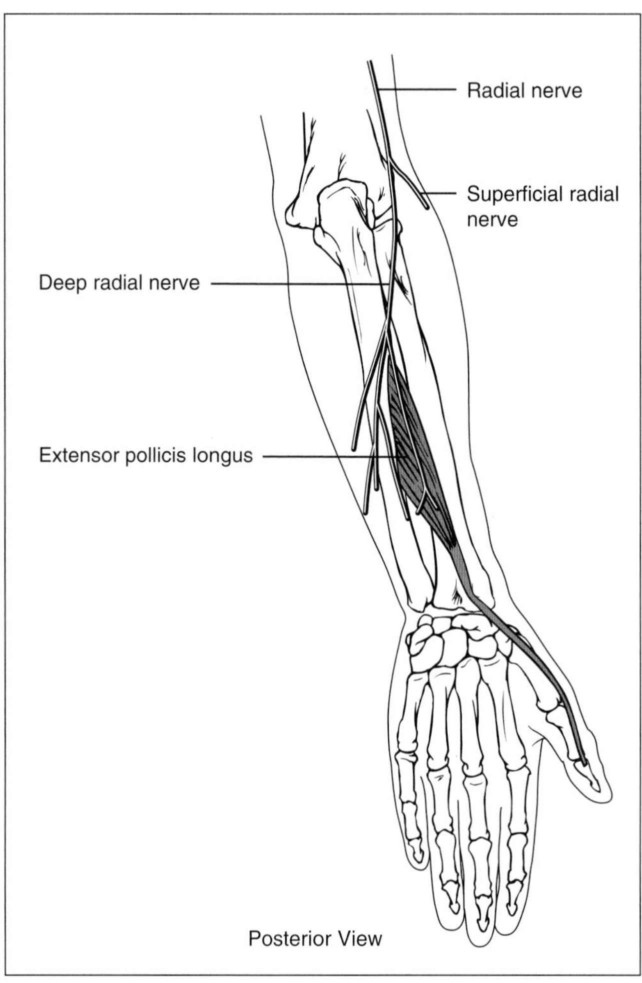

	ATTACHMENTS	NERVE SUPPLY	FUNCTION
Extensor pollicis longus	Origin: Dorsolateral surface of the ulna; interosseous membrane Insertion: Base of the distal phalanx of the thumb	Peripheral nerve: Deep radial nerve Nerve root: C6–C8	Extension of the IP joint of the thumb; assists in extending the MCP and CMC joints of the thumb

Grades 5 and 4

Patient position: Seated with forearm in neutral rotation (halfway between pronation and supination) and supported on a flat surface, wrist in neutral position, MCP and IP joints of thumb slightly flexed (Fig. 2-175).

Fig. 2-175.

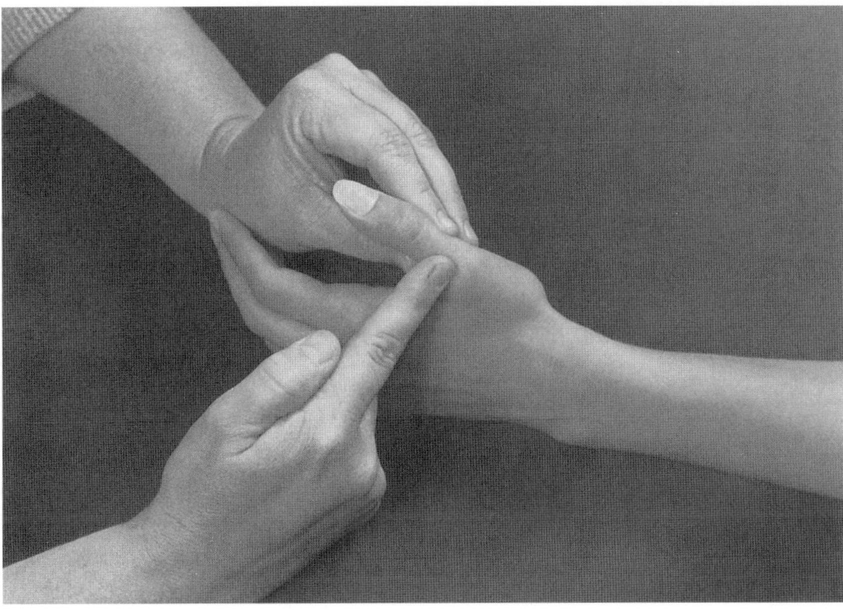

Stabilization/palpation: Stabilize sides of proximal phalanx of thumb. Palpate tendon of extensor pollicis longus on dorsal surface of first metacarpal and proximal phalanx of thumb, just to ulnar side of extensor pollicis brevis tendon (Fig. 2-175).

Examiner action: While instructing patient in motion desired, extend IP joint of patient's thumb. Return patient to starting position. Performing passive movement allows determination of patient's available ROM and shows patient exact motion desired.

Patient action: Patient extends IP joint of thumb. (Note: Patient will be unable to extend IP joint without also extending MCP joint unless firm stabilization is used.) examiner maintains stabilization of proximal phalanx and palpates extensor pollicis longus tendon during active movement by patient (Fig. 2-176).

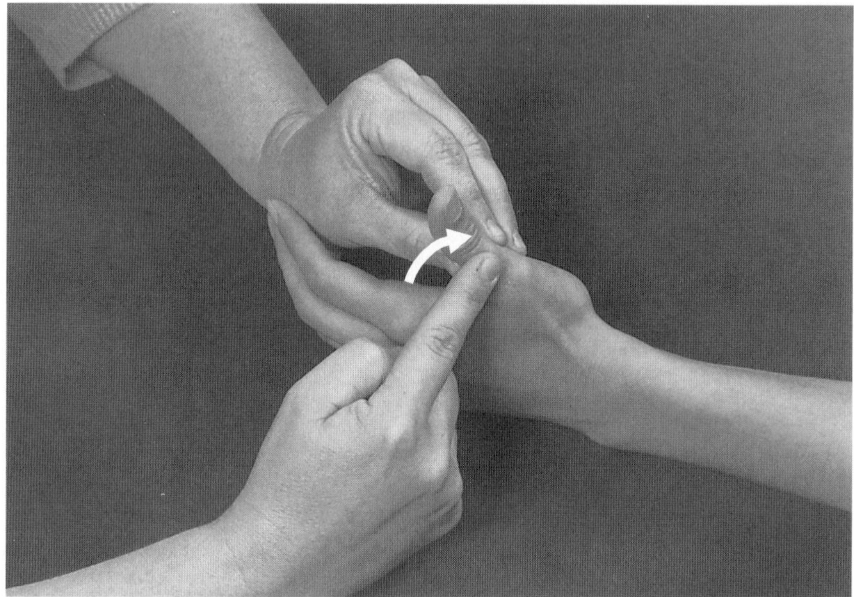

Fig. 2-176. Arrow indicates direction of movement.

Resistance: Use one finger to apply resistance along dorsal surface of distal phalanx of thumb in direction of IP flexion. Palpating hand is moved to distal phalanx to apply resistance (Fig. 2-177).

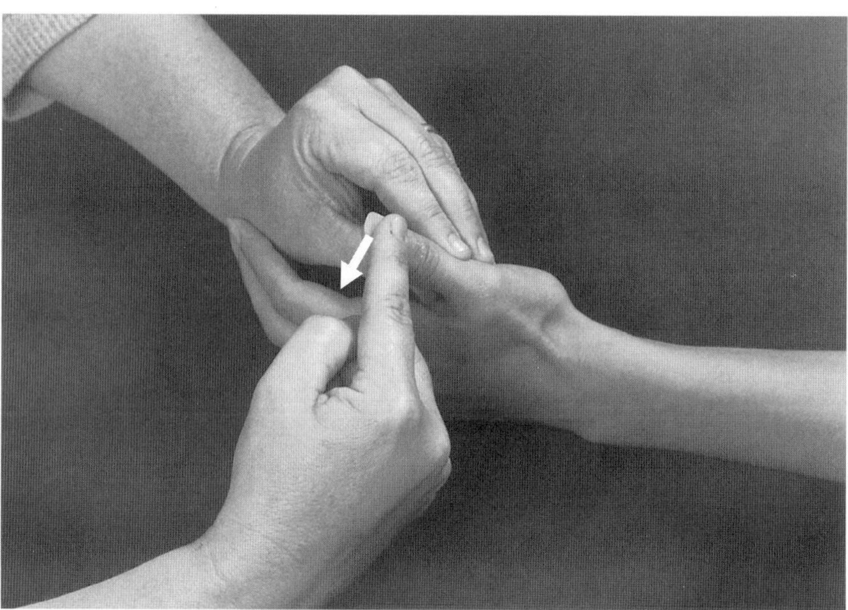

Fig. 2-177. Arrow indicates direction of resistance.

Grades 3 and Below

There is no separate test of this muscle for grades below 3. Grading is altered as follows to accommodate lack of a gravity-eliminated position.

For grade 3: Patient extends joint through full ROM without resistance.

For grade 2: Patient extends joint through partial ROM.

For grade 1: No motion, but a palpable contraction is present. Palpation occurs as described earlier (see Fig. 2-175).

For grade 0: No motion or contraction is present.

■ THUMB ABDUCTION

ABDUCTOR POLLICIS LONGUS AND BREVIS (Figs. 2-178 and 2-179)

Fig. 2-178.

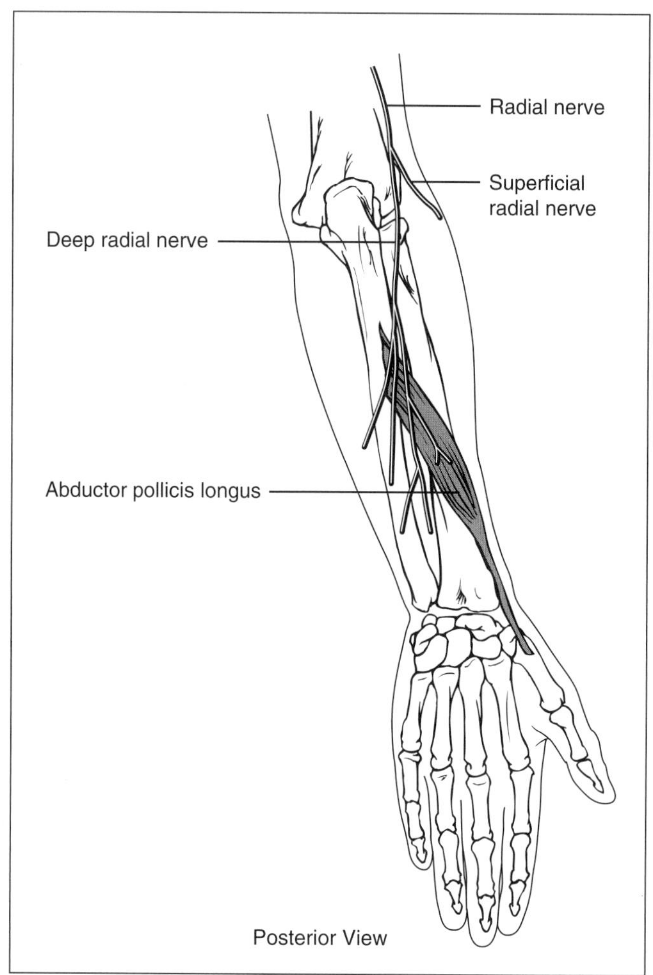

Fig. 2-179.

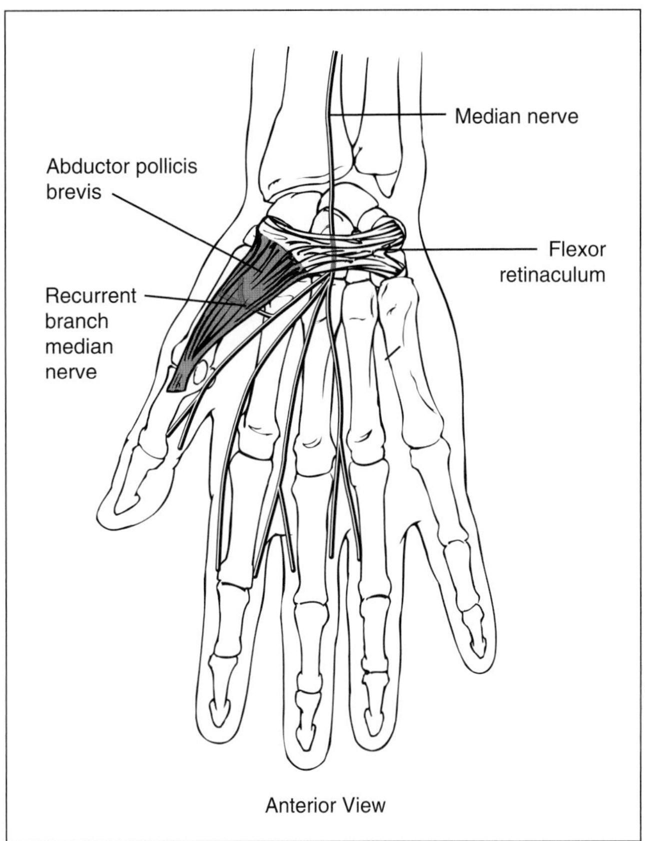

	ATTACHMENTS	NERVE SUPPLY	FUNCTION
Abductor pollicis longus	Origin: Posterior surface of the ulna and radius; interosseous membrane Insertion: Radial side of the base of the 1st metacarpal bone	Peripheral nerve: Deep radial nerve Nerve root: C6, C7	Abduction and extension of the CMC joint of the thumb; assists in abduction (radial deviation) and flexion of the wrist
Abductor pollicis brevis	Origin: Flexor retinaculum; scaphoid, trapezium Insertion: Radial side of the base of the proximal phalanx of the thumb	Peripheral nerve: Median nerve Nerve root: C8, T1	Abduction of the CMC and MCP joints of the thumb

Grades 5 and 4

Patient position: Seated with forearm supinated and supported on a flat surface, wrist in neutral position, thumb adducted (Fig. 2-180).

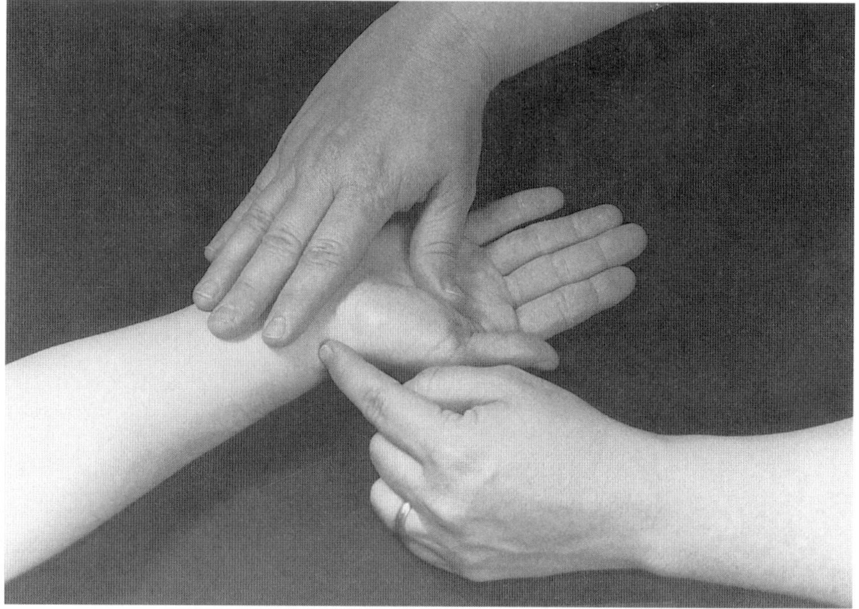

Fig. 2-180. Palpation is of abductor pollicis longus tendon.

Stabilization/palpation: Stabilize volar surface of wrist and second through fifth metacarpals. Palpate tendon of abductor pollicis longus at base of first metacarpal directly adjacent to tendon of extensor pollicis brevis (Fig. 2-180). Abductor pollicis brevis is palpable on lateral aspect of thenar eminence (Fig. 2-181).

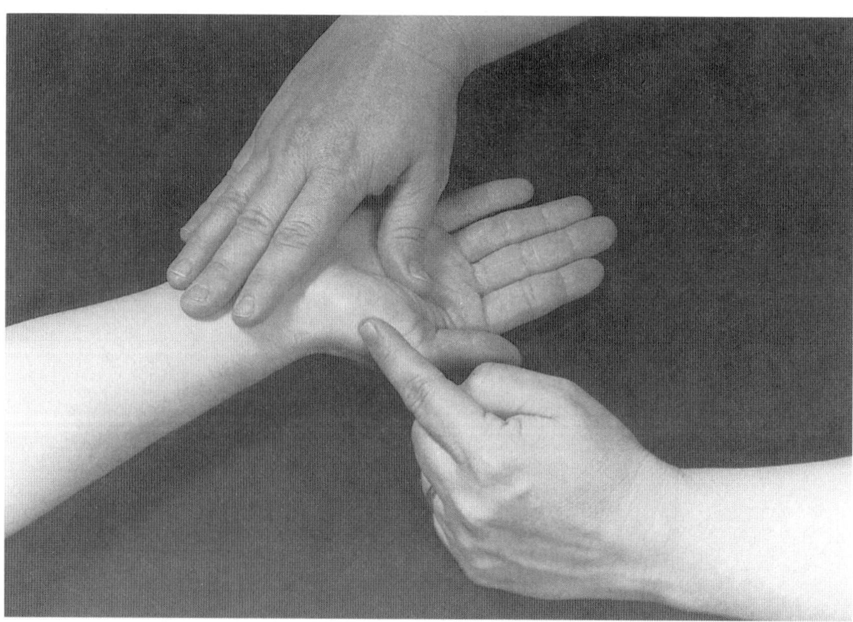

Fig. 2-181. Palpation is of abductor pollicis brevis.

Examiner action: While instructing patient in motion desired, abduct patient's thumb. Return patient to starting position. Performing passive movement allows determination of patient's available ROM and shows patient exact motion desired.

Patient action: Patient abducts thumb through full ROM while examiner maintains stabilization of wrist and metacarpals and palpation of thumb abductor tendons (Fig. 2-182).

Resistance: For abductor pollicis longus: Use one finger to apply resistance along lateral aspect of first metacarpal bone in direction of carpometacarpal adduction. Palpating hand is moved to metacarpal to apply resistance (Fig. 2-182).

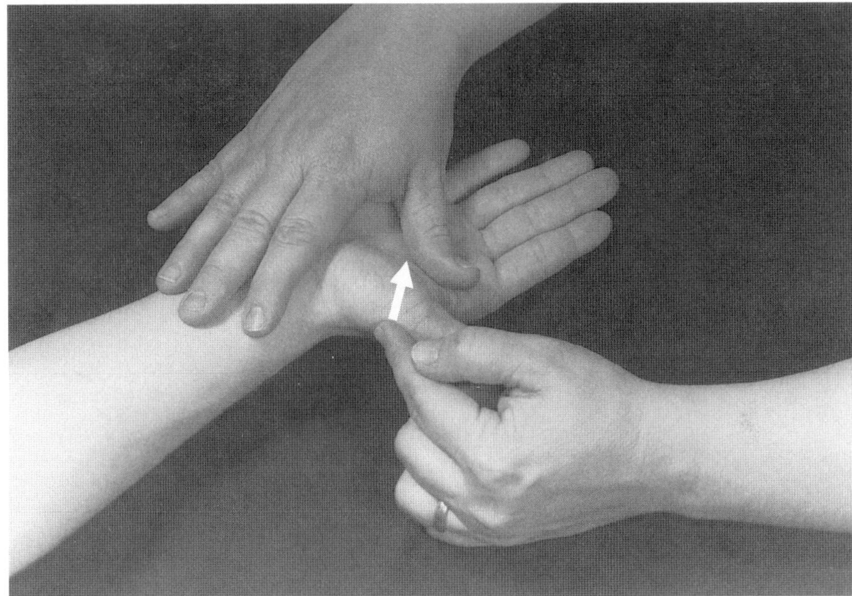

Fig. 2-182. Arrow indicates direction of resistance.

For abductor pollicis brevis: Use one finger to apply resistance along lateral aspect of proximal phalanx of thumb in direction of MCP adduction. Palpating hand is moved to proximal phalanx to apply resistance (Fig. 2-183).

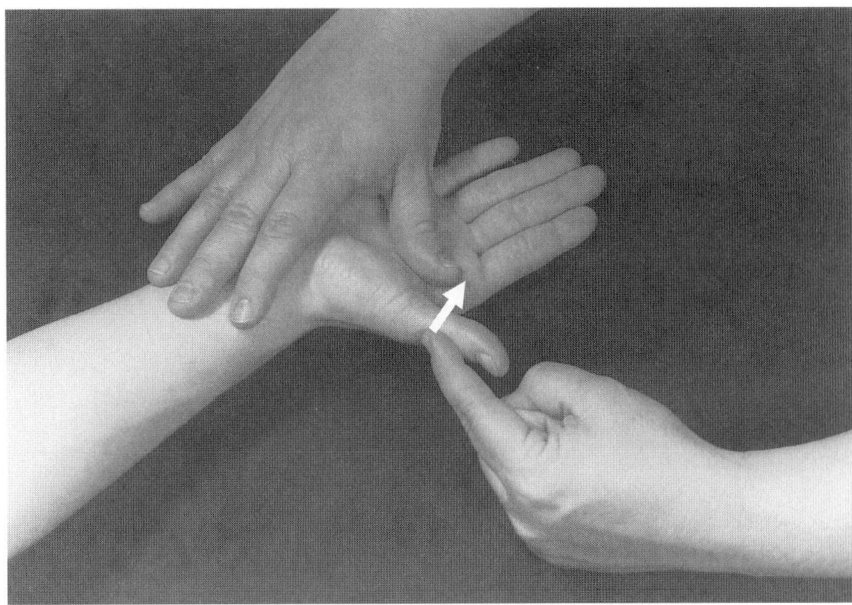

Fig. 2-183. Arrow indicates direction of resistance.

Grades 3 and below

There is no separate test of these muscles for grades below 3. Grading is altered as follows to accommodate lack of a gravity-eliminated position.

For grade 3: Patient abducts joint through full ROM without resistance.

For grade 2: Patient abducts joint through partial ROM.

For grade 1: No motion, but a palpable contraction is present. Palpation occurs as described earlier (see Figs. 2-180 and 2-181).

For grade 0: No motion or contraction is present.

■ THUMB ADDUCTION

ADDUCTOR POLLICIS (Fig. 2-184)

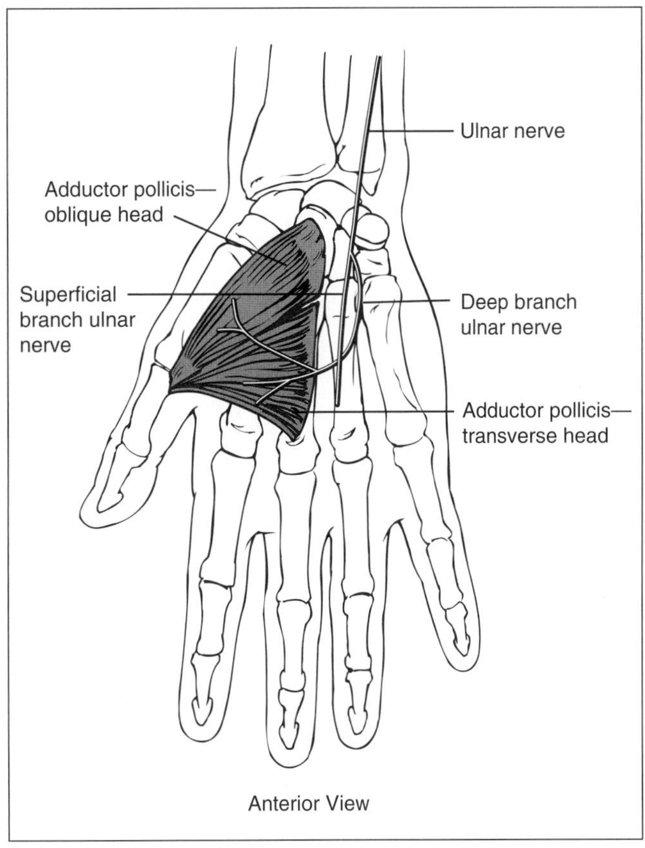

Fig. 2-184.

	ATTACHMENTS	NERVE SUPPLY	FUNCTION
Adductor pollicis	Origin: Oblique head: Capitate, trapezoid, trapezium, metacarpals 1–4* Transverse head: Palmar surface of the 3rd metacarpal bone Insertion: Ulnar side of the base of the proximal phalanx of the thumb	Peripheral nerve: Ulnar nerve Nerve root: C8, T1	Adduction of the thumb

*Anatomic information derived from Chang and Blair (1985).

Grades 5 and 4

Patient position: Seated with forearm pronated and supported on a flat surface, wrist in neutral position, hand and thumb extending beyond supporting surface, thumb abducted at CMC joint (Fig. 2-185).

Fig. 2-185.

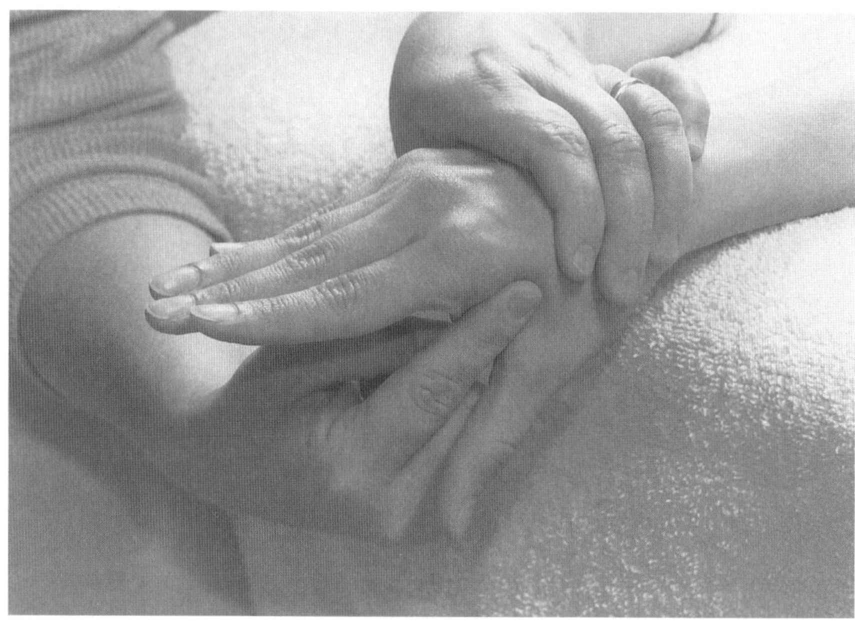

Stabilization/palpation: Stabilize dorsum of wrist and second through fifth metacarpals. Palpate adductor pollicis between first and second metacarpal bones (Fig. 2-185).

Examiner action: While instructing patient in motion desired, adduct patient's thumb. Return patient to starting position. Performing passive movement allows determination of patient's available ROM and shows patient exact motion desired.

Patient action:

Patient adducts thumb through full ROM while examiner maintains stabilization of wrist and metacarpals and palpation of adductor pollicis (Fig. 2-186).

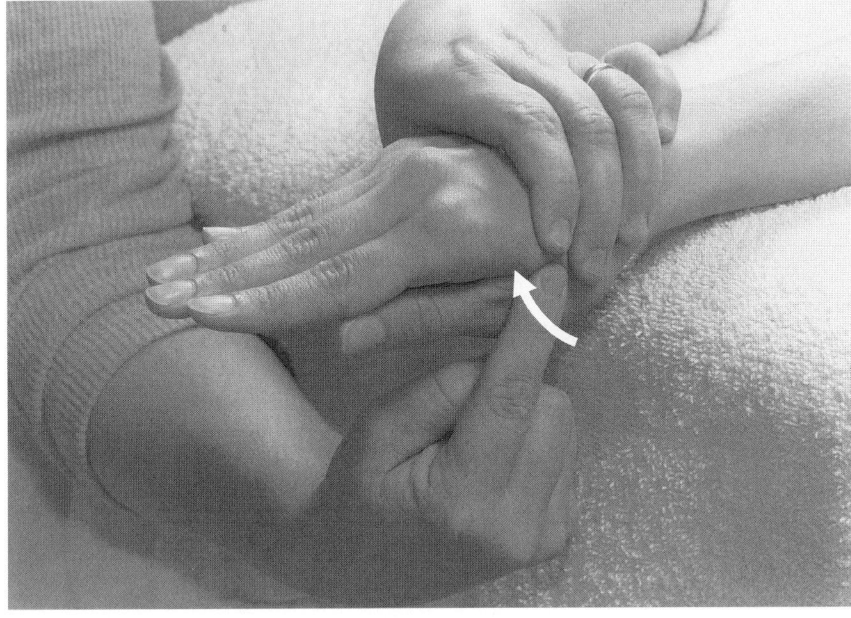

Fig. 2-186. Arrow indicates direction of movement.

Resistance:

Use one finger to apply resistance along medial surface of proximal phalanx of thumb in direction of CMC abduction. Palpating hand is moved to proximal phalanx to apply resistance (Fig. 2-187).

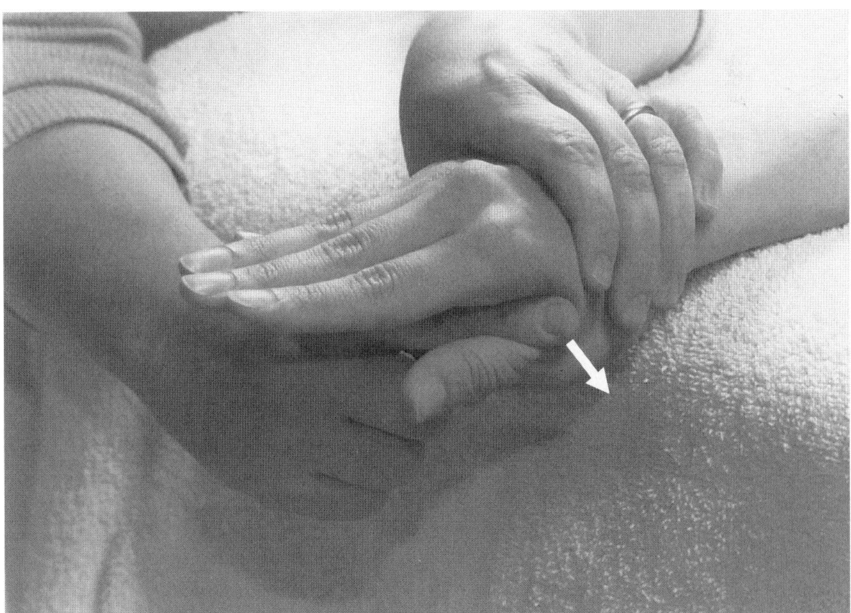

Fig. 2-187. Arrow indicates direction of resistance.

Grades 3 and Below

There is no separate test of this muscle for grades below 3. Grading is altered as follows to accommodate lack of a gravity-eliminated position.

For grade 3: Patient adducts joint through full ROM without resistance.

For grade 2: Patient adducts joint through partial ROM.

For grade 1: No motion, but a palpable contraction is present. Palpation occurs as described earlier (see Fig. 2-185).

For grade 0: No motion or contraction is present.

COMMON SUBSTITUTION

Flexor pollicis longus and brevis: Patient should adduct thumb without flexing MCP or IP joints of thumb to avoid substitution by thumb flexors.

■ OPPOSITION OF THUMB AND FIFTH DIGIT

OPPONENS POLLICIS: OPPONENS DIGITI MINIMI (Fig. 2-188)

Fig. 2-188.

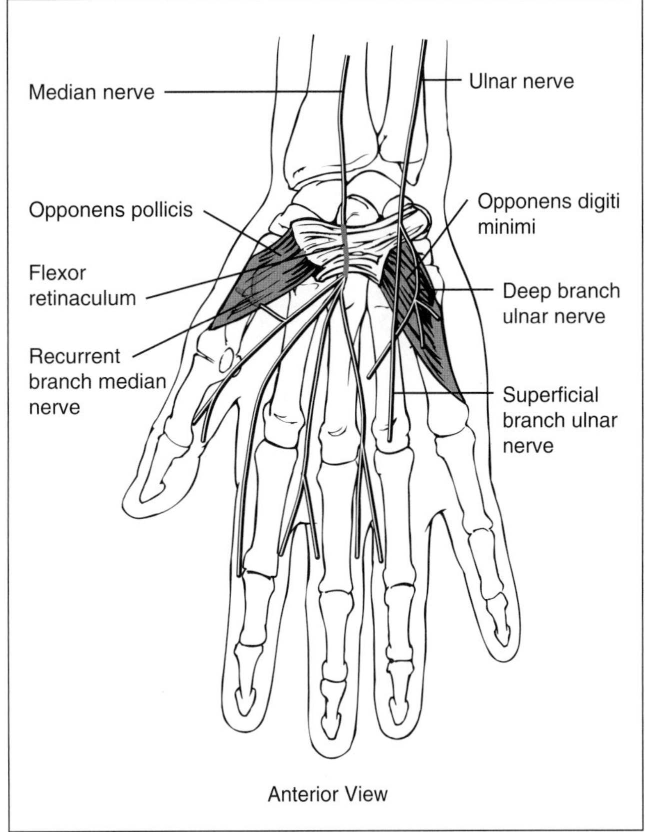

	ATTACHMENTS	NERVE SUPPLY	FUNCTION
Opponens pollicis	Origin: Flexor retinaculum; trapezium bone Insertion: Radial side of the 1st metacarpal bone	Peripheral nerve: Median nerve Nerve root: C8, T1	Opposition at the CMC joint of the thumb
Opponens digiti minimi	Origin: Flexor retinaculum; hook of the hamate Insertion: Ulnar side of the 5th metacarpal bone	Peripheral nerve: Ulnar nerve Nerve root: C8, T1	Opposition at the CMC joint of the 5th digit

Grades 5 and 4

Patient position: Seated with forearm supinated and supported on a flat surface, wrist in neutral position, fingers extended (Fig. 2-189).

Fig. 2-189.

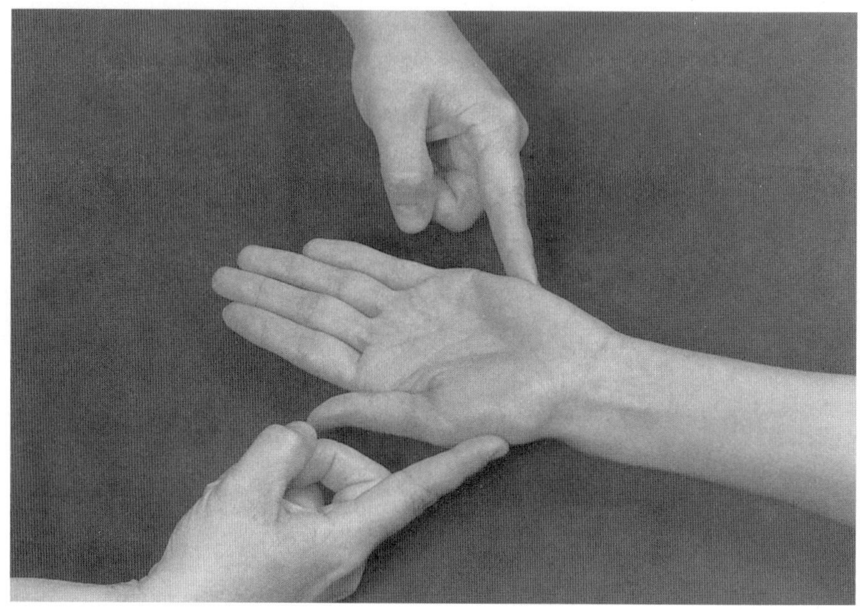

Stabilization/palpation: No stabilization necessary. Palpate opponens pollicis along radial border of first metacarpal. Opponens digiti minimi is palpable along ulnar border of fifth metacarpal (Fig. 2-189).

Examiner action: While instructing patient in motion desired, move patient's thumb and fifth digit into opposition. Return patient to starting position. Performing passive movement allows determination of patient's available ROM and shows patient exact motion desired.

Patient action: Patient opposes thumb and fifth digit simultaneously through full ROM while examiner maintains palpation of opponens muscles (Fig. 2-190).

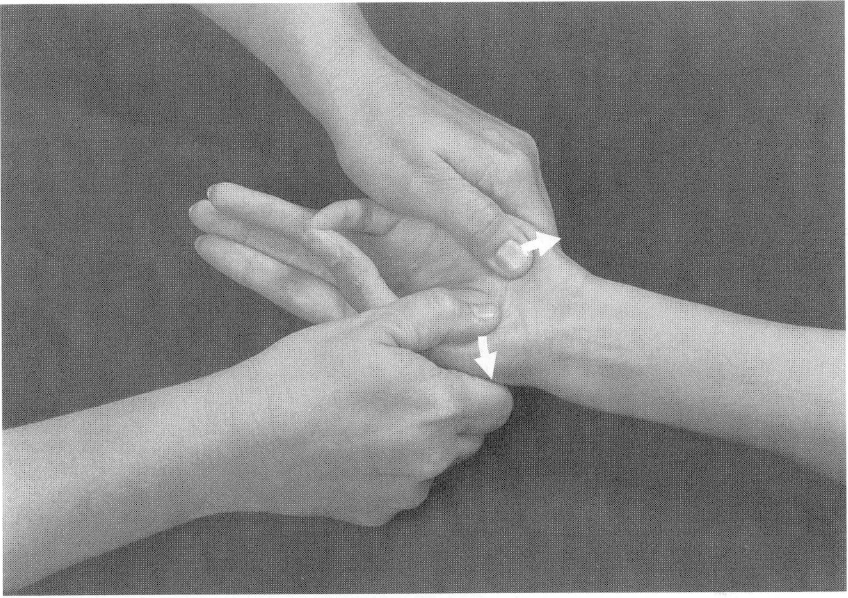

Fig. 2-190. Arrows indicate direction of resistance.

Resistance: Apply resistance simultaneously along volar shaft of first and fifth metacarpal bones, attempting to separate first and fifth digits (Fig. 2-190).

Grades 3 and Below

There is no separate test of these muscles for grades below 3. Grading is altered as follows to accommodate lack of a gravity-eliminated position.

For grade 3: Patient moves joint through full ROM without resistance.

For grade 2: Patient moves joint through partial ROM.

For grade 1: No motion, but a palpable contraction is present. Palpation occurs as described earlier (see Fig. 2-189).

For grade 0: No motion or contraction is present.

CASE 2-1 SPINAL CORD INJURY

Mr. Q is a 17-year-old male who suffered a fracture of the sixth cervical vertebra during a motor vehicle accident. Owing to compression of the spinal cord by the fracture fragments, he sustained an incomplete spinal cord injury at a C7 neurologic level. His fracture site has been completely stabilized, and he has been admitted to the rehabilitation unit at 3 months post injury due to multiple medical complications that delayed his transfer to rehabilitation. As a result of prolonged hospitalization, Mr. Q is unable to tolerate an upright position. You are planning your initial examination in which you must determine his level of motor and sensory functioning.

Answer the following questions regarding your examination of this patient. Note: This case is continued in Chapter 4: Techniques of Manual Muscle Testing: Lower Extremity and in Chapter 8: Techniques of the Sensory Examination.

1. Given that this patient's injury is at the C7 spinal level, which muscles would you expect to be free from motor weakness?
2. How would you need to alter the following muscle tests to accommodate for the patient's inability to maintain an upright position?
   a. Biceps brachii—gravity resisted
   b. Middle deltoid—gravity resisted
   c. Extensor carpi radialis longus and brevis—gravity resisted
   d. Upper trapezius—gravity resisted
   e. Pectoralis major—gravity eliminated
3. How would you alter your documentation to accommodate the changes in patient positioning described in your answer to question number 2?

CASE 2-2 PERIPHERAL NERVE INJURY

Dr. J is a 52-year-old dentist who suffered a midshaft fracture of the humerus in a motorcycle accident 5 days earlier. Damage to the radial nerve was evident following the fracture, and the fracture site was stabilized with an external fixation device. Dr. J now presents to your clinic for rehabilitation and assistance with activities of daily living (ADLs). He brings no information with him regarding the exact fracture site, and he has not had electrodiagnostic testing to determine the extent of radial nerve damage. You are not completely certain what this patient's functional limitations will be, but have a fairly good idea based on your knowledge of the anatomy of the radial nerve and related structures.

Answer the following questions regarding your examination of this patient (you may want to refer to an anatomy text to assist with your answers). Note: This case is continued in Chapter 8: Techniques of the Sensory Examination.

1. Provide a rationale for radial nerve damage in this patient based on the anatomy of the radial nerve.
2. Which muscles will you need to test to determine the level and extent of radial nerve damage?
3. If this patient's radial nerve is functionally severed above the elbow, what muscles would you expect to be weak? Nonfunctional?
4. What movements will the patient be unable to perform due to the muscle weakness/paralysis expected?

CASE 2-3 **MANUAL MUSCLE TESTING AND MUSCULOSKELETAL EXAMINATION**

Ms. B is a 34-year-old college tennis coach who is referred to you for shoulder pain. After listening to Ms. B's patient history, you conclude that one objective of your examination will be to rule out injury to the rotator cuff. Answer the following questions regarding examination of the muscles of the rotator cuff:

1. What muscles make up the rotator cuff?
2. What is the innervation and action of each of the cuff muscles?
3. How is strength assessed in rotator cuff muscles using manual muscle testing techniques?
4. How are the muscles of the rotator cuff assessed using musculoskeletal examination techniques (i.e., special tests)?
5. What does the literature say about isolating the action of the rotator cuff muscles during strength testing and exercise? (Hint: See references in the Bibliography for Chapter 2.)
6. How do the techniques described in the answer to question number 5 compare with the testing procedures described in this text (similarities and differences)? Give examples of when each technique would be more appropriate.
7. Can traditional manual muscle test grades be used to grade muscles assessed using the techniques described in the answer to question number 5? Why or why not?

References

1. Chang L, Blair WF. The origin and innervation of the adductor pollicis muscle. *J Anat* 1985;140:381–388.
2. Clemente CD. *Gray's Anatomy, 30th American ed.* Philadelphia: Lea & Febiger, 1985.
3. Kendall FP, McCreary EK, Provance PG. *Muscles: Testing and Function,* 4th ed. Baltimore: Williams & Wilkins, 1993.

Bibliography

American Spinal Injury Association. *International Standards for Neurological Classification of Spinal Cord Injury.* Revised, 2002. Chicago: ASIA, 2002.

Bagg SD, Forrest WJ. Electromyographic study of scapular rotators during arm abduction in the scapular plane. *Am J Phys Med* 1986;65:111–124.

Basmajian JV, DeLuca CJ. *Muscles Alive: Their Function Revealed by Electromyography,* 5th ed. Baltimore: Williams & Wilkins, 1985.

Bohannon RW. Make and break tests of elbow flexor muscle strength. *Phys Ther* 1988;68:193–194.

Brandsma JW, Schreuders TAR, Birke JA, et al. Intraobserver and interobserver reliabilities for the intrinsic muscles of the hand. *J Hand Ther* 1995;8:185–190.

Brandsma JW, Schreuders TAR. Sensible manual muscle strength testing to evaluate and monitor strength of the intrinsic muscles of the hand: a commentary. *J Hand Ther* 2001;14:273–278.

Broome HL, Basmajian JV. The function of the teres major muscle: an electromyographic study. *Anat Rec* 1970;170:309–310.

Brown JMM, Solomon C, Paton M. Further evidence of functional differentiation within biceps brachii. *Electromyogr Clin Neurophysiol* 1993;33:301–309.

Chang L, Blair WF. The origin and innervation of the adductor pollicis muscle. *J Anat* 1985;140:381–388.

Clarkson HM. *Musculoskeletal Assessment: Joint Range of Motion and Manual Muscle Strength,* 2nd ed. Philadelphia: Lippincott, Williams & Wilkins, 2000.

Daniels L, Worthingham C. *Muscle Testing: Techniques of Manual Examination,* 5th ed. Philadelphia: WB Saunders, 1986.

de Freitas V, Vitti M, Furlani J. Electromyographic analysis of the levator scapulae and rhomboideus major muscle in movements of the shoulder. *Electromyogr Clin Neurophysiol* 1979;19:335–342.

Decker MF, et al. Subscapularis muscle activity during selected rehabilitation exercises. *Am J Sports Med* 2003;31:126–134.

Devinsky O, Feldmann E. *Examination of the Cranial and Peripheral Nerves.* New York: Churchill Livingstone, 1988.

Filho JG, de Freitas V, Furlani J. Electromyographic study of the trapezius muscle in free movements of the shoulder. *Electromyogr Clin Neurophysiol* 1994;34:279–283.

Florence JM, Pandya S, King WM, et al. Intrarater reliability of manual muscle test (Medical Research Council scale) grades in Duchenne's muscular dystrophy. *Phys Ther* 1992;72:115–126.

Frese E, Brown M, Norton BJ. Clinical reliability of manual muscle testing: Middle trapezius and gluteus medius muscles. *Phys Ther* 1987;67:1072–1076.

Furlani J. Electromyographic study of the m. biceps brachii in movements at the glenohumeral joint. *Acta Anat* 1976;96:270–284.

Gandevia SC, McKenzie DK. Activation of human muscles at short muscle lengths during maximal static efforts. *J Physiology* 1988;407:599–613.

Hellwig EV, Perrin DH. A comparison of two positions for assessing shoulder rotator peak torque: the traditional frontal plane versus the plane of the scapula. *Isokinet Exerc Sci* 1991;1:202–206.

Hollister A, Giurintano DJ: Thumb movements, motions and moments. *J Hand Ther* 1995;8:106–114.

Hoppenfeld S. *Physical Examination of the Spine and Extremities.* New York: Appleton-Century-Crofts, 1976.

Howell JW, Rothstein JM, Lamb RL, et al. An experimental investigation of the validity of the manual muscle test positions for the extensor pollicis longus and flexor pollicis brevis muscles. *J Hand Ther* 1989;2:20–28.

Jamison JC, Caldwell GE. Muscle synergies and isometric torque production: Influence of supination and pronation level on elbow flexion. *J Neurophys* 1993;70:947–960.

Kelly BT, et al. Optimal normalization tests for shoulder muscle activation: an electromyographic study. *J Orthopaedic Res* 1996;14:647–653.

Kelly BT, Kadrmas WR, Speer KP. The manual muscle examination for rotator cuff strength. *Am J Sports Med* 1996;24:581–588.

Kilbreath SL, Gandevia SC. Limited independent flexion of the thumb and fingers in human subjects. *J Physiol (Lond)* 1994;479:487–497.

Levy AS, et al. Function of the long head of the biceps at the shoulder: electromyographic analysis. *J Shoulder Elbow Surg* 2001;10:250–255.

Liu F, Carlson L, Watson HK. Quantitative abductor pollicis brevis strength testing: reliability and normative values. *J Hand Surg* 2000;25A:752–759.

Malanga GA, Jenp Y, Growney ES, et al. EMG analysis of shoulder positioning in testing and strengthening the supraspinatus. *Med Sci Sports Exerc* 1996;28:661–664.

Michiels I, Boden F. The deltoid muscle: an electromyographical analysis of its activity in arm abduction in various body postures. *Int Orthop* 1992;16:268–271.

Moseley JB, et al. EMG analysis of the scapular muscles during a shoulder rehabilitation program. *Am J Sports Med* 1992;20;128–134.

Paton ME, Brown JMM. Functional differentiation within latissimus dorsi. *Electromyogr Clin Neurophysiol* 1995;35:301–309.

Ranney D, Wells R. Lumbrical muscle function as revealed by a new and physiological approach. *Anat Rec* 1988;222:110–114.

Rasch PJ. Effect of position of forearm on strength of elbow flexion. *Res Q* 1956;27:333–337.

Reider B. *The Orthopaedic Physical Examination*. Philadelphia: WB Saunders, 1999.

Ringelberg JA. EMG and force production of some human shoulder muscles during isometric abduction. *J Biomechanics* 1985;18:939–947.

Schreuders TAR, Stam HJ. Strength measurements of the lumbrical muscles. *J Hand Ther* 1996;9:303–305.

Shevlin MG, Lehmann JF, Lucci JA. Electromyographic study of the function of some muscles crossing the glenohumeral joint. *Arch Phys Med Rehabil* 1969;50:264–270.

Tis LL, Maxwell T. The effect of positioning on shoulder isokinetic measures in females. *Med Sci Sports Exerc* 1996;28:1188–1192.

van Oudenaarde E, Brandsma JW, Oostendorp RAB. The influence of forearm, hand and thumb positions on extensor carpi ulnarix and abductor pollicis longus activity. *Acta Anat* 1997;158:296–302.

Wadsworth CT, Krishnan R, Sear M, et al. Intrarater reliability of manual muscle testing and hand-held dynametric testing. *Phys Ther* 1987;67:1342–1347.

Worrell TW, Corey BJ, York SL, et al. An analysis of supraspinatus EMG activity and shoulder isometric force development. *Med Sci Sports Exerc* 1992;24:744–748.

Wintz MM. Variations in current manual muscle testing. *Phys Ther Rev* 1959;39:466–475.

3

TECHNIQUES of MANUAL MUSCLE TESTING: HEAD, NECK, and TRUNK

■ NECK FLEXION

LONGUS CAPITIS, LONGUS COLLI, RECTUS CAPITIS ANTERIOR, ANTERIOR SCALENE, STERNOCLEIDOMASTOID (Fig. 3-1)

Fig. 3-1.

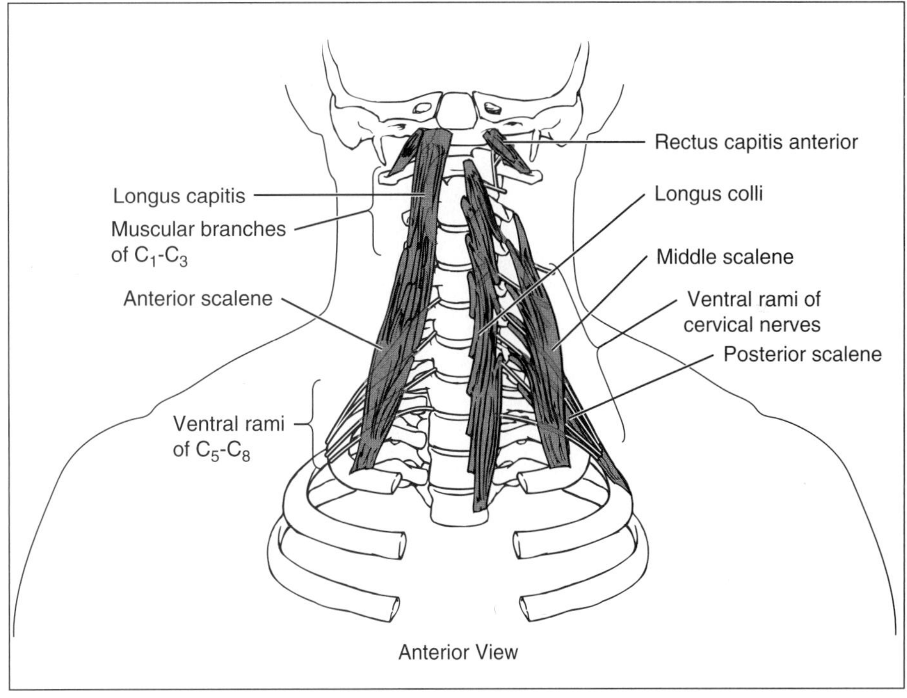

	ATTACHMENTS	NERVE SUPPLY	FUNCTION
Longus capitis	Origin: Transverse processes of C3–C6 Insertion: Basilar part of the occipital bone	First three cervical nerves	Bilateral action: Flexion of the head on the atlas; flexion of the cervical spine Unilateral action: Lateral flexion and rotation of the cervical spine to the same side
Longus colli	Origin: Transverse processes of C3–C5 and the anterolateral surface of C5–C7 and T1–T3 Insertion: Anterior arch of the atlas; anterior surface of C2–C4 and transverse processes of C5, C6	Ventral rami of C2–C6	Bilateral action: Flexion of the cervical spine Unilateral action: Lateral flexion and rotation of the cervical spine to the same side
Rectus capitis anterior	Origin: Lateral aspect and transverse process of the atlas Insertion: Basilar part of the occipital bone	Ventral rami of C1, C2	Flexion of the head on the atlas
Anterir scalene	Origin: Transverse processes of C3–C6 Insertion: Upper surface of the first rib	Ventral rami of C5, C6	Bilateral action: Flexion of the cervical spine Unilateral action: Lateral flexion and rotation of the cervical spine to the same side
Sternocleido-mastoid	Origin: Sternal head: Anterior aspect of the manubrium of the sternum Clavicular head: Medial ⅓ of the clavicle Insertion: Mastoid process of the skull	Accessory nerve (cranial nerve XI); ventral rami of C2, C3	Bilateral action: Flexion of the cervical spine; in the absence of cervical vertebral stabilizers, it extends the head on the atlas Unilateral action: Lateral flexion of the cervical spine to the same side; rotation of the cervical spine to the opposite side

Grades 5 and 4

Patient position: Supine with shoulders abducted to 90°, elbows flexed to 90°, dorsal forearms resting on table (Fig. 3-2).

Fig. 3-2.

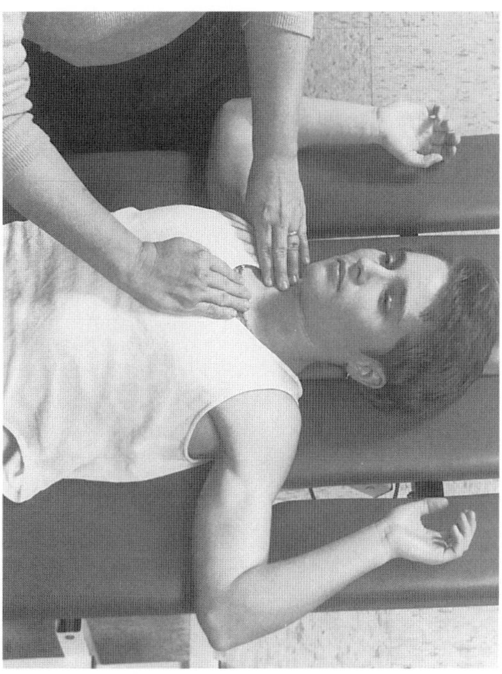

Examiner action: While instructing patient in motion desired, tuck patient's chin toward chest and flex cervical spine through full available range of motion (ROM). Return patient to starting position. Performing passive movement allows determination of patient's available ROM and shows patient exact motion desired.

Stabilization/palpation: Stabilization normally is supplied by patient's abdominal muscles via fixating action on thorax. In patients with weak abdominals, stabilize over anterior aspect of thorax. With opposite hand, palpate sternocleidomastoid (SCM) from mastoid process to attachment on sternum and medial aspect of clavicle; longus capitis and longus colli on anterolateral surface of cervical vertebrae deep to SCM; and anterior scalene above clavicle posterior to SCM (Fig. 3-2). Rectus capitis anterior is too deep to palpate.

Patient action:

Patient flexes head and neck through full ROM, initiating motion by tucking chin toward chest, then flexing cervical spine (see common substitution for gravity-eliminated test). Examiner stabilizes thorax (if needed) and palpates neck flexors during patient's active movement (Fig. 3-3).

Fig. 3-3. Arrow indicates direction of movement.

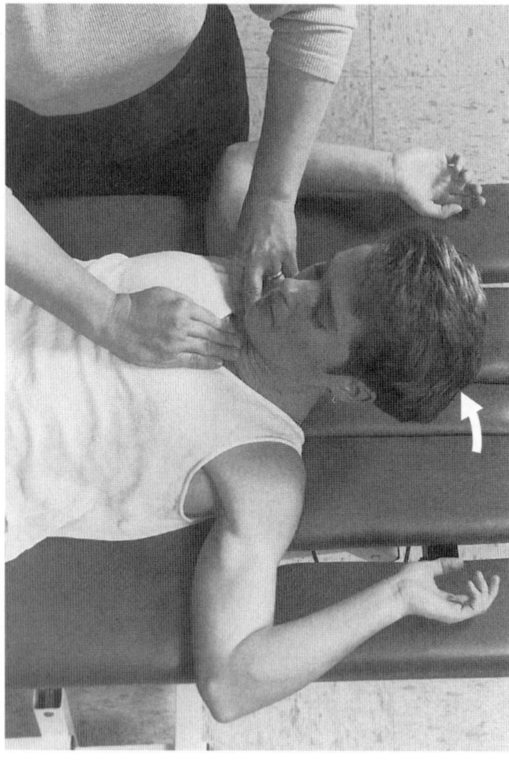

Resistance:

Apply resistance over forehead in direction of neck extension (Fig. 3-4).

Fig. 3-4. Arrow indicates direction of resistance.

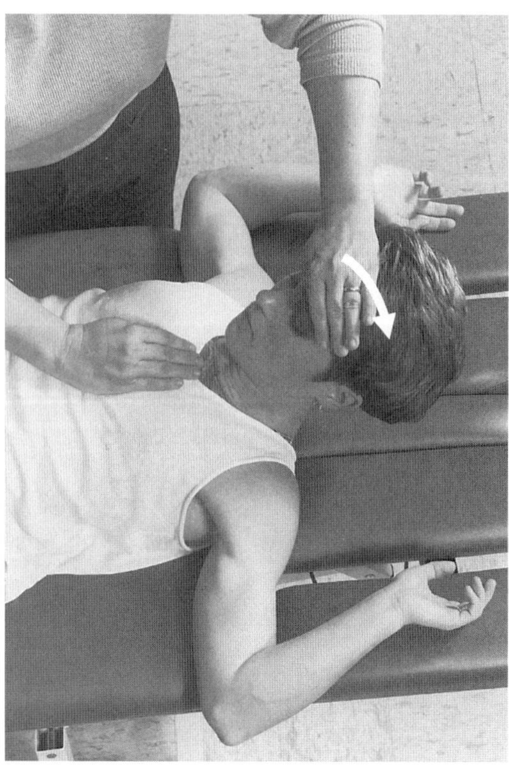

Grades 3 and Below

There is no separate test of these muscles for grades below 3. Grading is altered as follows to accommodate lack of a gravity-eliminated position.

For grade 3: Patient flexes head and neck through full ROM without resistance.

For grade 2: Patient flexes head and neck through partial ROM.

For grade 1: No motion, but a palpable contraction is present. Palpation occurs as in gravity-resisted test (Fig. 3-2).

For grade 0: No motion or contraction is present.

COMMON SUBSTITUTION

SCM; see Clinical Comment: "SCM as a substitute for weak neck flexors" (Fig. 3-5).

CLINICAL COMMENT: SCM AS A SUBSTITUTE FOR WEAK NECK FLEXORS

Patients with weak anterior neck flexors may attempt neck flexion using the sternocleidomastoid (SCM) exclusively. In such cases, the patient will be unable to maintain a tucked chin and will flex the neck with the chin pointed toward the ceiling. Such an action is due to the fact that the SCM flexes the lower cervical spine and also (because of its attachment on the mastoid process of the skull) extends the head on the atlas, an action that will become evident when anterior cervical stabilizers are weak.

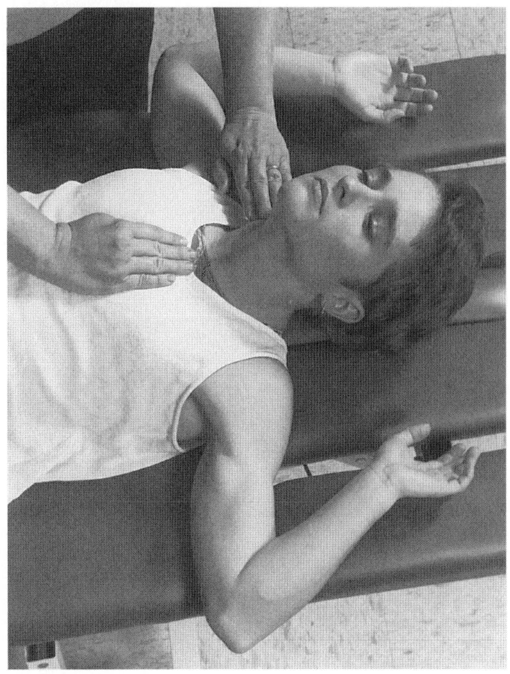

Fig. 3-5. Substitution by sternocleidomastoid.

■ ANTEROLATERAL NECK FLEXION

STERNOCLEIDOMASTOID (Fig. 3-6)

Fig. 3-6.

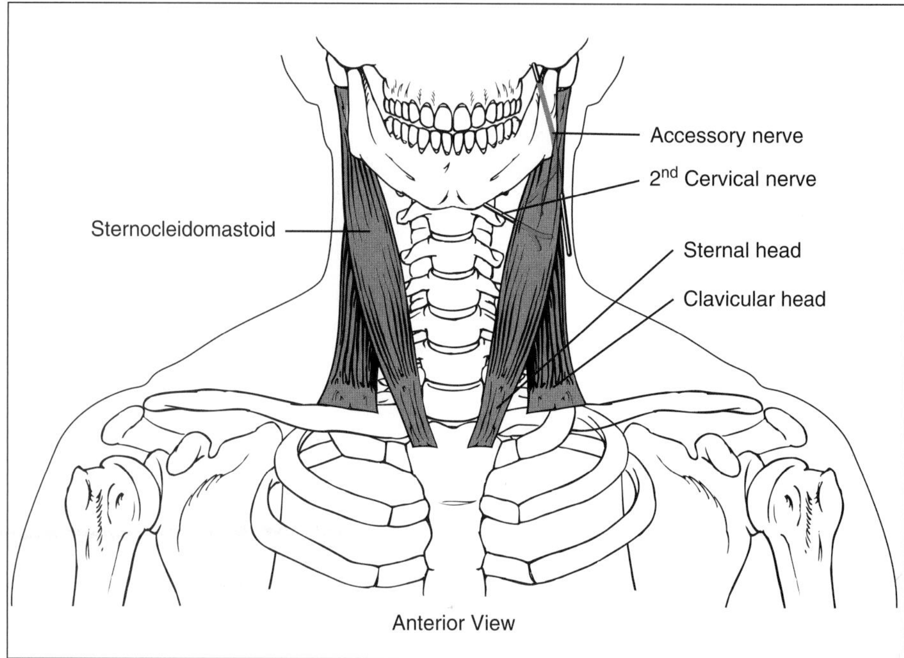

	ATTACHMENTS	NERVE SUPPLY	FUNCTION
Sternocleido-mastoid	Origin: Sternal head: Anterior aspect of the manubrium of the sternum Clavicular head: Medial ⅓ of the clavicle Insertion: Mastoid process of the skull	Accessory nerve (cranial nerve XI); ventral rami of C2, C3	Bilateral action: Flexion of the cervical spine; in the absence of cervical vertebral stabilizers, it extends the head on the atlas Unilateral action: Lateral flexion of the cervical spine to the same side; rotation of the cervical spine to the opposite side

Grades 5 and 4

Patient position: Supine with head turned to contralateral side, shoulders abducted to 90°, elbows flexed to 90°, dorsal forearms resting on table (Fig. 3-7).

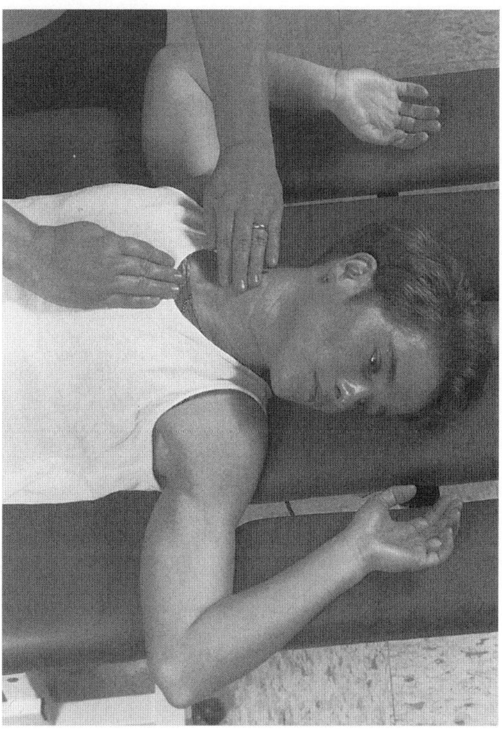

Fig. 3-7.

Examiner action: While instructing patient in motion desired, laterally flex patient's neck while keeping head turned to side (see clinical comment: "cervical spine motion and vertebral artery patency"). Return patient to starting position. Performing passive movement allows determination of patient's available ROM and shows patient exact motion desired.

Stabilization/palpation: Stabilization normally is supplied by patient's abdominals via fixating action on thorax. For patients with weak abdominals, stabilize over anterior aspect of thorax. With opposite hand, palpate SCM from mastoid process to attachment on sternum and medial aspect of clavicle (Fig. 3-7).

Patient action: Patient laterally flexes neck to same side while keeping head rotated to opposite side. Examiner stabilizes thorax (if needed) and palpates SCM during patient's active movement (Fig. 3-8).

Fig. 3-8. Arrow indicates direction of movement.

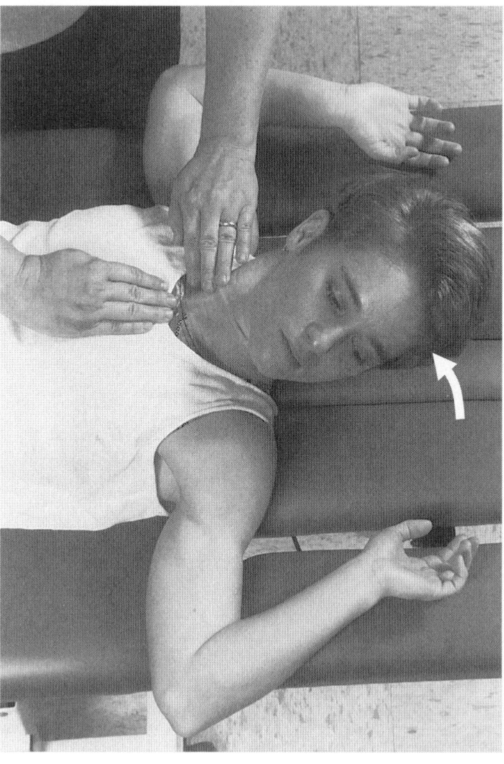

Resistance: Apply resistance over lateral aspect of skull toward examining table (Fig. 3-9).

Fig. 3-9. Arrow indicates direction of resistance.

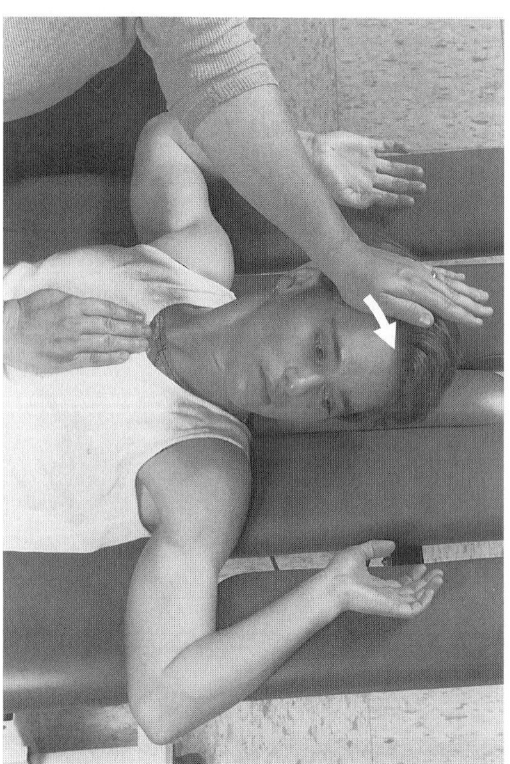

Grades 3 and Below

There is no separate test of this muscle for grades below 3. Grading is altered as follows to accommodate lack of a gravity-eliminated position.

For grade 3: Patient laterally flexes neck through full ROM without resistance.

For grade 2: Patient laterally flexes neck through partial ROM.

For grade 1: No motion, but a palpable contraction is present. Palpation occurs as in gravity-resisted test (see Fig. 3-7).

For grade 0: No motion or contraction is present.

CLINICAL COMMENT: CERVICAL SPINE MOTION AND VERTEBRAL ARTERY PATENCY

The vertebral arteries travel through the transverse foramina of the first six cervical vertebrae and enter the cranial cavity through the foramen magnum. These two arteries provide the main blood supply to the posterior aspects of the brain, including the brain stem. Movements of the cervical spine can compromise blood flow through these arteries, particularly if there is atherosclerosis present. Movements that may compromise patency of the vertebral arteries include rotation, either alone or in combination with flexion or extension, and, to a lesser extent, lateral flexion. Symptoms of decreased blood flow through the vertebral system include dizziness, visual disturbances, nystagmus, or lightheadedness. Caution should be taken when performing any examination procedure involving the cervical spine that involves movements affecting the vertebral arteries. Pre-testing the vertebral arteries for signs of compromised blood flow has been advocated prior to undertaking such procedures.

■ NECK EXTENSION

ERECTOR SPINAE (CERVICAL PORTION), OBLIQUUS CAPITIS SUPERIOR, RECTUS CAPITIS POSTERIOR MAJOR AND MINOR, SEMISPINALIS CAPITIS AND CERVICIS, SPLENIUS CAPITIS AND CERVICIS, UPPER TRAPEZIUS (Figs. 3-10 and 3-11)

Fig. 3-10.

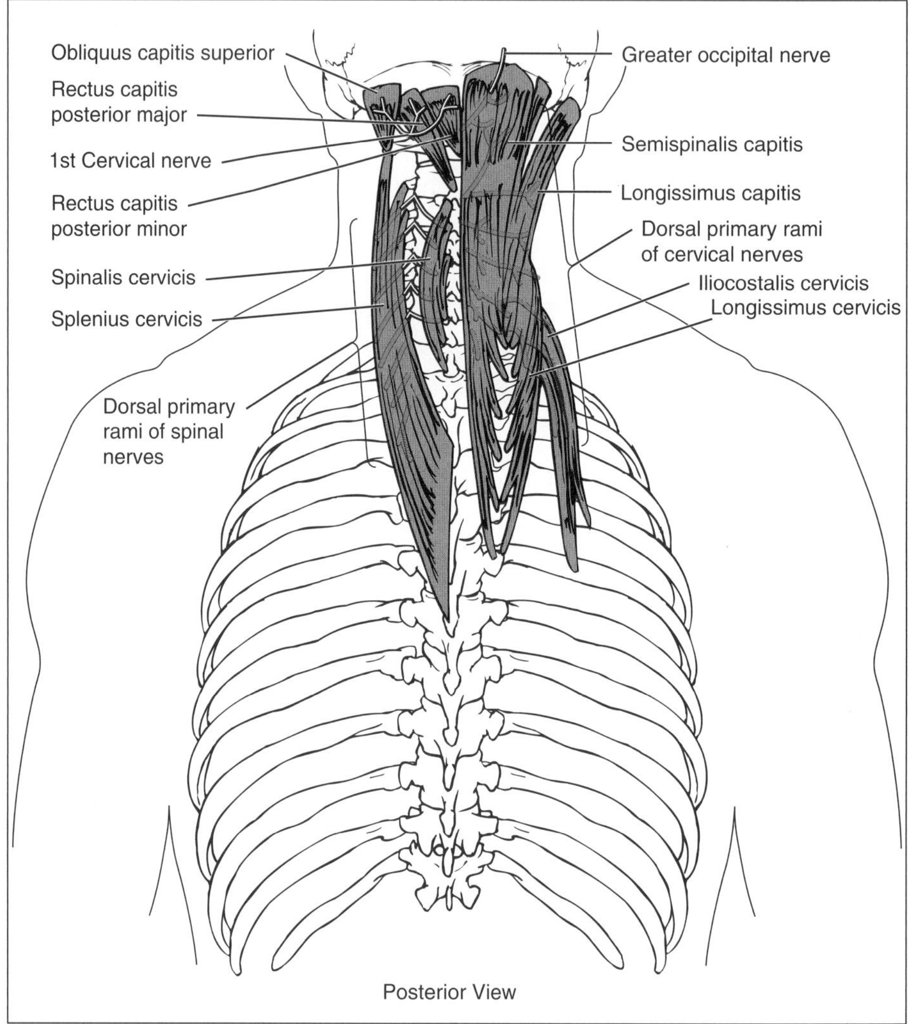

Fig. 3-11.

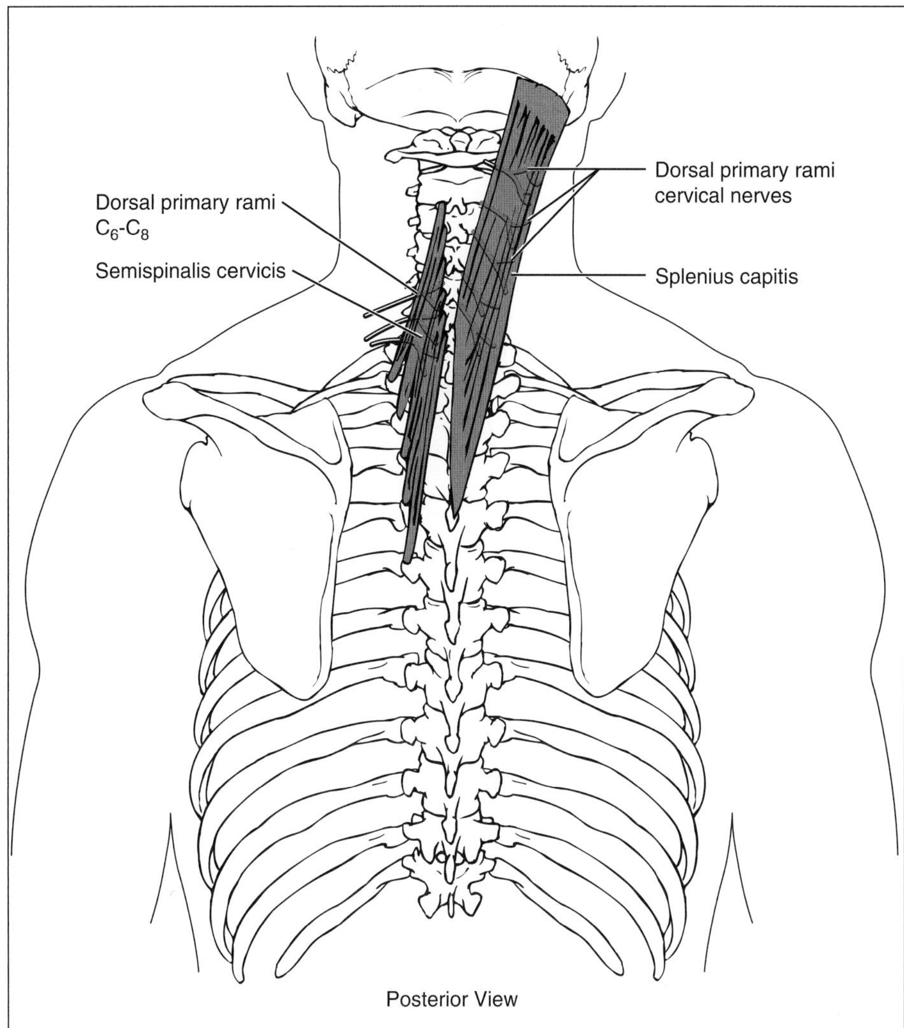

	ATTACHMENTS	NERVE SUPPLY	FUNCTION
Iliocostalis cervicis	Origin: Angles of ribs 3–6 Insertion: Transverse processes of C4–C6	Dorsal primary rami of the spinal nerves	Bilateral action: Extension of the cervical spine Unilateral action: Lateral flexion of the cervical spine
Longissimus capitis	Origin: Articular processes of the last 3–4 cervical vertebrae and the transverse processes of the upper 4–5 thoracic vertebrae Insertion: Posterior aspect of the mastoid process	Dorsal primary rami of the middle and lower cervical nerves	Bilateral action: Extension of the head on the atlas Unilateral action: Lateral flexion and rotation of the cervical spine to the same side

	ATTACHMENTS	NERVE SUPPLY	FUNCTION
Longissimus cervicis	Origin: Transverse processes of the upper 4–5 thoracic vertebrae Insertion: Transverse processes of C2–C6	Dorsal primary rami of the spinal nerves	Bilateral action: Extension of the cervical spine Unilateral action: Lateral flexion of the cervical spine
Obliquus capitis superior	Origin: Transverse process of the atlas Insertion: Occipital bone	Suboccipital nerve (C1)	Bilateral action: Extension of the head on the atlas Unilateral action: Lateral flexion of the head on the atlas (minor)
Rectus capitis posterior major	Origin: Spinous process of the axis Insertion: Inferior nuchal line of the occipital bone (the lateral aspect)	Suboccipital nerve (C1)	Bilateral action: Extension of the head on the atlas Unilateral action: Rotation of the upper cervical spine
Rectus capitis posterior minor	Origin: Posterior tubercle of the axis Insertion: Inferior nuchal line of the occipital bone (the medial aspect)	Suboccipital nerve (C1)	Extension of the head on the atlas
Semispinalis capitis	Origin: Transverse processes of the 7th cervical and the first 6–7 thoracic vertebrae and the articular processes of C4–C6 Insertion: Occipital bone between the superior and inferior nuchal lines	Dorsal primary rami of the first six cervical nerves	Bilateral action: Extension of the head and the cervical spine Unilateral action: Rotation of the cervical spine to the opposite side
Semispinalis cervicis	Origin: Transverse processes of the first 5–6 thoracic vertebrae Insertion: Spinous processes of the first five cervical vertebrae	Dorsal primary rami of the lower three cervical nerves	Bilateral action: Extension of the cervical spine Unilateral action: Rotation of the cervical spine to the opposite side
Spinalis capitis	Origin: Transverse processes of the 7th cervical and the first 6–7 thoracic vertebrae and the articular processes of C4–C6 Insertion: Occipital bone between the superior and inferior nuchal lines	Dorsal primary rami of the spinal nerves	Extension of the cervical spine
Spinalis cervicis	Origin: Ligamentum nuchae, spinous processes of C7, T1, T2 Insertion: Spinous process of the axis	Dorsal primary rami of the spinal nerves	Extension of the cervical spine
Splenius capitis	Origin: Ligamentum nuchae, spinous processes of C7, T1–T3 Insertion: Lateral aspect of the superior nuchal line and the mastoid process	Dorsal primary rami of the middle cervical nerves	Bilateral action: Extension of the head and cervical spine Unilateral action: Lateral flexion and rotation of the cervical spine to the same side
Splenius cervicis	Origin: Spinous processes of T3–T6 Insertion: Transverse processes of the upper 2–3 cervical vertebrae	Dorsal primary rami of the lower cervical nerves	Bilateral action: Extension of the cervical spine Unilateral action: Lateral flexion and rotation of the cervical spine to the same side
Upper trapezius	Origin: External occipital protuberance, medial ⅓ of the superior nuchal line, ligamentum nuchae, the spinous process of the 7th cervical vertebra Insertion: Lateral ⅓ of the clavicle	Accessory nerve (cranial nerve XI); ventral rami of C3, C4	Bilateral action: With insertion fixed, it extends the cervical spine and head Unilateral action: Lateral flexion of the cervical spine; rotation of the cervical spine to the opposite side

Grades 5 and 4

Patient position: Prone with head in neutral rotation, shoulders abducted to 90°, elbows flexed, ventral forearms resting on table (Fig. 3-12).

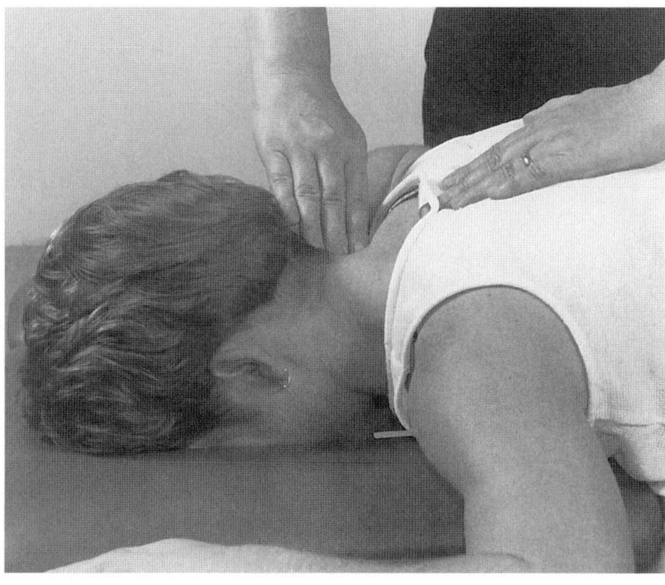

Fig. 3-12.

Examiner action: While instructing patient in motion desired, extend patient's cervical spine through full available ROM. Return patient to starting position. Performing passive movement allows determination of patient's available ROM and shows patient exact motion desired.

Stabilization/palpation: Stabilize upper thorax. With opposite hand, palpate neck extensors over posterior cervical spine (see Fig. 3-12).

Patient action: Patient extends head and neck through full ROM while examiner palpates neck extensors and stabilizes thorax (Fig. 3-13).

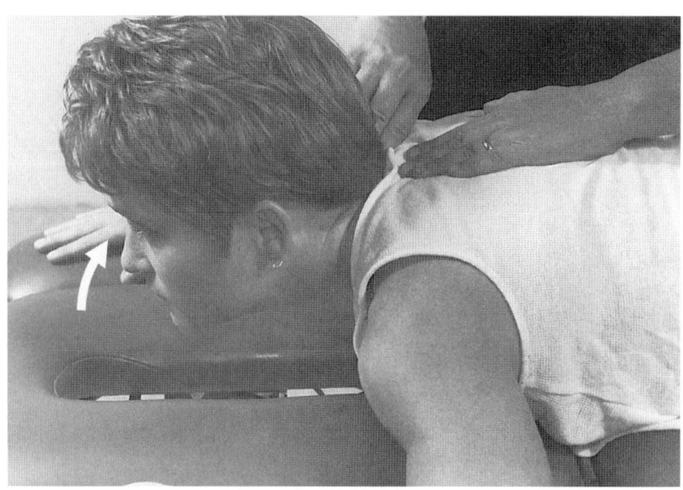

Fig. 3-13. Arrow indicates direction of movement.

Resistance: Apply resistance over occiput in direction of neck flexion (Fig. 3-14).

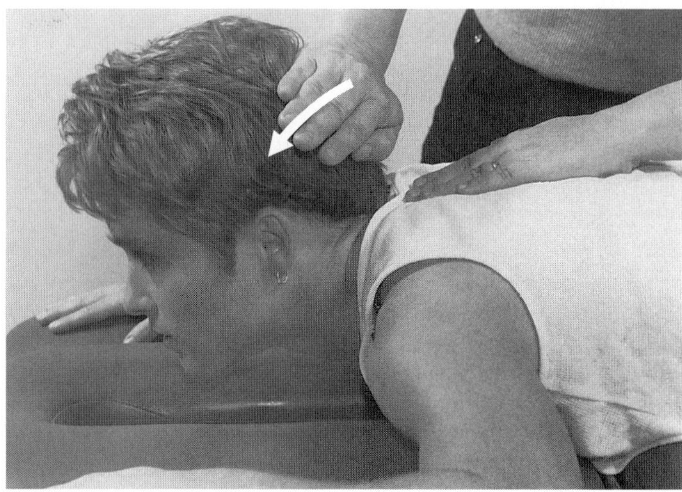

Fig. 3-14. Arrow indicates direction of resistance.

Grades 3 and Below

There is no separate test of these muscles for grades below 3. Grading is altered as follows to accommodate lack of a gravity-eliminated position.

For grade 3: Patient extends head and neck through full ROM without resistance.

For grade 2: Patient extends head and neck through partial ROM.

For grade 1: No motion, but a palpable contraction is present. Palpation occurs as in gravity-resisted test (see Fig. 3-12).

For grade 0: No motion or contraction is present.

TRUNK FLEXION

RECTUS ABDOMINIS (Fig. 3-15)

Fig. 3-15.

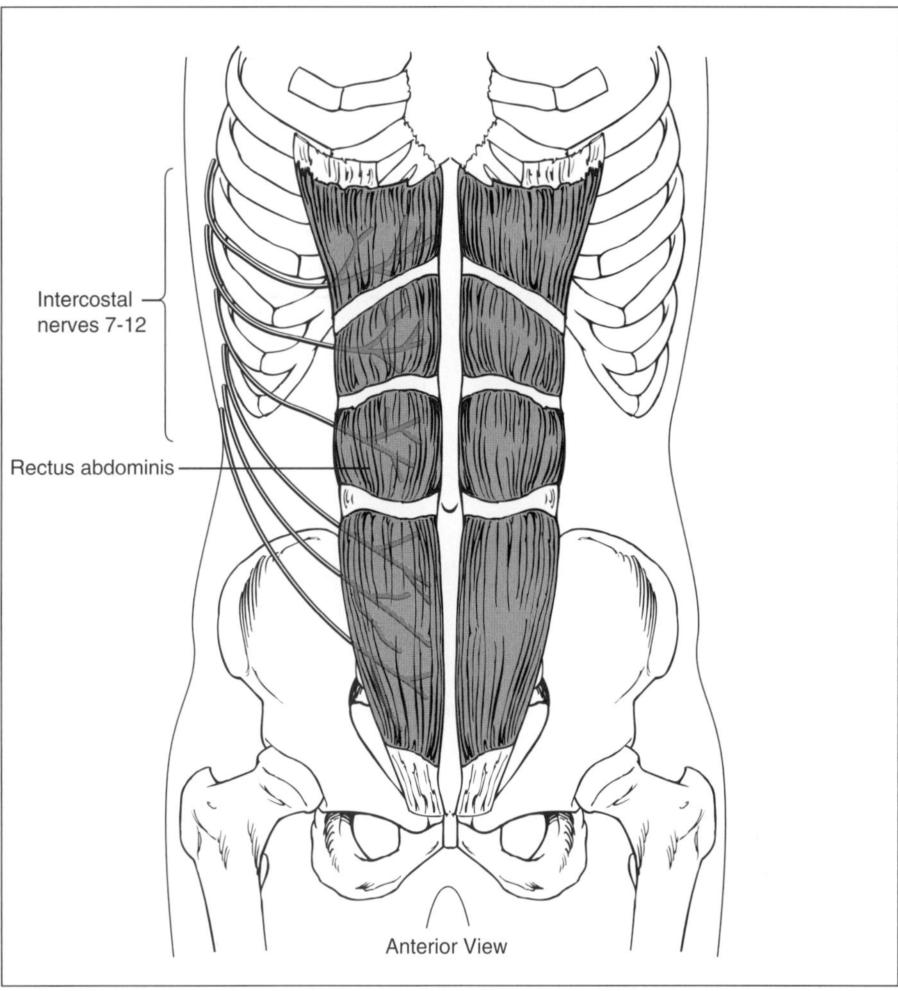

	ATTACHMENTS	NERVE SUPPLY	FUNCTION
Rectus abdominis	Origin: Pubic crest and symphysis pubis Insertion: Costal cartilage of ribs 5–7; xiphoid process	Intercostal nerves 7–12	Flexion of the vertebral column, particularly the lumbar spine

Grade 5

Patient position:

Supine with hands behind neck, lower extremities fully extended, pelvis tilted posteriorly (lumbar spine should be flat against examining table). If hip flexor tightness prevents flattening of lumbar spine, hips may be flexed passively (maintained by a pillow under knees) until lumbar spine is flat (Fig. 3-16; passive flexing not shown).

Fig. 3-16.

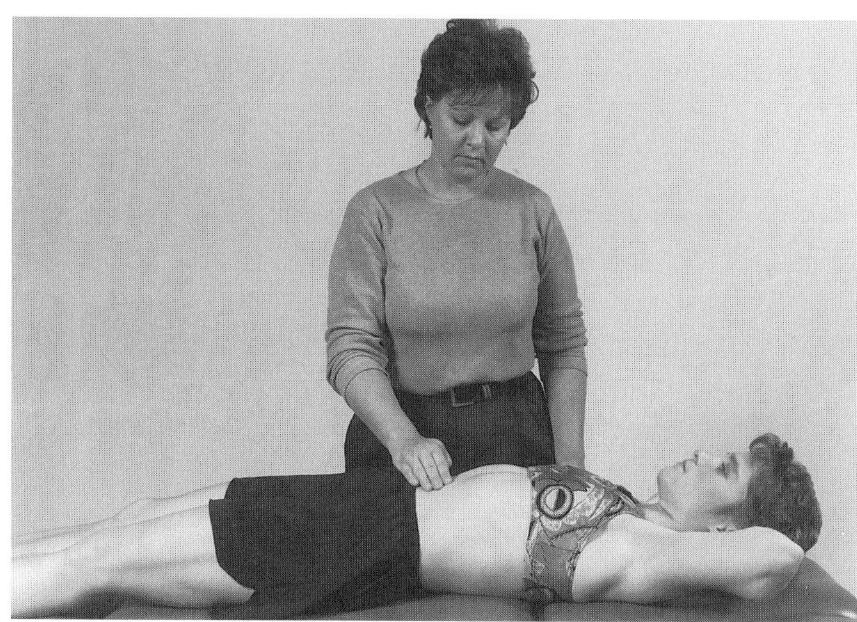

Examiner action:

While instructing patient in motion desired, assist patient in flexing trunk forward until scapulae have cleared table (or as far forward as patient is able to flex if weakness prevents flexion to point of clearing scapulae). Return patient to starting position. Performing passive movement allows determination of patient's available ROM and shows patient exact motion desired.

Stabilization/palpation:

No stabilization is necessary, stabilization may in fact allow substitution by hip flexors (see Clinical comment: "Rectus abdominis test"). Palpate rectus abdominis over anterior aspect of trunk just lateral to midline (Fig. 3-16).

Patient action: Patient flexes trunk while maintaining posterior pelvic tilt until inferior angles of both scapulae have cleared table. Examiner palpates rectus abdominis during patient's active movement (Fig. 3-17).

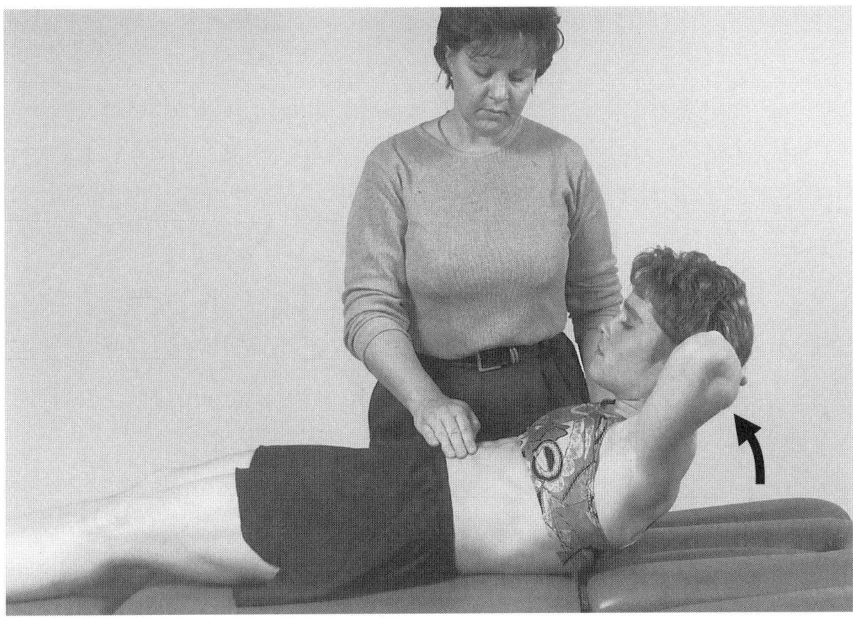

Fig. 3-17. Arrow indicates direction of movement.

Resistance: No resistance is needed.

Grades 4 and Below

There is no separate test of this muscle for grades below 5. Assignment of grades below 5 depends on upper extremity position as follows.

For grade 4: Patient completes above test with arms folded across chest (Fig. 3-18).

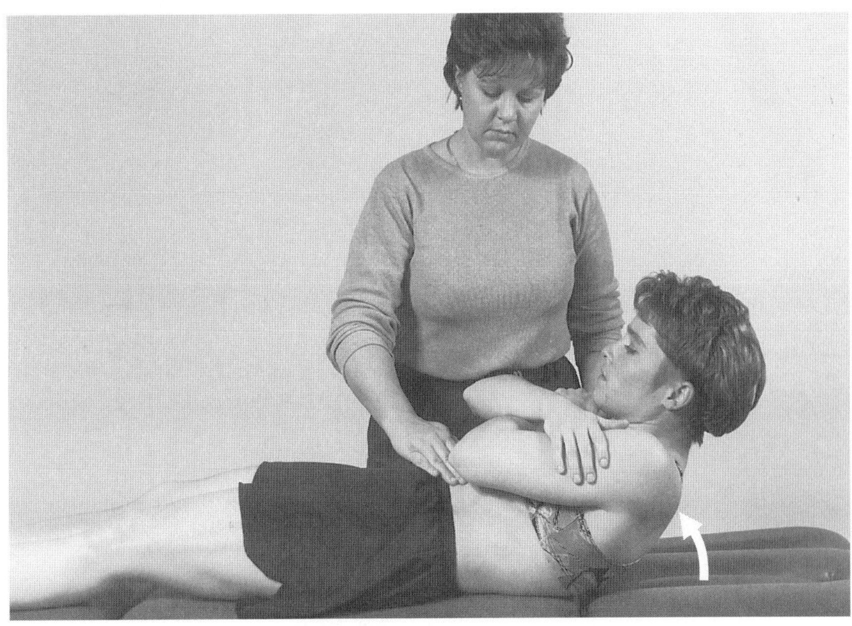

Fig. 3-18. Arrow indicates direction of movement.

For grade 3+:

Patient completes above test with arms at sides (Fig. 3-19).

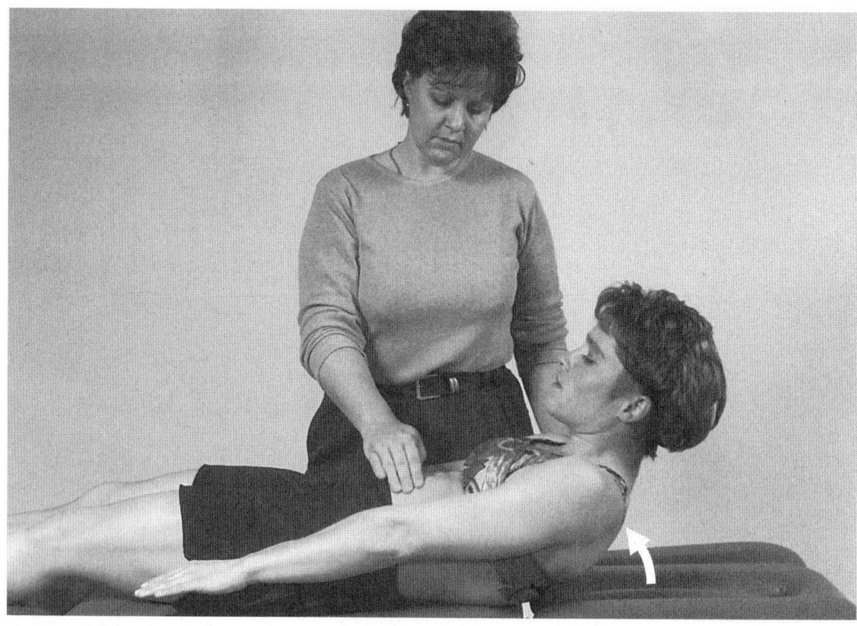

Fig. 3-19. Arrow indicates direction of movement.

For grade 3:

With arms at sides, patient raises head and spine until upper portion of scapulae have cleared table. Inferior angles of scapulae remain in contact with surface (Fig. 3-20).

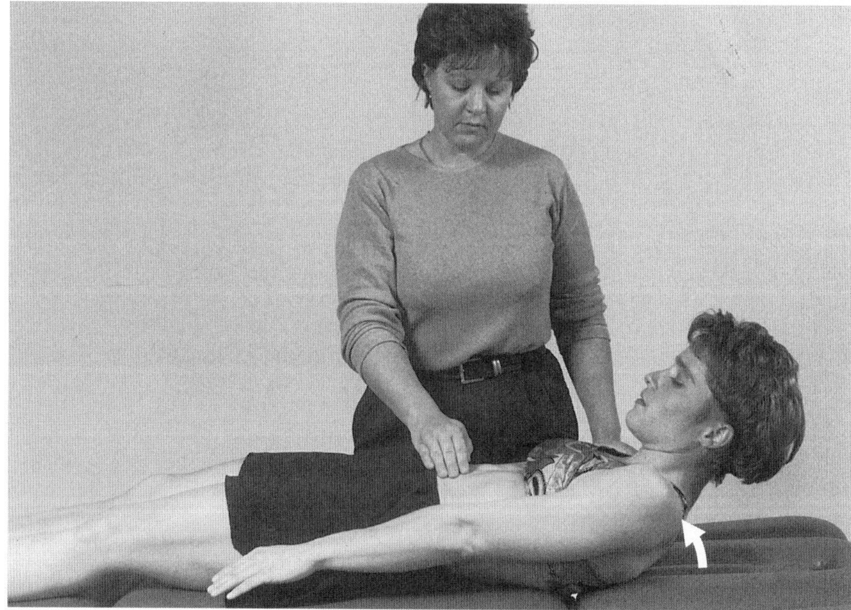

Fig. 3-20. Arrow indicates direction of movement.

For grade 2: With arms at sides, patient raises head and cervical spine from table. All of scapulae remain in contact with surface (Fig. 3-21).

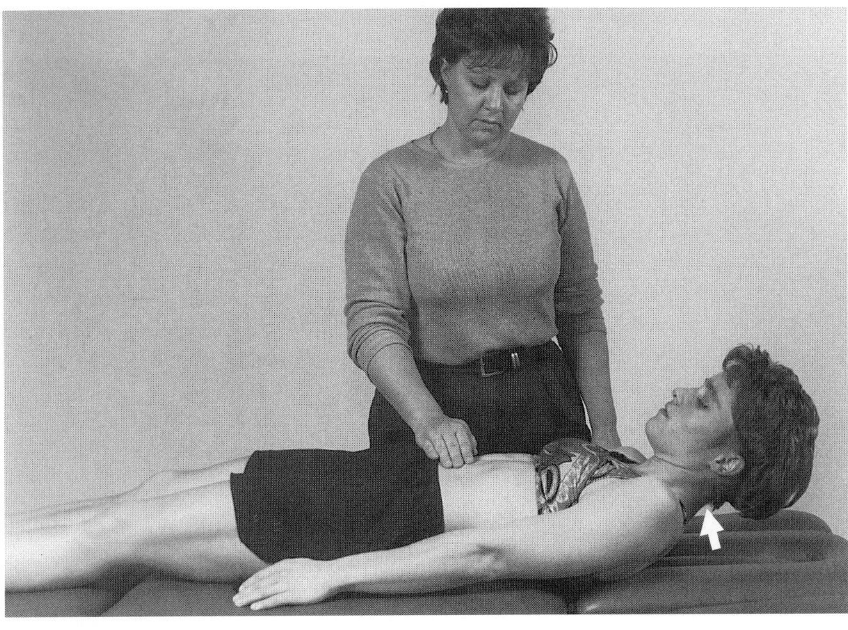

Fig. 3-21. Arrow indicates direction of movement.

For grade 1: No motion, but a palpable contraction is present. Palpation occurs as described earlier (see Fig. 3-16).

For grade 0: No motion or contraction is present.

CLINICAL COMMENT: RECTUS ABDOMINIS MUSCLE TEST

The partial sit-up, which is used to assess strength of the rectus abdominis muscle, also is used as an abdominal strengthening exercise. Frequently, one may observe individuals performing sit-ups with the feet being stabilized by a second person or an immoveable object. Stabilization of the feet during a sit-up causes increased activity in the hip flexors, allowing hip flexor strength to substitute for abdominal weakness. Whether using the sit-up as a strengthening tool or an examination device, the feet should be left unstabilized during the movement.

▪ TRUNK FLEXION—ALTERNATIVE TEST: LEG LOWERING

RECTUS ABDOMINIS, EXTERNAL ABDOMINAL OBLIQUE

All Grades

Patient position: Supine with arms across chest, hips flexed to 90°, knees extended (Fig. 3-22).

Fig. 3-22.

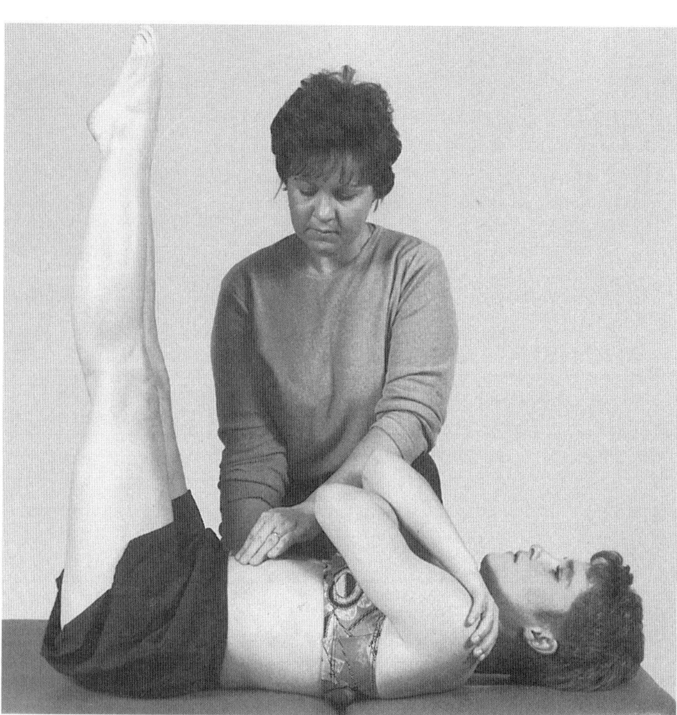

Examiner action: While instructing patient in motion desired, place one hand beneath patient's back and slowly lower patient's legs toward table, instructing patient to keep back pressed into table. Return patient to starting position.

Stabilization/palpation: No stabilization is performed. Examiner places one hand under patient's lumbar spine to detect arching of low back while palpating rectus abdominis (over anterior aspect of trunk just lateral to midline) with other hand (Fig. 3-22).

Patient action:

Patient slowly lowers legs toward table, keeping knees extended and back flat against examiner's hand. Examiner palpates rectus abdominis and lumbar spine during patient's active movement (Fig. 3-23).

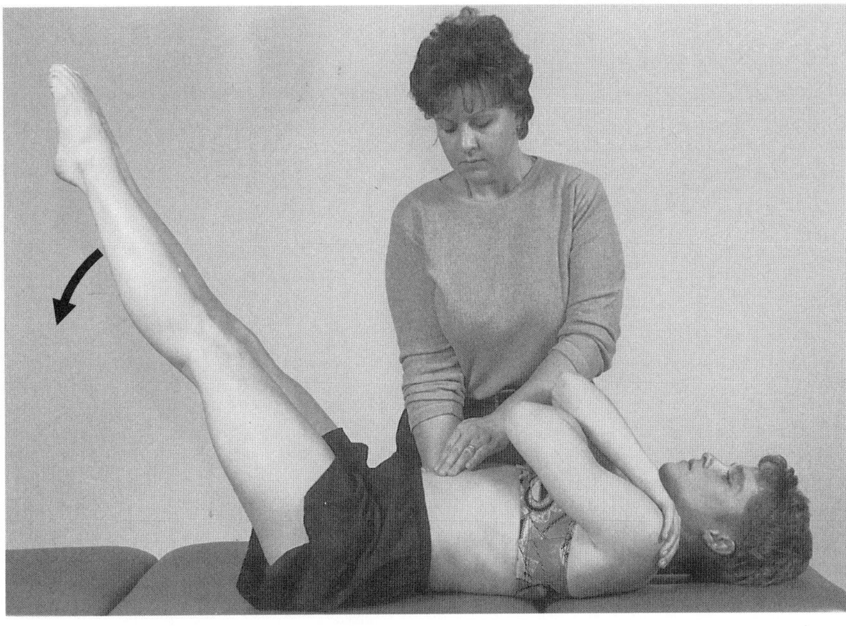

Fig. 3-23. Arrow indicates direction of movement.

Resistance:

No resistance is needed. Examiner notes point where lumbar spine begins to arch.

GRADING

Grading is based on point where patient is no longer able to maintain a posterior pelvic tilt. At that point, weight of lower extremities has overcome ability of abdominals to fixate pelvis. Grade is assigned based on angle of lower extremities with table when posterior pelvic tilt is lost (lumbar spine begins to arch).

For grade 5:

Angle between lower extremities and table is 0°. Patient is able to lower legs completely to table without losing posterior pelvic tilt (Fig. 3-24).

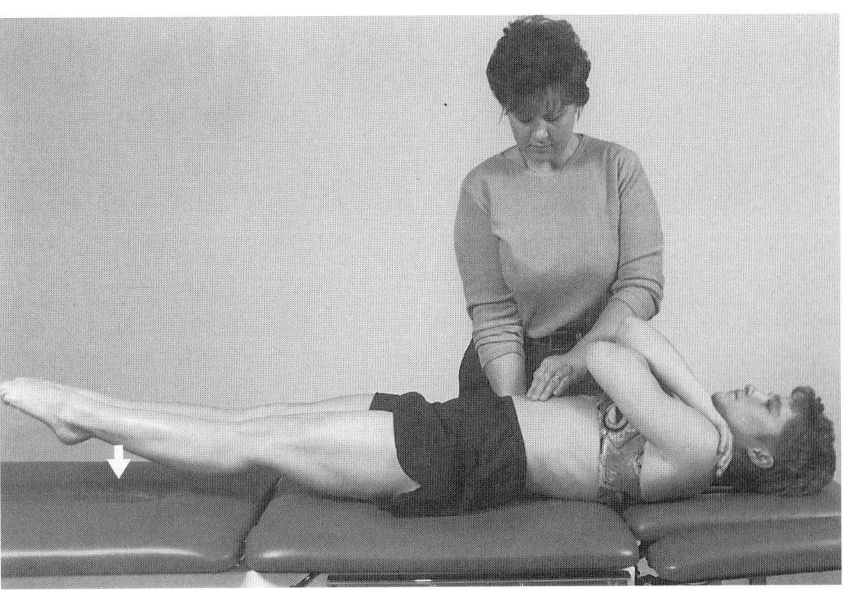

Fig. 3-24. Arrow indicates direction of movement.

For grade 4+: Angle between lower extremities and table is 15° when posterior pelvic tilt is lost.

For grade 4: Angle between lower extremities and table is 30° when posterior pelvic tilt is lost (Fig. 3-25).

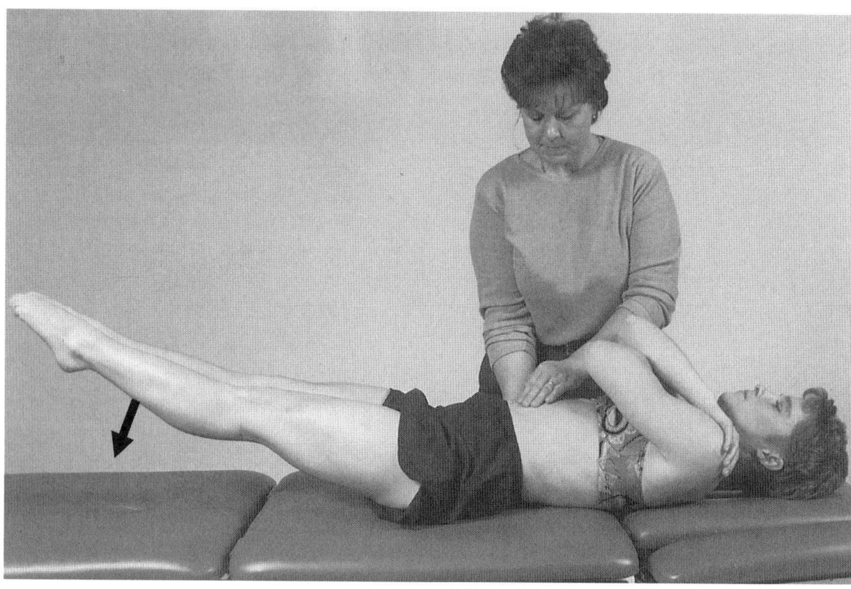

Fig. 3-25. Arrow indicates direction of movement.

For grade 4–: Angle between lower extremities and table is 45° when posterior pelvic tilt is lost.

For grade 3+: Angle between lower extremities and table is 60° when posterior pelvic tilt is lost.

For grade 3: Angle between lower extremities and table is 70° when posterior pelvic tilt is lost (Fig. 3-26).

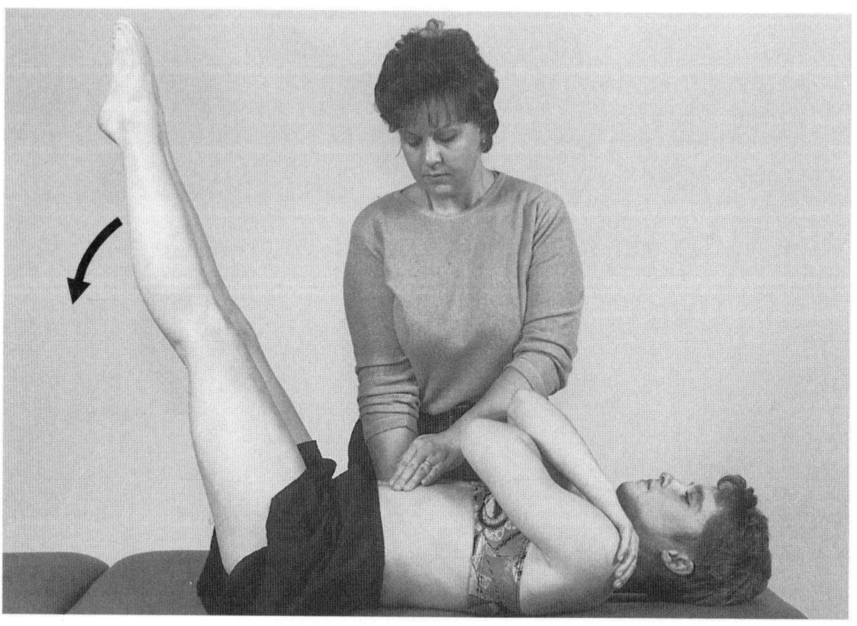

Fig. 3-26. Arrow indicates direction of movement.

For grade 2:

Angle between lower extremities and table is greater than 75° when posterior pelvic tilt is lost (Fig. 3-27).

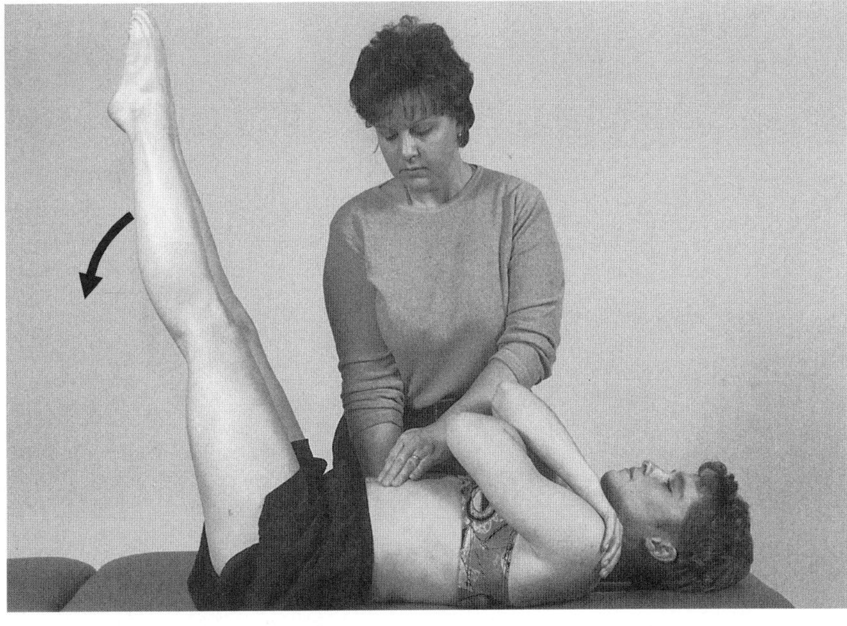

Fig. 3-27. Arrow indicates direction of movement.

For grade 1:

Patient is unable to assume or maintain position, but palpable contraction of rectus abdominis is present. Palpation occurs as described earlier (Fig. 3-28).

Note: Test was adapted from test by Kendall et al. (1993) for "lower" abdominals.

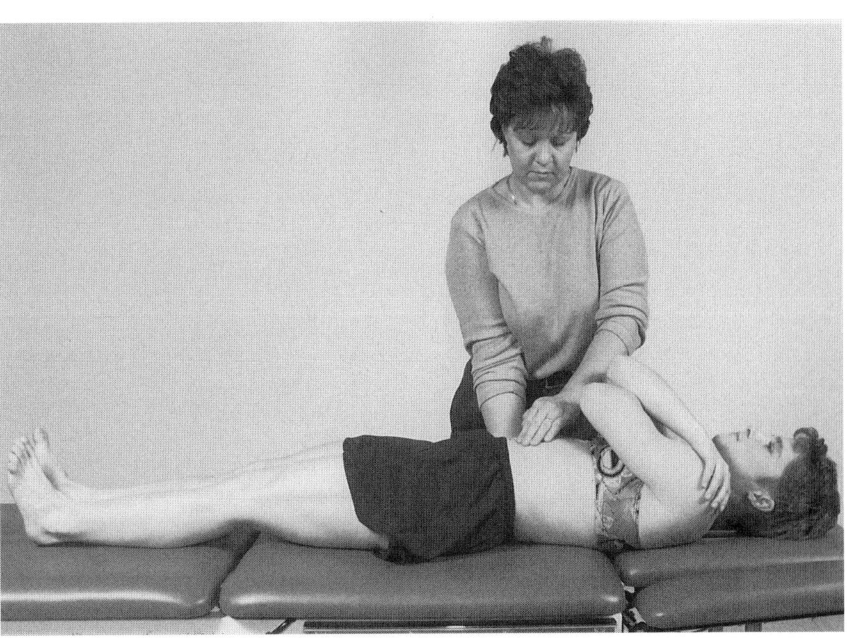

Fig. 3-28.

■ TRUNK ROTATION

EXTERNAL AND INTERNAL ABDOMINAL OBLIQUES (Fig. 3-29)

Fig. 3-29.

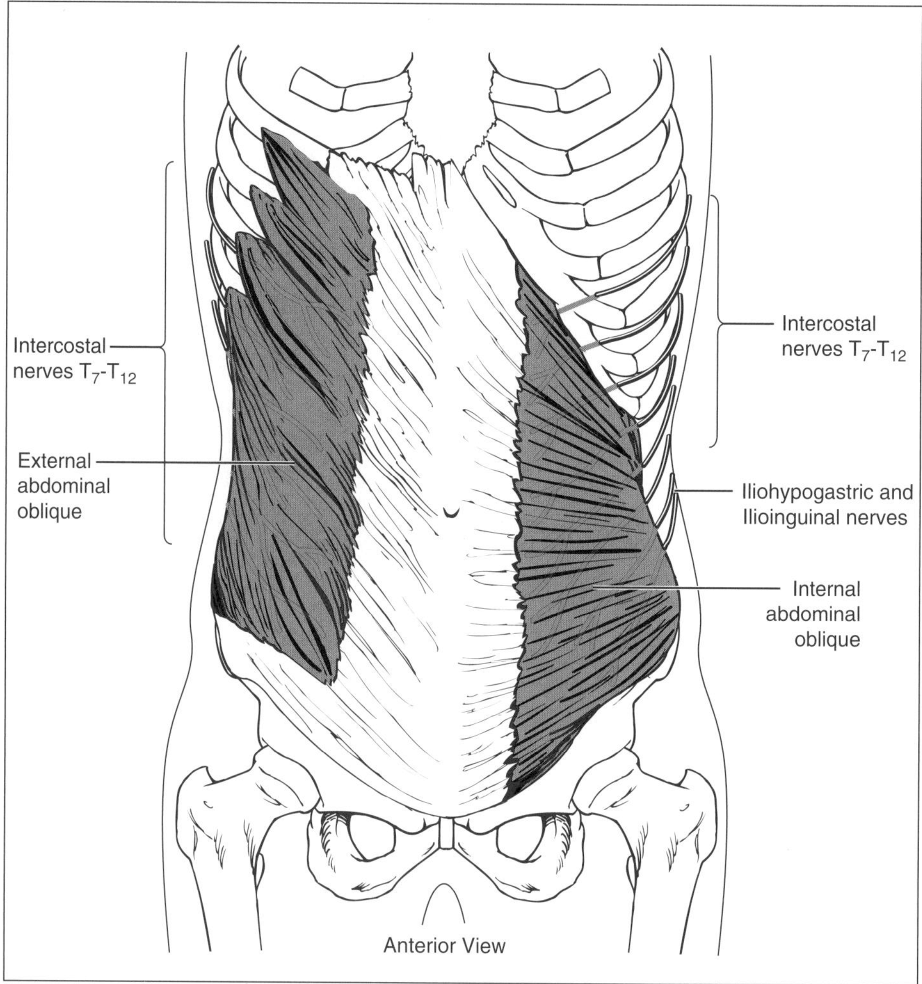

	ATTACHMENTS	NERVE SUPPLY	FUNCTION
External abdominal oblique	Origin: By interdigitating slips from the external surfaces of the lower 8 ribs Insertion: Abdominal aponeurosis, anterior aspect of the outer lip of the iliac crest	Intercostal nerves 7–12	Bilateral action: Flexion of the vertebral column Unilateral action: Lateral flexion and rotation of the vertebral column toward the opposite side
Internal abdominal oblique	Origin: Thoracolumbar fascia, anterior ⅔ of the middle lip of the iliac crest, the lateral ½ of the inguinal ligament Insertion: Inferior aspect of the costal cartilages of the last 3–4 ribs, via aponeurosis into the rectus sheath, pectineal line of the pubic bone	Intercostal nerves 8–12, iliohypogastric nerve, ilioinguinal nerve	Bilateral action: Flexion of the vertebral column Unilateral action: Lateral flexion and rotation of the vertebral column toward the same side

Gravity-Resisted Test (Grade 5)

Patient position: Supine with hands behind neck, lower extremities fully extended (Fig. 3-30).

Fig. 3-30.

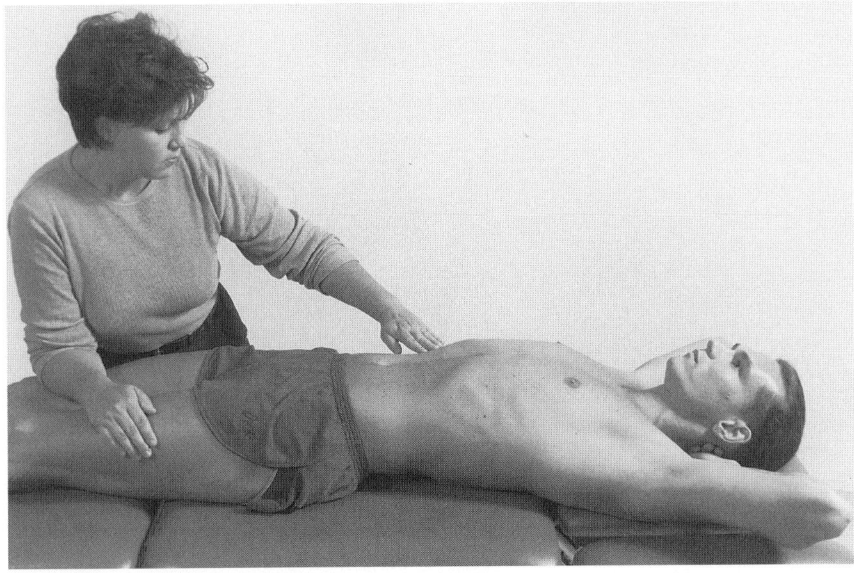

Examiner action: While instructing patient in motion desired, assist patient in trunk rotation and forward flexion until both scapulae have cleared table (or as far forward as patient is able to flex if weakness prevents flexion to point of clearing scapulae). Return patient to starting position. Performing passive movement allows determination of available ROM and shows patient exact motion desired.

Stabilization/palpation: Stabilize with one forearm over anterior aspect of patient's lower extremities. With opposite hand, palpate external oblique on anterolateral aspect of trunk (Fig. 3-30).

Patient action:

Patient flexes and rotates trunk just until both scapulae completely clear table. Rotation of trunk to one side results in contraction of ipsilateral internal oblique and contralateral external oblique. Examiner stabilizes lower extremities and palpates external oblique during patient's active movement (Fig. 3-31).

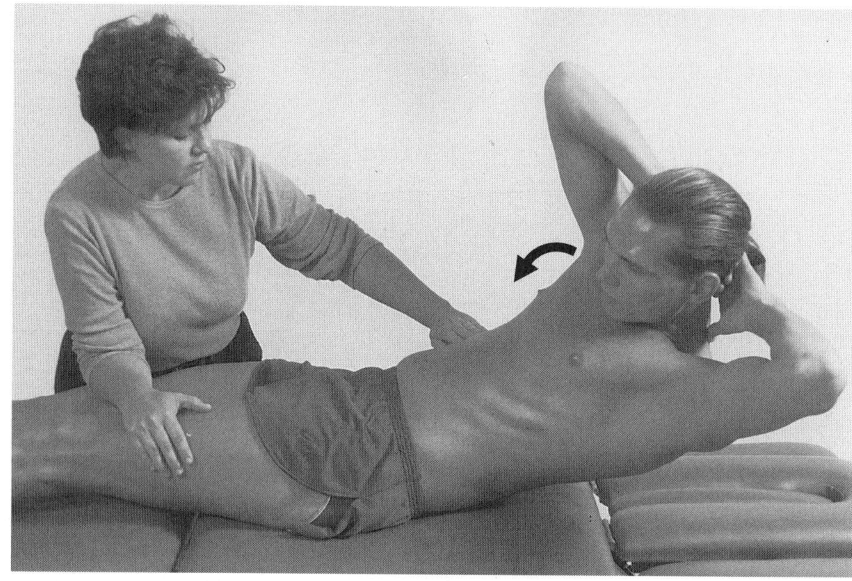

Fig. 3-31. Arrow indicates direction of movement.

Resistance:

No resistance is needed.

Gravity-Resisted Test (Grades 4 and 3)

Grading for grades 4 and 3 depends on upper extremity position. Stabilization, palpation, patient action are same as those for grade 5 test.

For grade 4:

Patient flexes and rotates trunk through full ROM with arms folded across chest (Fig. 3-32).

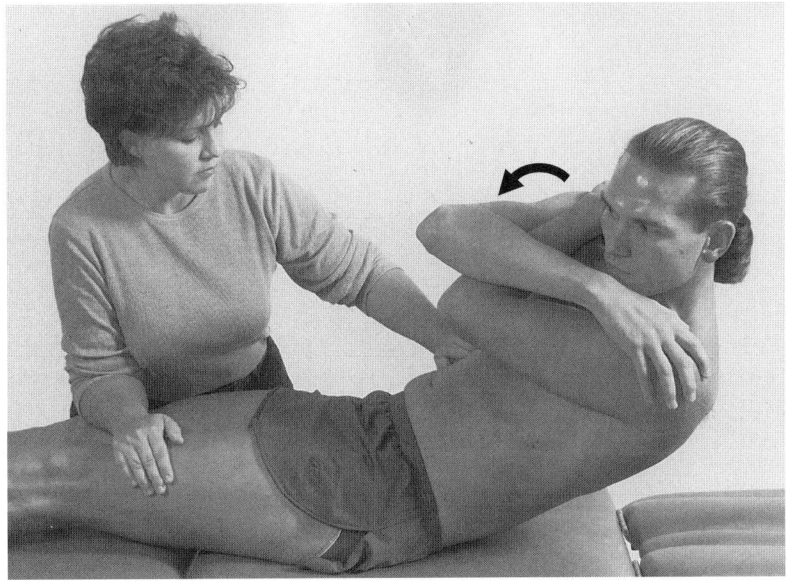

Fig. 3-32. Arrow indicates direction of movement.

For grade 3:

Patient flexes and rotates trunk through full ROM with arms at sides (Fig. 3-33).

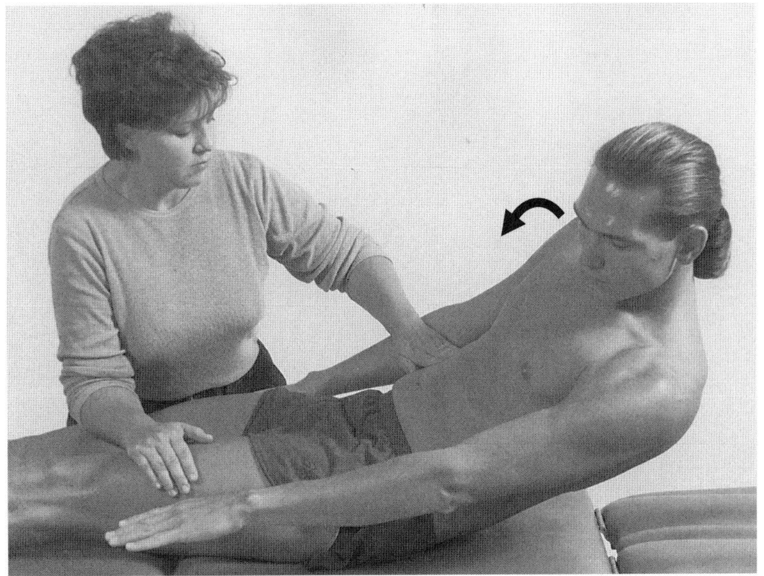

Fig. 3-33. Arrow indicates direction of movement.

Gravity-Eliminated Test (Grades Below 3)

Patient position: Seated with arms at sides. Hands should not be allowed to grip table (Fig. 3-34).

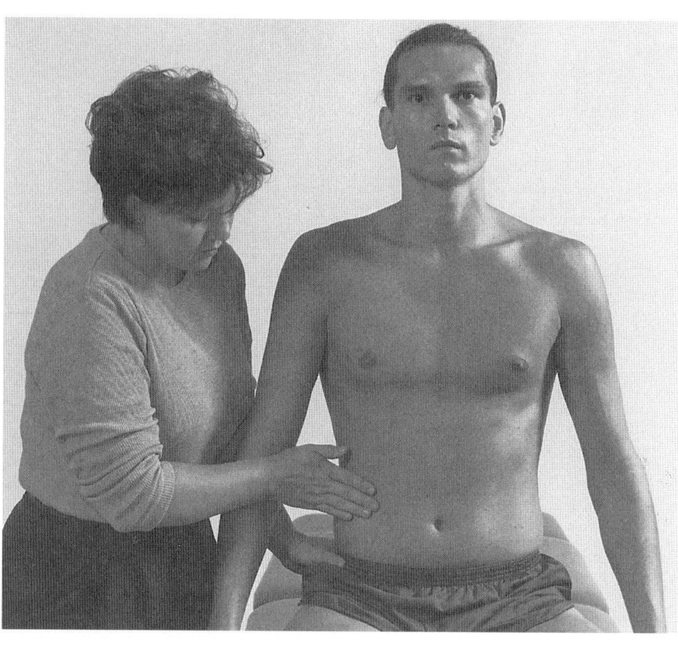

Fig. 3-34.

Examiner action: While instructing patient in motion desired, rotate patient's trunk to appropriate side through full available ROM. Return patient to starting position. Performing passive movement allows determination of patient's available ROM and shows patient exact motion desired.

Stabilization/palpation: Examiner stabilizes pelvis while palpating external oblique with fingertips. Palpation occurs as in gravity-resisted test (Fig. 3-34).

Patient action: Patient rotates trunk through full ROM while examiner stabilizes pelvis and palpates external oblique (Fig. 3-35).

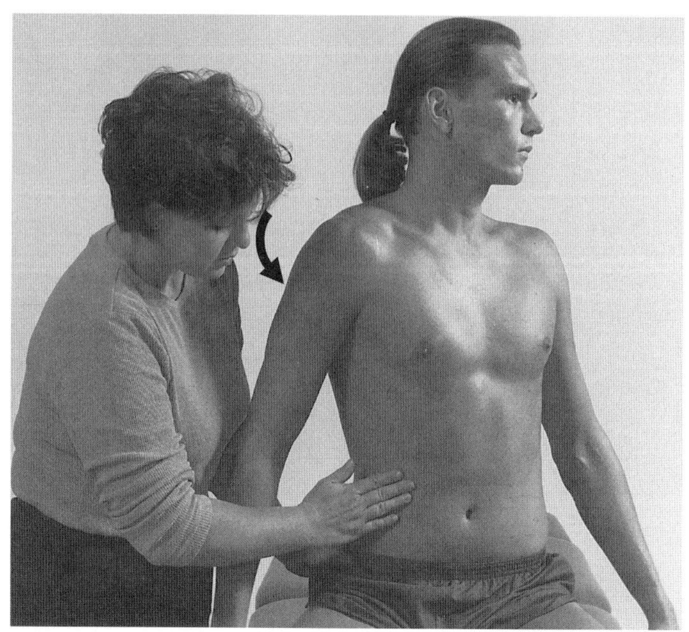

Fig. 3-35. Arrow indicates direction of movement.

■ TRUNK EXTENSION

ERECTOR SPINAE (THORACIC AND LUMBAR PORTIONS), MULTIFIDUS, SEMISPINALIS THORACIS, QUADRATUS LUMBORUM (Fig. 3-36)

Fig. 3-36.

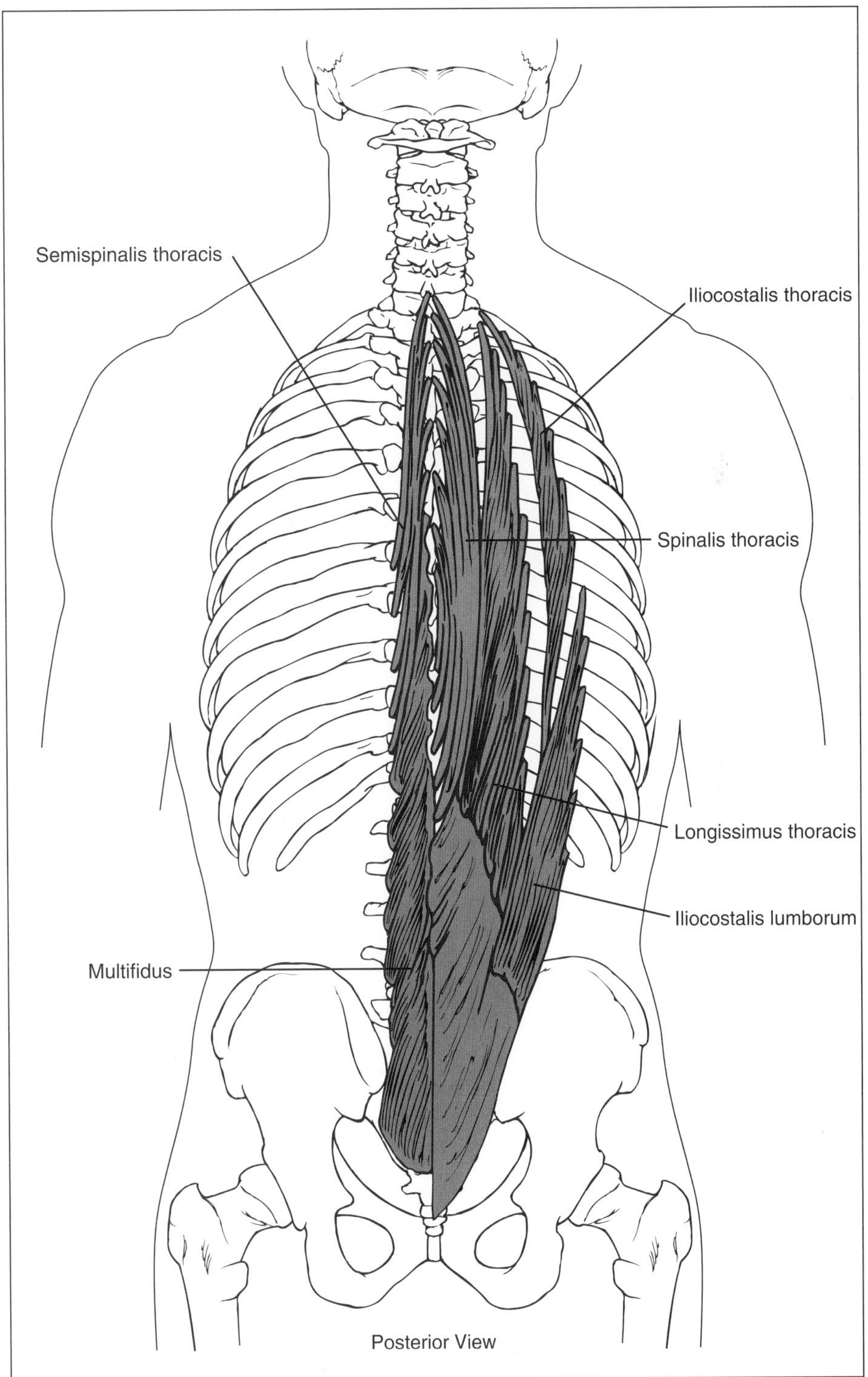

	ATTACHMENTS	NERVE SUPPLY	FUNCTION
Iliocostalis thoracis	Origin: Angles of ribs 7–12 Insertion: Angles of ribs 1–6; transverse process of C7	Dorsal primary rami of the spinal nerves	Bilateral action: Extension of the vertebral column Unilateral action: Lateral flexion and rotation of the vertebral column
Iliocostalis lumborum	Origin: Common erector spinae tendon from the median sacral crest, spinous processes of all lumbar and lower two thoracic vertebrae, dorsum of the iliac crests, lateral crest of the sacrum, sacrotuberous and posterior sacroiliac ligaments Insertion: Angles of the last 6–7 ribs	Dorsal primary rami of the spinal nerves	Bilateral action: Extension of the vertebral column Unilateral action: Lateral flexion and rotation of the vertebral column; elevation of the pelvis
Longissimus thoracis	Origin: Transverse processes of lumbar vertebrae, thoracolumbar fascia Insertion: Between tubercles and angles of the lower 9–10 ribs; transverse processes of the thoracic vertebrae	Dorsal primary rami of the spinal nerves	Bilateral action: Extension of the vertebral column Unilateral action: Lateral flexion of the vertebral column
Multifidus	Origin: Posterior aspect of the sacrum, posterior superior iliac spine, posterior sacroiliac ligament, mamillary processes of the lumbar vertebrae, transverse processes of the thoracic vertebrae, articular processes of the lower four cervical vertebrae Insertion: Spinous processes of the lumbar, thoracic, and cervical vertebrae	Dorsal primary rami of the spinal nerves	Bilateral action: Extension of the vertebral column Unilateral action: Lateral flexion of the vertebral column; rotation of the vertebral column to the opposite side
Semispinalis thoracis	Origin: Transverse processes of T6–T10 Insertion: Spinous processes of C6–T4	Dorsal primary rami of T1–T6	Bilateral action: Extension of the vertebral column Unilateral action: Rotation of the vertebral column to the opposite side
Spinalis thoracis	Origin: Spinous processes of T11–L2 Insertion: Spinous processes of the upper 4–8 thoracic vertebrae	Dorsal primary rami of the spinal nerves	Extension of the vertebral column
Quadratus lumborum	Origin: Iliac crest, iliolumbar ligament Insertion: Transverse processes of L2–L4; inferior border of the 12th rib	12th thoracic and upper 3–4 lumbar nerves	Bilateral action: Extension of the lumbar spine Unilateral action: Lateral flexion of the lumbar spine; elevation of the pelvis

Grade 5

Patient position: Prone with hands behind neck, pillow under abdomen, lower extremities extended (Fig. 3-37; pillow not shown).

Fig. 3-37.

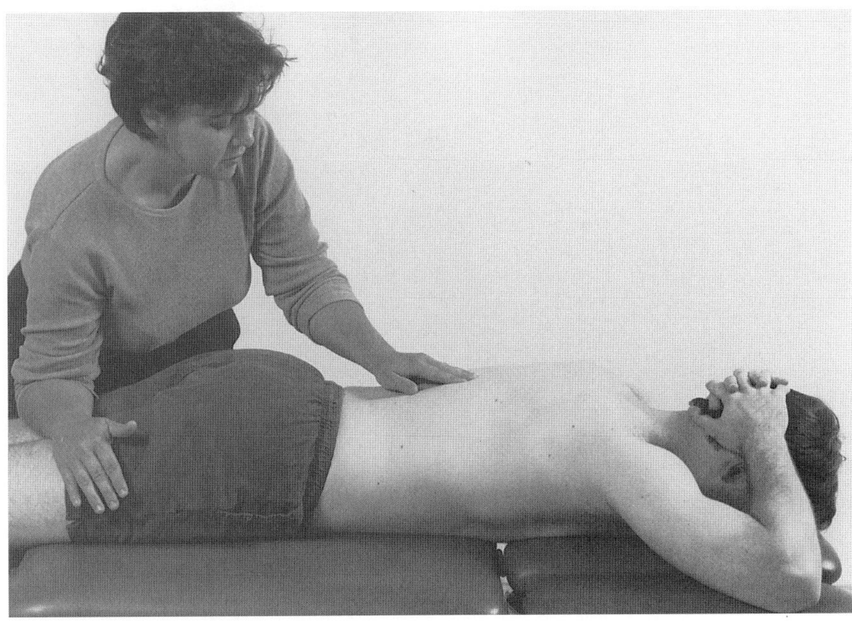

Examiner action: While instructing patient in movement desired, assist patient in extending spine through full available ROM. Return patient to starting position. Performing passive movement allows determination of patient's available ROM and shows patient exact motion desired.

Stabilization/palpation: Stabilize over posterior aspect of patient's thighs and pelvis with forearm. With opposite hand, palpate erector spinae lateral to spinous processes of lumbar and thoracic vertebrae (Fig. 3-37).

Patient action:

Patient extends trunk through full ROM (entire sternum, including xiphoid process, should clear table) while examiner stabilizes posterior pelvis and thighs and palpates erector spinae (Fig. 3-38).

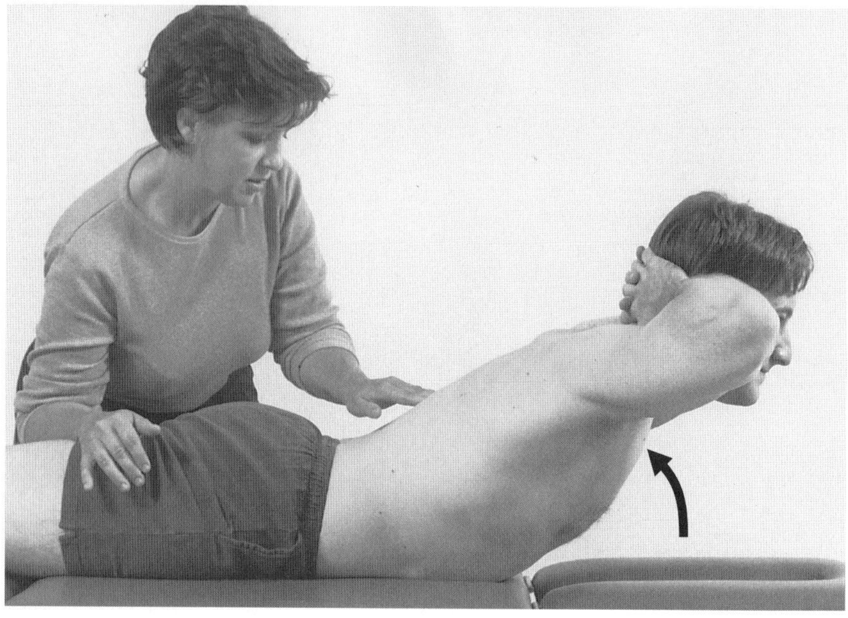

Fig. 3-38. Arrow indicates direction of movement.

Resistance:

No resistance is needed.

Grades 4 and Below

There is no separate test of these muscles for grades below 5. Assignment of grades below 5 depends on upper extremity position as follows.

For grade 4:

Patient extends trunk through full ROM with arms folded behind back (Fig. 3-39).

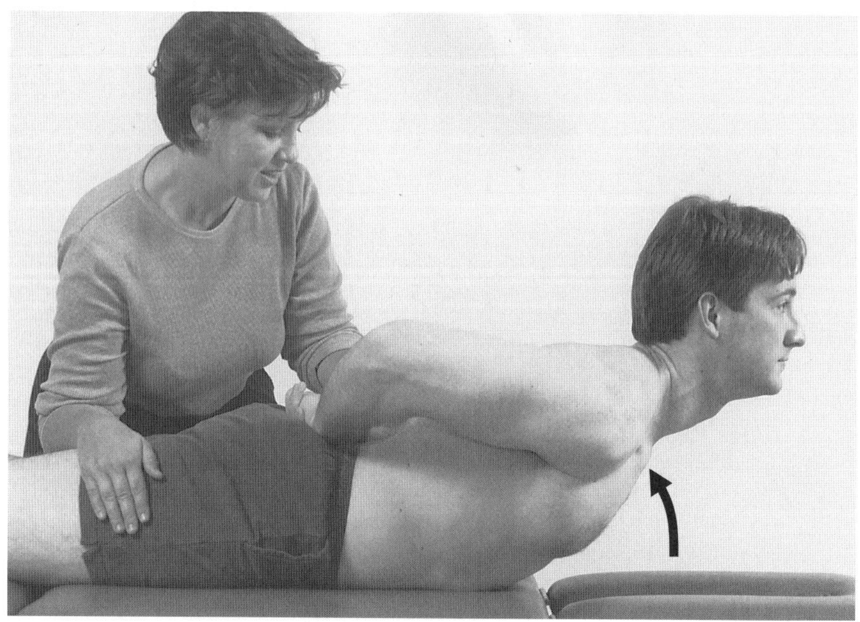

Fig. 3-39. Arrow indicates direction of movement.

For grade 3:

Patient extends trunk through full ROM with arms at sides (Fig. 3-40).

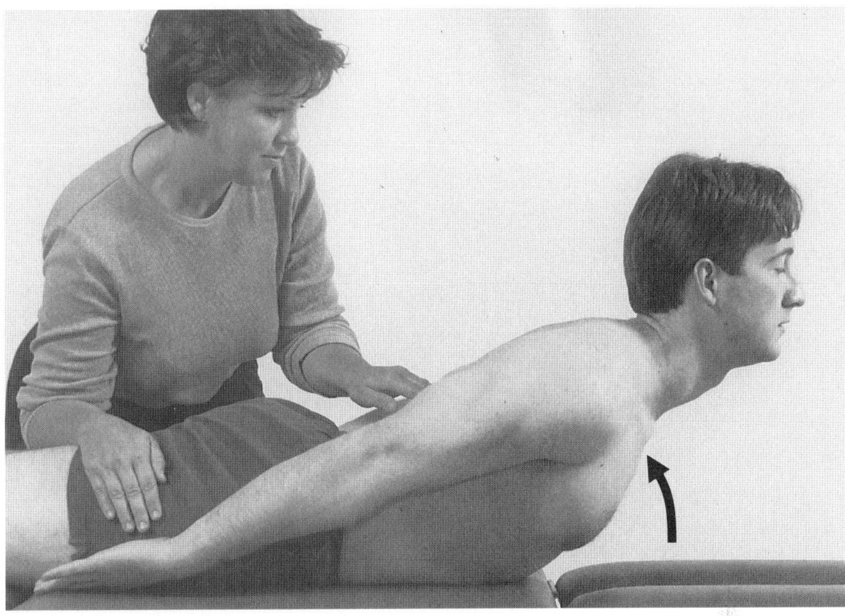

Fig. 3-40. Arrow indicates direction of movement.

For grade 2:

Patient extends trunk through partial ROM with arms at sides (Fig. 3-41).

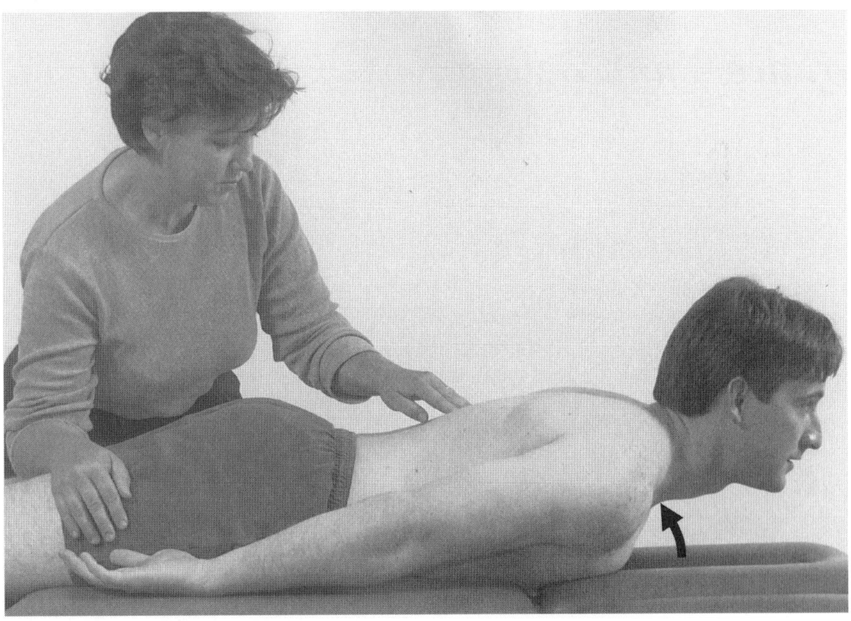

Fig. 3-41. Arrow indicates direction of movement.

For grade 1:

No motion, but a palpable contraction is present. Palpation occurs as described earlier (see Fig. 3-37).

For grade 0:

No motion or contraction is present.

■ PELVIC ELEVATION

QUADRATUS LUMBORUM, ILIOCOSTALIS LUMBORUM (Fig. 3-42)

Fig. 3-42.

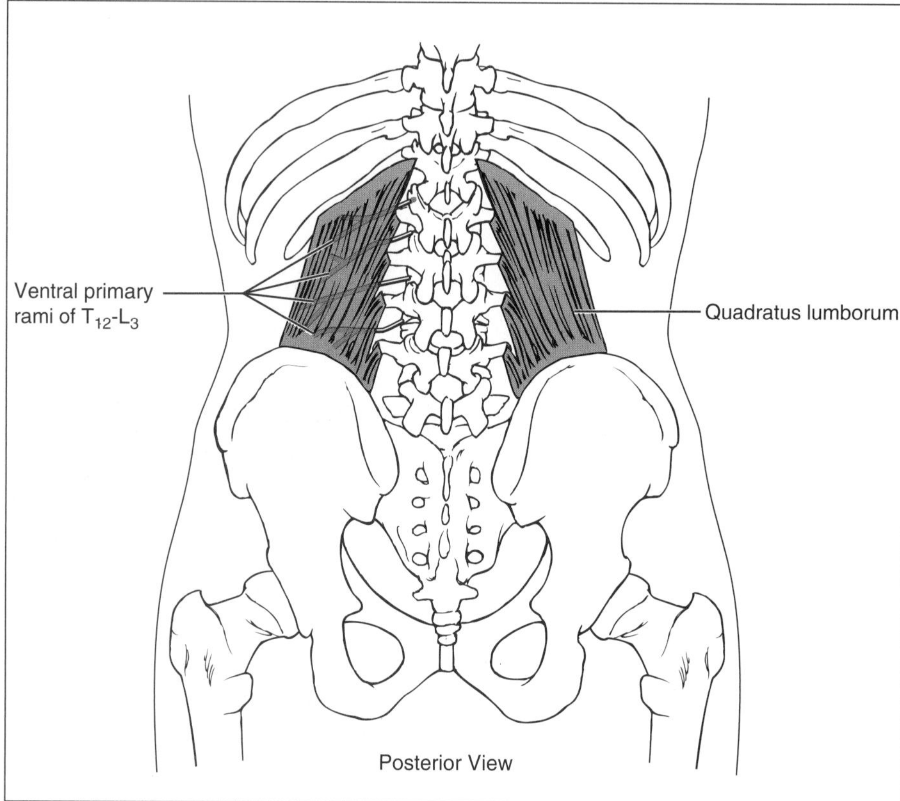

	ATTACHMENTS	NERVE SUPPLY	FUNCTION
Quadratus lumborum	Origin: Iliac crest, iliolumbar ligament Insertion: Transverse processes of L1–L4; inferior border of the 12th rib	12th thoracic and upper 3–4 lumbar nerves	Bilateral action: Extension of the lumbar spine Unilateral action: Lateral flexion of the lumbar spine; elevation of the pelvis
Iliocostalis lumborum	Origin: Common erector spinae tendon from the median sacral crest, spinous processes of all lumbar and the lower two thoracic vertebrae, dorsum of the iliac crests, lateral crest of the sacrum, sacrotuberous and posterior sacroiliac ligaments Insertion: Angles of the last 6–7 ribs	Dorsal primary rami of the spinal nerves	Bilateral action: Extension of the vertebral column Unilateral action: Lateral flexion and rotation of the vertebral column; elevation of the pelvis

All Grades

Patient position: Supine (or prone) with hip on side to be tested in slight abduction and feet off end of table (Fig. 3-43).

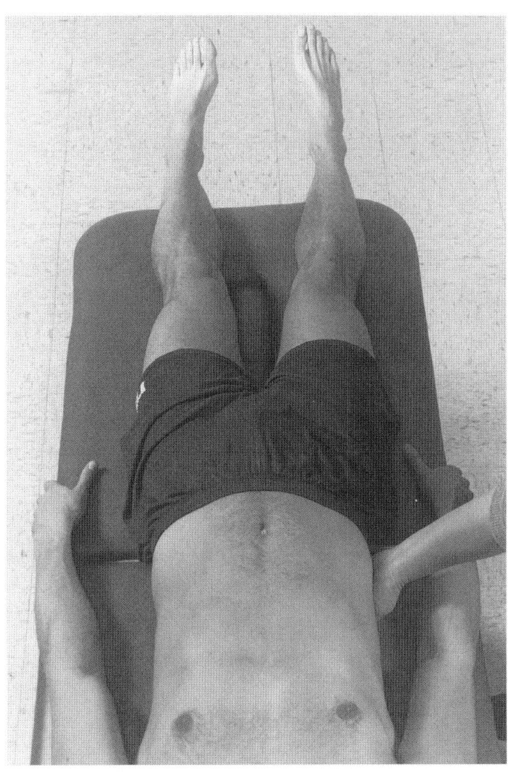

Fig. 3-43.

Examiner action: While instructing patient in movement desired, elevate patient's pelvis on side to be tested through full available ROM. Return patient to starting position. Performing passive movement allows determination of patient's available ROM and shows patient exact motion desired.

Stabilization/palpation: Patient holds edge of table to stabilize thorax. Quadratus lumborum is difficult to palpate but may be felt just above posterior iliac crest lateral to erector spinae when patient is supine (Fig. 3-43).

Patient action: Patient elevates ipsilateral pelvis through full ROM (Fig. 3-44).

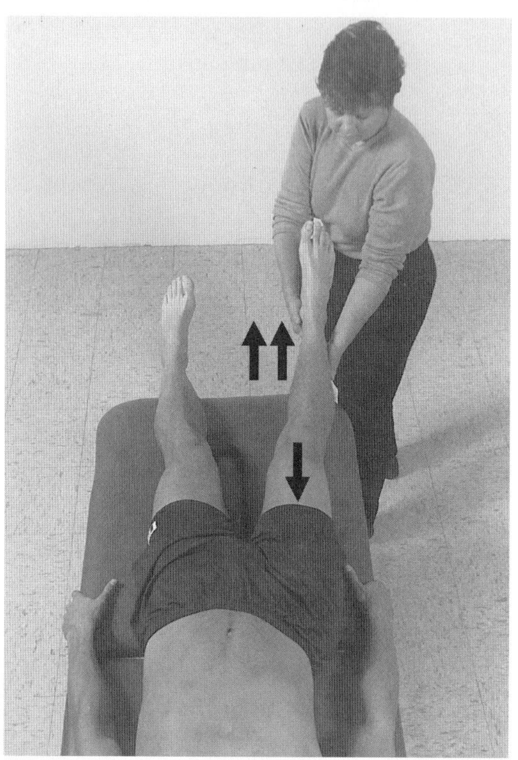

Fig. 3-44. Single arrow indicates direction of movement; double arrows indicate direction of resistance.

Resistance: Apply resistance just proximal to ankle by inferior (caudal) pull on lower extremity (Fig. 3-44).

GRADING

Grading for this test is altered slightly from standard grading and occurs as follows.

For grade 5: Patient maintains pelvic elevation against maximum resistance.

For grade 4: Patient maintains pelvic elevation against moderate resistance.

For grade 3: Patient maintains pelvic elevation against minimum resistance.

For grade 2: Patient elevates pelvis through full ROM without resistance.

For grade 1: No motion, but a palpable contraction is present. Palpation occurs as described above (see Fig. 3-43).

For grade 0: No motion or contraction is present.

COMMON SUBSTITUTION

Patient may flex trunk to contralateral side in attempt to elevate ipsilateral pelvis. Care should be taken to prevent lateral flexion of trunk.

MUSCLES OF MASTICATION

MASSETER, MEDIAL PTERYGOID, LATERAL PTERYGOID, TEMPORALIS (Figs. 3-45 and 3-46)

Fig. 3-45.

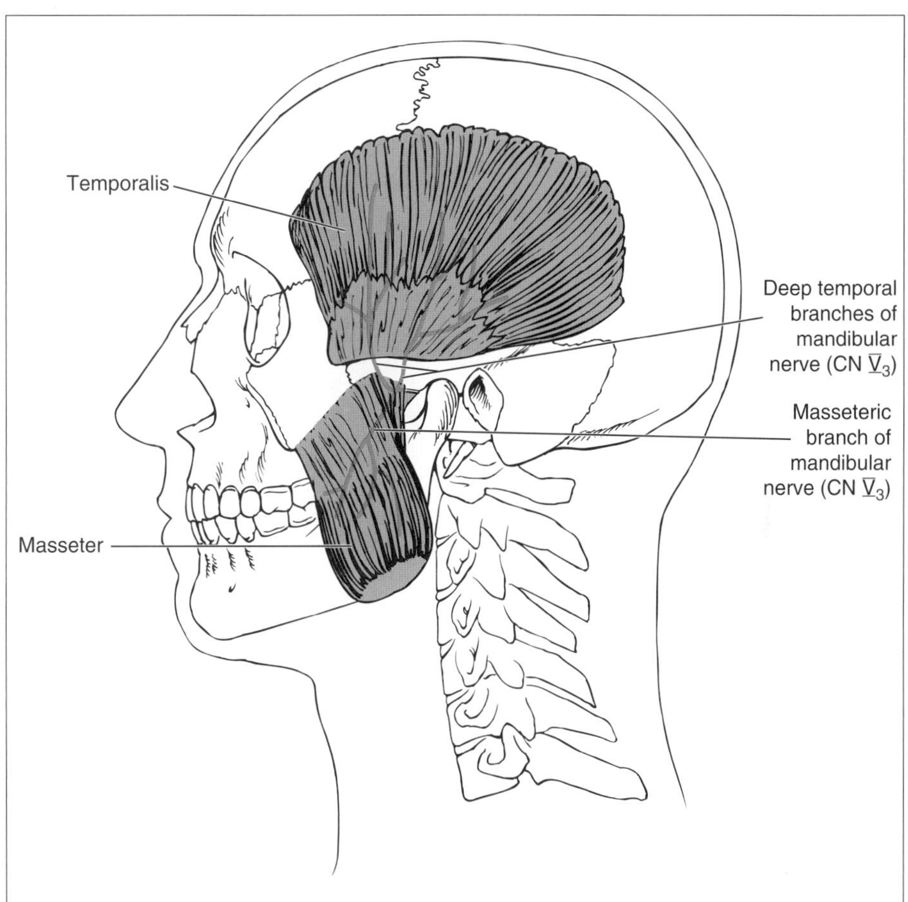

Fig. 3-46.

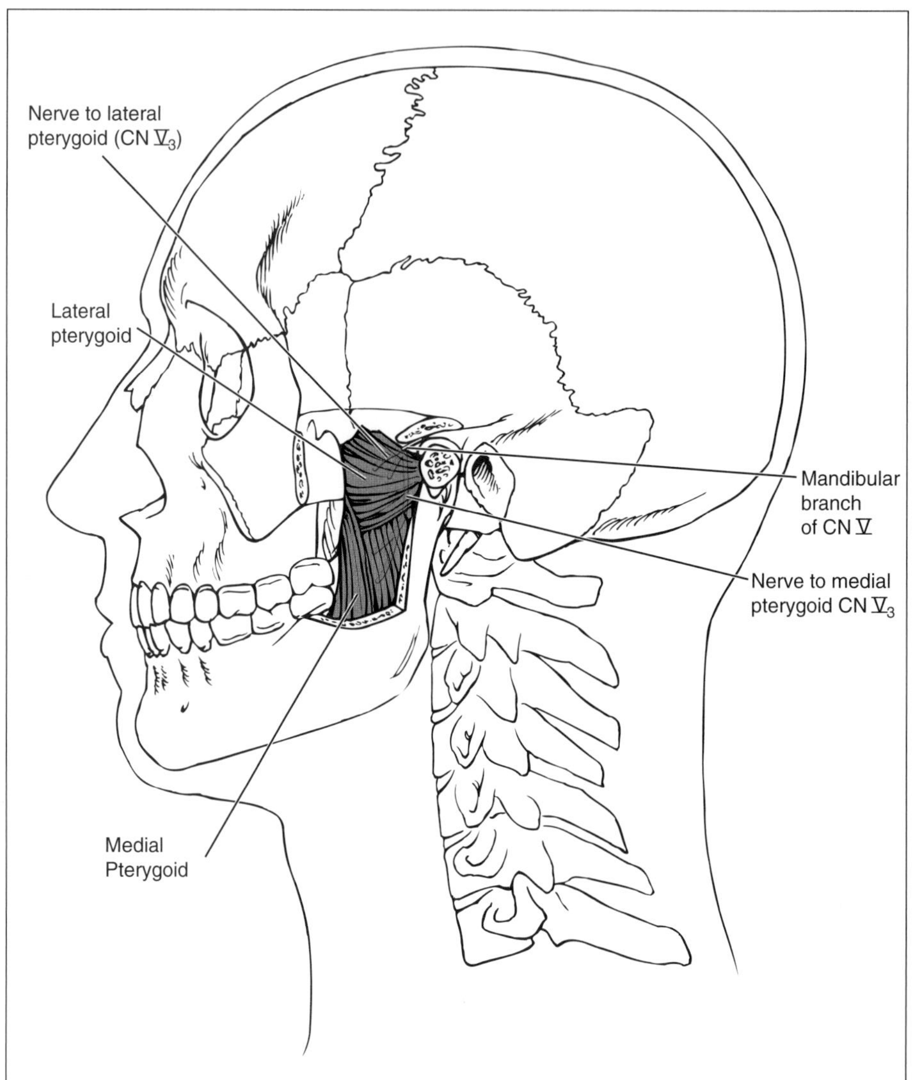
Nerve to lateral pterygoid (CN V3)
Lateral pterygoid
Mandibular branch of CN V
Nerve to medial pterygoid CN V3
Medial Pterygoid

	ATTACHMENTS	NERVE SUPPLY	FUNCTION
Masseter	Origin: Zygomatic process of the maxilla, zygomatic arch Insertion: Angle and lateral surface of the ramus of the mandible, coronoid process of the mandible	Mandibular division of the trigeminal nerve (cranial nerve V)	Elevates the mandible (closes the jaw); assists in mandibular protraction
Medial pterygoid	Origin: Medial surface of the lateral pterygoid plate, pyramidal process of the palatine bone, tuberosity of the maxilla Insertion: Medial surface of the ramus and the angle of the mandible	Mandibular division of the trigeminal nerve (cranial nerve V)	Unilateral action: Protracts and deviates the mandible to the opposite side Bilateral action: Elevates the mandible (closes the jaw)
Lateral pterygoid	Origin: Upper head: Infratemporal crest and the lateral surface of the greater wing of the sphenoid bone Inferior head: Lateral surface of the lateral pterygoid plate Insertion: Anterior aspect of the neck of the mandibular condyle and the anterior aspect of the articular disc of the temporomandibular joint	Mandibular division of the trigeminal nerve (cranial nerve V)	Protracts and depresses the mandible (opens the jaw)
Temporalis	Origin: Temporal fossa of the skull Insertion: Coronoid process and ramus of the mandible	Mandibular division of the trigeminal nerve (cranial nerve V)	Retracts and elevates the mandible (closes the jaw)

For following muscle tests, patient performs motion described and depicted in corresponding figure. No resistance is needed. Grading for these muscles is described at end of this section.

MASSETER, MEDIAL PTERYGOID, TEMPORALIS

Patient closes jaw firmly, clenching teeth. Examiner palpates masseter and temporalis bilaterally for symmetry of contraction (Fig. 3-47).

Fig. 3-47. Palpation of masseter and temporalis.

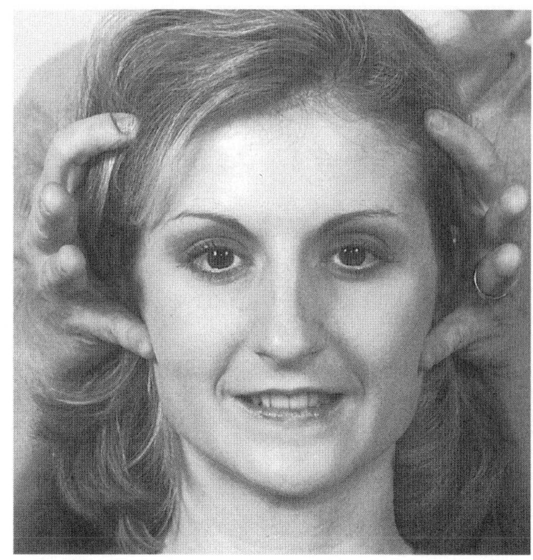

MEDIAL PTERYGOID

Patient protrudes jaw, deviating mandible to contralateral side (Fig. 3-48).

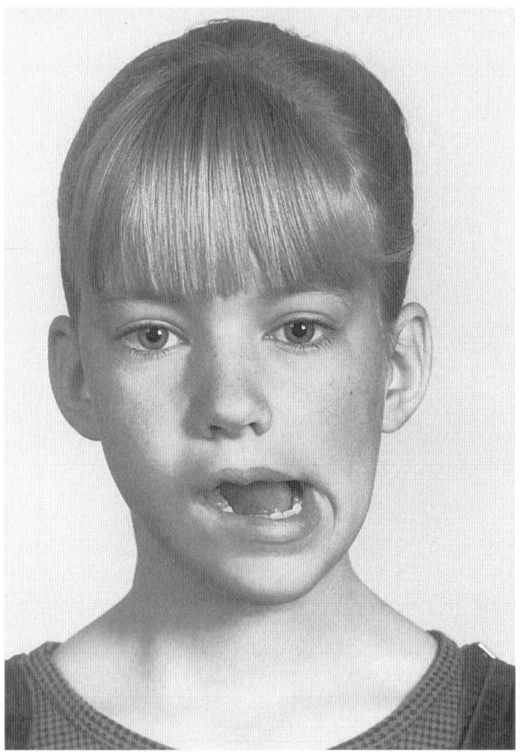

Fig. 3-48. Medial pterygoid.

LATERAL PTERYGOID

Patient opens mouth (Fig. 3-49).

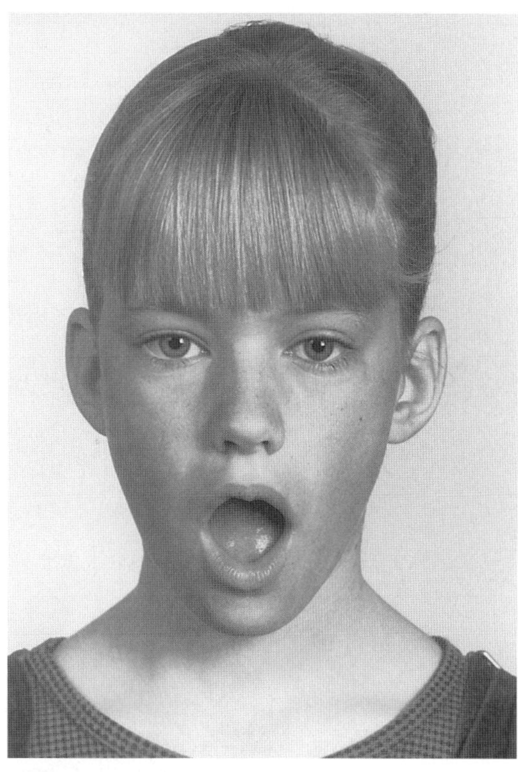

Fig. 3-49. Lateral pterygoid.

GRADING

Following muscle test grades should be used when evaluating muscles of mastication.

For grade 5: Patient performs motion through full available ROM without difficulty.

For grade 3: Motion is performed but with difficulty, or only a partial ROM is completed.

For grade 1: No motion, but a palpable contraction is present.

For grade 0: No motion or contraction is present.

■ MUSCLES OF FACIAL EXPRESSION

OCCIPITOFRONTALIS (FRONTAL BELLY), CORRUGATOR SUPERCILII, ORBICULARIS OCULI, PROCERUS, NASALIS, LEVATOR LABII SUPERIORIS, LEVATOR ANGULI ORIS, ZYGOMATICUS MAJOR, ORBICULARIS ORIS, RISORIUS, BUCCINATOR, DEPRESSOR LABII INFERIORIS, MENTALIS, DEPRESSOR ANGULI ORIS, PLATYSMA

For following muscle tests, patient mimics facial expression described and depicted in corresponding figure. No resistance is needed. Grading for these muscles is described at end of this section (Fig. 3-50).

Fig. 3-50.

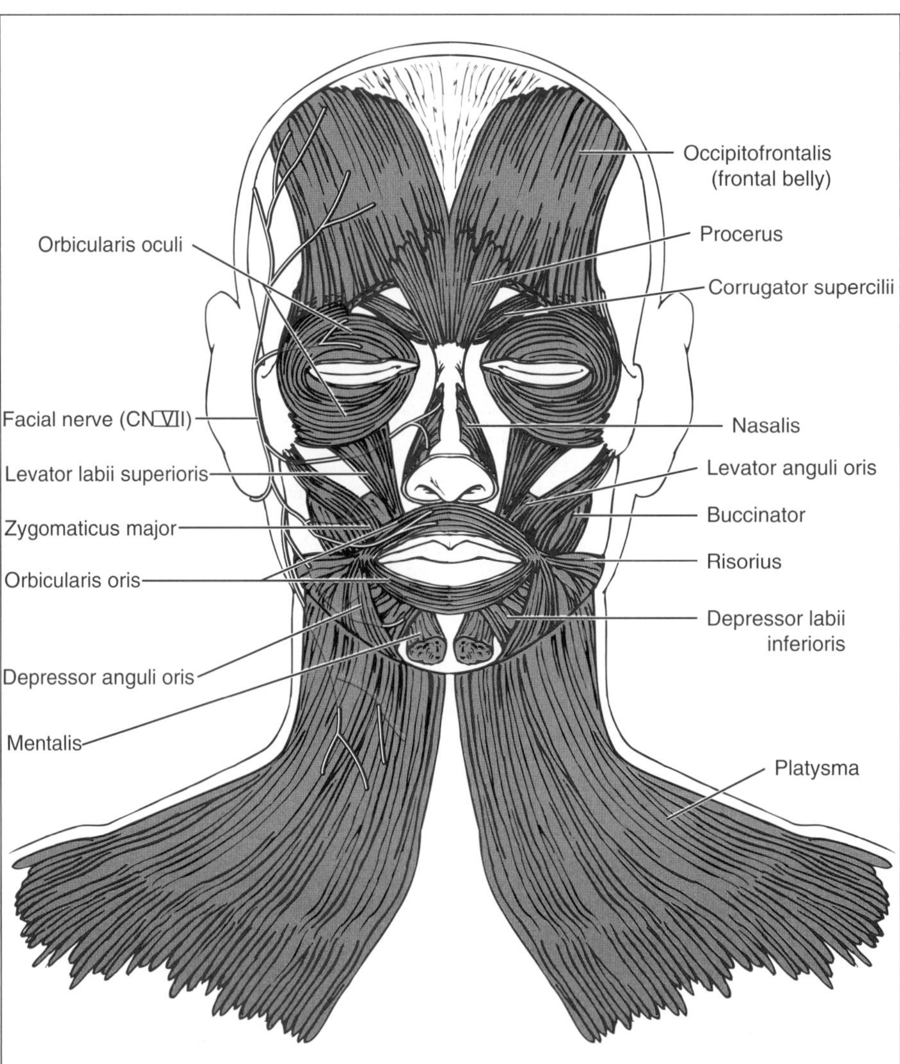

	ATTACHMENTS	NERVE SUPPLY	FUNCTION
Occipitofrontalis (frontal belly)	Origin: Gale aponeurotica Insertion: Skin of the eyebrows and root of the nose	Facial nerve (cranial nerve VII)	Elevates the eyebrows
Corrugator supercilii	Origin: Medial aspect of the superciliary arch Insertion: Skin of the medial half of the eyebrow	Facial nerve (cranial nerve VII)	Draws the eyebrows medially

	ATTACHMENTS	NERVE SUPPLY	FUNCTION
Orbicularis oculi	Origin: Nasal part of the frontal bone, frontal process of the maxilla, medial palpebral ligament Insertion: Lateral palpebral raphe, corrugator supercilii and frontal belly of the occipitofrontalis muscle, skin of the eyebrow	Facial nerve (cranial nerve VII)	Closes the eye
Procerus	Origin: Lateral nasal cartilage and lower part of the nasal bone Insertion: Skin over the lower part of the forehead between the two eyebrows	Facial nerve (cranial nerve VII)	Draws the medial angle of the eyebrows down
Nasalis	Origin: Medial aspect of the maxilla Insertion: Aponeurosis of procerus and contralateral nasalis muscles, alar cartilage	Facial nerve (cranial nerve VII)	Dilates the nasal aperture
Levator labii superioris	Origin: Inferior margin of the orbit Insertion: Lateral one half of the upper lip	Facial nerve (cranial nerve VII)	Raises the upper lip
Levator anguli oris	Origin: Canine fossa of the maxilla Insertion: Angle of the mouth	Facial nerve (cranial nerve VII)	Elevates the angle of the mouth
Zygomaticus major	Origin: Zygomatic bone Insertion: Angle of the mouth	Facial nerve (cranial nerve VII)	Draws the angle of the mouth upward and backward as in smiling or laughing
Orbicularis oris	Origin: Other facial muscles, primarily the buccinator, levator anguli oris, and depressor anguli oris; maxilla; septum of the nose; mandible Insertion: Skin and mucous membrane surrounding the mouth	Facial nerve (cranial nerve VII)	Approximates and protrudes the lips
Risorius	Origin: Parotid fascia overlying the masseter muscle Insertion: Skin of the angle of the mouth	Facial nerve (cranial nerve VII)	Retracts the angle of the mouth
Buccinator	Origin: Alveolar processes of the maxilla and mandible, opposite three molar teeth; pterygomandibular raphe Insertion: Angle of the lips	Facial nerve (cranial nerve VII)	Compresses the cheek
Depressor labii inferioris	Origin: Oblique line of the mandible Insertion: Skin of the lower lip	Facial nerve (cranial nerve VII)	Depresses the angle of the mouth
Mentalis	Origin: Incisive fossa of the mandible Insertion: Skin of the chin	Facial nerve (cranial nerve VII)	Raises and protrudes the lower lip; wrinkles the skin of the chin
Depressor anguli oris	Origin: Oblique line of the mandible Insertion: Angle of the mouth	Facial nerve (cranial nerve VII)	Depresses the angle of the mouth
Platysma	Origin: Fascia covering the deltoid and pectoralis Insertion: Mandible, skin of the lower part of the face	Facial nerve (cranial nerve VII)	Draws the lower lip and corner of the mouth laterally and inferiorly

OCCIPITOFRONTALIS (FRONTAL BELLY)

Patient raises eyebrows, wrinkling forehead (Fig. 3-51).

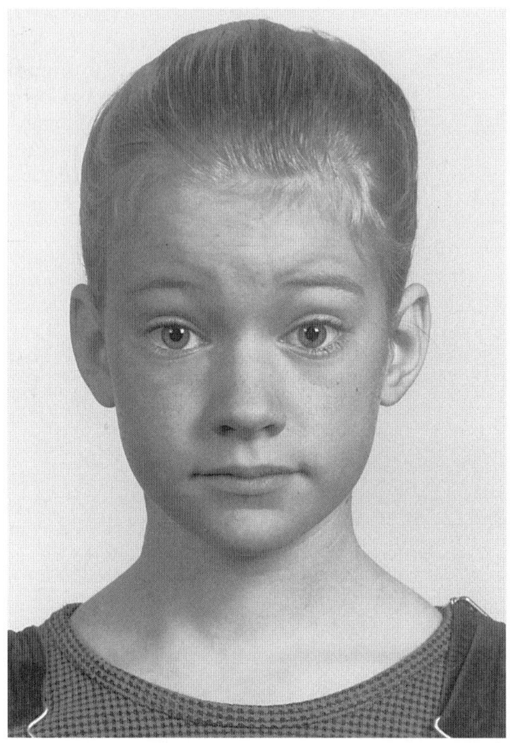

Fig. 3-51. Occipitofrontalis (frontal belly).

CORRUGATOR SUPERCILII

Patient pulls eyebrows together in midline as in frowning or squinting (Fig. 3-52).

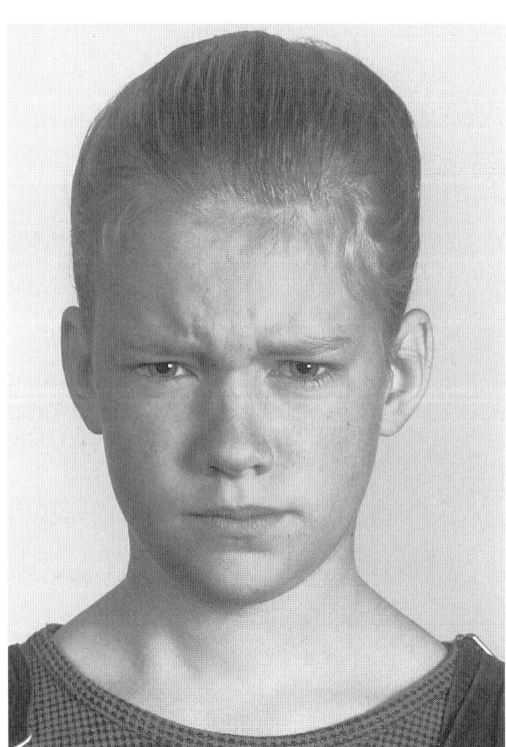

Fig. 3-52. Corrugator supercilii.

ORBICULARIS OCULI

Patient closes eyes tightly (Fig. 3-53).

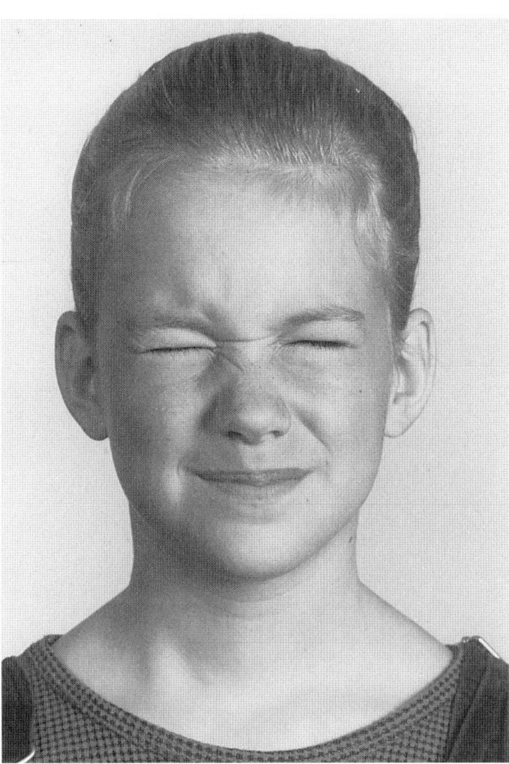

Fig. 3-53. Orbicularis oculi.

PROCERUS

Patient raises skin of nose toward forehead while pulling eyebrows medially (expression of distaste). Skin over bridge of nose should wrinkle horizontally (Fig. 3-54).

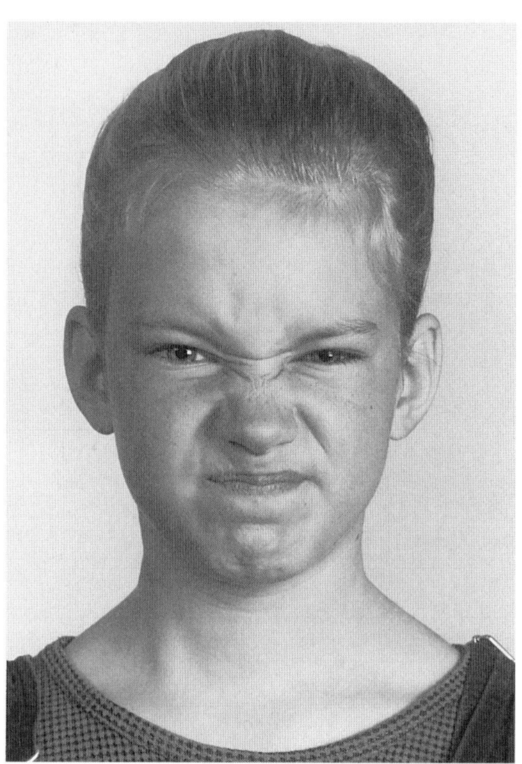

Fig. 3-54. Procerus.

NASALIS

Patient widens nostrils as in breathing in deeply (Fig. 3-55).

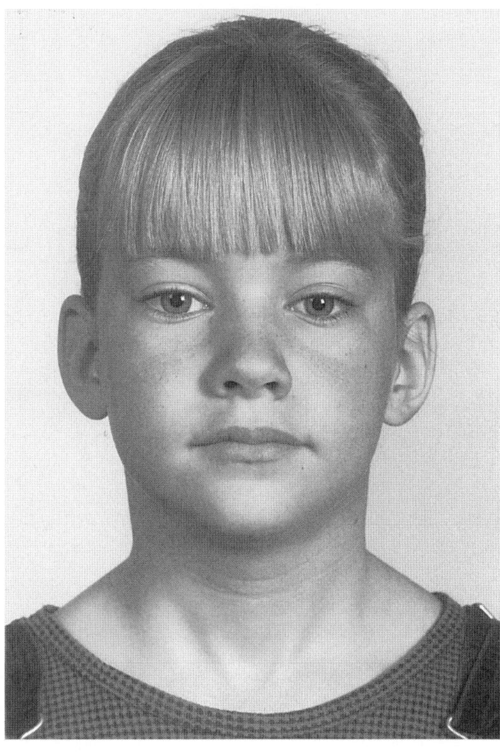

Fig. 3-55. Nasalis.

LEVATOR LABII SUPERIORIS

Patient raises upper lip as in showing upper teeth and gums (Fig. 3-56).

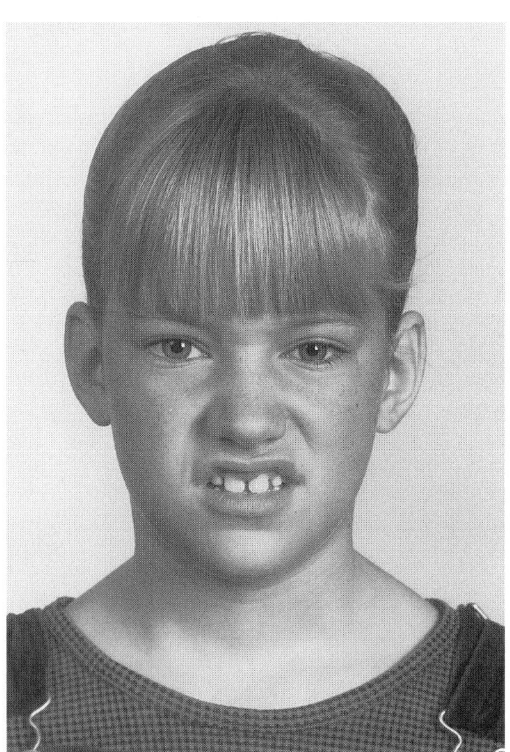

Fig. 3-56. Levator labii superioris.

LEVATOR ANGULI ORIS

Patient raises one side of upper lip as in sneering (Fig. 3-57).

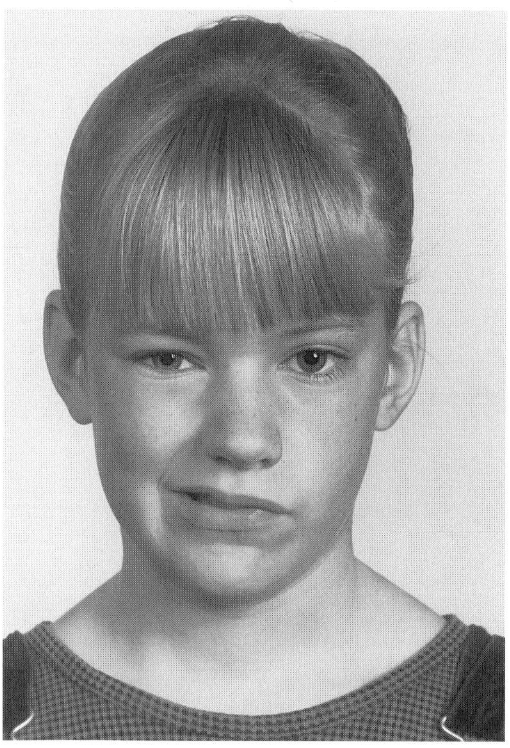

Fig. 3-57. Levator anguli oris.

ZYGOMATICUS MAJOR

Patient smiles (Fig. 3-58).

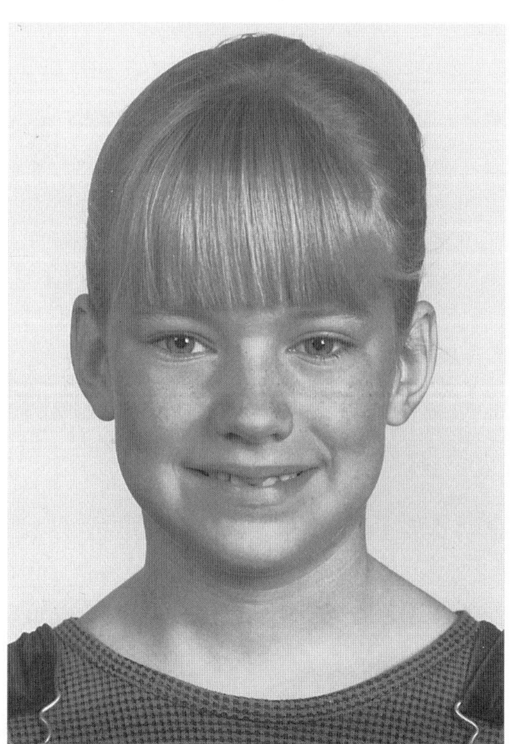

Fig. 3-58. Zygomaticus major.

ORBICULARIS ORIS

Patient compresses and protrudes lips as in whistling (Fig. 3-59).

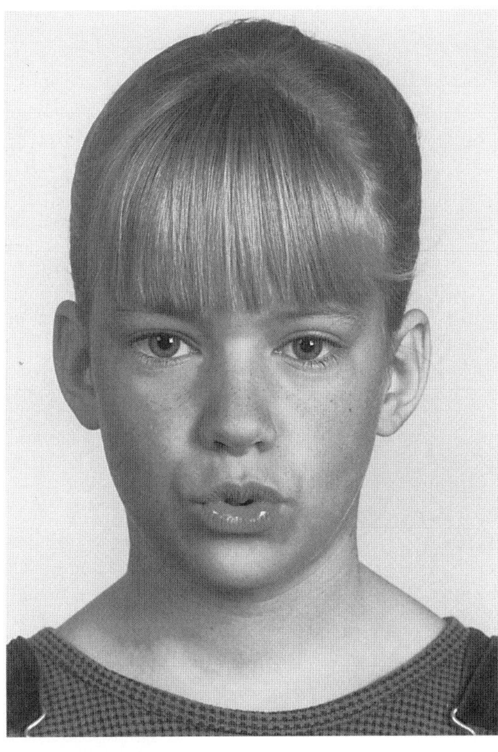

Fig. 3-59. Orbicularis oris.

RISORIUS

Patient pulls lateral angle of lips directly backward (Fig. 3-60).

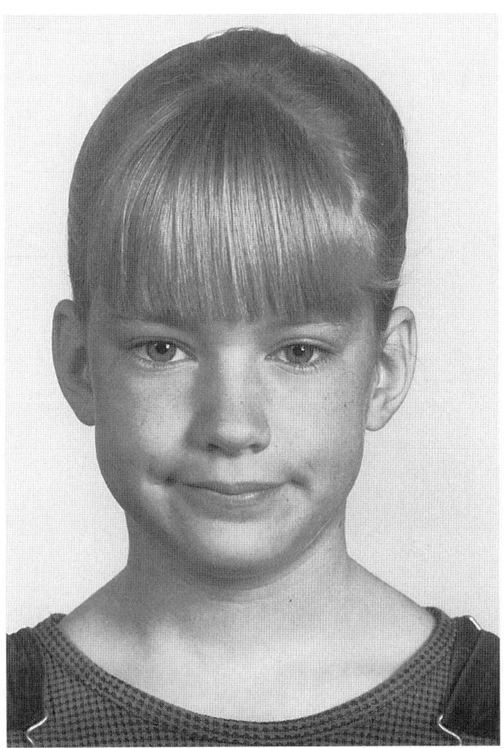

Fig. 3-60. Risorius.

BUCCINATOR

Patient pulls cheeks in against molars and pulls angle of mouth directly backward, as in blowing a flute or trumpet (Fig. 3-61).

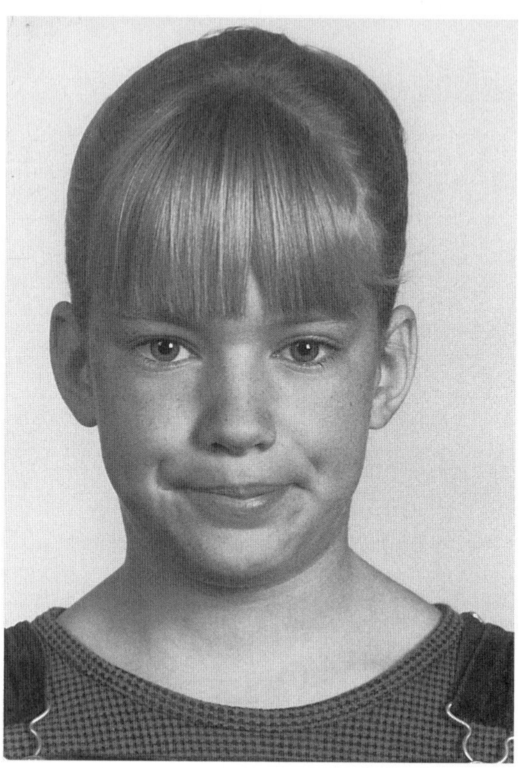

Fig. 3-61. Buccinator.

DEPRESSOR ANGULI ORIS

Patient pulls lateral angle of lips downward (Fig. 3-62).

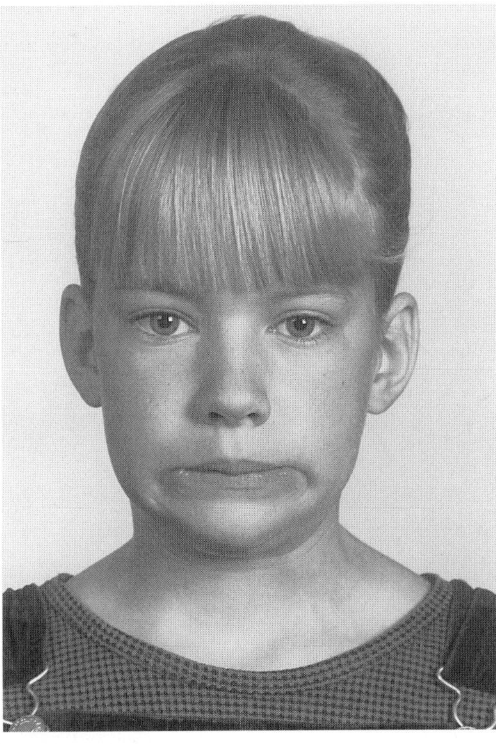

Fig. 3-62. Depressor anguli oris.

MENTALIS

Patient raises skin of chin while protruding lower lip (Fig. 3-63).

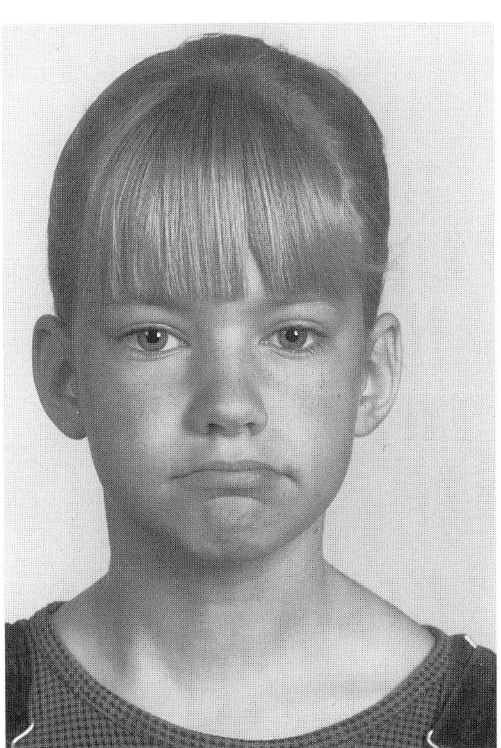

Fig. 3-63. Mentalis.

DEPRESSOR LABII INFERIORIS AND PLATYSMA

Patient pulls lateral angle of lips downward and backward while tensing skin of neck (Fig. 3-64).

Fig. 3-64. Depressor labii inferioris and platysma.

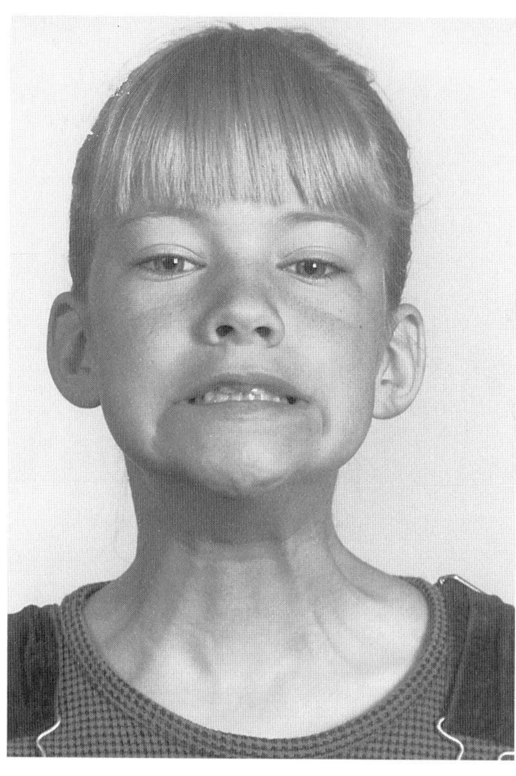

GRADING

Following muscle test grades should be used when evaluating muscles of facial expression.

For grade 5: Patient performs motion through full available ROM without difficulty.

For grade 3: Motion is performed but with difficulty, or only a partial ROM is completed.

For grade 1: No motion, but a palpable contraction is present.

For grade 0: No motion or contraction is present.

CLINICAL COMMENT: FACIAL WEAKNESS

When examining patients with facial weakness, function of the muscles of the forehead should be closely examined. Patients with LMN lesions (ex. Bell's palsy) will be unable to raise the eyebrow on the affected side or to close the eye tightly on that side. A patient with an UMN lesion has no such deficit of forehead movement (can raise both eyebrows). Eye closure ability is variable, as the number of ipsilateral corticobulbar fibers that innervate orbicularis oculi motor neurons is variable from person to person.

CASE 3-1 LUMBOSACRAL STRAIN

Ms. R is a 16-year-old high-school volleyball player who has complaints of left-sided lumbosacral pain following an intensive weekend volleyball tournament. During volleyball participation, the patient engages in forceful movements involving trunk rotation combined with flexion or extension. Pain is present when the patient is active or seated. The patient has excessive hamstring length secondary to a 12-year history of dance (ballet and jazz) and slightly tight quadriceps bilaterally. An essential part of your examination is a strength assessment of the trunk stabilizers.

Answer the following questions regarding your examination of this patient (you may want to refer to a kinesiologic textbook to assist with your answers). Note: This case is continued in Chapter 4: Techniques of Manual Muscle Testing: Lower Extremity.

1. What muscles are stabilizers of the lumbar spine? Provide the action(s) of each muscle listed in your answer.
2. How do the abdominal muscles assist in stabilization of the spine and pelvis?
3. Which abdominal muscles produce forceful rotation of the trunk to the left? Which muscles of the spine assist in this motion?
4. How is strength assessment of the trunk stabilizers accomplished? Contrast methods described in this text with those found in texts aimed at musculoskeletal assessment. Which methods would be most appropriate for this patient? Why?

CASE 3-2 FACIAL WEAKNESS

Mr. S is your 64-year-old neighbor who awoke one morning with weakness and drooping on the right side of his face. His wife, not sure what to do, and knowing you "knew about stuff like that," called and asked you to come see about her husband. She told you little over the telephone, other than her husband "couldn't move his mouth right." On the basis of the little that you know, you believe your neighbor's husband has suffered some pathology along the facial nerve or in the fibers from the cerebrum that control the facial nucleus.

Answer the following questions regarding this case (you may want to refer to an anatomy text to assist with your answers). Note: This case is continued in Chapter 9: Techniques of the Remainder of the Neurologic Examination.

1. What is the course of the facial nerve within the skull? Where does it exit?
2. After the facial nerve enters the parotid gland, it divides into five main branches. Name these branches and describe their general distribution.
3. How much of the patient's face would demonstrate weakness if the entire facial nerve were damaged during its course through the skull?
4. What is the disorder described in question number 3 commonly called?

Reference

Kendall FP, McCreary EK, Provance PG. *Muscles: Testing and Function*, 4th ed. Baltimore: Williams & Wilkins, 1993.

Bibliography

American Spinal Injury Association. *International Standards for Neurological Classification of Spinal Cord Injury*. Revised, 2002. Chicago: ASIA, 2002.

Andersson EA, Nilsson J, Ma Z, et al. Abdominal and hip flexor muscle activation during various training exercises. *Eur J Appl Physiol* 1997;75:115–123.

Aspden RM. Review of the functional anatomy of the spinal ligaments and the lumbar erector spinae muscles. *Clin Anat* 1992;5:372–387.

Basmajian JV, DeLuca CJ. *Muscles Alive: Their Function Revealed by Electromyography,* 5th ed. Baltimore: Williams & Wilkins, 1985.

Beimborn DS, Morrissey MC. A review of the literature related to trunk muscle performance. *Spine* 1988;13:655–660.

Bruintjes TD, Olphen AF, Hillen B, et al. Electromyography of the human nasal muscles. *Eur Arch Otorhinolaryngol* 1996;253:464–469.

Cacou C, Greenfield BE, Hunt NP, et al. Patterns of coordinated lower facial muscle function and their importance in facial reanimation. *Br J Plast Surg* 1996;49:274–280.

Carman DJ, Blanton PL, Biggs NL. Electromyographic study of the anterolateral abdominal musculature utilizing indwelling electrodes. *Am J Phys Med* 1972;51:113–129.

Clarkson HM: *Musculoskeletal Assessment: Joint Range of Motion and Manual Muscle Strength,* 2nd ed. Philadelphia: Lippincott, Williams & Wilkins, 2000.

Clemente CD. *Gray's Anatomy, 30th American ed.* Philadelphia: Lea & Febiger, 1985.

Daniels L, Worthingham C. *Muscle Testing: Techniques of Manual Examination,* 5th ed. Philadelphia: WB Saunders, 1986.

Devinsky O, Feldmann E. *Examination of the Cranial and Peripheral Nerves.* New York: Churchill Livingstone, 1988.

Donisch EW, Basmajian JV. Electromyography of deep back muscles in man. *Am J Anat* 1972;133:25–36.

Florence JM, Pandya S, King WM, et al. Intrarater reliability of manual muscle test (Medical Research Council scale) grades in Duchenne's muscular dystrophy. *Phys Ther* 1992;72:115–126.

Floyd WF, Silver PHS. The function of the erectors spinae muscles in certain movements and postures in man. *J Physiol* 1955;129:184–203.

Gilleard WL, Brown JM. An electromyographic validation of an abdominal muscle test. *Arch Phys Med Rehabil* 1994;75:1002–1006.

Haynes, MJ. Doppler studies comparing the effects of cervical rotation and lateral flexion on vertebral artery blood flow. *J Manip Physiol Ther* 1996;19:378–384.

Hoppenfeld S. *Physical Examination of the Spine and Extremities.* New York: Appleton-Century-Crofts, 1976.

Isley CL, Basmajian JV. Electromyography of the human cheeks and lips. *Anat Rec* 1973;176: 143–147.

Juker D, McGill S, Kropf P, et al. Quantitative intramuscular myoelectric activity of lumbar portions of psoas and the abdominal wall during a wide variety of tasks. *Med Sci Sports Exerc* 1998;30:301–310.

Keagy RD, Brumlik J, Bergan JJ. Direct electromyography of the psoas major muscle in man. *J Bone Joint Surg* 1966;48A:1377–1382.

Kumar S, Narayan Y, Zedka M. An electromyographic study of unresisted trunk rotation with normal velocity among healthy subjects. *Spine* 1996;21:1500–1512.

Lehman GJ, McGill SM. Quantification of the differences in electromyographic activity magnitude between the upper and lower portions of the rectus abdominis muscles during selected trunk exercises. *Phys Ther* 2001;81:1096–1101.

Lefkof MB. Trunk flexion in healthy children aged 3 to 7 years. *Phys Ther* 1986;66:39–44.

Macintosh JE, Bogduk N. The attachments of the lumbar erector spinae. *Spine* 1991;16:763–792.

Magee DJ. *Orthopedic Physical Assessment*, 4th ed. Philadelphia: WB Saunders, 2002.

Mahan PE, et al. Superior and inferior bellies of the lateral pterygoid muscle EMG activity at basic jaw positions. *J Prosthet Dent* 1983;50:710–718.

McNamara JA. The independent functions of the two heads of lateral pterygoid muscle. *Am J Anat* 1973;138:197–206.

Reider B. *The Orthopaedic Physical Examination*. Philadelphia: WB Saunders, 1999.

Sarti MA, Monfort M, Fuster MA, et al. Muscle activity in upper and lower rectus abdominus during abdominal exercises. *Arch Phys Med Rehabil* 1996;77:1293–1297.

Shields RK, Heiss DG. An electromyographic comparison of abdominal muscle synergies during curl and double straight leg lowering exercises with control of the pelvic position. *Spine* 1997;22:1873–1879.

Smidt GL, Amundsen LR, Dostal WF. Muscle strength at the trunk. *J Orthop Sports Phys Ther* 1980;1:165–170.

Smidt GL, Blanpied PR, Anderson MA, et al. Comparison of clinical and objective methods of assessing trunk muscle strength: an experimental approach. *Spine* 1987;12:1020–1024.

Smidt GL, Blanpied PR. Analysis of strength test and resistive exercises commonly used for low-back disorders. *Spine* 1987;12:1025–1034.

Vitti M, Fujiwara M, Basmajian V, et al. The integrated roles of longus colli and sternocleidomastoid muscles: an electromyographic study. *Anat Rec* 1973;177:471–484.

4

TECHNIQUES of MANUAL MUSCLE TESTING: LOWER EXTREMITY

■ HIP FLEXION

ILIACUS AND PSOAS MAJOR (Fig. 4-1)

Fig. 4-1.

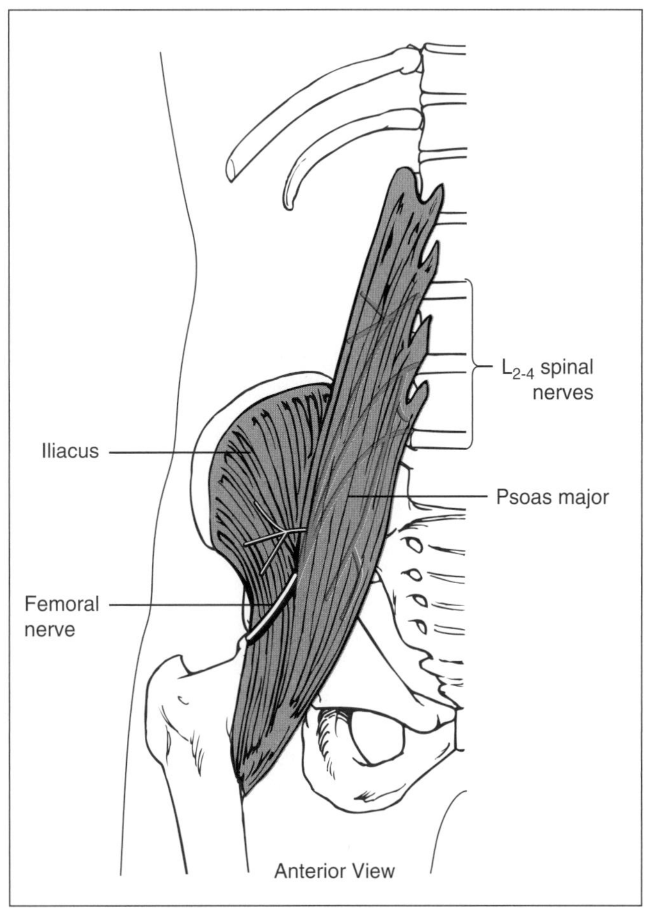

	ATTACHMENTS	NERVE SUPPLY	FUNCTION
Iliacus	Origin: Superior ⅔ of the iliac fossa, iliac crest, anterior sacroiliac and iliolumbar ligaments, ala of sacrum Insertion: Tendon of the psoas major, body of the femur	Peripheral nerve: Femoral nerve Nerve root: L2–L3	Flexion of the hip
Psoas major	Origin: Sides of the vertebral bodies and corresponding intervertebral discs of T12–L5 and transverse processes of L1–L5 Insertion: Lesser trochanter of the femur	Peripheral nerve: N/A Nerve root: L2–L4	Unilateral action: Flexion of the hip Bilateral action: With the thigh fixed, the psoas major flexes the trunk

Gravity-Resisted Test (Grades 5, 4, and 3)

Patient position: Seated with legs off side of treatment table, holding on to table edge with hands (Fig. 4-2).

Fig. 4-2.

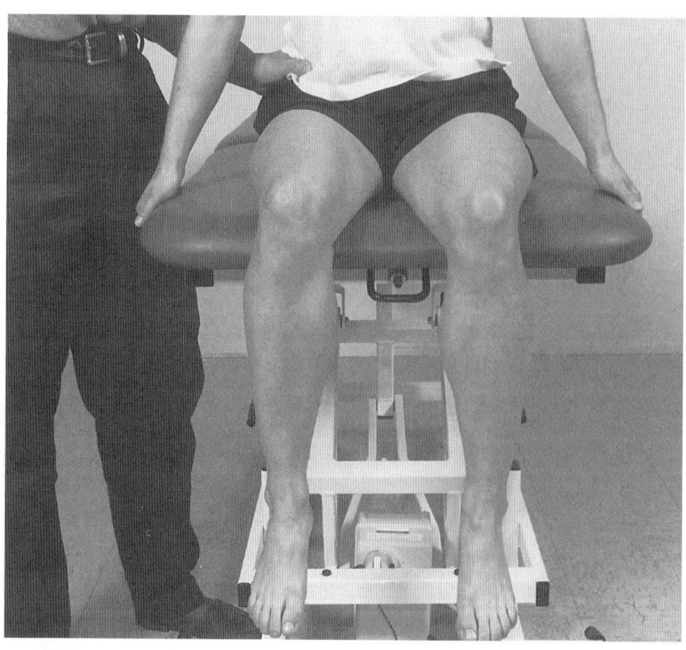

Stabilization/palpation: Stabilize pelvis over ipsilateral iliac crest (Fig. 4-2). Iliacus and psoas major are deep and very difficult to palpate.

Examiner action: While instructing patient in motion desired, flex patient's hip through full available range of motion (ROM), keeping knee flexed. Return limb to starting position. Performing passive movement allows determination of patient's available ROM and shows patient exact motion desired.

Patient action:

Patient flexes hip through full available ROM while keeping knee flexed. Examiner stabilizes pelvis during patient's active movement (Fig. 4-3).

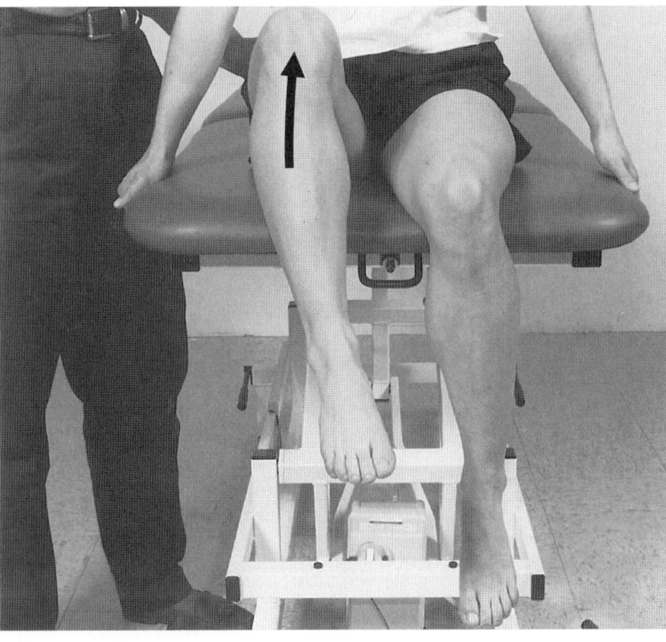

Fig. 4-3. Arrow indicates direction of movement.

Resistance:

Apply resistance over anterior aspect of distal thigh in direction of hip extension (Fig. 4-4).

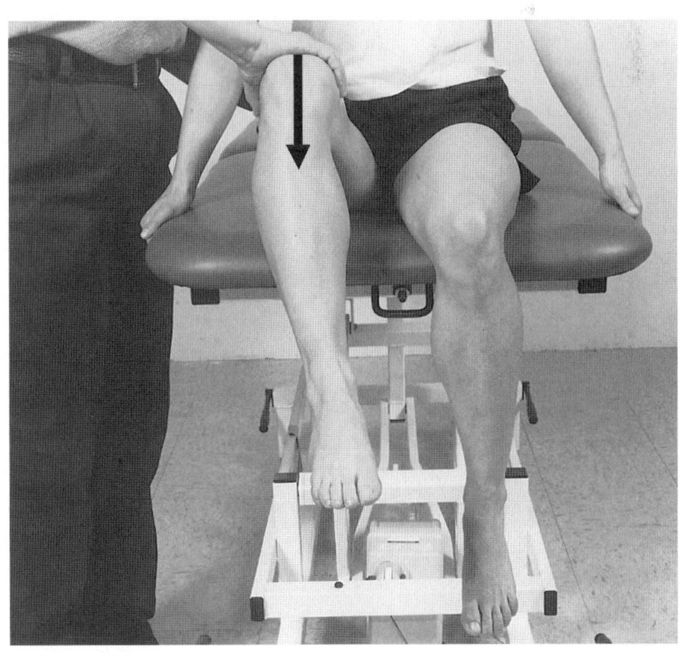

Fig. 4-4. Arrow indicates direction of resistance.

Gravity-Eliminated Test (Grades Below 3)

For patients unable to move through available ROM against gravity.

Patient position: Side lying on side of lower extremity to be tested, hip extended, knee flexed. Talcum powder and a cloth may be placed between limb and supporting surface to reduce friction (Fig. 4-5; starting position of extremity not shown).

Fig. 4-5. Arrow indicates direction of movement.

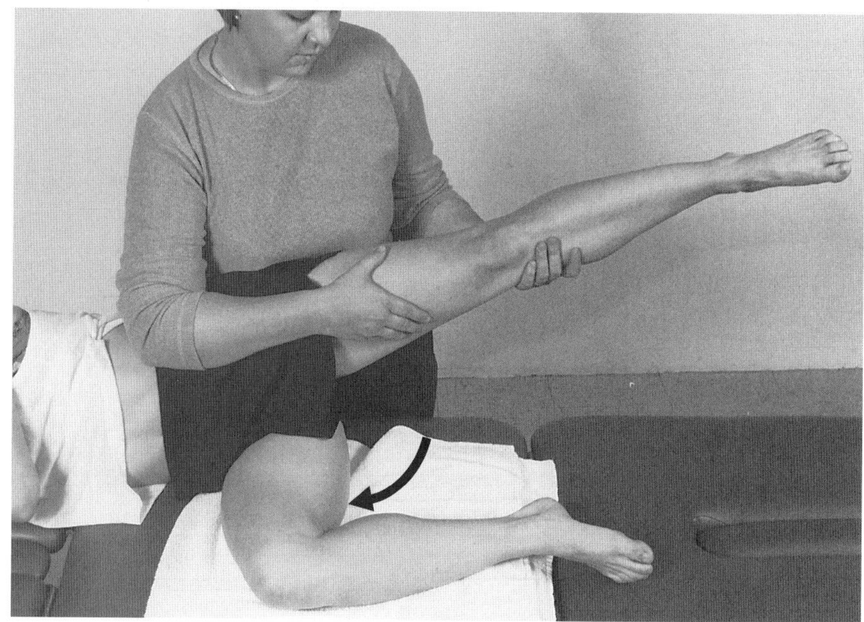

Stabilization/palpation: Stabilize pelvis and support uppermost lower extremity by standing behind patient (Fig. 4-5).

Examiner action: As in gravity-resisted test.

Patient action: Patient flexes hip of lower limb through full available ROM while keeping knee flexed. Examiner stabilizes pelvis during patient's active movement (Fig. 4-5).

COMMON SUBSTITUTIONS

1. Sartorius: Patient may substitute with sartorius by abducting hip and rotating it laterally during hip flexion in gravity-resisted position (Fig. 4-6).
2. Rectus femoris: Patients attempting to substitute with rectus femoris will demonstrate knee extension during hip flexion.

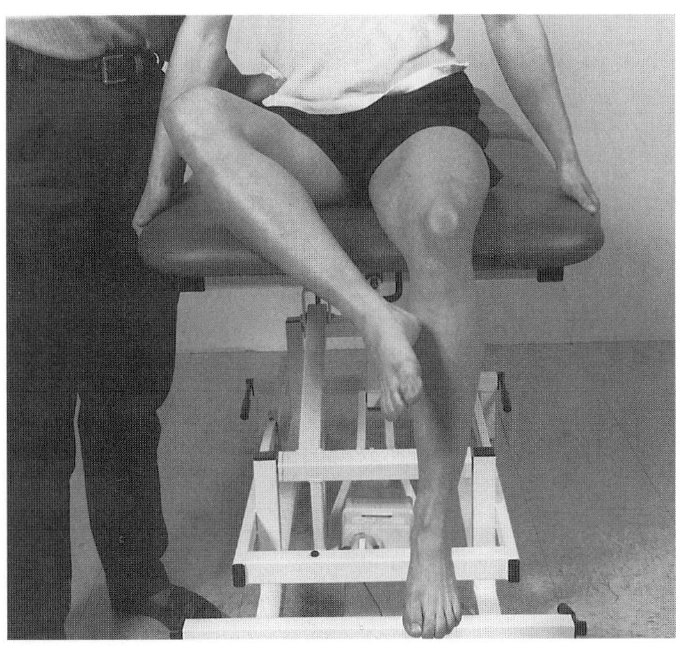

Fig. 4-6. Substitution by sartorius.

CLINICAL COMMENT: ILIOPSOAS MUSCLE AND L1 NEUROLOGIC ASSESSMENT

The iliopsoas muscle is a key muscle for examining the integrity of the L1 and L2 spinal nerves or neurologic segments of the spinal cord. Complete assessment of the L1 neurologic level includes:

Strength assessment of:
Iliopsoas (pp. 254-256)

Sensory testing of:
Skin just below inguinal ligament (L1 dermatome; pp. 528-532)

■ HIP FLEXION, ABDUCTION AND LATERAL ROTATION

SARTORIUS (Fig. 4-7)

Fig. 4-7.

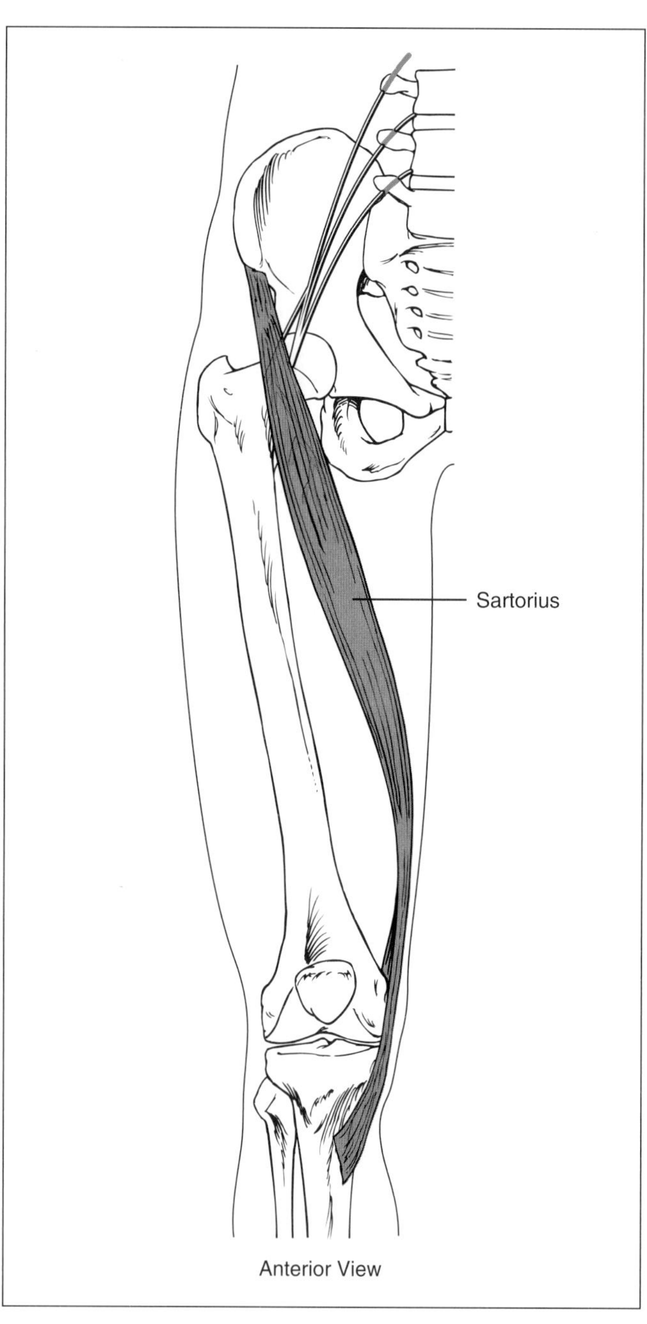

	ATTACHMENTS	NERVE SUPPLY	FUNCTION
Sartorius	Origin: Anterior superior iliac spine, upper aspect of the iliac notch Insertion: Proximal aspect of the medial surface of the tibia	Peripheral nerve: Femoral nerve Nerve root: L2, L3	Flexion, abduction, and lateral rotation of the hip, flexion of the knee

Gravity-Resisted Test (Grades 5, 4, and 3)

Patient position: Seated with legs off side of treatment table, holding on to table edge with hands (Fig. 4-8).

Fig. 4-8.

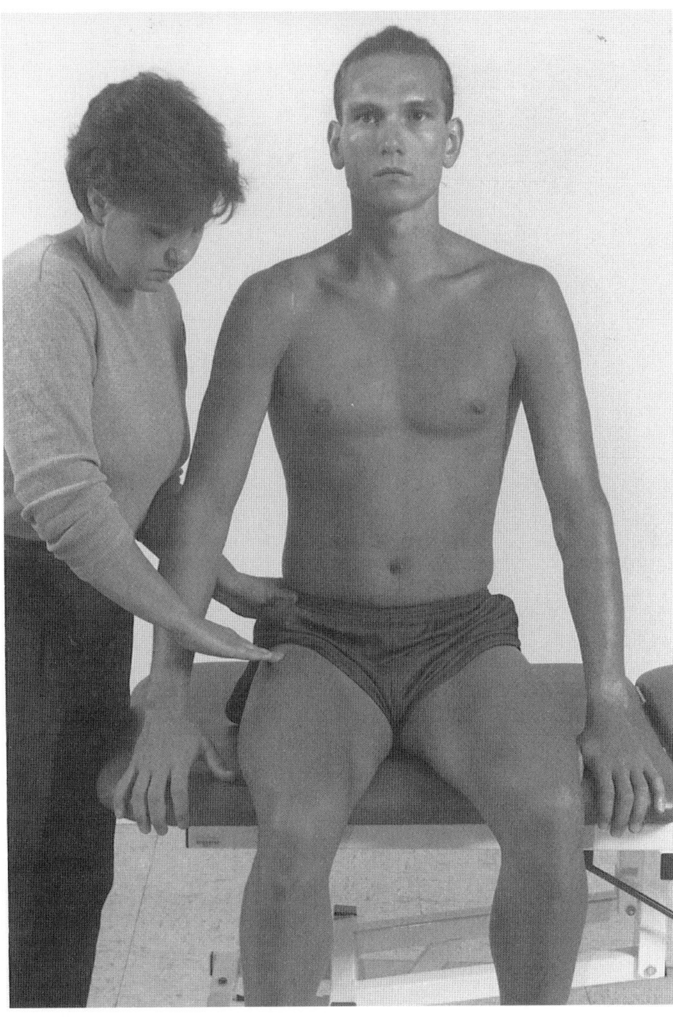

Stabilization/palpation: Stabilize pelvis over ipsilateral iliac crest with one hand. With opposite hand, palpate sartorius beginning just distal to anterosuperior iliac spine (Fig. 4-8).

Examiner action: While instructing patient in motion desired, flex, abduct, and laterally rotate patient's hip, while flexing knee (instruct patient to slide heel of limb being tested up shin of opposite leg). Return limb to starting position. Performing passive movement allows determination of patient's available ROM and shows patient exact motion desired.

Patient action:

Patient flexes, abducts, and laterally rotates hip while flexing knee. Examiner stabilizes pelvis and palpates sartorius during patient's active movement (Fig. 4-9).

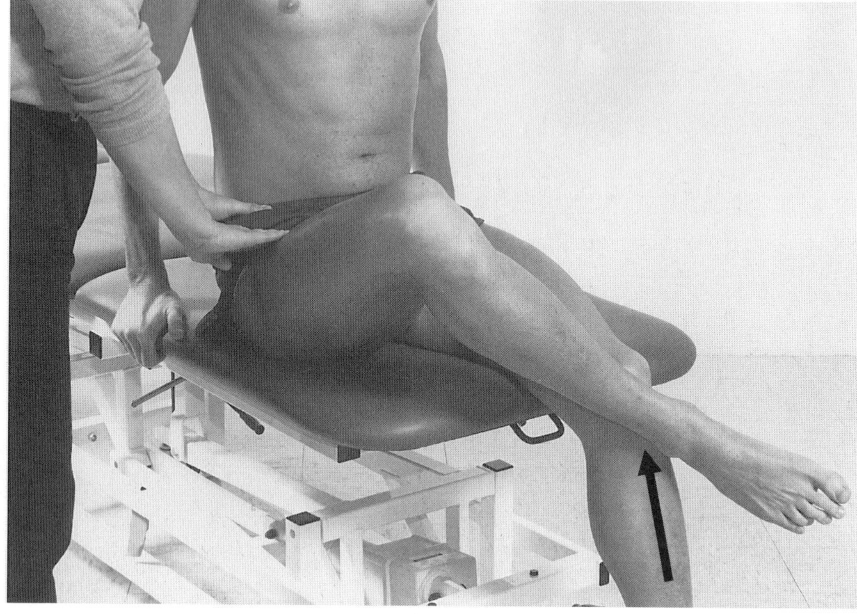

Fig. 4-9. Arrow indicates direction of movement of heel.

Resistance:

Apply resistance by moving palpating and stabilizing hands to ankle and anterolateral thigh. One hand applies resistance over anterolateral aspect of thigh in direction of hip extension and adduction while other hand applies resistance on medial side of ankle in direction of hip medial rotation and knee extension (Fig. 4-10).

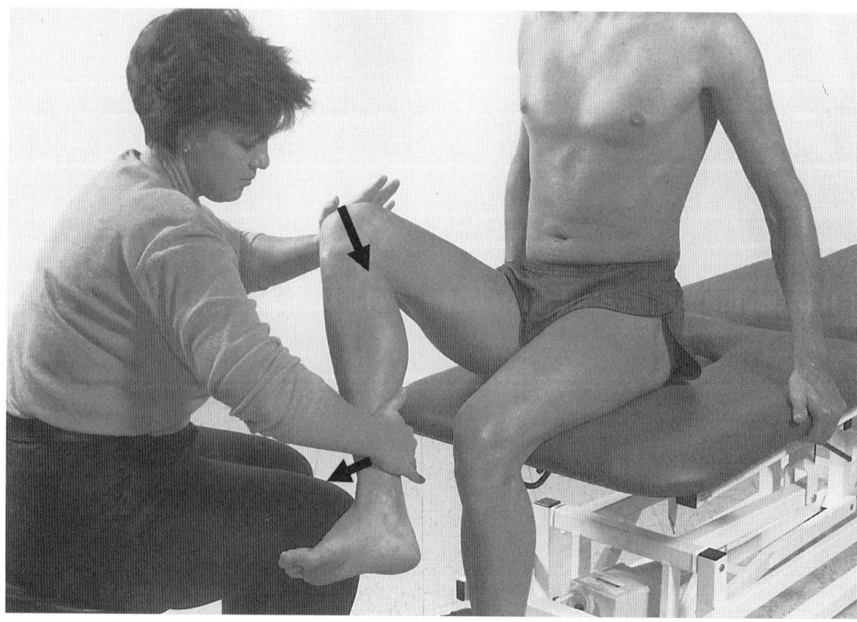

Fig. 4-10. Arrows indicate direction of resistance.

Gravity-Eliminated Test (Grades Below 3)

For patients unable to move through available ROM against gravity.

Patient position: Supine with heel of lower extremity to be tested on ventral surface of contralateral ankle, contralateral lower extremity extended (Fig. 4-11; starting position of test limb not shown).

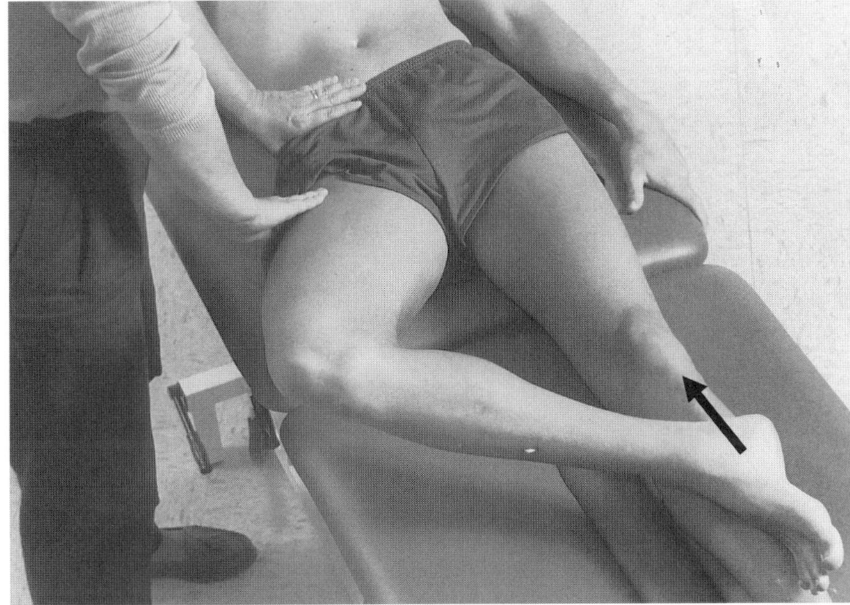

Fig. 4-11. Arrow indicates direction of movement of heel.

Stabilization/palpation: Stabilize ipsilateral pelvis. With opposite hand, palpate sartorius (as in gravity-resisted test) (Fig. 4-11).

Examiner action: As in gravity-resisted test

Patient action: Patient slides heel of limb to be tested up shin of opposite leg. Examiner stabilizes pelvis and palpates sartorius during patient's active movement (Fig. 4-11).

COMMON SUBSTITUTIONS

Iliopsoas or rectus femoris: Patient will flex hip without accompanying abduction or lateral rotation (see Fig. 4-3). If patient attempts to substitute with rectus femoris, knee extension will occur.

CLINICAL COMMENT: ILIOPSOAS MUSCLE AND L2 NEUROLOGIC ASSESSMENT

The iliopsoas muscle is a key muscle for examining the integrity of the L1 and L2 spinal nerves or neurologic segments of the spinal cord. Complete assessment of the L2 neurologic level includes:

Strength assessment of:
Iliopsoas (pp. 254-256)

Sensory testing of:
Skin over anterior aspect of thigh (L2 dermatome; pp. 528-532)

■ HIP EXTENSION

GLUTEUS MAXIMUS, SEMITENDINOSUS, SEMIMEMBRANOSUS, AND BICEPS FEMORIS (Figs. 4-12 and 4-13)

Fig. 4-12.

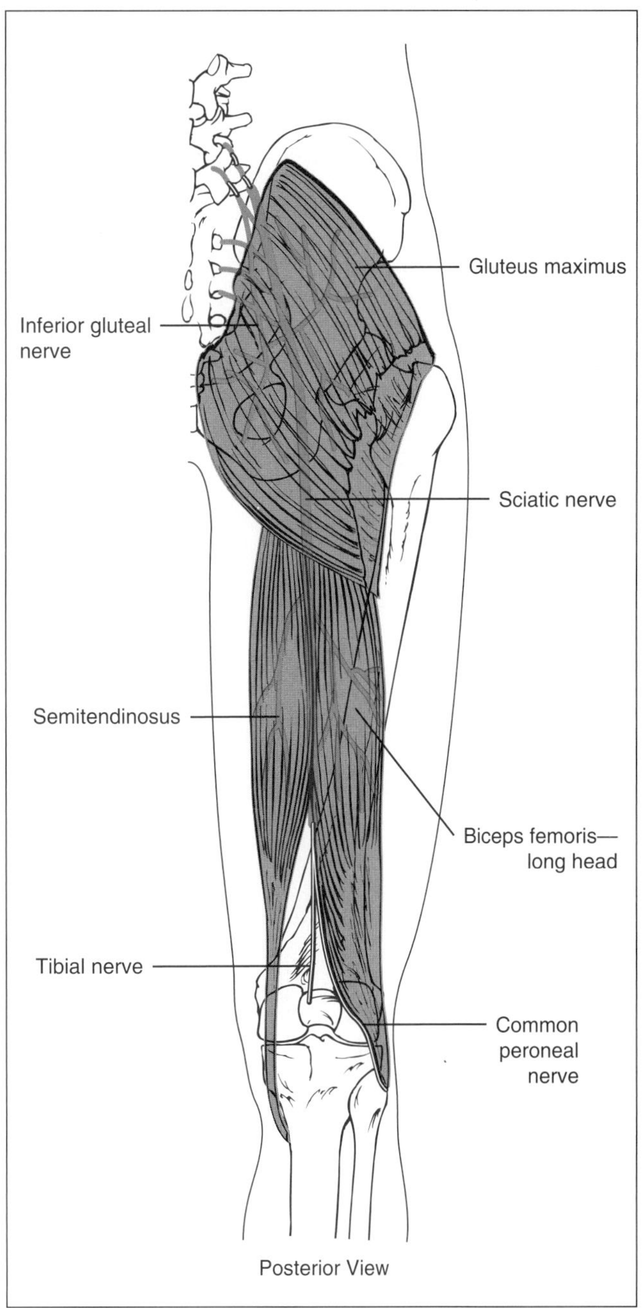

Fig. 4-13.

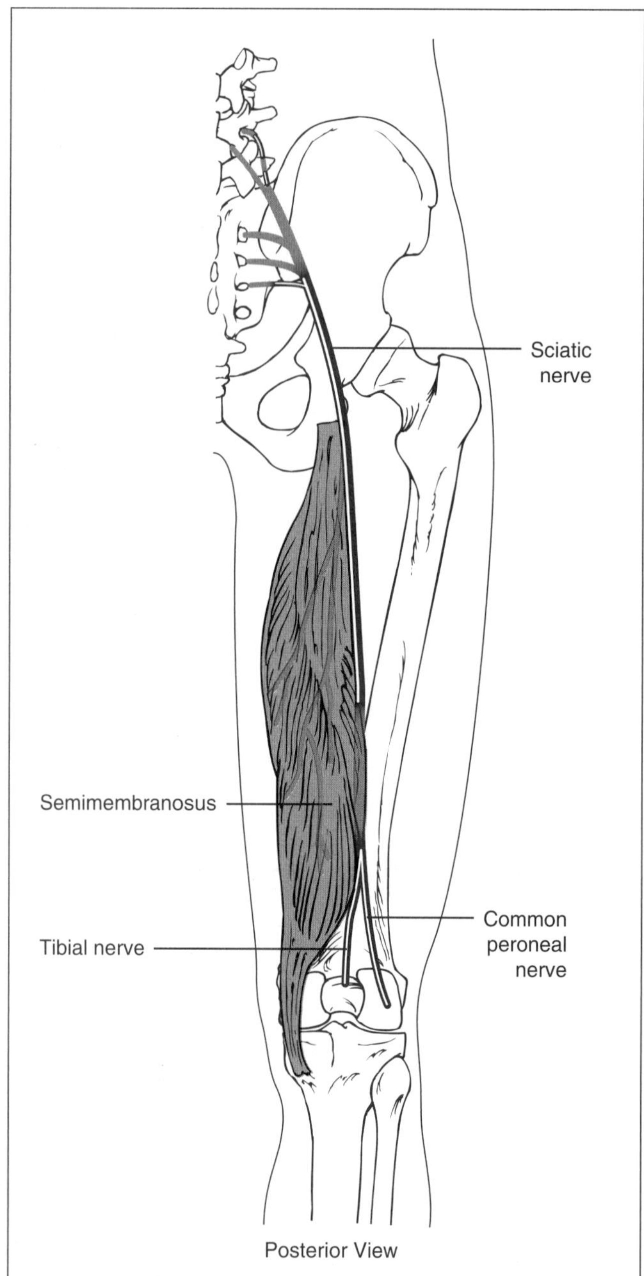
Sciatic nerve
Semimembranosus
Common peroneal nerve
Tibial nerve
Posterior View

	ATTACHMENTS	NERVE SUPPLY	FUNCTION
Gluteus maximus	Origin: Posterior gluteal line of the ilium, iliac crest, dorsum of the sacrum and coccyx, sacrotuberous ligament Insertion: Iliotibial tract, gluteal tuberosity of the femur	Peripheral nerve: Inferior gluteal nerve Nerve root: L5, S1, S2	Extension and lateral rotation of the hip
Semitendinosus	Origin: Ischial tuberosity Insertion: Proximal aspect of the medial surface of the tibia	Peripheral nerve: Tibial portion of the sciatic nerve Nerve root: L5, S1, S2	Extension of the hip, flexion and medial rotation of the knee
Semimembranosus	Origin: Ischial tuberosity Insertion: Medial condyle of the tibia	Peripheral nerve: Tibial portion of the sciatic nerve	Extension of the hip, flexion and medial rotation of the knee
Biceps femoris	Origin: Long head: Ischial tuberosity Short head: Lateral lip of the linea aspera of the femur and the lateral intermuscular septum Insertion: Lateral aspect of the head of the fibula	Peripheral nerve: Long head: Tibial portion of the sciatic nerve Short head: Peroneal portion of the sciatic nerve Nerve root: L5, S1, S2	Extension of the hip, flexion and lateral rotation of the knee

Gravity-Resisted Test (Grades 5, 4, and 3)

Patient position: Prone with lower extremities extended (Fig. 4-14).

Fig. 4-14.

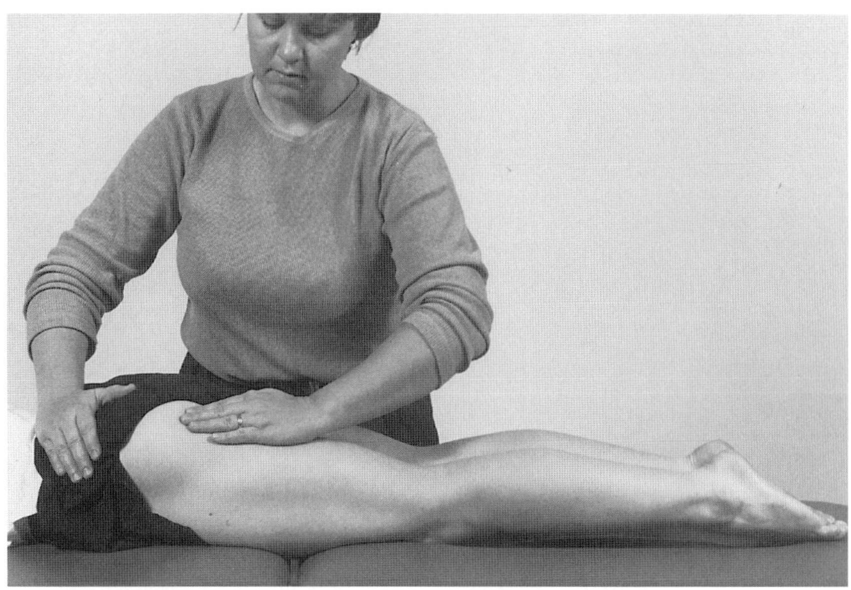

Stabilization/palpation: Stabilize with one hand over posterosuperior aspect of pelvis. With opposite hand, palpate gluteus maximus and proximal hamstrings over posteroinferior pelvis and posterosuperior thigh (Fig. 4-14).

Examiner action:

While instructing patient in motion desired, extend patient's hip through full available ROM while keeping knee extended. Return limb to starting position. Performing passive movement allows determination of patient's available ROM and shows patient exact motion desired.

Patient action:

Patient extends hip through full available ROM, keeping knee extended. Examiner stabilizes pelvis and palpates hip extensors during patient's active movement (Fig. 4-15).

Fig. 4-15. Arrow indicates direction of movement.

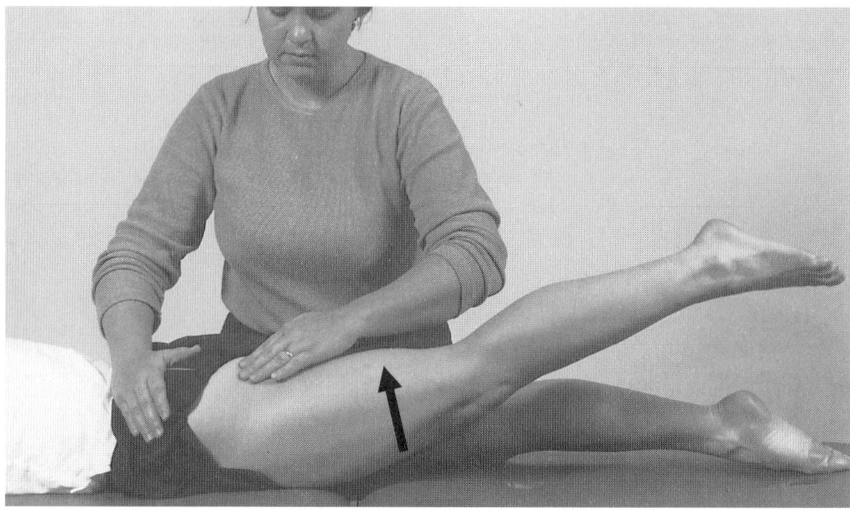

Resistance:

Apply resistance over posterior aspect of distal thigh in direction of hip flexion. Palpating hand is moved to posterior thigh to apply resistance (Fig. 4-16).

Fig. 4-16. Arrow indicates direction of resistance.

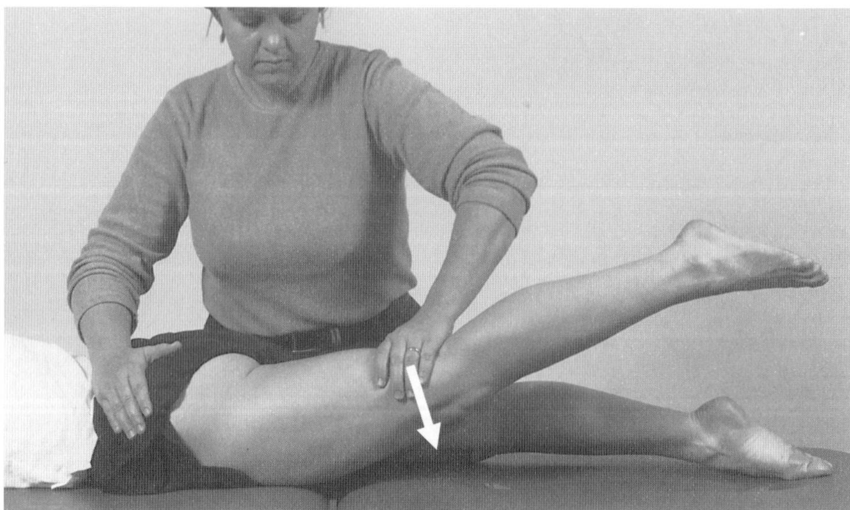

Gravity-Eliminated Test (Grades Below 3)

For patients unable to move through available ROM against gravity.

Patient position:

Side lying on side of lower extremity to be tested, hip of lowermost limb in slight flexion, patient's pelvis close to examiner's trunk for stabilization. Talcum powder and a cloth may be placed between lower extremity and supporting surface to reduce friction (Fig. 4-17; starting position of test limb not shown).

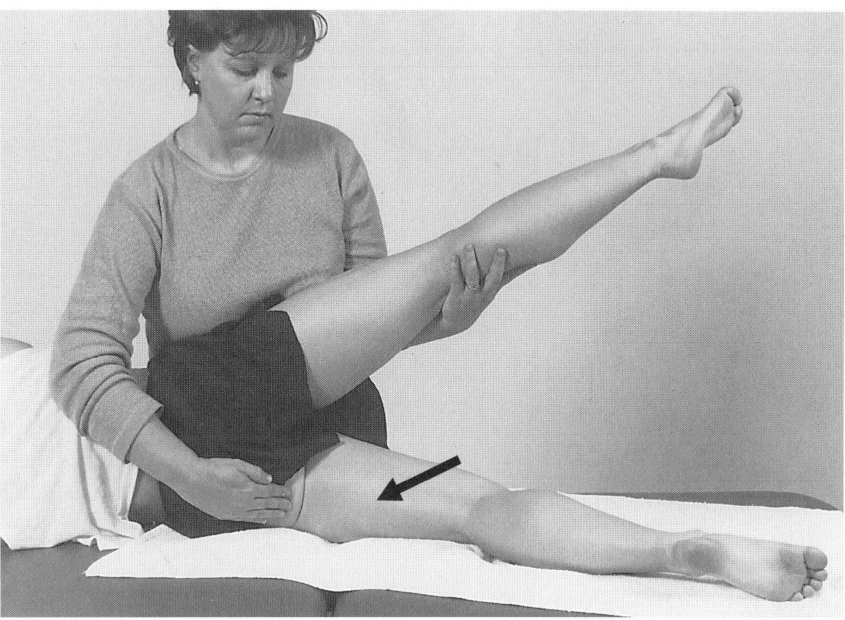

Fig. 4-17. Arrow indicates direction of movement.

Stabilization/palpation:

Stand directly in front of patient's pelvis, support uppermost lower extremity, and stabilize pelvis with one hand. With opposite hand, palpate gluteus maximus (as in gravity-resisted test) (Fig. 4-17).

Examiner action:

As in gravity-resisted test.

Patient action:

Patient extends hip through full available ROM while examiner stabilizes pelvis and palpates hip extensors (Fig. 4-17).

CLINICAL COMMENT: GLUTEUS MAXIMUS MUSCLE AND S1 NEUROLOGIC ASSESSMENT

The gluteus maximus muscle is a key muscle for examining the integrity of the S1 spinal nerve or neurologic segment of the spinal cord. Complete assessment of the S1 neurologic level includes:

Strength assessment of:
Gluteus maximus (pp. 265-267)
Gastrocnemius (pp. 317-321)
Soleus (pp. 317-321)
Peroneus longus and brevis (pp. 339-342)

Reflex testing of:
Achilles reflex (p. 551)

Sensory testing of:
Skin over the plantar surface of the foot and little toe (S1 dermatome; pp. 528-532)

■ HIP EXTENSION—ALTERNATIVE TESTS

GLUTEUS MAXIMUS: OPTION I

Gluteus maximus extends and laterally rotates hip.[1,2,3] Stronger activation of muscle occurs when both actions are combined. Test described below examines both extension and lateral rotation functions of gluteus maximus.

Gravity-Resisted Test (Grades 5 and 4)

Patient position: Prone with hip of limb to be tested in full lateral rotation, knee extended (Fig. 4-18).

Fig. 4-18.

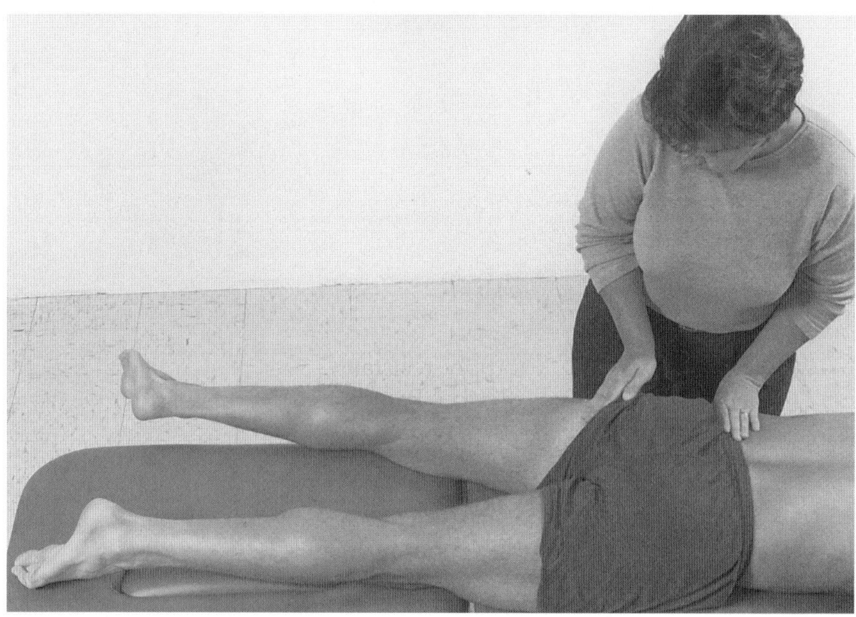

Stabilization/palpation: Stabilize over posterosuperior aspect of pelvis. With opposite hand, palpate gluteus maximus over posteroinferior aspect of pelvis (Fig. 4-18).

Examiner action: While instructing patient in motion desired, extend patient's hip through full available ROM, maintaining hip in lateral rotation and knee in extension. Return limb to starting position. Performing passive movement allows determination of patient's available ROM and shows patient exact motion desired.

Patient action:

Patient extends hip through full available ROM while maintaining hip in full lateral rotation. Examiner stabilizes pelvis and palpates gluteus maximus during patient's active movement (Fig. 4-19).

Fig. 4-19. Arrow indicates direction of movement.

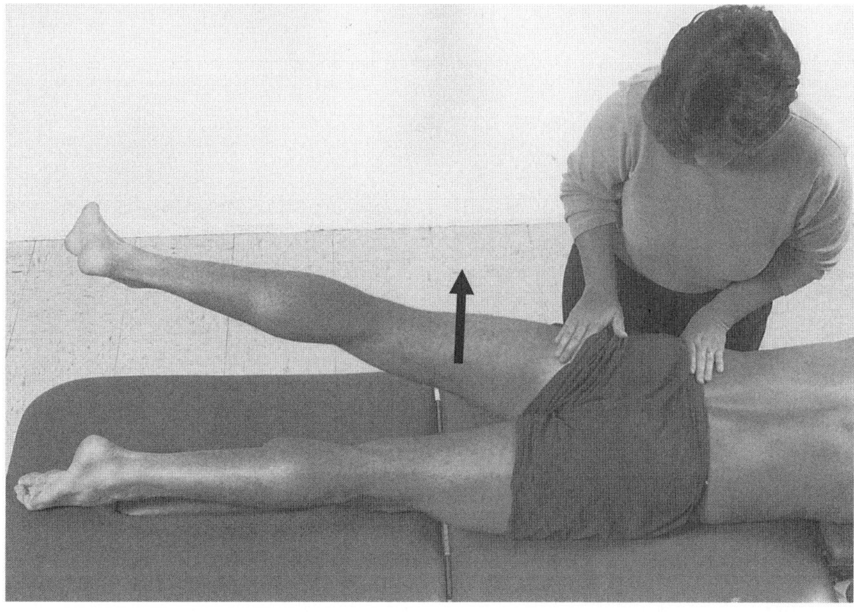

Resistance:

Apply resistance over posterolateral aspect of distal thigh in direction of hip flexion. Palpating hand is moved to distal thigh to apply resistance (Fig. 4-20).

Fig. 4-20. Arrow indicates direction of resistance.

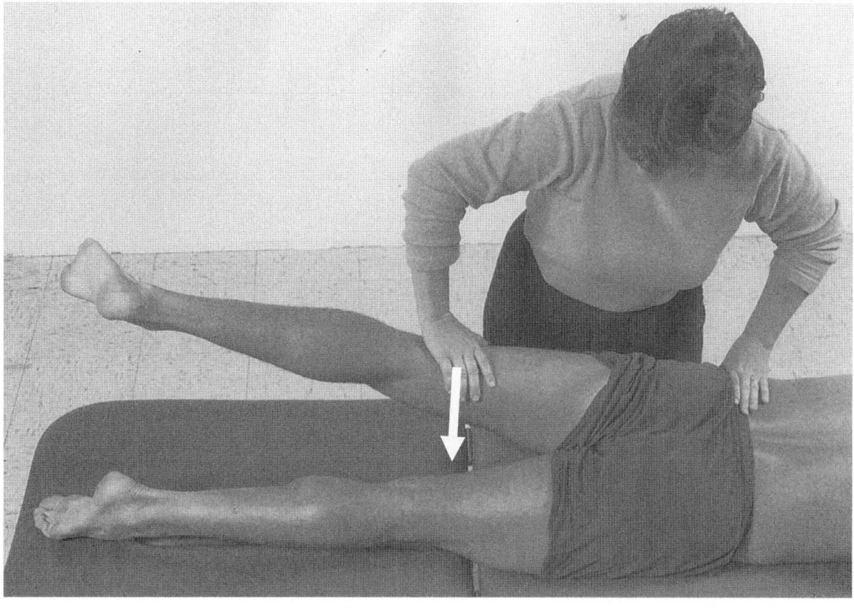

Grades 3 and Below

For patients unable to move through available ROM against gravity.

There is no separate test of this muscle for grades below 3. Grading is altered as follows to accommodate lack of a gravity-eliminated position.

For grade 3: Patient moves joint through full ROM without resistance.

For grade 2: Patient moves joint through partial ROM.

For grade 1: No motion, but a palpable contraction is present (see Fig. 4-18).

For grade 0: No motion or contraction is present.

GLUTEUS MAXIMUS: OPTION II

Positioning for this test reflects effort to decrease participation of hamstring muscles in action of hip extension. By flexing knee, hamstrings are placed in shortened position, reducing their effectiveness as hip extensors. Examiner should be aware that cramping of hamstrings can occur during resisted hip extension with knee flexed.

Gravity-Resisted Test (Grades 5, 4, and 3)

Patient position: Prone with hips in extension, knee of limb to be tested in 90° flexion (Fig. 4-21).

Fig. 4-21.

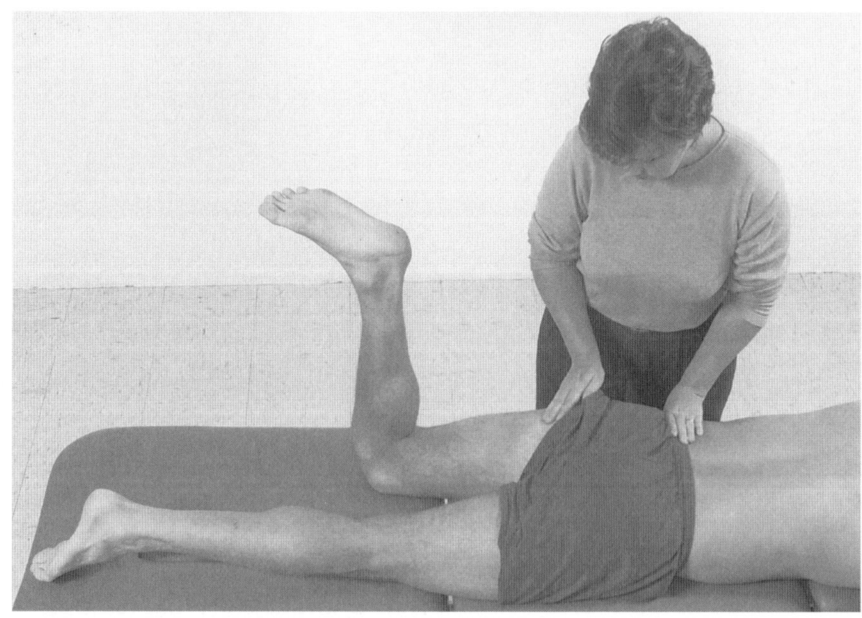

Stabilization/palpation: Stabilize over posterosuperior aspect of pelvis. With opposite hand, palpate gluteus maximus over posteroinferior aspect of pelvis (Fig. 4-21).

Examiner action:

While instructing patient in motion desired, extend patient's hip through full available ROM, keeping knee flexed. Return limb to starting position. Performing passive movement allows determination of patient's available ROM and shows patient exact motion desired.

Patient action:

Patient extends hip through full available ROM while maintaining knee in 90° flexion. Examiner stabilizes pelvis and palpates gluteus maximus during patient's active movement (Fig. 4-22).

Fig. 4-22. Arrow indicates direction of movement.

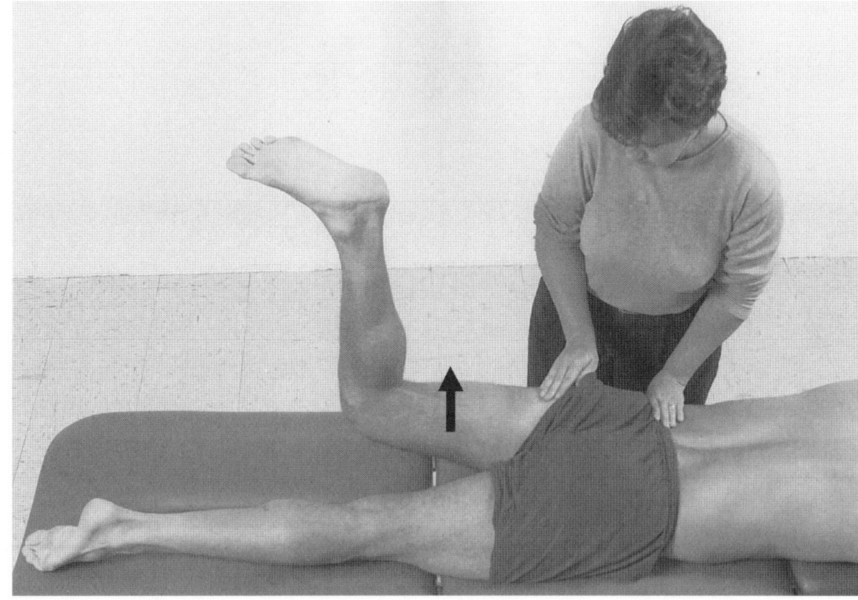

Resistance:

Apply resistance over posterior aspect of distal thigh in direction of hip flexion. Palpating hand is moved to distal thigh to apply resistance (Fig. 4-23).

Fig. 4-23. Arrow indicates direction of resistance.

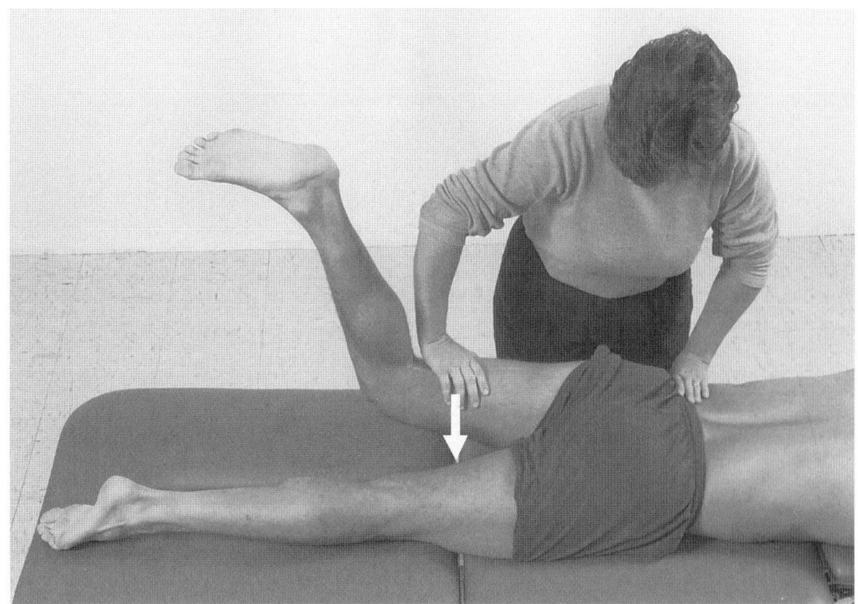

Gravity-Eliminated Test (Grades Below 3)

For patients unable to move through available ROM against gravity.

Patient position: Side lying on side of limb to be tested with hip of test limb in slight flexion, knee of test limb flexed to 90°, patient's pelvis close to examiner's trunk for stabilization. Talcum powder and a cloth may be placed between limb and supporting surface to reduce friction (Fig. 4-24; starting hip position of test limb not shown).

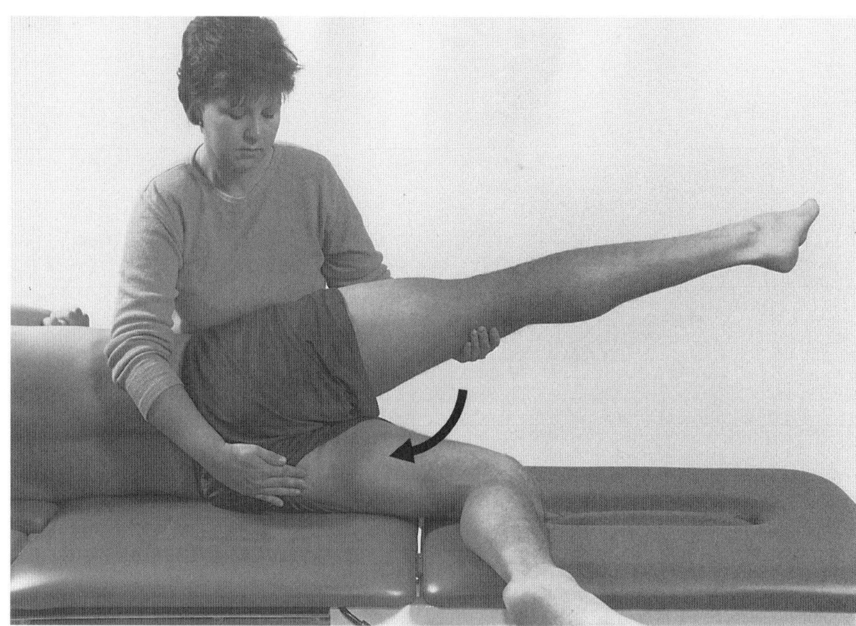

Fig. 4-24. Arrow indicates direction of movement.

Stabilization/palpation: Stand directly in front of patient's pelvis, support uppermost lower extremity and stabilize pelvis with one hand. With opposite hand, palpate gluteus maximus (e.g., as in gravity-resisted test) of limb to be tested (Fig. 4-24).

Examiner action: As in gravity-resisted test.

Patient action: Patient extends hip through full available ROM without extending knee. Examiner stabilizes pelvis and palpates gluteus maximus during patient's active movement (Fig. 4-24).

HIP ABDUCTION

GLUTEUS MEDIUS AND MINIMUS (Figs. 4-25 and 4-26)

Fig. 4-25.

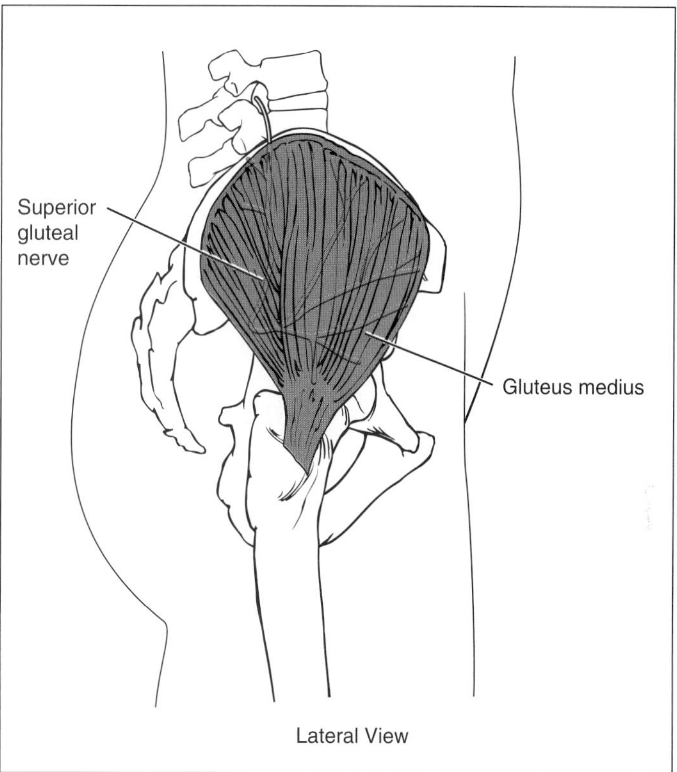

Fig. 4-26.

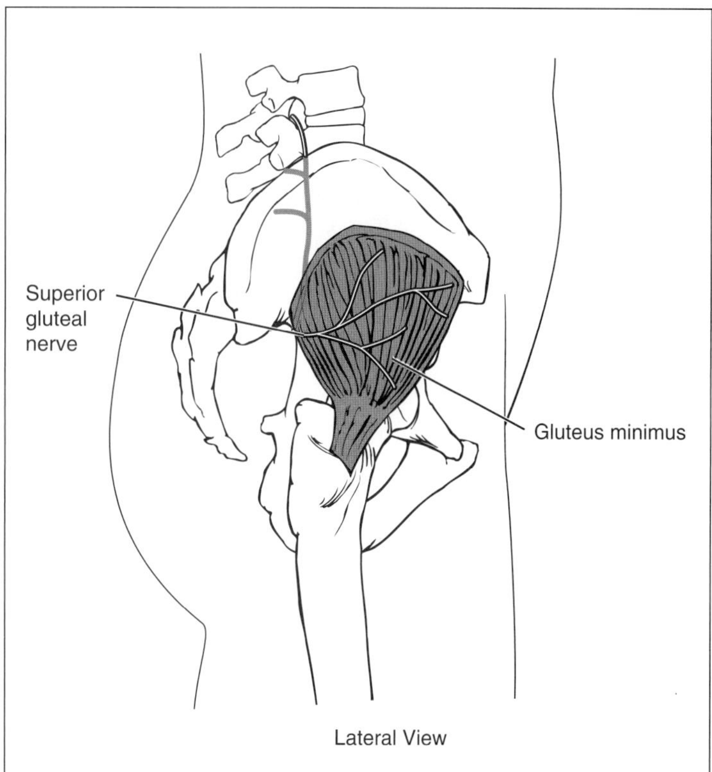

	ATTACHMENTS	NERVE SUPPLY	FUNCTION
Gluteus medius	Origin: Outer surface of the ilium between the anterior and posterior gluteal lines Insertion: Greater trochanter of the femur	Peripheral nerve: Superior gluteal nerve Nerve root: L4, L5, S1	Abduction and medial rotation of the hip
Gluteus minimus	Origin: Outer surface of the ilium between the anterior and inferior gluteal lines Insertion: Greater trochanter of the femur	Peripheral nerve: Superior gluteal nerve Nerve root: L4, L5, S1	Abduction and medial rotation of the hip

Gravity-Resisted Test (Grades 5, 4, and 3)

Patient position: Side lying with limb to be tested uppermost, pelvis facing directly forward, hip of uppermost lower extremity slightly extended and in neutral rotation, patient's pelvis close to examiner's trunk for stabilization. Lowermost limb may be flexed at hip and knee for balance, comfort, and stabilization (Fig. 4-27).

Fig. 4-27.

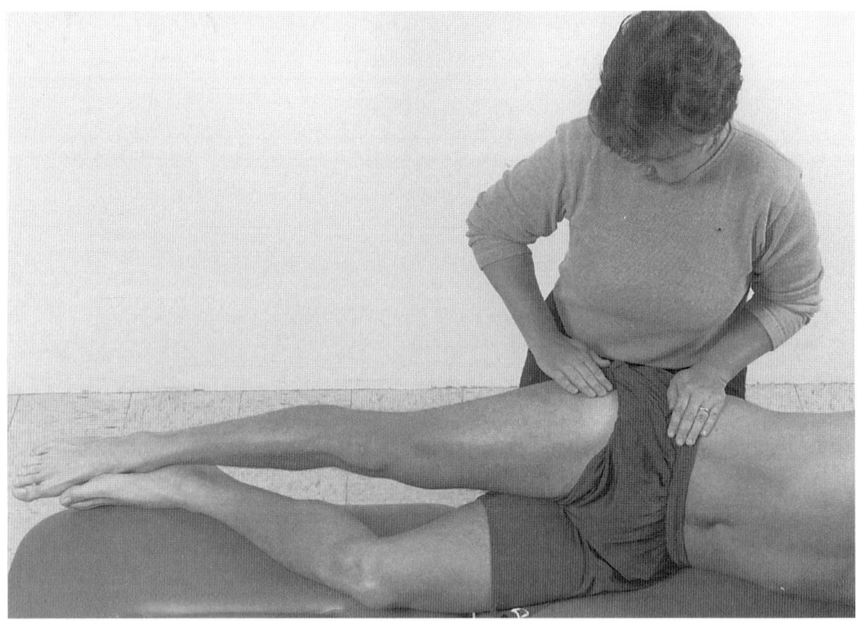

Stabilization/palpation: Stand directly behind patient's pelvis and stabilize lateral aspect of pelvis. With opposite hand, palpate gluteus medius just above greater trochanter on lateral side of pelvis (Fig. 4-27).

Examiner action: While instructing patient in motion desired, abduct patient's hip through full available ROM. Return limb to starting position. Performing passive movement allows determination of patient's available ROM and shows patient exact motion desired.

Patient action:

Patient abducts hip through full available ROM without rotating femur or allowing pelvis to deviate from neutral position. Examiner stabilizes pelvis and palpates gluteus medius during patient's active movement (Fig. 4-28).

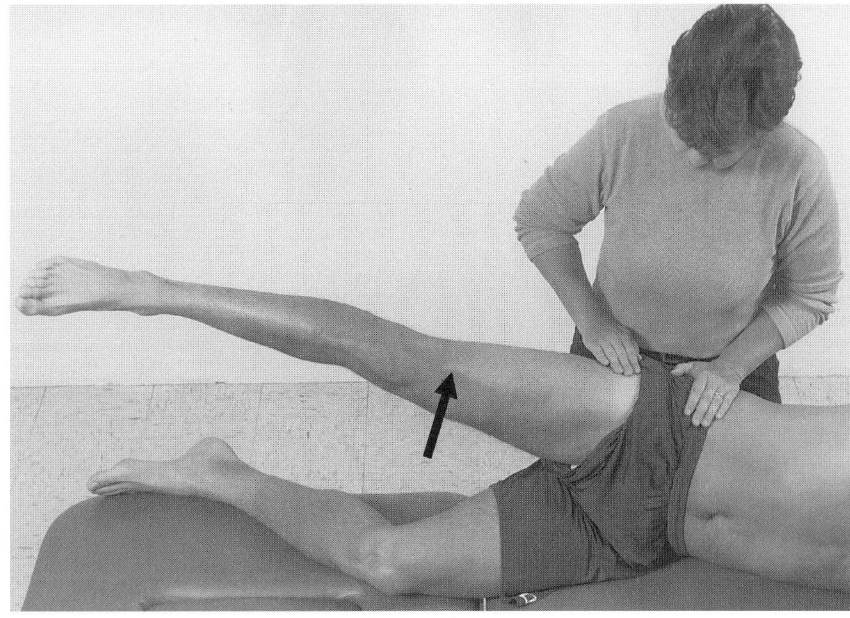

Fig. 4-28. Arrow indicates direction of movement.

Resistance:

Apply resistance over lateral aspect of distal thigh in direction of hip adduction. Palpating hand is moved to distal thigh to apply resistance (Fig. 4-29).

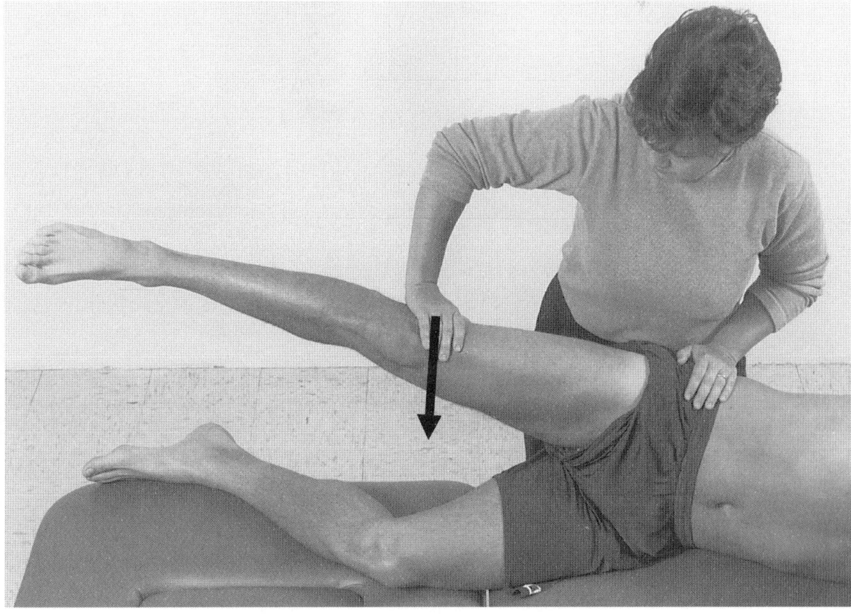

Fig. 4-29. Arrow indicates direction of resistance.

Gravity-Eliminated Test (Grades Below 3)

For patients unable to move completely through available ROM against gravity.

Patient position: Supine with hips fully adducted, knees extended (Fig. 4-30; starting position of test hip not shown).

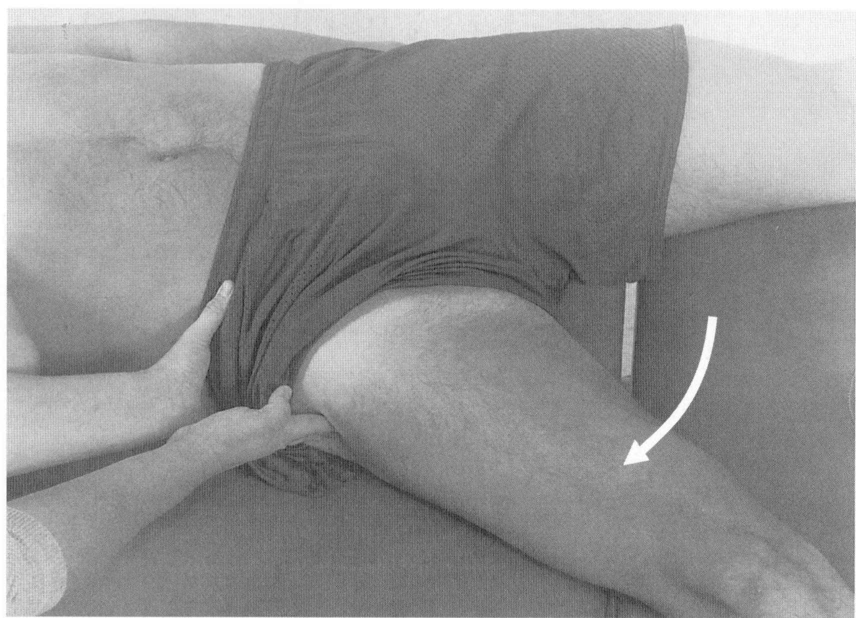

Fig. 4-30. Arrow indicates direction of movement.

Stabilization/palpation: Stabilize over anterolateral aspect of ipsilateral pelvis. With opposite hand, palpate gluteus medius (as in gravity-resisted test) (Fig. 4-30).

Examiner action: As in gravity-resisted test.

Patient action: Patient abducts hip through full available ROM. Examiner stabilizes pelvis and palpates gluteus medius during patient's active movement (Fig. 4-30).

COMMON SUBSTITUTIONS

1. Tensor fascia lata: Posterior rotation of pelvis during side-lying test allows substitution by tensor fascia lata (Fig. 4-31). Care should be taken to maintain pelvis in neutral rotation during test.

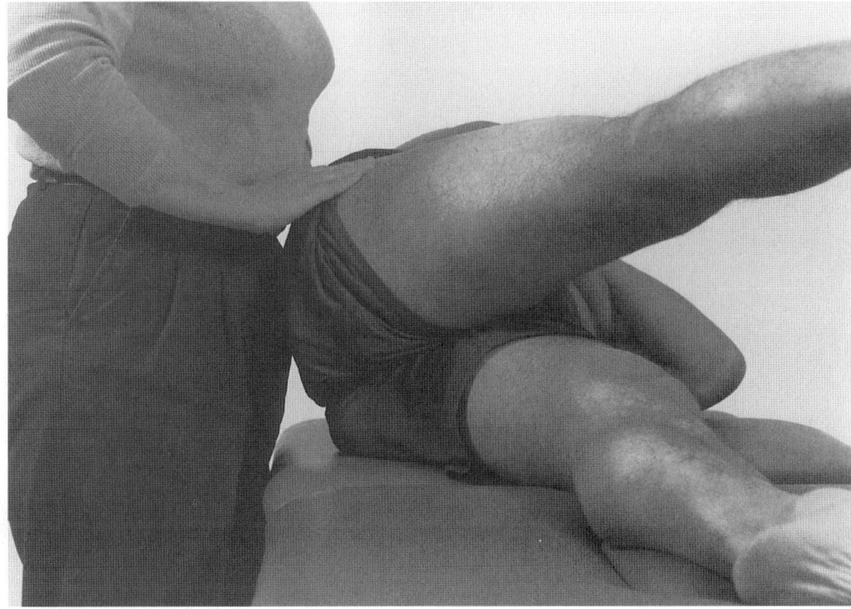

Fig. 4-31. Substitution by tensor fascia lata.

2. Hip flexors: Lateral rotation of hip during gravity-eliminated test allows substitution by hip flexors. Care should be taken to maintain hip in neutral rotation during test.

CLINICAL COMMENT: HIP ABDUCTOR MUSCLES AND L5 NEUROLOGIC ASSESSMENT

The hip abductor muscles (gluteus medius and tensor fascia lata) are key muscles for examining the integrity of the L5 spinal nerve or neurologic segment of the spinal cord. Complete assessment of the L5 neurologic level includes:

Strength assessment of:
Extensor hallucis longus (pp. 358-360)
Extensor digitorum longus (pp. 354-356)
Hip abductors (pp. 274-276)

Sensory testing of:
Skin over the lateral side of the leg and dorsum of the foot (L5 dermatome; pp. 528-532)

■ HIP ABDUCTION WITH FLEXION

TENSOR FASCIA LATA: OPTION I (Fig. 4-32)

During this test (traditionally attributed to Daniels and Worthingham[4]), examiner resists abduction component of tensor fascia lata while patient maintains hip in flexion.

Fig. 4-32.

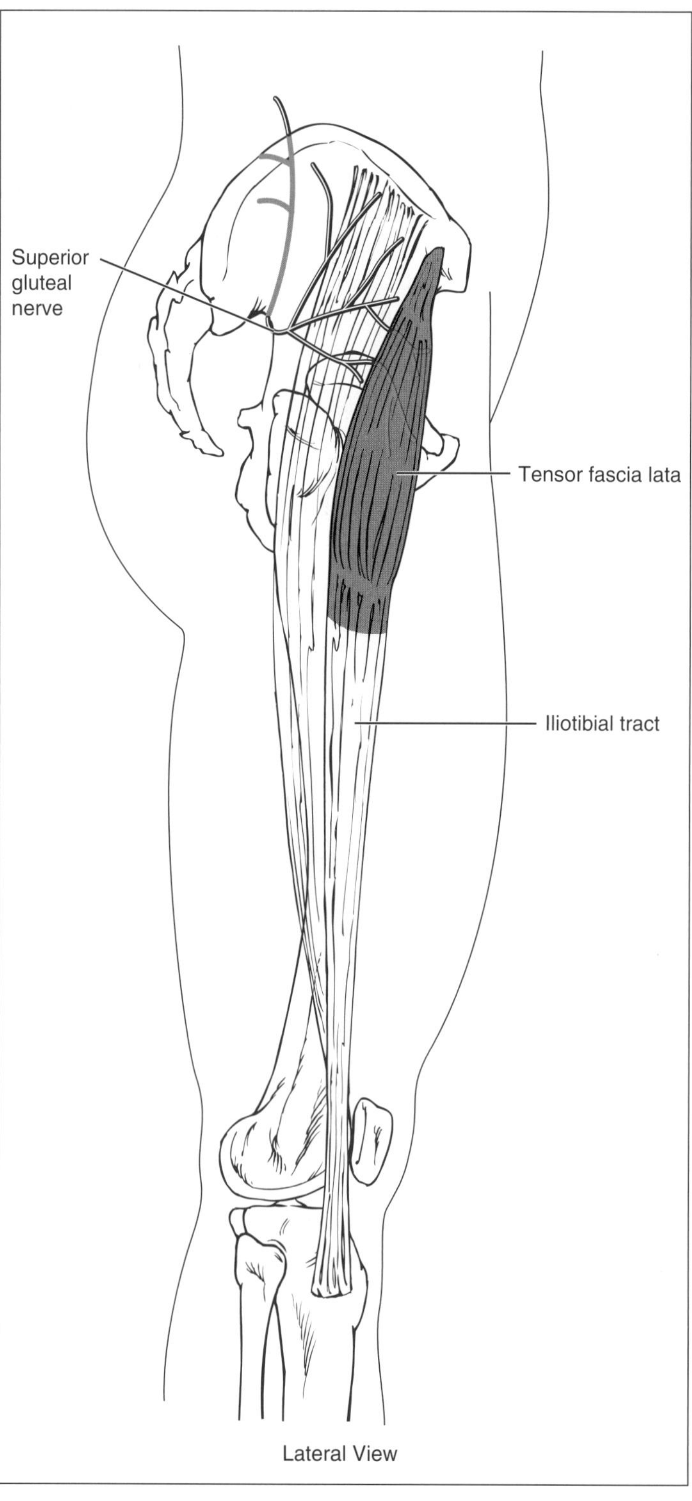

	ATTACHMENTS	NERVE SUPPLY	FUNCTION
Tensor fascia lata	Origin: Anterior superior iliac spine, anterior aspect of the outer lip of the iliac crest Insertion: Iliotibial tract approximately ⅓ down the thigh	Peripheral nerve: Superior gluteal nerve Nerve root: L4, L5, S1	Abduction, flexion, and medial rotation of the hip; extension of the knee

Gravity-Resisted Test (Grades 5, 4, and 3)

Patient position: Side lying with limb to be tested uppermost, pelvis facing directly forward and close to examiner's trunk, hip of upper limb in 45° flexion and neutral rotation, lower limb flexed for balance and comfort (Fig. 4-33).

Fig. 4-33.

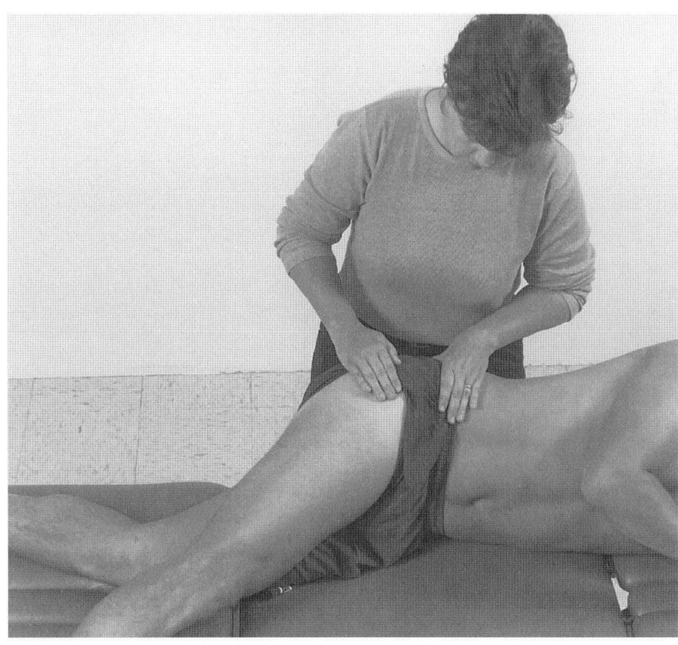

Stabilization/palpation: Stand directly behind patient's pelvis and stabilize lateral aspect of pelvis. With opposite hand, palpate tensor fascia lata just distal to anterior superior iliac spine, lateral to proximal end of sartorius (Fig. 4-33).

Examiner action: While instructing patient in motion desired, abduct patient's hip approximately 30°, maintaining hip in 45° flexion. Return limb to starting position. Performing passive movement allows determination of patient's available ROM and shows patient exact motion desired.

Patient action:

Patient abducts hip through approximately 30° of motion, hip flexed to 45° and pelvis and femur maintained in neutral position (not allowed to rotate). Examiner stabilizes pelvis and palpates tensor fascia lata during patient's active movement (Fig. 4-34).

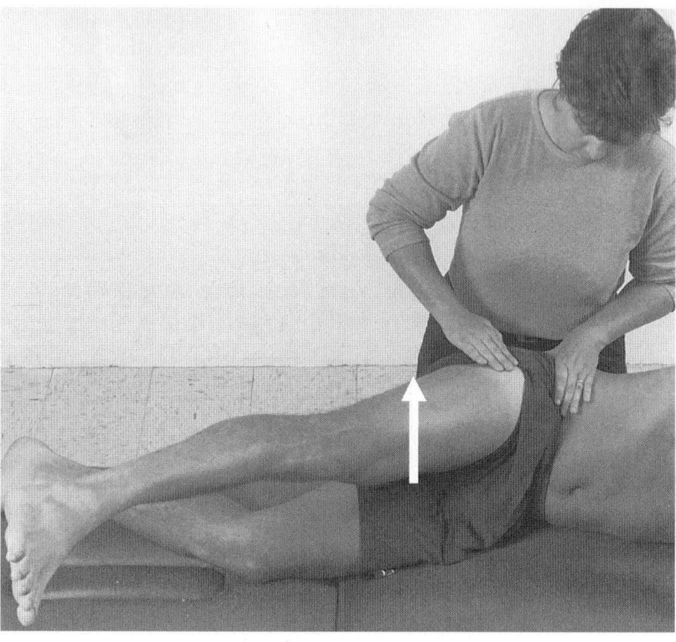

Fig. 4-34. Arrow indicates direction of movement.

Resistance:

Apply resistance over lateral aspect of distal thigh in direction of hip adduction. Palpating hand is moved to distal thigh to apply resistance (Fig. 4-35).

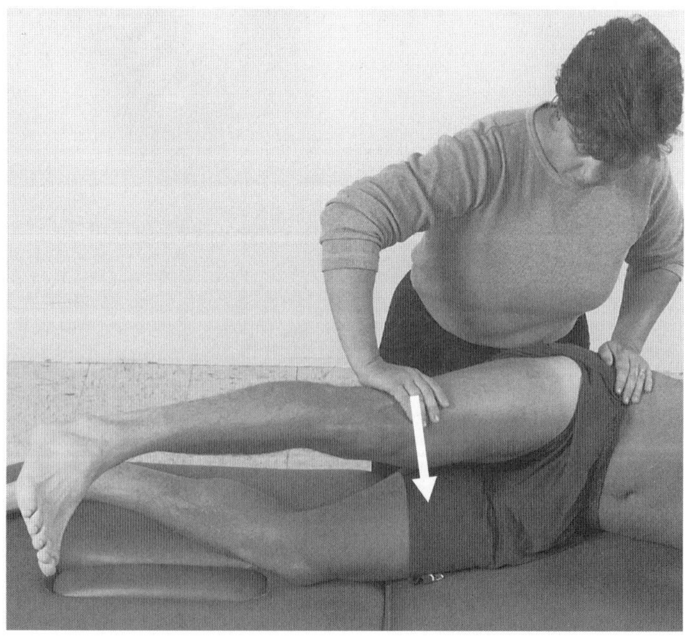

Fig. 4-35. Arrow indicates direction of resistance.

Gravity-Eliminated Test (Grades Below 3)

For patients unable to move completely through available ROM against gravity.

Patient position: Long-sitting, hips flexed to 45°, knees extended. Patient supports trunk by leaning back on extended arms. For patients with weak upper extremities, trunk may be supported by a wedge.

Stabilization/palpation: Stabilize anterolateral aspect of pelvis while palpating tensor fascia lata (as in gravity-resisted test) with opposite hand (Fig. 4-36).

Fig. 4-36. Arrow indicates direction of movement.

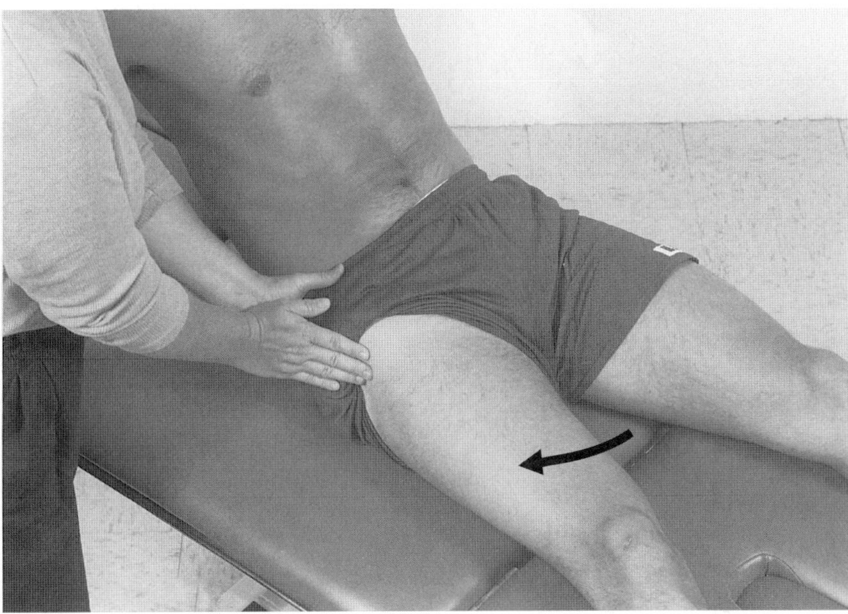

Examiner action: As in gravity-resisted test.

Patient action: Patient abducts hip through full available ROM while examiner stabilizes pelvis and palpates tensor fascia lata (Fig. 4-36).

COMMON SUBSTITUTIONS

Hip flexors: Lateral rotation of hip during gravity-eliminated test allows substitution by hip flexors. Care should be taken to maintain hip in neutral (or medial) rotation during test.

TENSOR FASCIA LATA: OPTION II

During this test (advocated by Kendall et al.[5]), examiner resists flexion and abduction components of tensor fascia lata while patient maintains hip in medial rotation.

Gravity-Resisted Test (Grades 5 and 4)

Patient position: Supine with test limb in partial hip abduction and full medial rotation, knee extended. Patient may grasp sides of table for stability (Fig. 4-37).

Fig. 4-37.

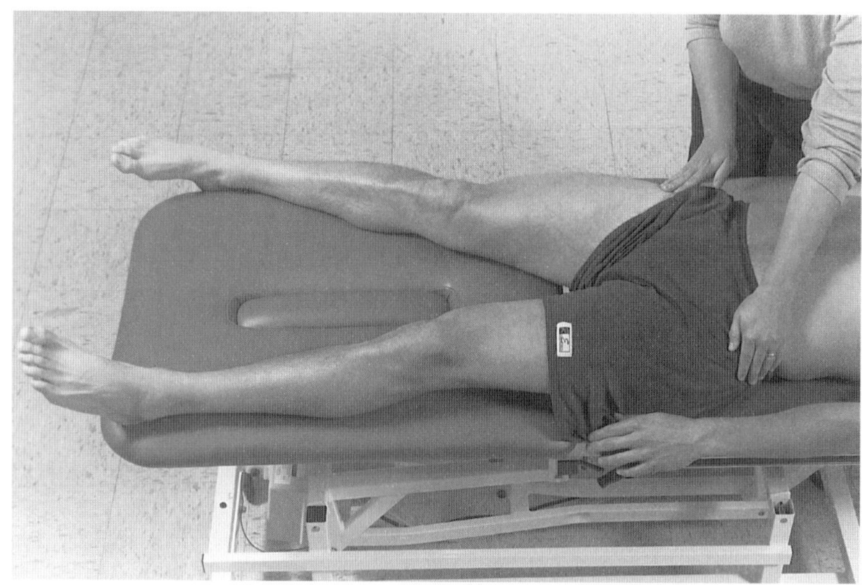

Stabilization/palpation: Stabilize over anterior aspect of contralateral pelvis. With opposite hand, palpate tensor fascia lata just distal to anterior superior iliac spine, lateral to proximal end of sartorius (Fig. 4-37).

Examiner action: While instructing patient in motion desired, flex patient's hip approximately 45°, maintaining hip in abduction and medial rotation and knee in extension. Return limb to starting position. Performing passive movement allows determination of patient's available ROM and shows patient exact motion desired.

Patient action:

Patient raises thigh into approximately 45° hip flexion while maintaining abduction and medial rotation of hip and extension of knee. Examiner stabilizes pelvis and palpates tensor fascia lata during patient's active movement (Fig. 4-38).

Fig. 4-38. Arrow indicates direction of movement.

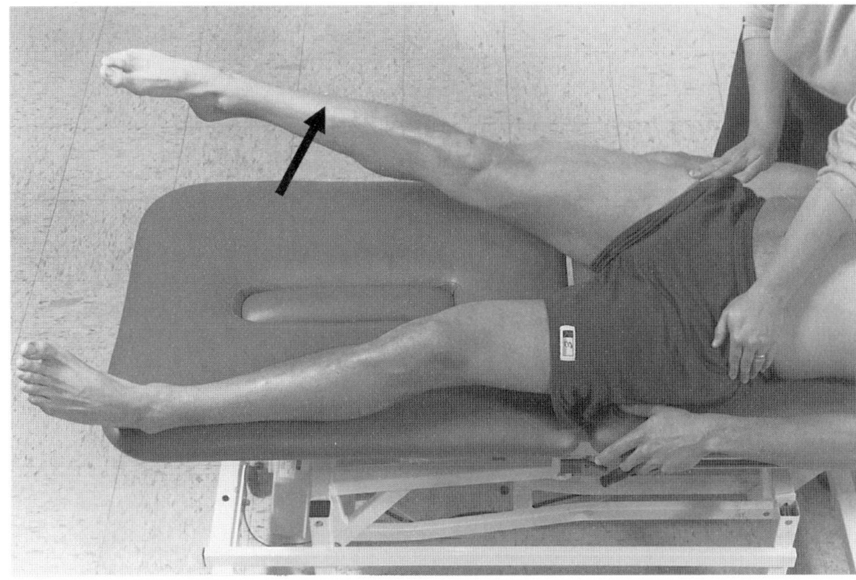

Resistance:

Apply resistance over anterolateral aspect of leg in direction of hip extension and adduction. Palpating hand is moved to anterolateral aspect of leg to apply resistance (Fig. 4-39).

Fig. 4-39. Arrow indicates direction of resistance.

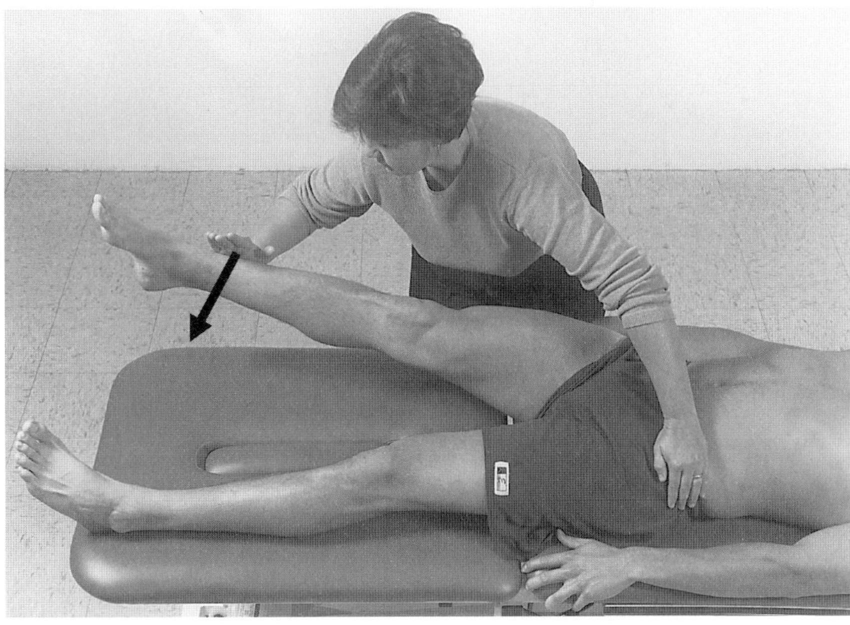

Grades 3 and Below

There is no separate test of this muscle for grades below 3. Grading is altered as follows to accommodate lack of a gravity-eliminated position.

For grade 3: Patient moves hip into 45° flexion while maintaining hip abduction, hip medial rotation, and knee extension, but is unable to maintain position against any resistance.

For grade 2: Patient moves hip through less than 45° flexion.

For grade 1: No motion, but a palpable contraction is present. Palpation occurs as in gravity-resisted test (see Fig. 4-37).

For grade 0: No motion or contraction is present.

■ HIP ADDUCTION

ADDUCTOR MAGNUS, ADDUCTOR LONGUS, ADDUCTOR BREVIS, PECTINEUS, AND GRACILIS (Figs. 4-40 and 4-41)

Fig. 4-40.

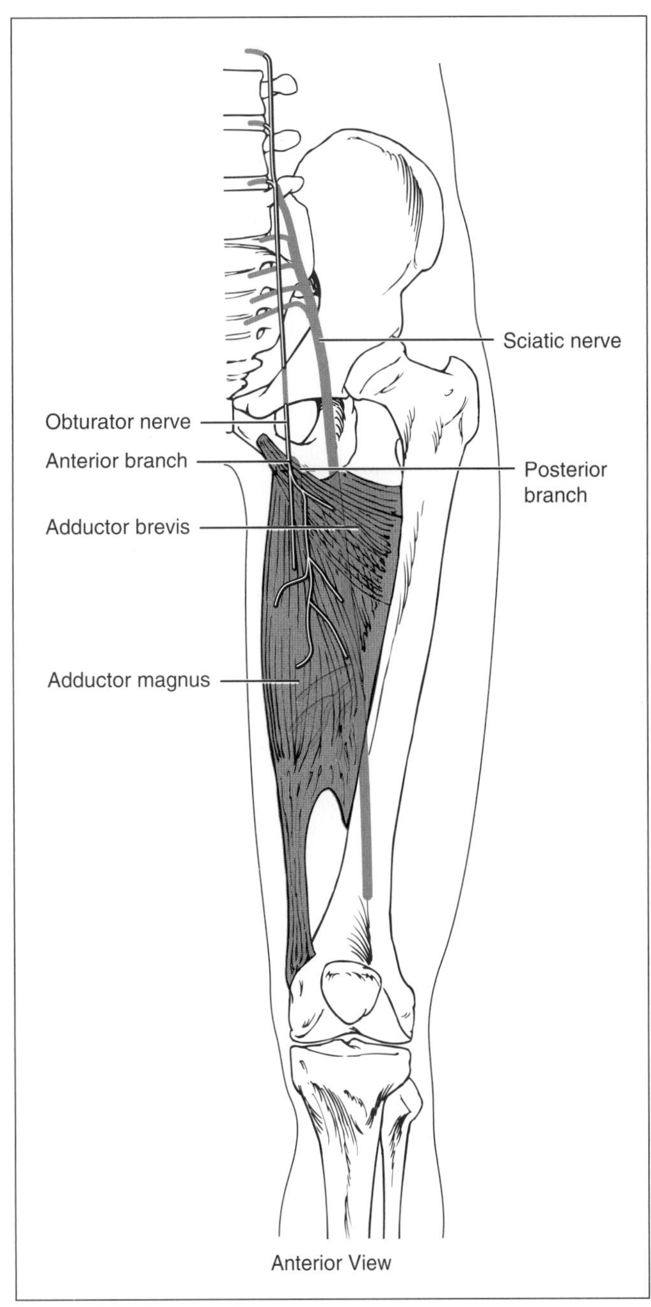

Fig. 4-41.

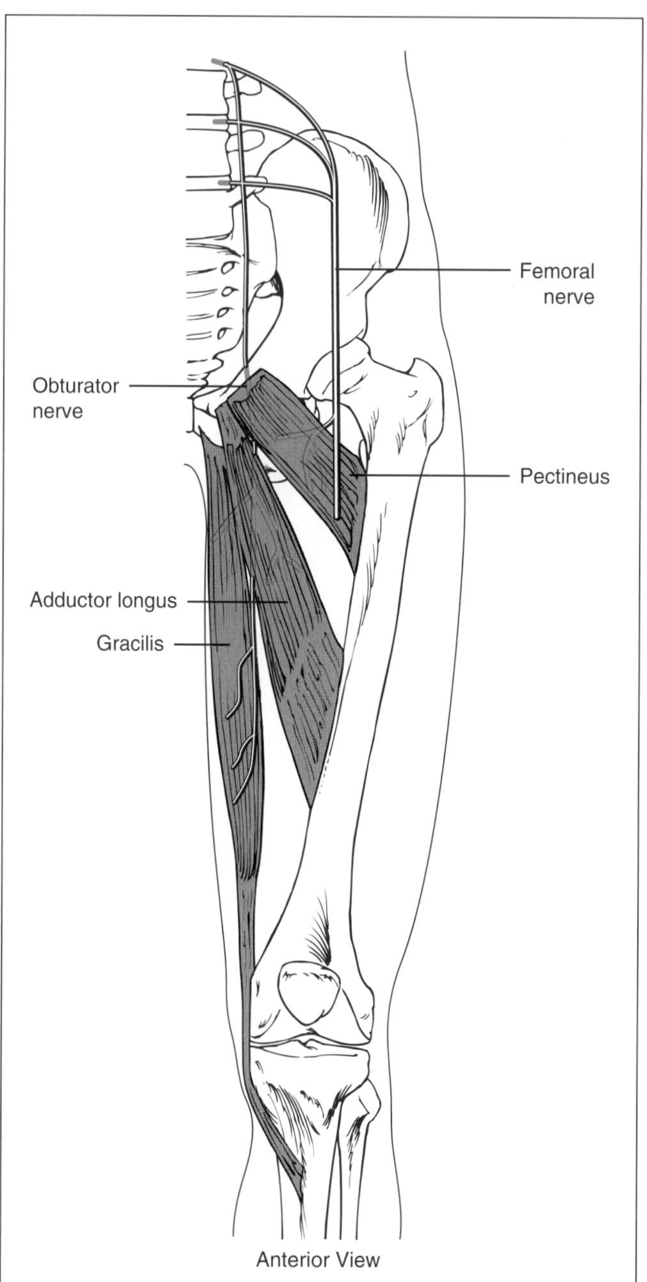
Femoral nerve
Obturator nerve
Pectineus
Adductor longus
Gracilis
Anterior View

	ATTACHMENTS	NERVE SUPPLY	FUNCTION
Adductor magnus	Origin: Inferior rami of the pubis and ischium, ischial tuberosity Insertion: A line from the greater trochanter to the linea aspera of the femur, linea aspera, adductor tubercle, medial supracondylar line of the femur	Peripheral nerve: Obturator and sciatic nerves Nerve root: L2–L4	Adduction of the hip; upper portion of muscle assists in hip flexion, lower portion assists in hip extension
Adductor longus	Origin: Anterior aspect of the pubis Insertion: Linea aspera along the middle ⅓ of the femur	Peripheral nerve: Obturator nerve Nerve root: L2–L4	Adduction and flexion of the hip
Adductor brevis	Origin: Inferior ramus of the pubis Insertion: A line from the lesser trochanter to the linea aspera, upper portion of the linea aspera	Peripheral nerve: Obturator nerve Nerve root: L2–L4	Adduction, flexion, and medial rotation of the hip
Pectineus	Origin: Pectineal line of the pubis Insertion: A line from the lesser trochanter to the linea aspera	Peripheral nerve: Femoral nerve Nerve root: L2–L4	Adduction, flexion, and medial rotation of the hip
Gracilis	Origin: Body and ramus of the pubis Insertion: Proximal aspect of the medial surface of the tibia	Peripheral nerve: Obturator nerve Nerve root: L2, L3	Adduction of the hip, flexion, and medial rotation of the knee

Gravity-Resisted Test (Grades 5, 4, and 3)

Patient position: Side lying on side of limb to be tested, pelvis facing directly forward and close to examiner's trunk, hip of lowermost limb in neutral position. Patient may hold edge of table for support (Fig. 4-42).

Fig. 4-42.

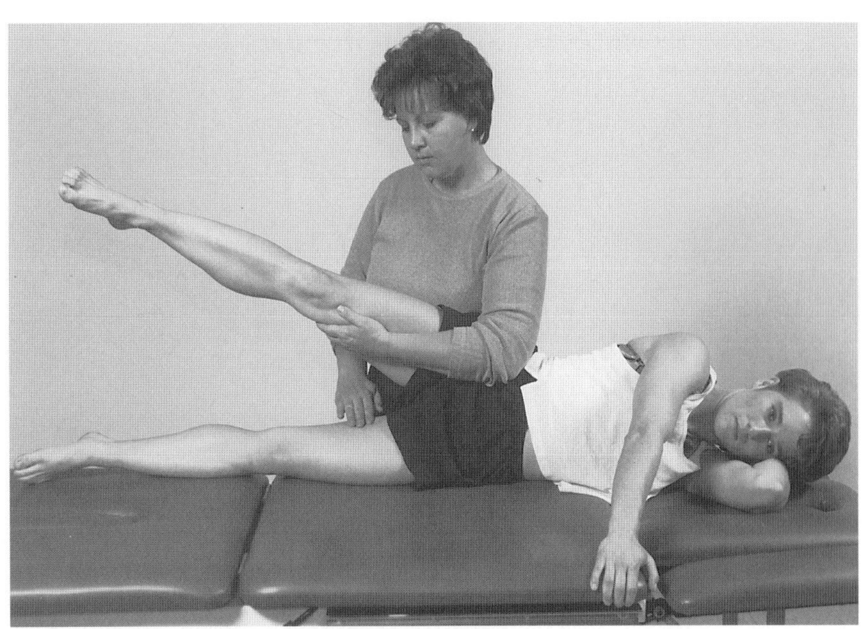

Stabilization/palpation: Stand directly behind patient's pelvis, stabilize pelvis against examiner's trunk, and support uppermost lower extremity in 25° to 30° hip abduction. With opposite hand, palpate adductor muscles of test limb on medial aspect of thigh (Fig. 4-42).

Examiner action: While instructing patient in motion desired, adduct test hip through full available ROM. Return limb to starting position. Performing passive movement allows determination of patient's available ROM and shows patient exact motion desired.

Patient action: Patient adducts hip of test limb though full ROM (until it meets uppermost limb). Examiner stabilizes pelvis and palpates hip adductors during patient's active movement (Fig. 4-43).

Fig. 4-43. Arrow indicates direction of movement.

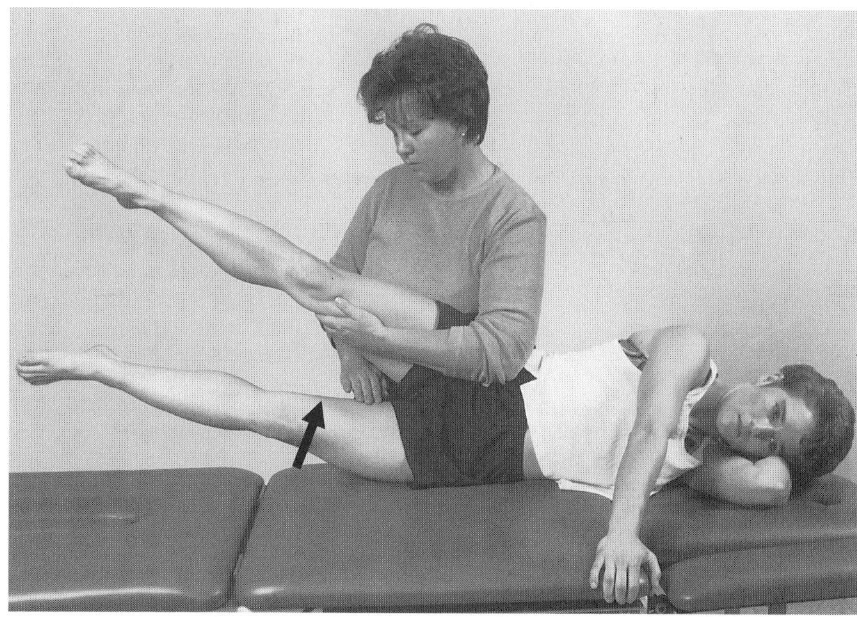

Resistance: Apply resistance on medial aspect of distal thigh, in direction of hip abduction. Palpating hand is moved to distal thigh to apply resistance (Fig. 4-44).

Fig. 4-44. Arrow indicates direction of resistance.

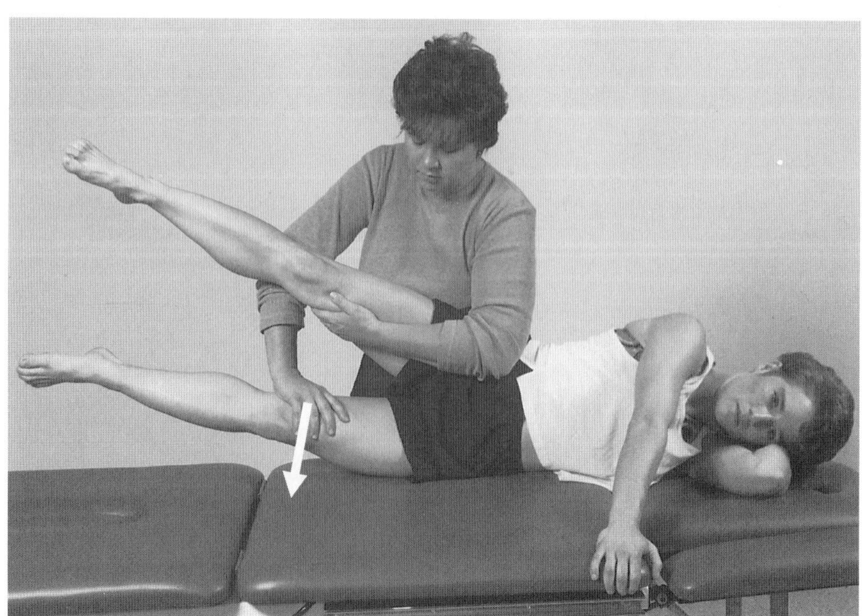

Gravity-Eliminated Test (Grades Below 3)

Patient position: Supine with non–test limb in full abduction, test limb in 0° adduction, pelvis level, knees extended. Talcum powder and a cloth may be placed between limb and supporting surface to reduce friction (Fig. 4-45; starting position of test limb not shown).

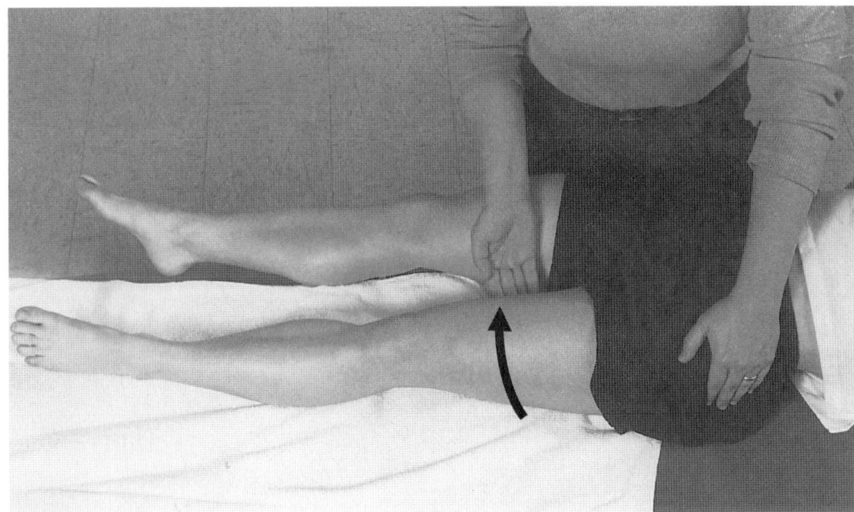

Fig. 4-45. Arrow indicates direction of movement.

Stabilization/palpation: Stabilize anterolateral aspect of ipsilateral pelvis while palpating adductors of test limb (as in gravity-resisted test) with opposite hand (Fig. 4-45).

Examiner action: As in gravity-resisted test.

Patient action: Patient adducts hip of test limb through full available ROM by sliding foot across table. Examiner stabilizes pelvis and palpates hip adductors during patient's active movement (Fig. 4-45).

COMMON SUBSTITUTIONS

1. Hip flexors: Posterior rotation of pelvis during side lying test allows substitution by hip flexors. Care should be taken to maintain pelvis in neutral rotation during test.
2. Hip extensors: Anterior rotation of pelvis during side lying test allows substitution by hip extensors. Care should be taken to maintain pelvis in neutral rotation during test.

■ HIP MEDIAL ROTATION

TENSOR FASCIA LATA, GLUTEUS MINIMUS, AND GLUTEUS MEDIUS (Fig. 4-46)

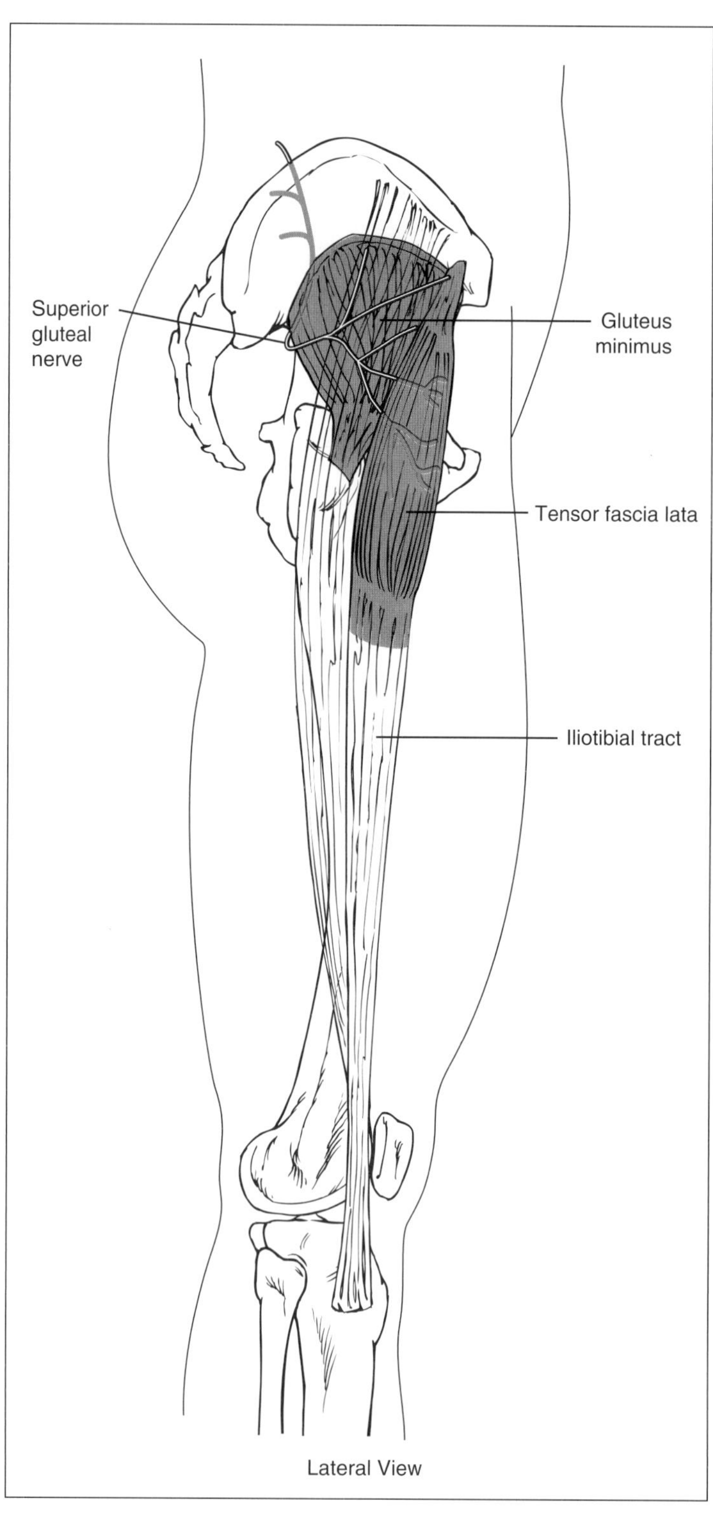

Fig. 4-46.

	ATTACHMENTS	NERVE SUPPLY	FUNCTION
Tensor fascia lata	Origin: Anterior superior iliac spine, anterior aspect of the outer lip of the iliac crest Insertion: Iliotibial tract approximately ⅓ down the thigh	Peripheral nerve: Superior gluteal nerve Nerve root: L4, L5, S1	Abduction, flexion, and medial rotation of the hip; extension of the knee
Gluteus minimus	Origin: Outer surface of the ilium between the anterior and inferior gluteal lines Insertion: Greater trochanter of the femur	Peripheral nerve: Superior gluteal nerve Nerve root: L4, L5, S1	Abduction and medial rotation of the hip
Gluteus medius (anterior fibers)	Origin: Outer surface of the ilium between the anterior and posterior gluteal lines Insertion: Greater trochanter of the femur	Peripheral nerve: Superior gluteal nerve Nerve root: L4, L5, S1	Abduction and medial rotation of the hip

Gravity-Resisted Test (Grades 5, 4, and 3)

Patient position: Seated with legs hanging off side of table, weight evenly distributed on both hips, a folded towel under knee of limb to be tested. Patient should hold on to sides of table to assist with stabilization (Fig. 4-47).

Fig. 4-47.

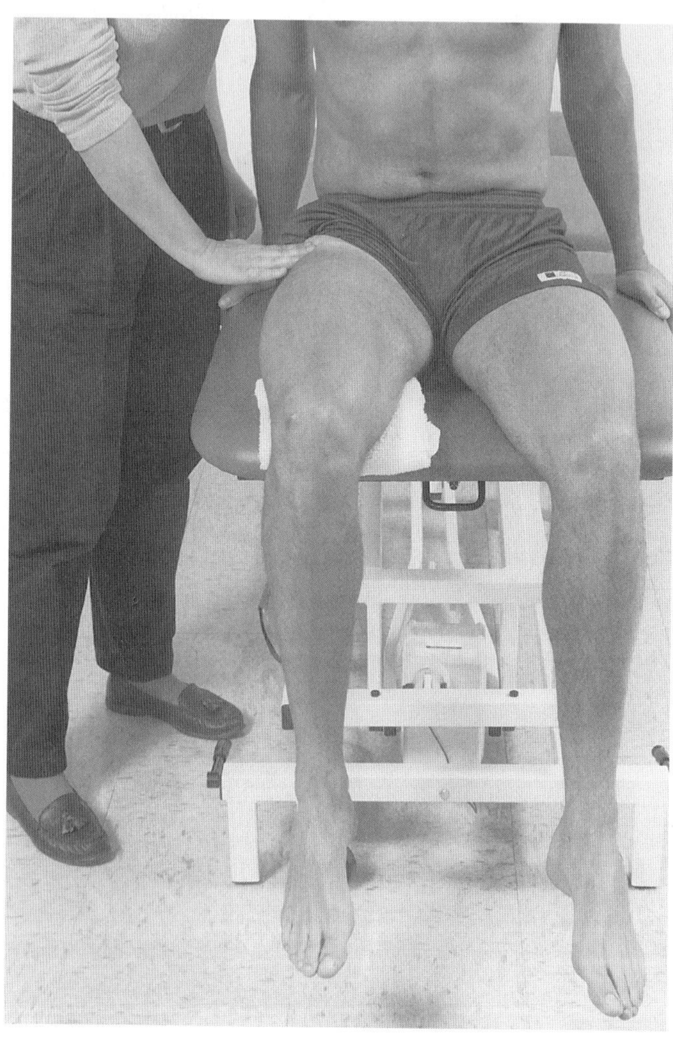

Stabilization/palpation: Weight of patient's trunk provides stabilization. Palpate anterior gluteus medius and tensor fascia lata on anterolateral aspect of pelvis, just lateral to proximal end of sartorius (tensor more anterior of two). Gluteus minimus is difficult to palpate (Fig. 4-47).

Examiner action: While instructing patient in motion desired, medially rotate patient's hip through full available ROM by moving foot laterally. Return limb to starting position. Performing passive movement allows determination of patient's available ROM and shows patient exact motion desired.

Patient action: Patient rotates hip medially through full available ROM by moving foot laterally. Examiner palpates medial rotators during patient's active movement (Fig. 4-48).

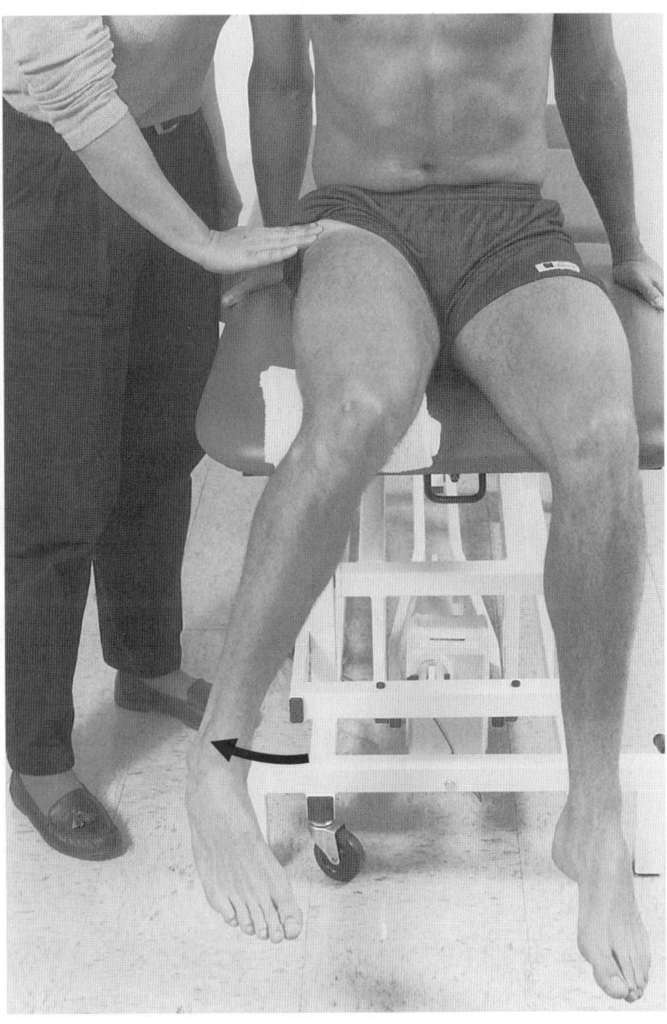

Fig. 4-48. Arrow indicates direction of movement.

Resistance: Examiner places one hand on anteromedial aspect of distal thigh and opposite hand on lateral aspect of distal leg. Resistance is applied in medial direction on lateral aspect of distal leg. Hand on distal thigh applies counterpressure during resistance (Fig. 4-49).

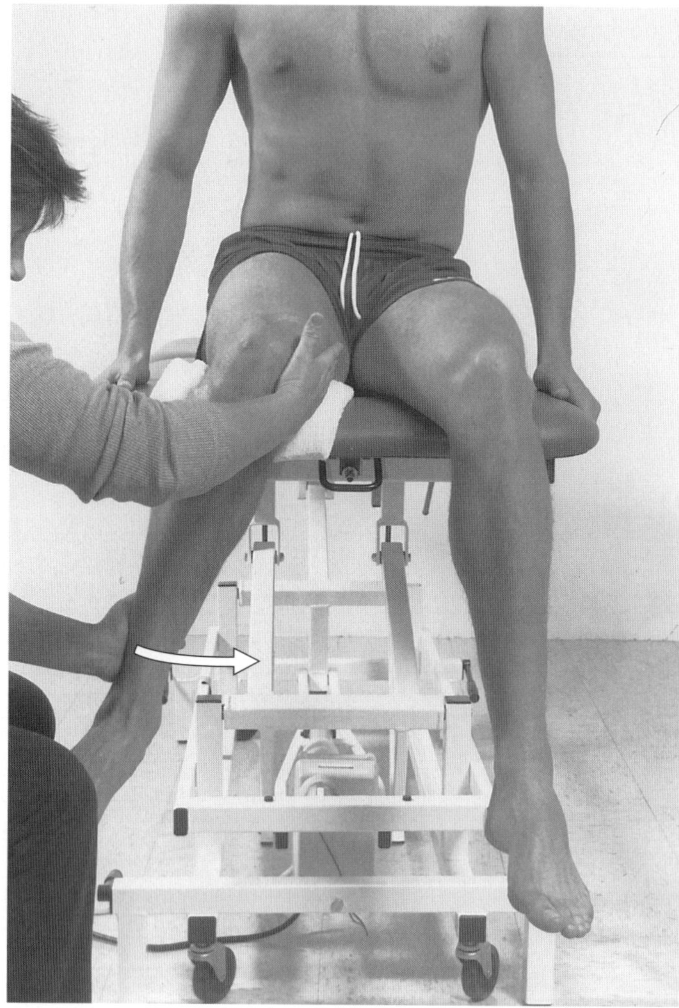

Fig. 4-49. Arrow indicates direction of resistance.

Gravity-Eliminated Test (Grades Below 3)

For patients unable to move completely through available ROM against gravity.

Patient position: Supine, with limb to be tested in full hip lateral rotation and extension, knee extended (Fig. 4-50).

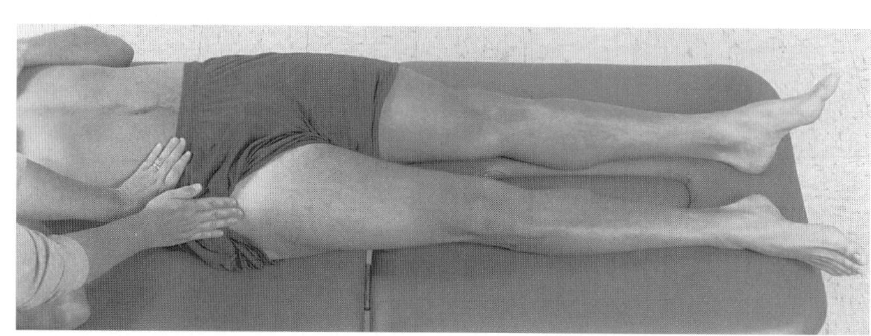

Fig. 4-50.

Stabilization/palpation: Stabilize over anterior aspect of ipsilateral pelvis while palpating tensor fascia lata and anterior gluteus medius (as in gravity-resisted test) with opposite hand (Fig. 4-50).

Examiner action: While instructing patient in motion desired, rotate patient's hip medially through full available ROM. Return limb to starting position. Performing passive movement allows determination of patient's available ROM and shows patient exact motion desired.

Patient action: Patient rotates hip medially through full available ROM. Examiner stabilizes pelvis and palpates hip medial rotators during patient's active movement (Fig. 4-51).

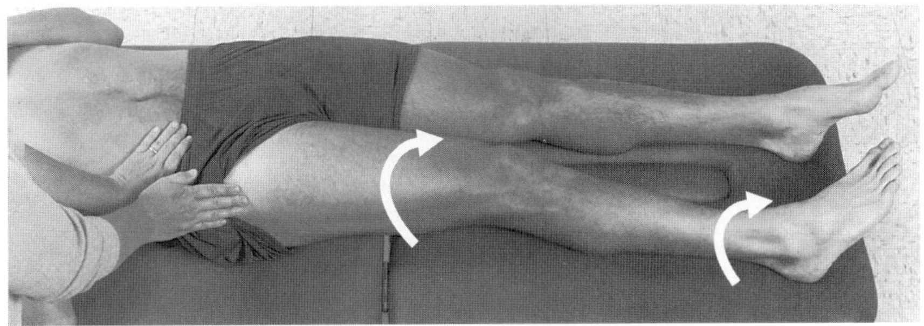

Fig. 4-51. Arrows indicate direction of movement.

COMMON SUBSTITUTION

Pelvic elevation: Patient should not be allowed to elevate pelvis on test side during gravity-resisted test. Shifting weight to nontest side during test can cause appearance of medial rotation on test side (Fig. 4-52).

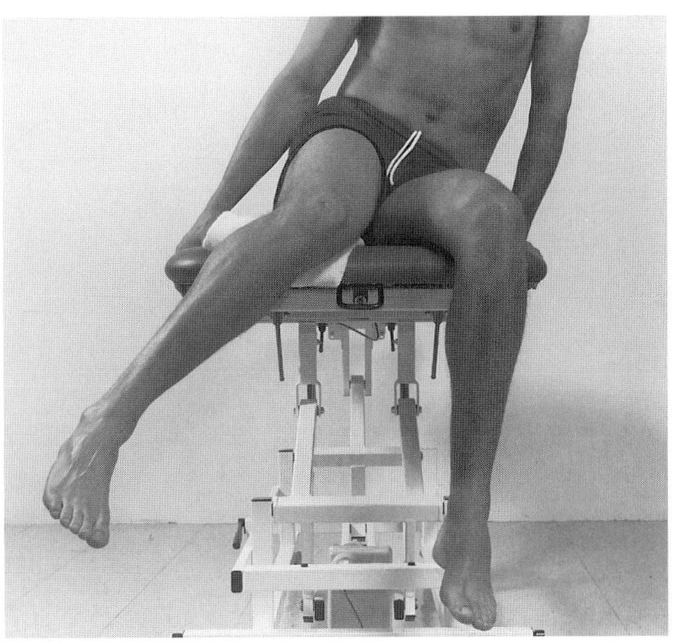

Fig. 4-52. Inappropriate trunk position during testing.

■ HIP LATERAL ROTATION

PIRIFORMIS, GEMELLUS SUPERIOR AND INFERIOR, OBTURATOR INTERNUS AND EXTERNUS, AND QUADRATUS FEMORIS (Figs. 4-53 and 4-54)

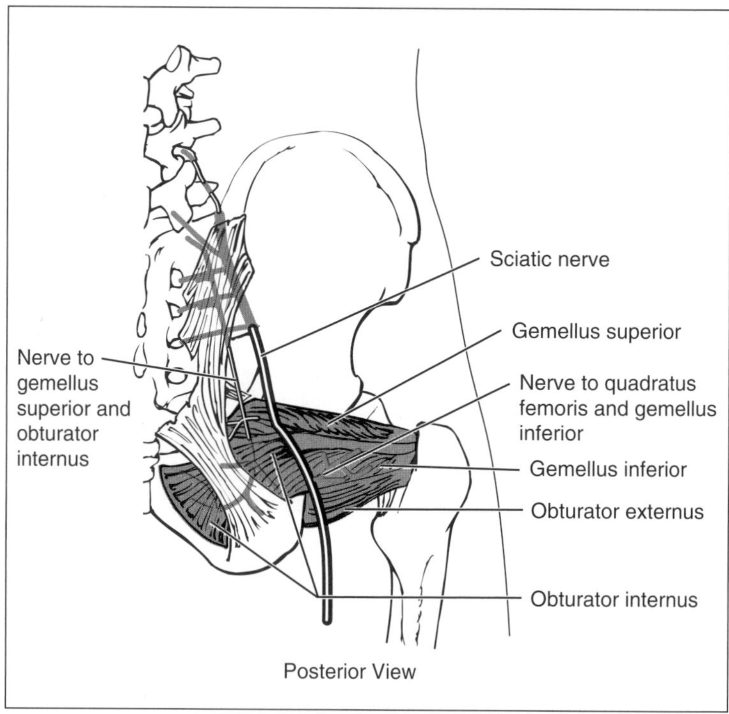

Fig. 4-53.

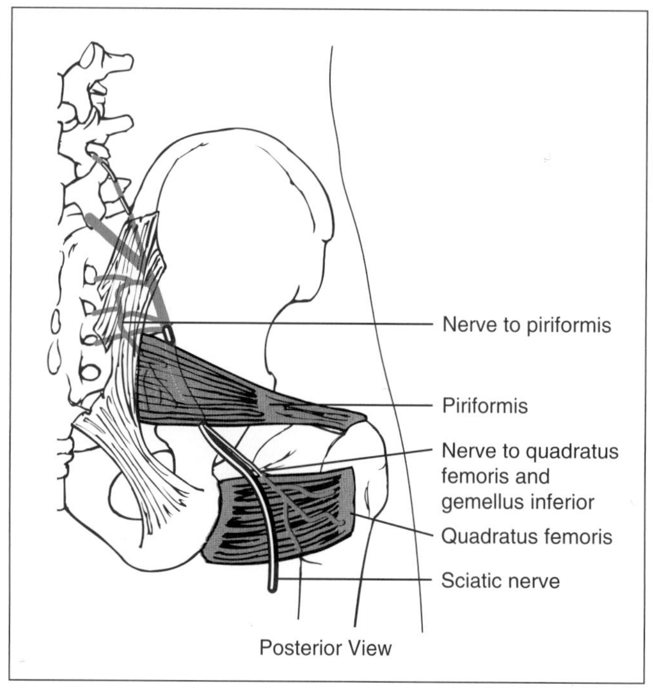

Fig. 4-54.

	ATTACHMENTS	NERVE SUPPLY	FUNCTION
Piriformis	Origin: Anterior surface of the sacrum, sacro-tuberous ligament Insertion: Greater trochanter of the femur	Sacral nerves 1 and 2	Lateral rotation of the hip, abduction of the flexed hip
Gemellus superior	Origin: Ischial spine Insertion: Greater trochanter of the femur	Peripheral nerve: Nerve to the obturator internus Nerve root: L5, S1, S2	Lateral rotation of the hip, abduction of the flexed hip
Gemellus inferior	Origin: Ischial tuberosity Insertion: Greater trochanter of the femur	Peripheral nerve: Nerve to the quadratus femoris Nerve root: L4, L5, S1	Lateral rotation of the hip, abduction of the flexed hip
Obturator internus	Origin: Obturator membrane and foramen, inner surface of the pelvis, inferior rami of the pubis and ischium Insertion: Greater trochanter of the femur	Peripheral nerve: Nerve to the obturator internus Nerve root: L5, S1, S2	Lateral rotation of the hip, abduction of the flexed hip
Obturator externus	Origin: Rami of the pubis and ischium, outer surface of the obturator membrane Insertion: Trochanteric fossa of the femur	Peripheral nerve: Obturator nerve Nerve root: L4, L5	Lateral rotation of the hip
Quadratus femoris	Origin: Ischial tuberosity Insertion: Quadrate tubercle of the femur	Peripheral nerve: Nerve to the quadratus femoris Nerve root: L4, L5, S1	Lateral rotation of the hip

Gravity-Resisted Test (Grades 5, 4, and 3)

Patient position: Seated with legs off side of table, weight distributed evenly on both hips, folded towel under knee of test limb. Patient should hold on to sides of table to assist with stabilization (Fig. 4-55).

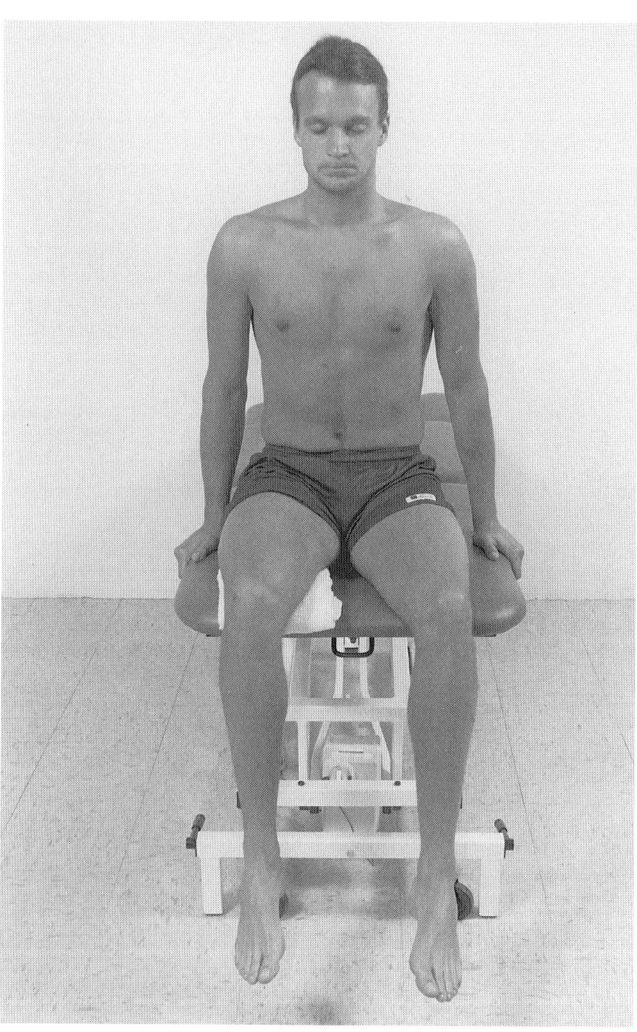

Fig. 4-55.

Stabilization/palpation: Weight of patient's trunk provides stabilization. Lateral rotators of hip are deep and very difficult to palpate. Piriformis may be palpable on posterior aspect of pelvis between sacrum and greater trochanter (not shown).

Examiner action: While instructing patient in motion desired, laterally rotate patient's hip through full available ROM by moving foot medially. Return limb to starting position. Performing passive movement allows determination of patient's available ROM and shows patient exact motion desired.

Patient action:

Patient rotates hip laterally through full available ROM by moving foot medially (Fig. 4-56).

Fig. 4-56.

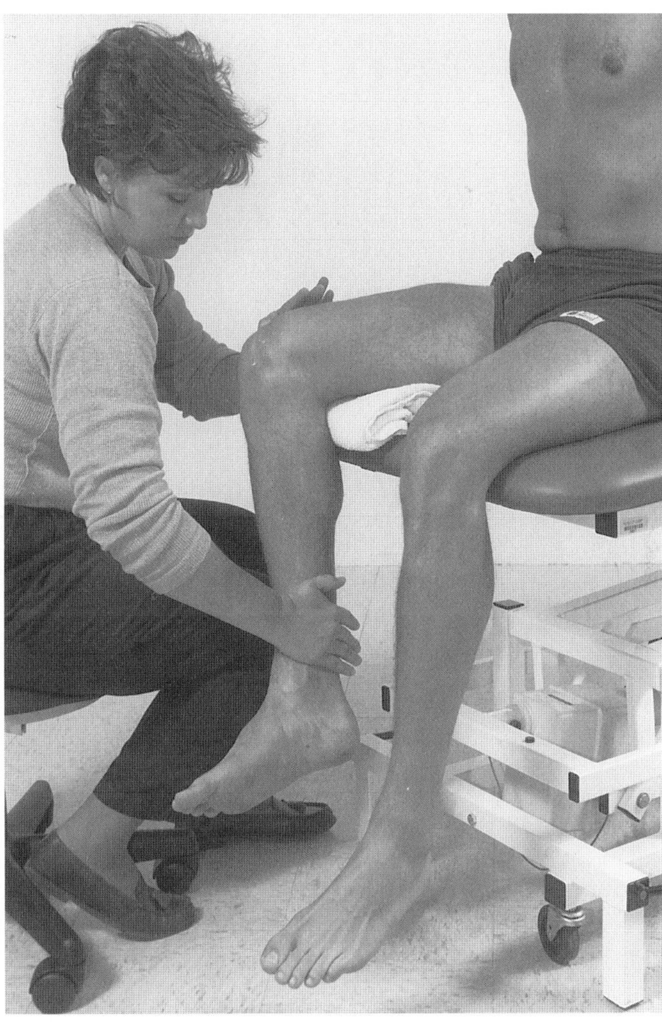

Resistance:

Examiner places one hand on anterolateral aspect of distal thigh and opposite hand on medial aspect of distal leg. Resistance is applied in lateral direction on medial aspect of distal leg. Hand on distal thigh applies counterpressure during resistance (Fig. 4-56).

Gravity-Eliminated Test (Grades Below 3)

For patients unable to move completely through available ROM against gravity.

Patient position: Supine with limb to be tested in full medial rotation at hip, with hip and knee extended (Fig. 4-57).

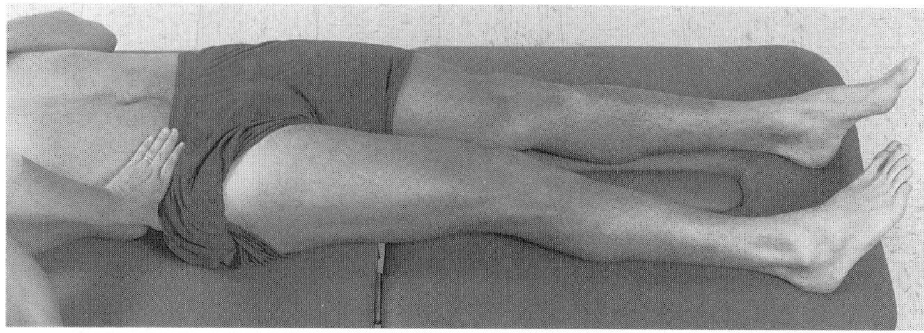

Fig. 4-57.

Stabilization/palpation: Stabilize over anterior aspect of ipsilateral pelvis (Fig. 4-57).

Examiner action: While instructing patient in motion desired, rotate patient's hip laterally through full available ROM. Return limb to starting position. Performing passive movement allows determination of patient's available ROM and shows patient exact motion desired.

Patient action: Patient rotates hip laterally through full available ROM, while examiner stabilizes pelvis (Fig. 4-58).

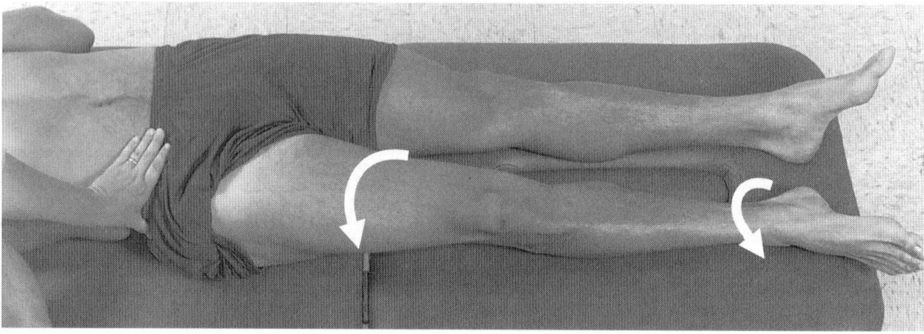

Fig. 4-58. Arrows indicate direction of movement.

COMMON SUBSTITUTION

Lateral trunk lean: Leaning of trunk toward test limb can substitute for lateral rotation of thigh (Fig. 4-59). Care should be taken to maintain an erect trunk during test.

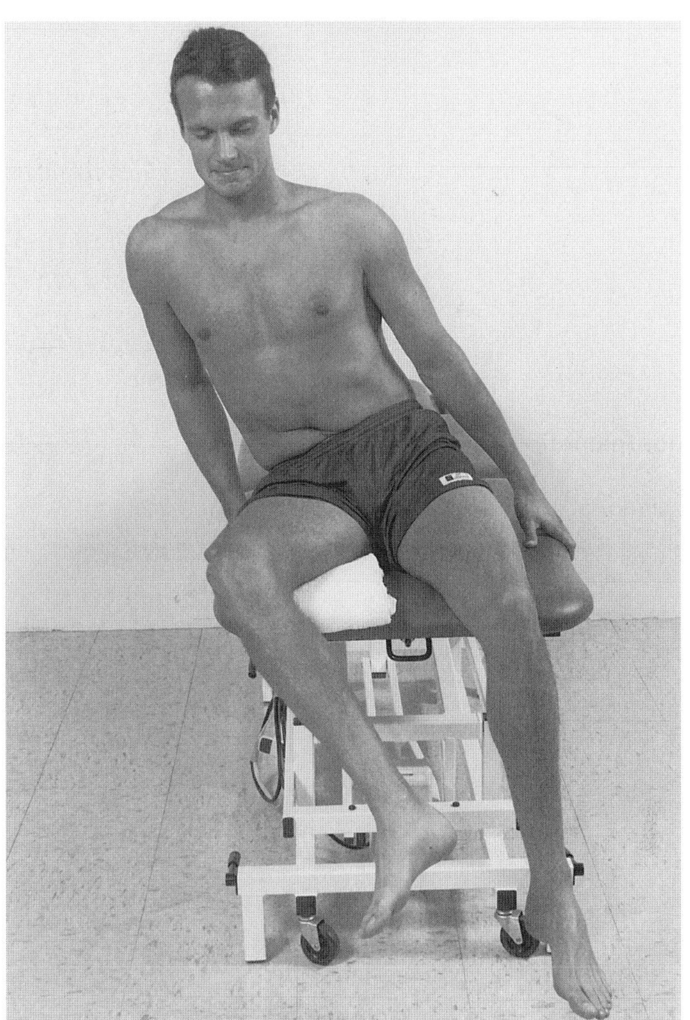

Fig. 4-59. Inappropriate trunk position during testing.

▪ KNEE EXTENSION

QUADRICEPS FEMORIS (Figs. 4-60 and 4-61)

Fig. 4-60.

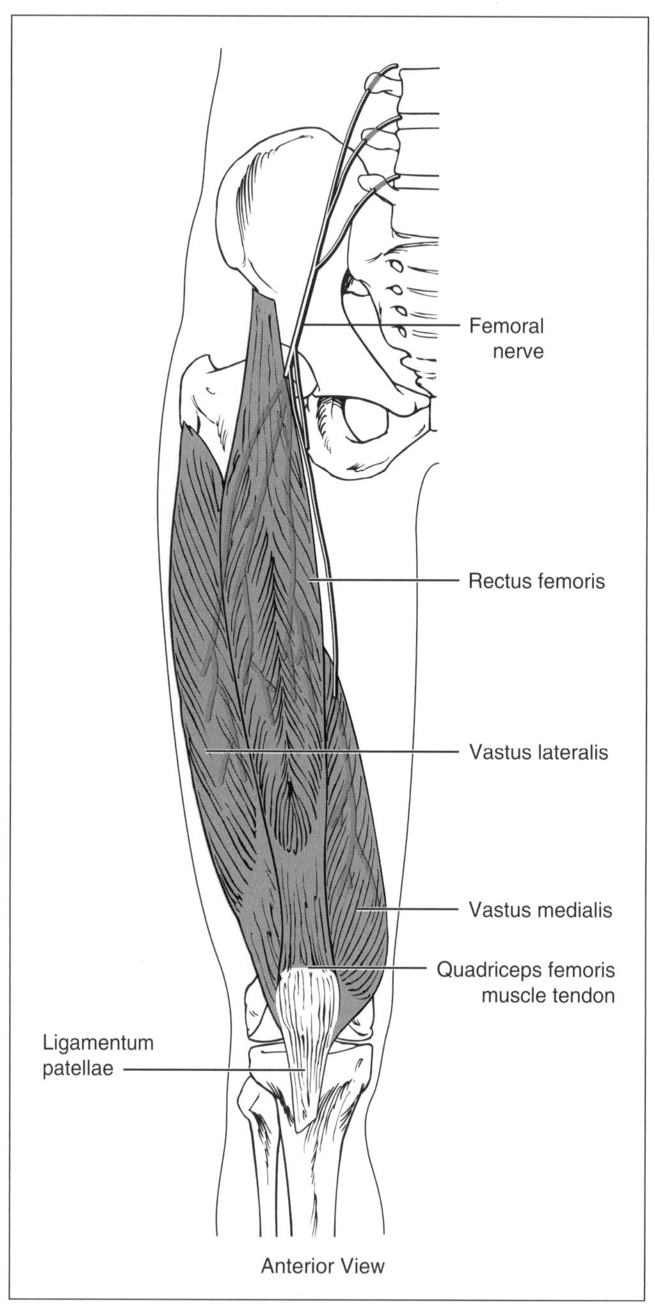

Fig. 4-61.

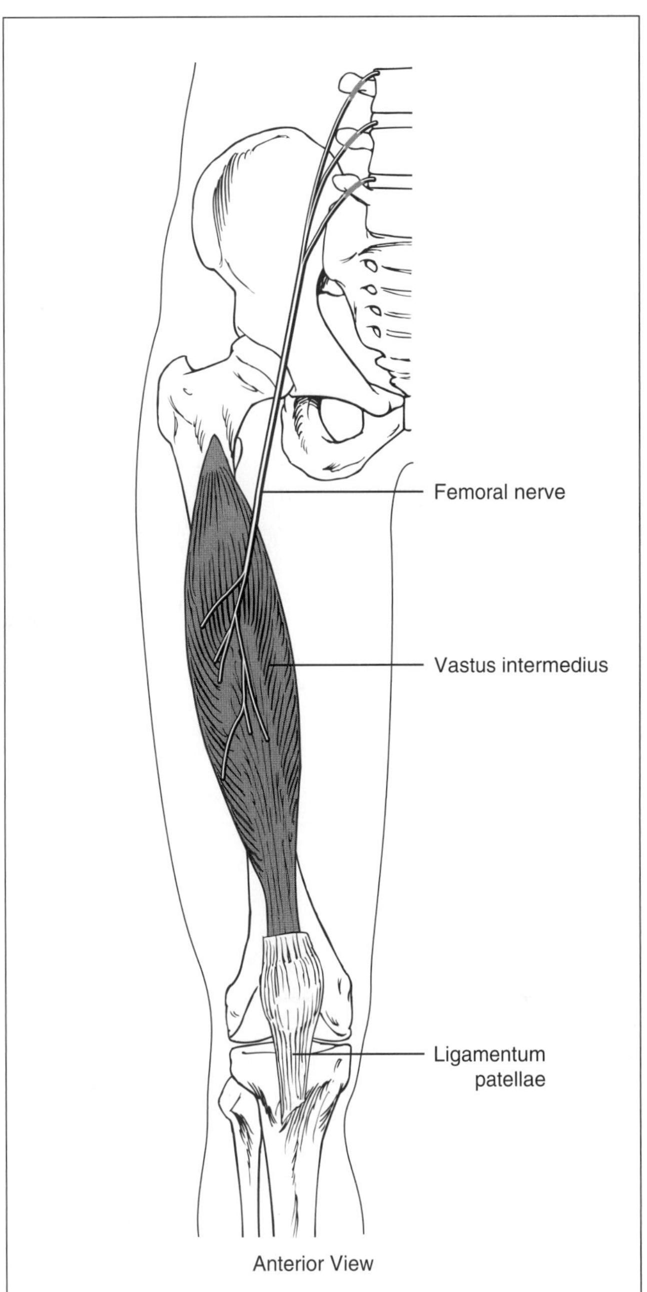
Femoral nerve
Vastus intermedius
Ligamentum patellae
Anterior View

	ATTACHMENTS	NERVE SUPPLY	FUNCTION
Rectus femoris	Origin: Anterior inferior iliac spine, groove above the posterior brim of the acetabulum Insertion: Base of the patella and via the ligamentum patellae into the tibial tuberosity	Peripheral nerve: Femoral nerve Nerve root: L2–L4	Extension of the knee, flexion of the hip
Vastus lateralis	Origin: Greater trochanter of the femur, intertrochanteric line, linea aspera, gluteal tuberosity Insertion: Lateral border of the patella and via the ligamentum patellae into the tibial tuberosity	Peripheral nerve: Femoral nerve Nerve root: L2–L4	Extension of the knee
Vastus medialis	Origin: Intertrochanteric line, linea aspera, medial supracondylar line of the femur Insertion: Medial border of the patella and via the ligamentum patellae into the tibial tuberosity	Peripheral nerve: Femoral nerve Nerve root: L2–L4	Extension of the knee
Vastus intermedius	Origin: Anterior and lateral surfaces of the upper ⅔ of the body of the femur Insertion: Base of the patella and via the ligamentum patellae into the tibial tuberosity	Peripheral nerve: Femoral nerve Nerve root: L2–L4	Extension of the knee

Gravity-Resisted Test (Grades 5, 4, and 3)

Patient position: Seated with legs off side of table, folded towel under knee of test limb. Patient grasps edges of table to assist in stability (Fig. 4-62).

Fig. 4-62.

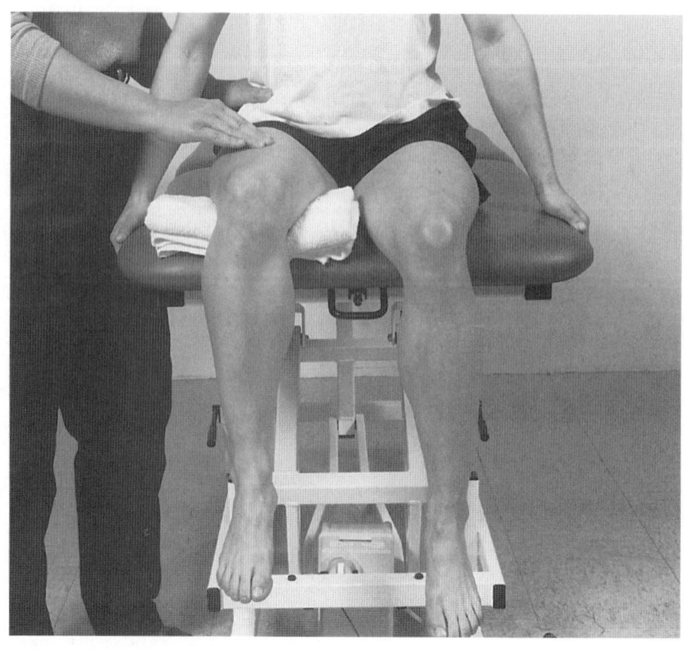

Stabilization/palpation: Stabilize anterior thigh over most proximal aspect, avoiding pressure over quadriceps muscles. With opposite hand, palpate quadriceps muscles over anterior aspect of thigh (Fig. 4-62).

Examiner action: While instructing patient in motion desired, extend patient's knee through full available ROM. Return limb to starting position. Performing passive movement allows determination of patient's available ROM and shows patient exact motion desired.

Patient action: Patient extends knee through full available ROM. Examiner stabilizes thigh and palpates quadriceps during patient's active movement (Fig. 4-63).

Fig. 4-63. Arrow indicates direction of movement.

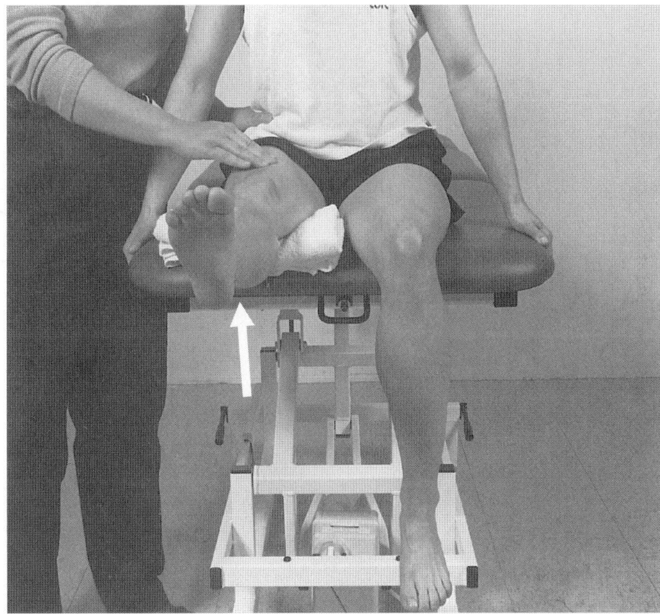

Resistance: Apply resistance over anterior aspect of distal leg in direction of knee flexion after first flexing knee slightly. Palpating hand is moved to distal leg to apply resistance (Fig. 4-64).

Fig. 4-64. Arrow indicates direction of resistance.

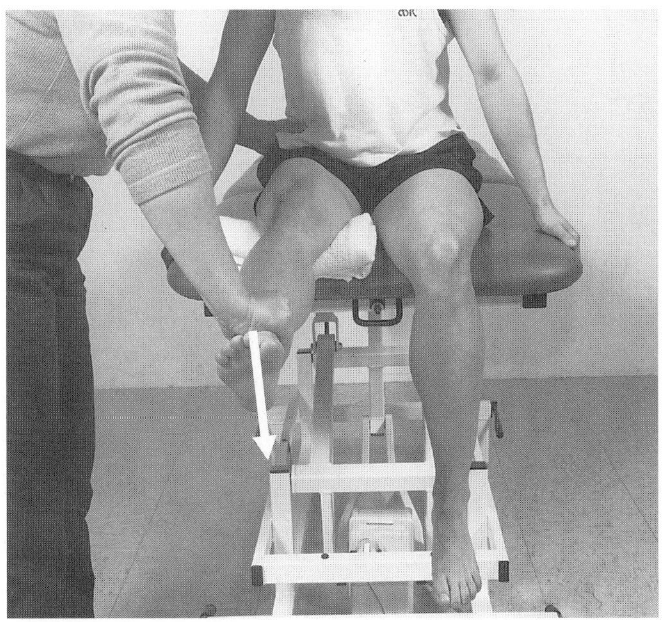

Gravity-Eliminated Test (Grades Below 3)

For patients unable to move completely through available ROM against gravity.

Patient position:

Side lying on side to be tested, patient's pelvis close to examiner's trunk, knee of lowermost limb fully flexed, hip extended. Talcum powder and a cloth may be placed between limb and supporting surface to reduce friction (Fig. 4-65; initial position of test knee not shown).

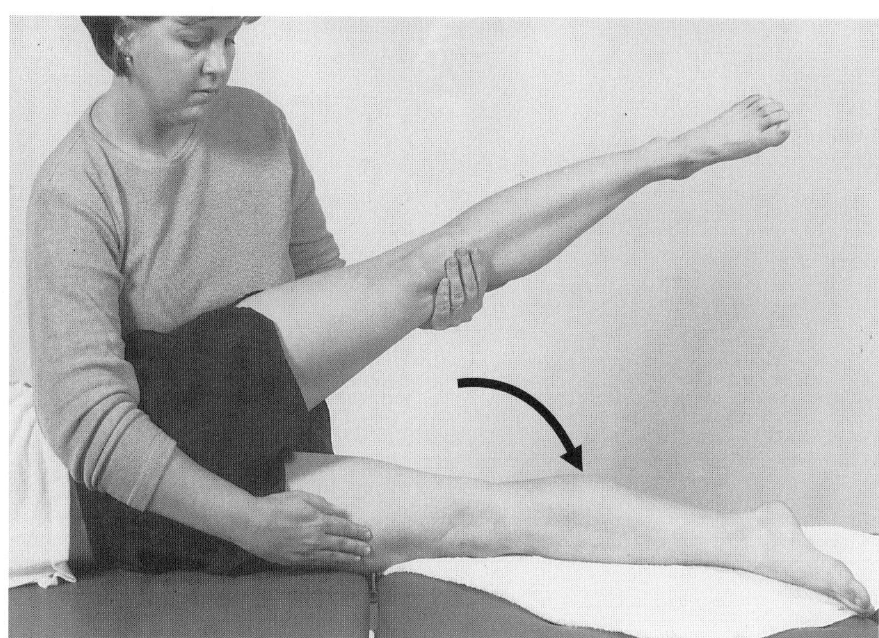

Fig. 4-65. Arrow indicates direction of movement.

Stabilization/palpation:

Stand directly behind patient's pelvis, stabilize pelvis with examiner's trunk, and support upper leg with one hand. With opposite hand, palpate quadriceps muscles (as in gravity-resisted test) (Fig. 4-65).

Examiner action:

As in gravity-resisted test.

Patient action:

Patient extends knee of test limb through full available ROM. Examiner stabilizes pelvis and palpates quadriceps during patient's active movement (Fig. 4-65).

COMMON SUBSTITUTION

Hip extension: If gravity-eliminated test is begun with test limb in hip flexion, patient may use hip extension to cause knee extension. Care should be taken to maintain hip in extension during gravity-eliminated test.

CLINICAL COMMENT: QUADRICEPS FEMORIS MUSCLE AND L3 NEUROLOGIC ASSESSMENT

The quadriceps femoris muscle is a key muscle for examining the integrity of the L3 spinal nerve or neurologic segment of the spinal cord. Complete assessment of the L3 neurologic level includes:

Strength assessment of:
Quadriceps femoris (pp. 304-306)
Hip adductors (pp. 287-289)

Reflex testing of:
Quadriceps (Patellar) tendon reflex (L2–L4; p. 550)

Sensory testing of:
Skin over anterior knee, just superior to patella (L3 dermatome; pp. 528-532)

■ KNEE FLEXION

BICEPS FEMORIS, SEMITENDINOSUS, AND SEMIMEMBRANOSUS (Figs. 4-66 and 4-67)

Fig. 4-66.

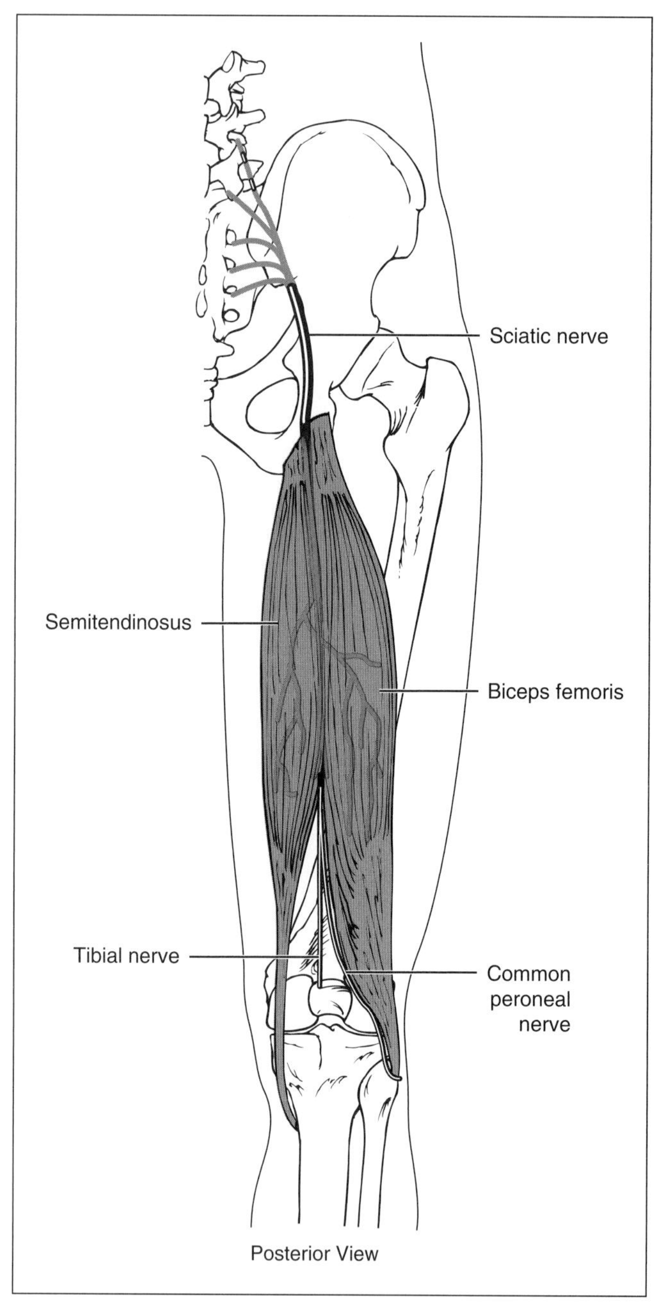

Fig. 4-67.

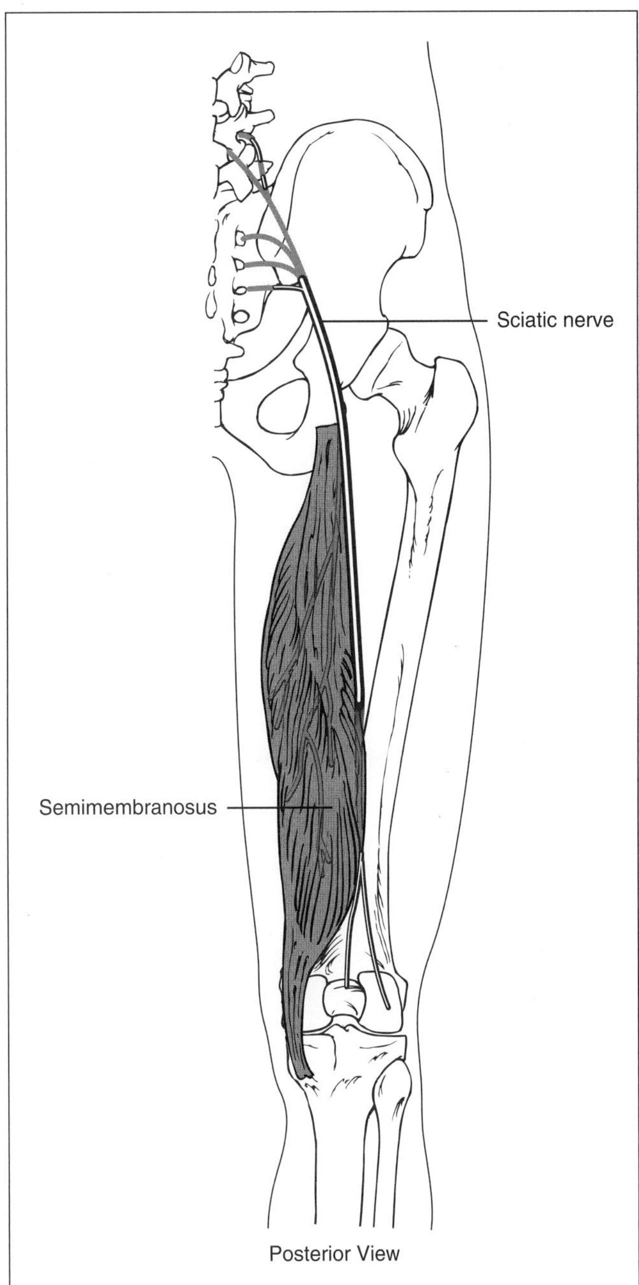

	ATTACHMENTS	NERVE SUPPLY	FUNCTION
Biceps femoris	Origin: Long head: Ischial tuberosity Short head: Lateral lip of the linea aspera of the femur and the lateral intermuscular septum Insertion: Lateral aspect of the head of the fibula	Peripheral nerve: Long head: Tibial portion of the sciatic nerve Short head: Peroneal portion of the sciatic nerve Nerve root: L5, S1, S2	Extension of the hip, flexion and lateral rotation of the knee
Semitendinosus	Origin: Ischial tuberosity Insertion: Proximal aspect of the medial surface of the tibia	Peripheral nerve: Tibial portion of the sciatic nerve Nerve root: L5, S1, S2	Extension of the hip, flexion and medial rotation of the knee
Semimembranosus	Origin: Ischial tuberosity Insertion: Medial condyle of the tibia	Peripheral nerve: Tibial portion of the sciatic nerve Nerve root: L5, S1, S2	Extension of the hip, flexion and medial rotation of the knee

Gravity-Resisted Test (Grades 5, 4, and 3)

BICEPS FEMORIS

Patient position: Prone with lower extremities extended (Fig. 4-68).

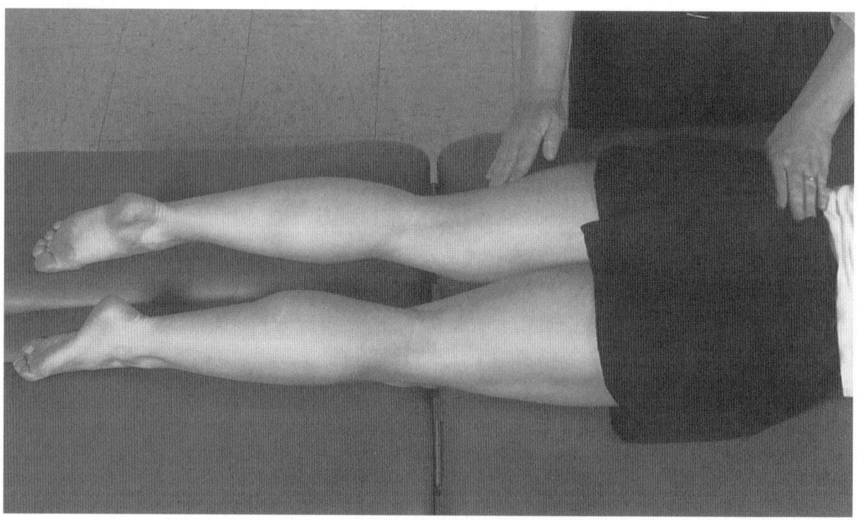

Fig. 4-68.

Stabilization/palpation: Stabilize over posterior aspect of pelvis. With opposite hand, palpate biceps femoris on lateral aspect of posterior thigh (Fig. 4-68).

Examiner action: While instructing patient in motion desired, flex patient's knee to 90°, rotating knee laterally. Return limb to starting position. Performing passive movement allows determination of patient's available ROM and shows patient exact motion desired.

Patient action:

Patient flexes knee to 90° while rotating knee laterally. Examiner stabilizes pelvis and palpates biceps femoris during patient's active movement (Fig. 4-69).

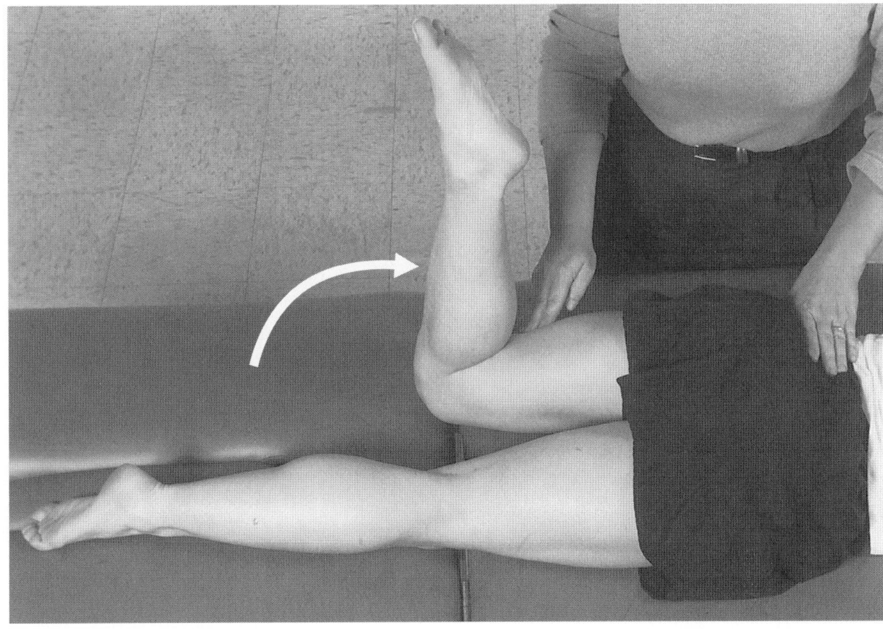

Fig. 4-69. Arrow indicates direction of movement.

Resistance:

Apply resistance over posterior aspect of distal leg in direction of knee extension. Palpating hand is moved to distal leg to apply resistance (Fig. 4-70).

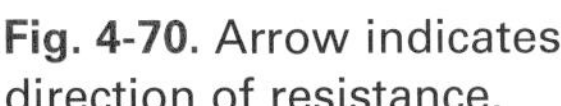

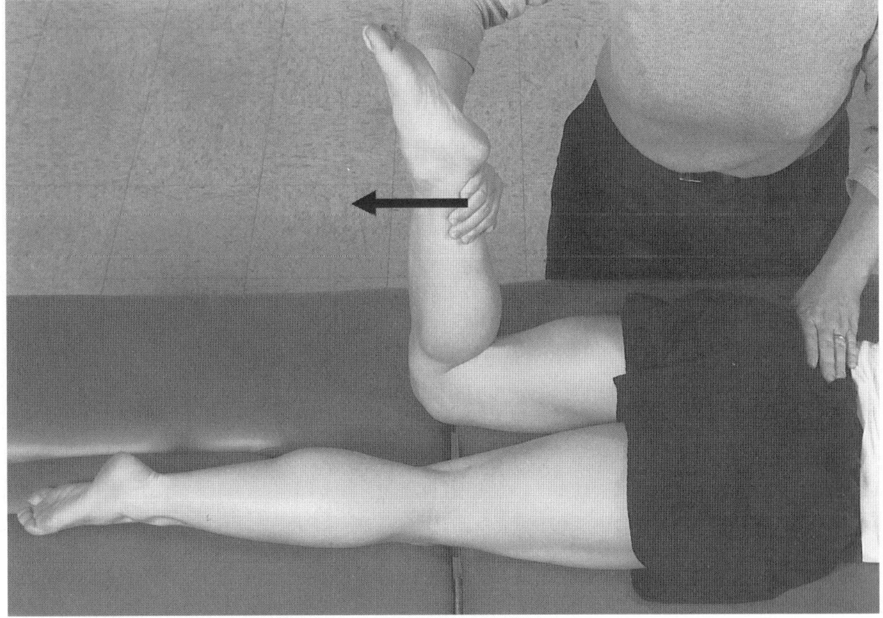

Fig. 4-70. Arrow indicates direction of resistance.

SEMITENDINOSUS AND SEMIMEMBRANOSUS

Patient position: Prone with lower extremities extended (Fig. 4-71).

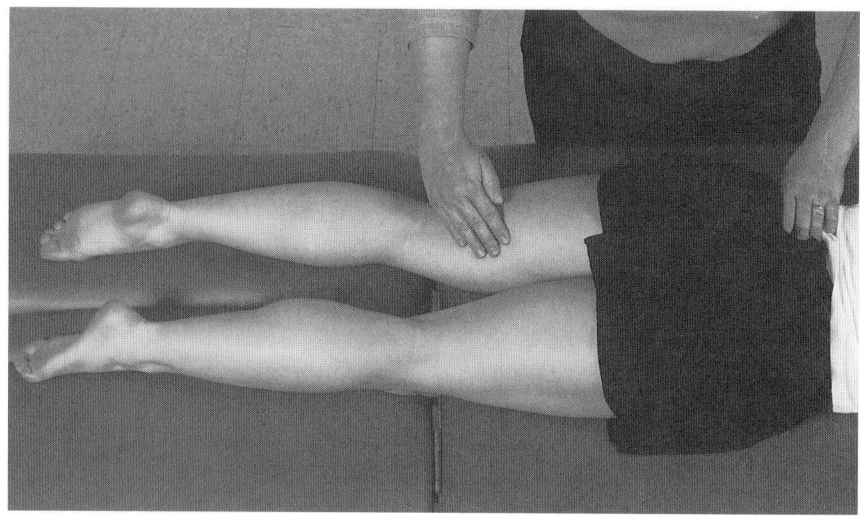

Fig. 4-71.

Stabilization/palpation: Stabilize over posterior aspect of pelvis. With opposite hand, palpate medial hamstrings over medial aspect of posterior thigh (Fig. 4-71).

Examiner action: While instructing patient in motion desired, flex patient's knee to 90°, rotating knee medially. Return limb to starting position. Performing passive movement allows determination of patient's available ROM and shows patient exact motion desired.

Patient action: Patient flexes leg to 90° while rotating knee medially. Examiner stabilizes pelvis and palpates medial hamstrings during patient's active movement (Fig. 4-72).

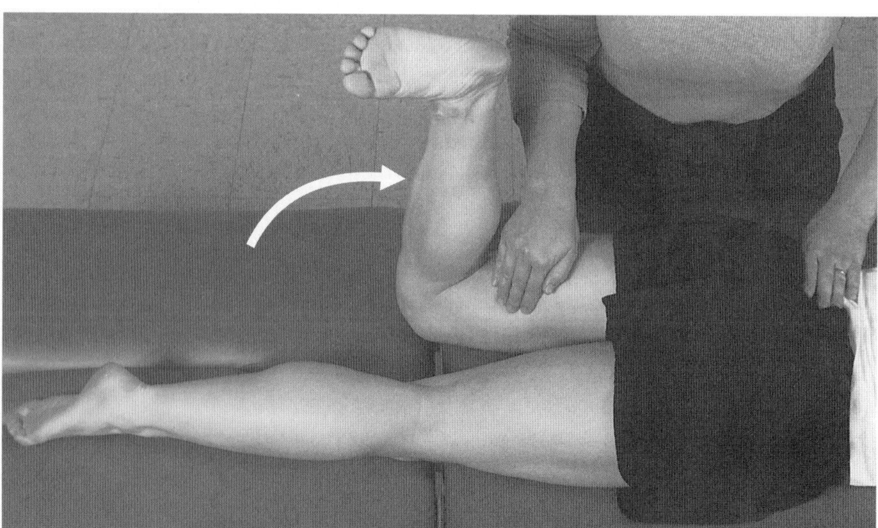

Fig. 4-72. Arrow indicates direction of movement.

Resistance: Apply resistance over posterior aspect of distal leg in direction of knee extension. Palpating hand is moved to distal leg to apply resistance (Fig. 4-73).

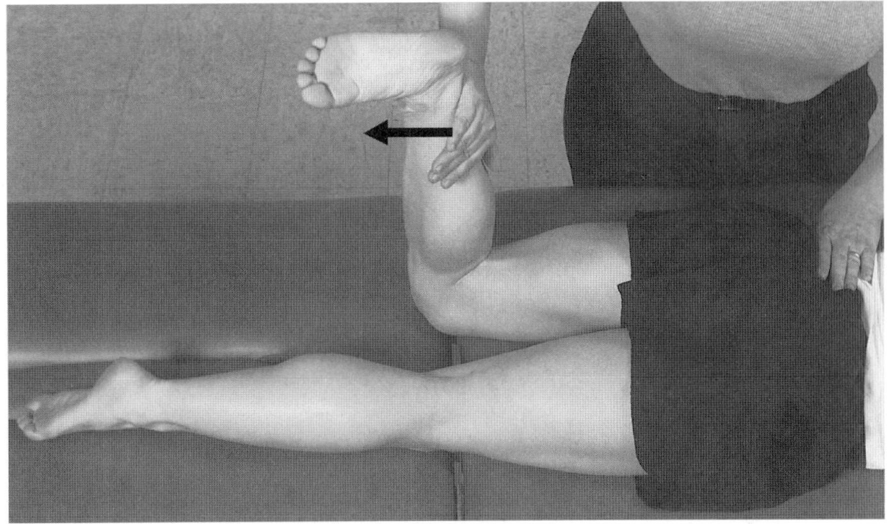

Fig. 4-73. Arrow indicates direction of resistance.

Gravity-Eliminated Test (Grades Below 3)

For patients unable to move completely through available ROM against gravity.

Patient position: Side lying on side to be tested, knee and hip of test limb fully extended. Talcum powder and a cloth may be placed between limb and supporting surface to reduce friction (Fig. 4-74; initial knee position of test limb not shown).

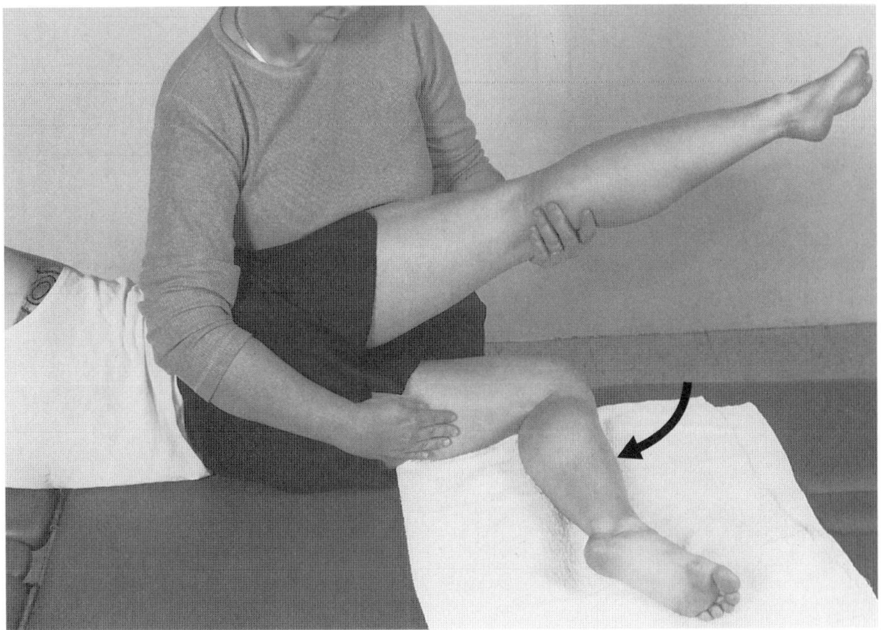

Fig. 4-74. Arrow indicates direction of movement.

Stabilization/palpation: Stand directly in front of patient's pelvis, stabilize pelvis with examiner's trunk, and support uppermost lower extremity with one hand. With opposite hand, palpate hamstring muscles (as in gravity-resisted test) (Fig. 4-74).

Examiner action: While instructing patient in motion desired, flex patient's knee through full available ROM. Return limb to starting position.

Patient action: Patient flexes knee of test limb through full available ROM. Examiner stabilizes pelvis and palpates hamstrings during patient's active movement (Fig. 4-74).

COMMON SUBSTITUTIONS

1. Hip flexors: Hip flexion, particularly as result of sartorius activity, may result in knee flexion without activity from hamstring muscles. Care should be taken to maintain hip in extension during test.
2. Gastrocnemius: Strong contraction of gastrocnemius may cause knee flexion. In such cases, ankle will be strongly plantar flexed.

■ ANKLE PLANTAR FLEXION: WEIGHT-BEARING TEST

GASTROCNEMIUS AND SOLEUS (Figs. 4-75 and 4-76)

Fig. 4-75.

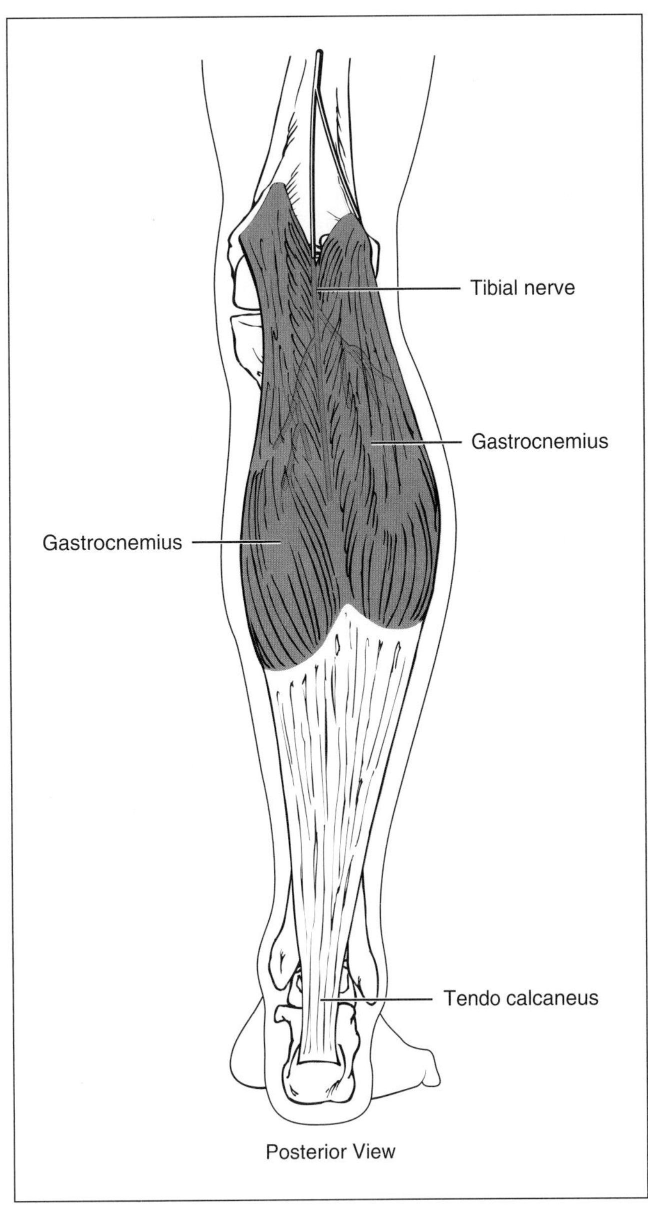

Fig. 4-76.

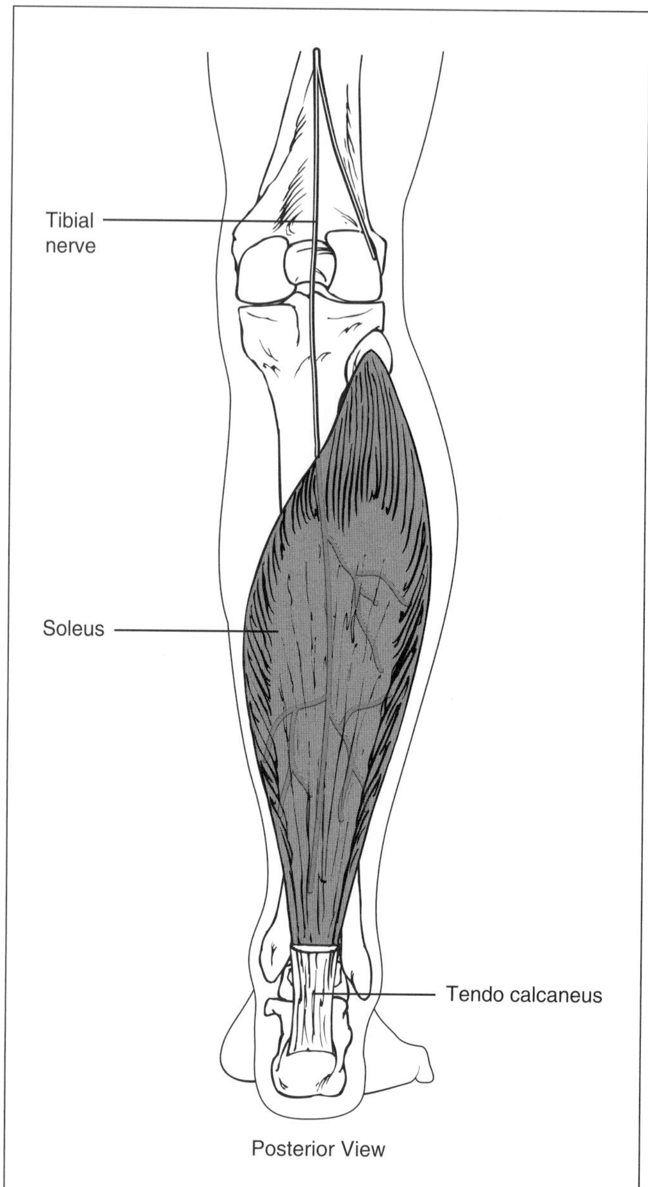

	ATTACHMENTS	NERVE SUPPLY	FUNCTION
Gastrocnemius	Origin: Medial head: Medial condyle and adjacent popliteal surface of the femur Lateral head: Lateral condyle of the femur Insertion: Via the tendo calcaneus into the posterior surface of the calcaneus	Peripheral nerve: Tibial nerve Nerve root: S1, S2	Plantar flexion of the ankle, flexion of the knee
Soleus	Origin: Posterior surface of the head and proximal ⅓ of the body of the fibula, soleal line and middle ⅓ of the medial border of the tibia Insertion: Via the tendo calcaneus into the posterior surface of the calcaneus	Peripheral nerve: Tibial nerve Nerve root: S1, S2	Plantar flexion of the ankle

Gravity-Resisted Test (Grades 5, 4, and 3)

GASTROCNEMIUS AND SOLEUS

Patient position: Standing on one leg (test limb), knee extended, foot flat on floor. Patient may rest one hand on table for balance only, not for weight support (Fig. 4-77).

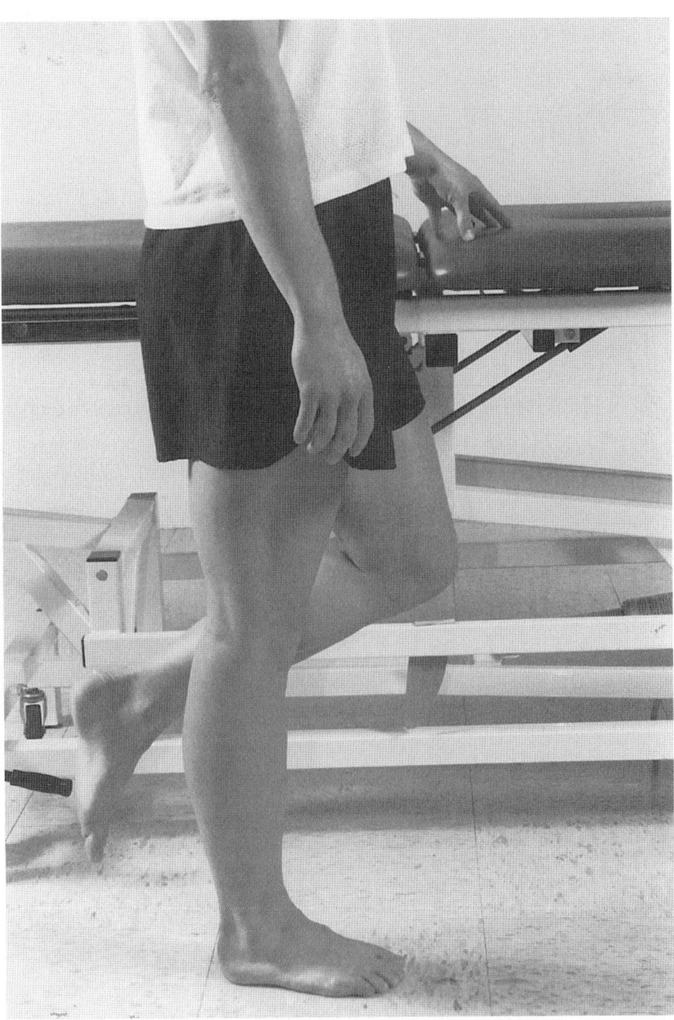

Fig. 4-77.

Stabilization/palpation: Patient's weight provides stabilization. Palpate gastrocnemius and soleus on posterior aspect of leg.

Examiner action: While instructing patient in motion desired, demonstrate movement of rising on toes with knee extended.

Patient action: Patient rises on toes of weight-bearing leg through full available range of ankle plantar flexion, keeping knee extended (Fig. 4-78). Patient repeats motion until fatigued or stopped by examiner.

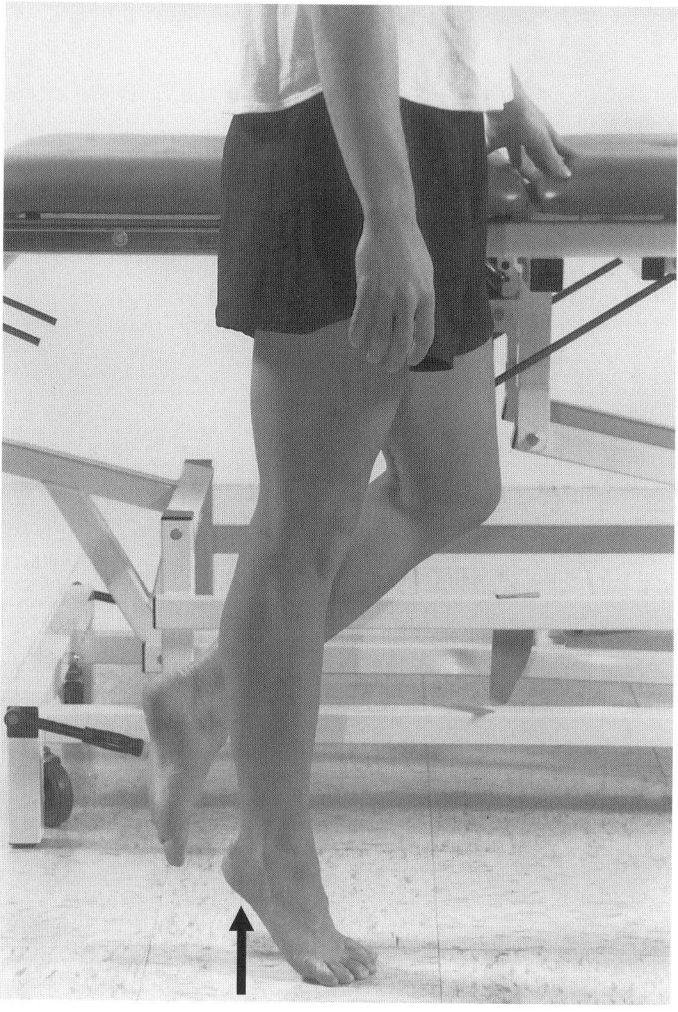

Fig. 4-78. Arrow indicates direction of movement.

Resistance: Patient's body weight and repetition provide resistance (see Grading, later in this section).

SOLEUS

Patient position: Patient is standing on one limb (test limb), knee flexed, foot flat on floor. Patient may rest one hand on table for balance only, not for weight support (Fig. 4-79).

Fig. 4-79.

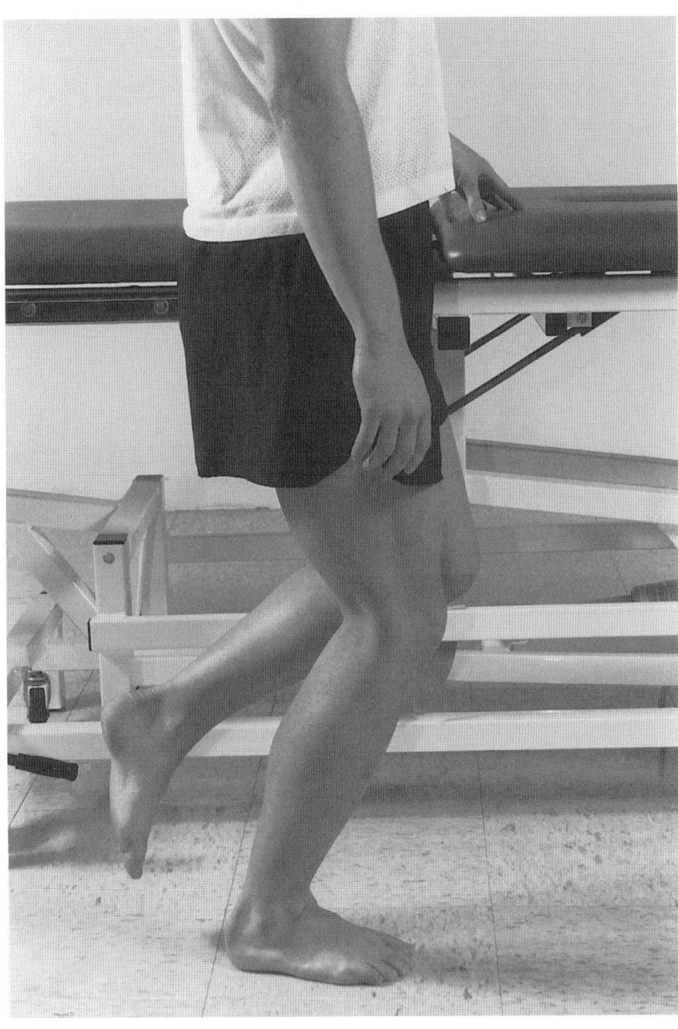

Stabilization/palpation: Patient's weight provides stabilization. Palpate soleus on distal aspect of posterior calf on sides of gastrocnemius.

Examiner action: While instructing patient in motion desired, demonstrate movement of rising on toes with knee flexed.

Patient action:

Patient rises on toes of weight-bearing leg through full available range of ankle plantar flexion, keeping knee flexed (Fig. 4-80). Patient repeats motion until fatigued or stopped by examiner.

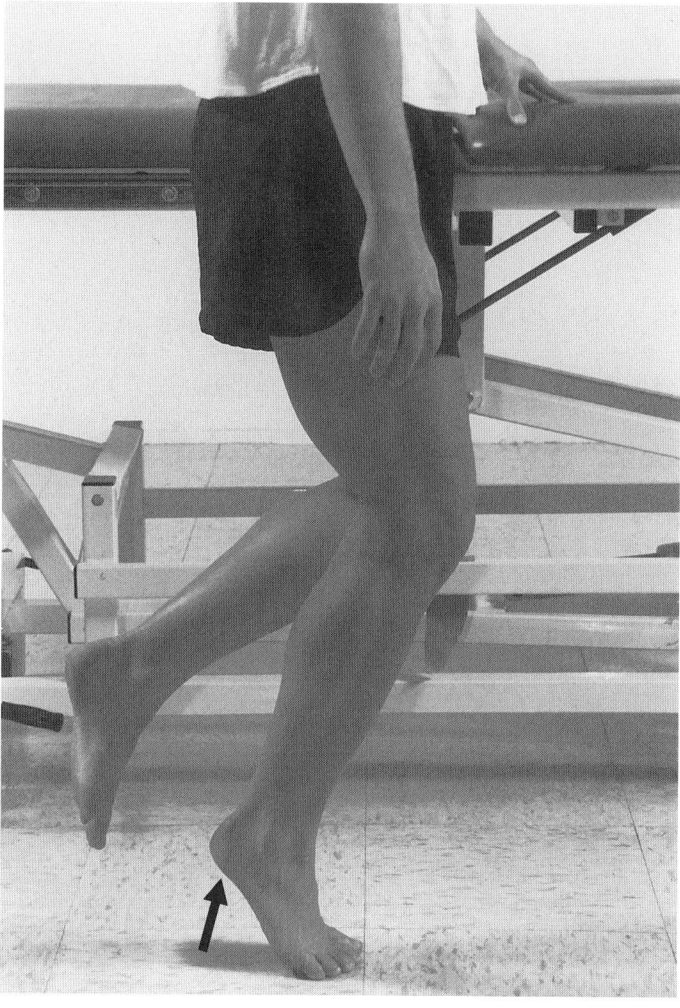

Fig. 4-80. Arrow indicates direction of movement.

Resistance:

Patient's body weight and repetition provide resistance (see Grading, later in this section).

Gravity-Eliminated Test (Grades Below 3)

Patient position: Side lying on side to be tested, test limb extended at hip and knee, ankle neutral (Fig. 4-81; starting position of ankle not shown).

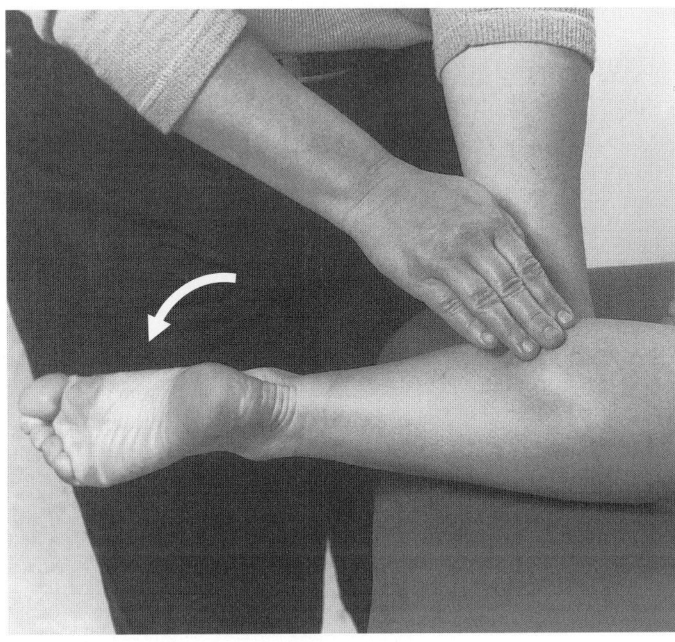

Fig. 4-81. Arrow indicates direction of movement.

Stabilization/palpation: Stabilize over anterior aspect of leg. With opposite hand, palpate gastrocnemius and soleus (as in gravity-resisted test) (Fig. 4-81).

Examiner action: While instructing patient in motion desired, plantar flex patient's ankle through full available ROM. Return limb to starting position. Performing passive movement allows determination of patient's available ROM and shows patient exact motion desired.

Patient action: Patient plantar flexes ankle through full available ROM while examiner stabilizes leg and palpates plantar flexors (Fig. 4-81).

GRADING

Criteria for grading weight-bearing test for gastrocnemius and soleus vary depending on source. Lunsford and Perry[4,6] proposed different grading criteria from those espoused by Daniels and Worthingham. Grading criteria delineated by Hislop and Montgomery's revision of Daniels and Worthingham text differ from both of previous sources[7]. All three sets of criteria are described below:

GRADE	DANIELS AND WORTHINGHAM	LUNSFORD AND PERRY	HISLOP AND MONTGOMERY
5	The patient raises the heel from the floor through full ROM 4–5 times	The patients raises the heel from the floor through full ROM 25 times	The patient raises the hell from the floor through full ROM 20 times
4	The patient raises the heel from the floor through full ROM 2–3 times	Not defined	The patient raises the heel from the floor through full ROM 10–19 times
3	The patient raises the heel from the floor through full ROM 1 time	The patient is "able to hold body weight once in heel-up position, but unable to raise body weight from neutral"	The patient raises the heel from the floor through full ROM 1–9 times

CLINICAL COMMENT: ANKLE PLANTAR FLEXOR MUSCLES AND S1 NEUROLOGIC ASSESSMENT

The ankle plantar flexor muscles (gastrocnemius and soleus) are key muscles for examining the integrity of the S1 spinal nerve or neurologic segment of the spinal cord. Complete assessment of the S1 neurologic level includes:

Strength assessment of:
Gluteus maximus (pp. 265-267)
Gastrocnemius (pp. 317-321)
Soleus (pp. 317-321)
Peroneus longus and brevis (pp. 339-342)
Reflex testing of:
Achilles reflex (p. 551)
Sensory testing of:
Skin over the plantar surface of the foot and the little toe (S1 dermatome; pp. 528-532)

ANKLE PLANTAR FLEXION: NON–WEIGHT-BEARING TEST

GASTROCNEMIUS AND SOLEUS

Patients unable to accomplish weight-bearing test for gastrocnemius and soleus strength due to problems with balance, general lower extremity weakness, or other factors can be tested in a non–weight-bearing position. However, non–weight-bearing testing should be avoided if possible, as muscle test grades above fair are suspect due to examiner's possible inability to apply sufficient force to adequately grade triceps surae group.

Gravity-Resisted Test (Grades 5, 4, and 3)

GASTROCNEMIUS AND SOLEUS

Patient position: Prone with knee extended, foot off end of table, ankle neutral (Fig. 4-82; starting position of ankle not shown).

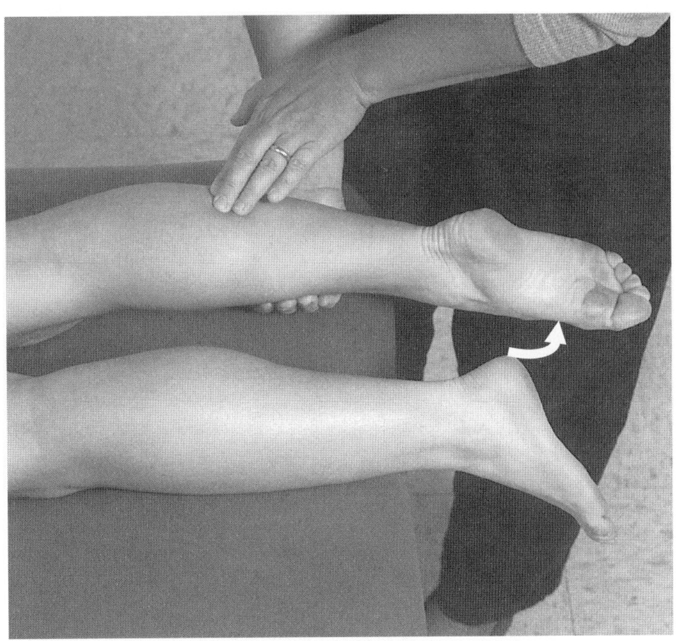

Fig. 4-82. Arrow indicates direction of movement.

Stabilization/palpation: Stabilize anterior aspect of distal leg, avoiding direct pressure over calcaneal tendon. With opposite hand, palpate gastrocnemius and soleus on posterior aspect of leg (Fig. 4-82).

Examiner action: While instructing patient in motion desired, plantar flex patient's ankle through full available ROM. Return limb to starting position. Performing passive movement allows determination of patient's available ROM and shows patient exact motion desired.

Patient action: Patient plantar flexes ankle through full available ROM while examiner stabilizes leg and palpates plantar flexors (Fig. 4-82).

Resistance:

Apply resistance on superoposterior aspect of calcaneus in direction of ankle dorsiflexion. Resistance may be supplemented by applying pressure against plantar surface of forefoot in direction of ankle dorsiflexion. When resistance is applied, palpating hand is moved to calcaneus to apply resistance while stabilizing hand remains in place (Fig. 4-83).

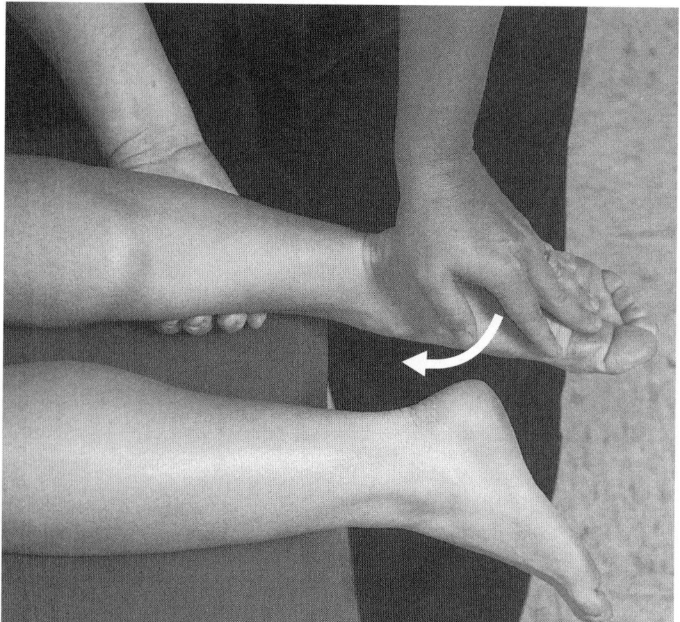

Fig. 4-83. Arrow indicates direction of resistance.

SOLEUS

Patient position: Prone with knee flexed to 90°, ankle neutral (Fig. 4-84; starting position of ankle not shown).

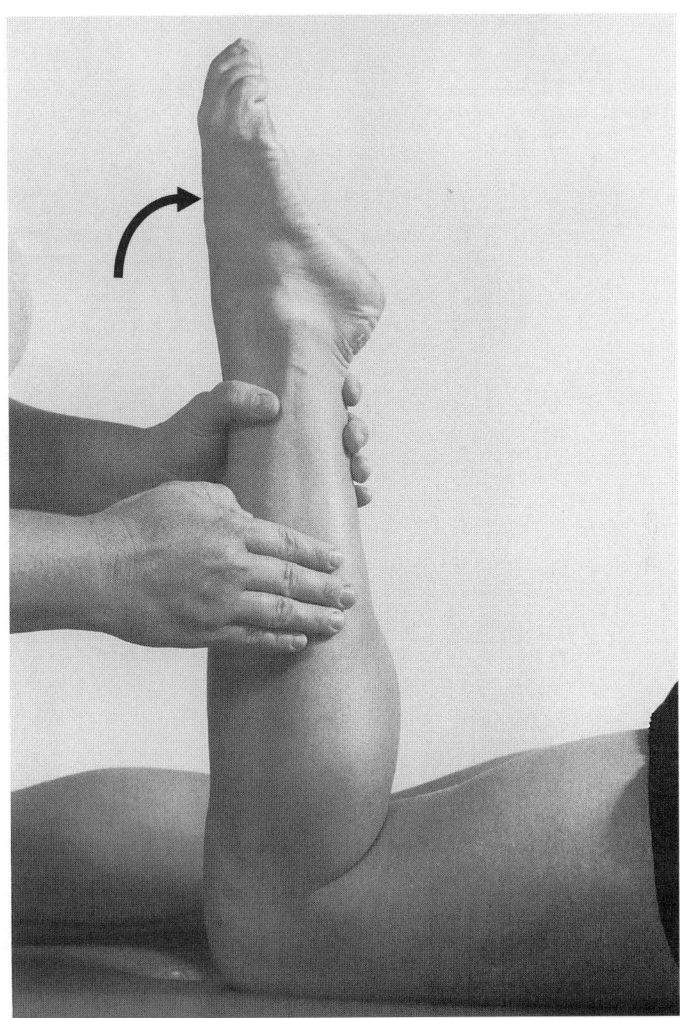

Fig. 4-84. Arrow indicates direction of movement.

Stabilization/palpation: Stabilize distal leg, avoiding direct pressure over calcaneal tendon. With opposite hand, palpate soleus on distal aspect of posterior calf at sides of gastrocnemius (Fig. 4-84).

Examiner action: While instructing patient in motion desired, plantar flex patient's ankle through full available ROM. Return limb to starting position. Performing passive movement allows determination of patient's available ROM and shows patient exact motion desired.

Patient action: Patient plantar flexes ankle through full available ROM, keeping knee flexed. Examiner stabilizes leg and palpates soleus during patient's active movement (Fig. 4-84).

Resistance: Apply resistance on superoposterior aspect of calcaneus in direction of ankle dorsiflexion. Resistance may be supplemented by applying pressure against plantar surface of forefoot in direction of ankle dorsiflexion. Palpating hand is moved to calcaneus to apply resistance while stabilizing hand remains in place (Fig. 4-85).

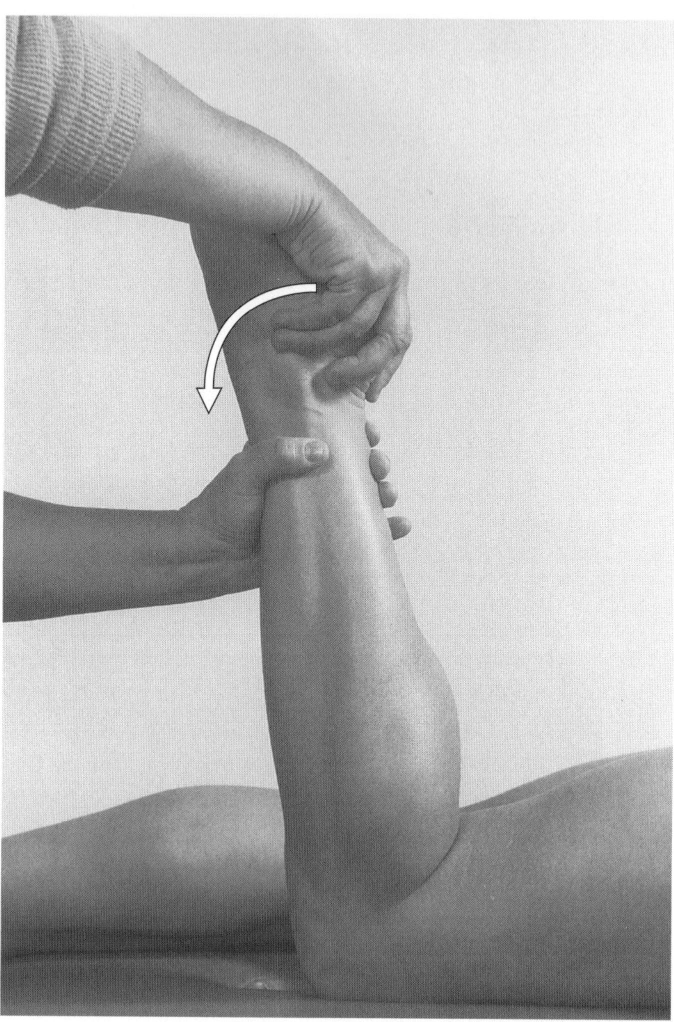

Fig. 4-85. Arrow indicates direction of resistance.

Gravity-Eliminated Test (Grades Below 3)

Gravity-eliminated test is same as that described in Ankle Plantar Flexion: Weight-Bearing Test.

■ ANKLE DORSIFLEXION AND SUBTALAR INVERSION

TIBIALIS ANTERIOR (Fig. 4-86)

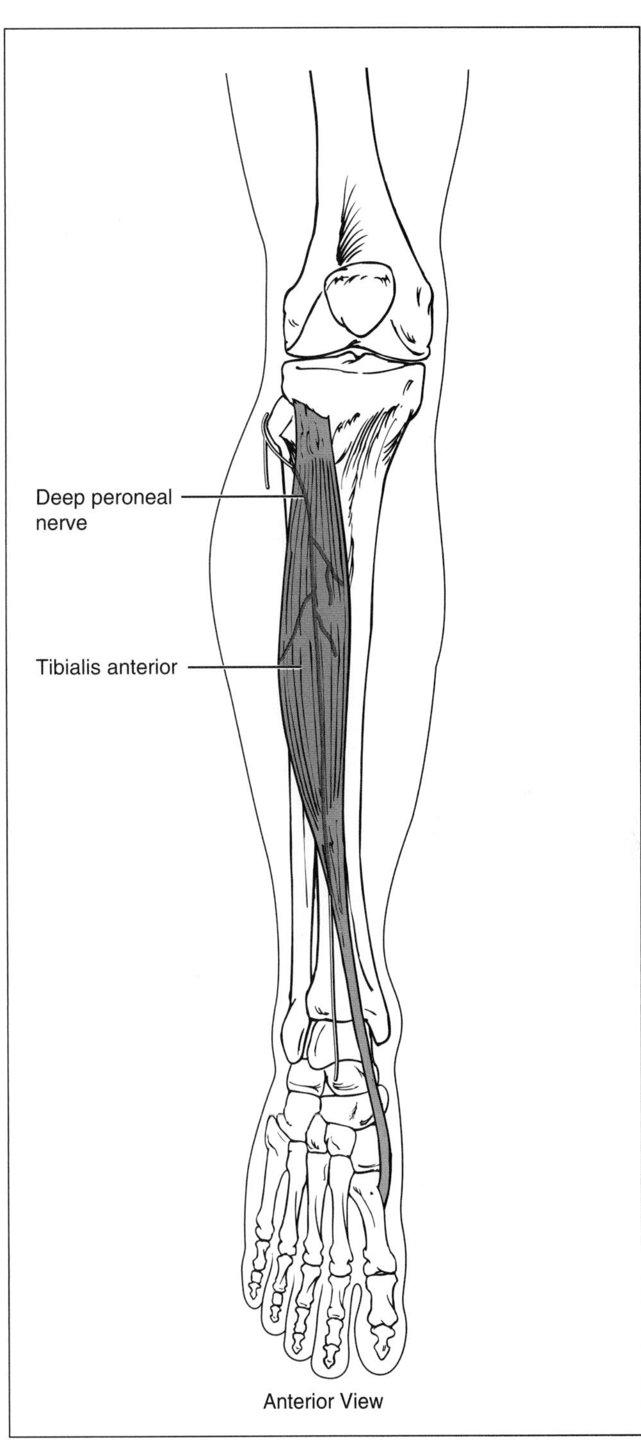

Fig. 4-86.

	ATTACHMENTS	NERVE SUPPLY	FUNCTION
Tibialis anterior	Origin: Lateral condyle and upper ⅔ of the lateral surface of the body of the tibia, interosseous membrane, deep crural fascia Insertion: Base of the 1st metatarsal, medial and plantar surfaces of the medial cuneiform bone	Peripheral nerve: Deep peroneal nerve Nerve root: L4, L5, S1	Dorsiflexion of the foot at the ankle, inversion of the foot at the subtalar and midtarsal joints

Gravity-Resisted Test (Grades 5, 4, and 3)

Patient position: Seated with legs off side of table, ankle neutral (Fig. 4-87).

Fig. 4-87.

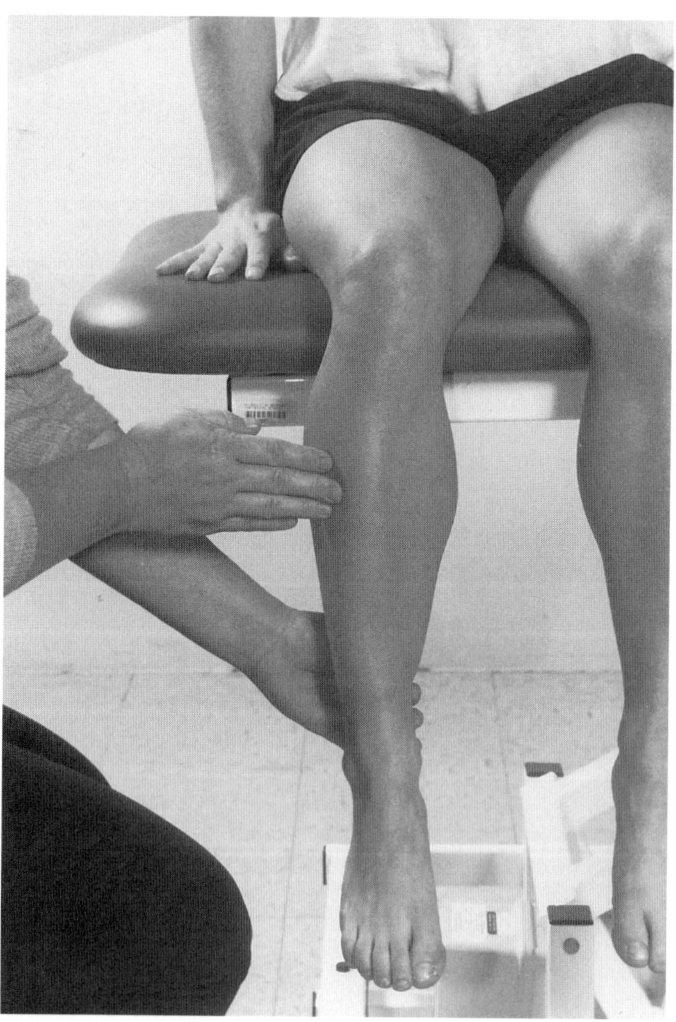

Stabilization/palpation: Stabilize over posterior aspect of distal leg. With opposite hand, palpate tibialis anterior on anterolateral aspect of tibia (Fig. 4-87).

Examiner action:

While instructing patient in motion desired, dorsiflex and invert patient's ankle through full available ROM. Return limb to starting position. Performing passive movement allows determination of patient's available ROM and shows patient exact motion desired.

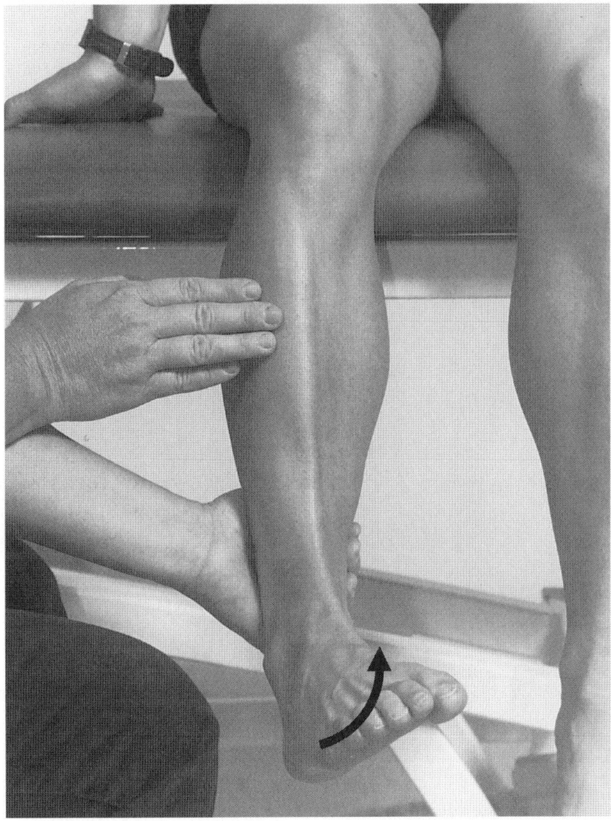

Fig. 4-88. Arrow indicates direction of movement.

Patient action:

Patient moves foot into dorsiflexion and inversion (toes should remain relaxed or flexed during movement). Examiner stabilizes distal leg and palpates tibialis anterior during patient's active movement (Fig. 4-88).

Resistance: Apply resistance over dorsal surface of medial side of foot in direction of plantar flexion and eversion. Palpating hand is moved to foot to apply resistance (Fig. 4-89).

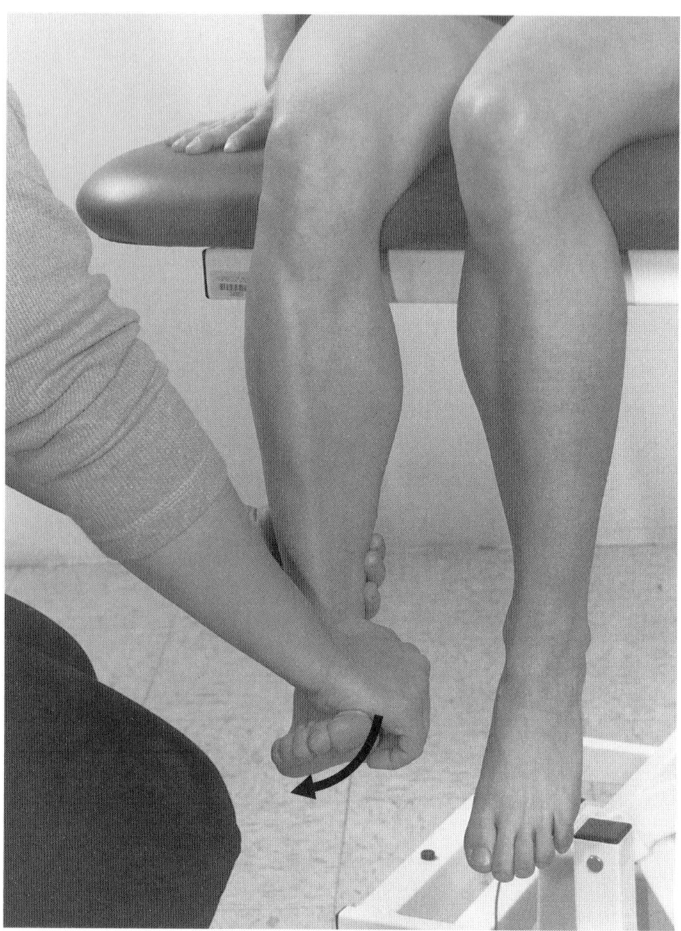

Fig. 4-89. Arrow indicates direction of resistance.

Gravity-Eliminated Test (Grades Below 3)

For patients unable to move completely through available ROM against gravity.

Patient position: Supine with lower extremities extended, ankle of test limb in neutral, foot extended beyond edge of table (Fig. 4-90; starting position of ankle not shown).

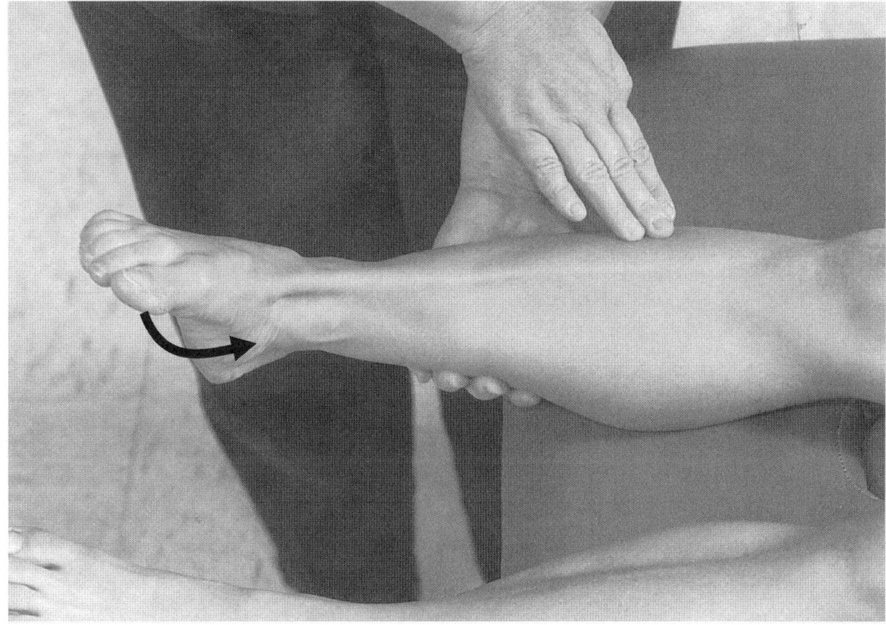

Fig. 4-90. Arrow indicates direction of movement.

Stabilization/palpation: As in gravity-resisted test (Fig. 4-90).

Examiner action: As in gravity-resisted test.

Patient action: Patient moves foot into dorsiflexion and inversion (toes should remain relaxed or flexed during movement). Examiner stabilizes distal leg and palpates tibialis anterior during patient's active movement (Fig. 4-90).

COMMON SUBSTITUTION

Long toe extensors: Substitution by long toe extensors results in extension of toes during dorsiflexion movement. Care should be taken to keep toes relaxed or flexed during movement.

CLINICAL COMMENT: TIBIALIS ANTERIOR MUSCLE AND L4 NEUROLOGIC ASSESSMENT

The tibialis anterior muscle is a key muscle for examining the integrity of the L4 spinal nerve or neurologic segment of the spinal cord. Complete assessment of the L4 neurologic level includes:

Strength assessment of:
Tibialis anterior (pp. 328-331)

Reflex testing of:
Quadriceps (Patellar) tendon reflex (p. 550)

Sensory testing of:
Skin over medial side of leg and medial malleolus (L4 dermatome; pp. 528-532)

■ SUBTALAR INVERSION

TIBIALIS POSTERIOR (Fig. 4-91)

Fig. 4-91.

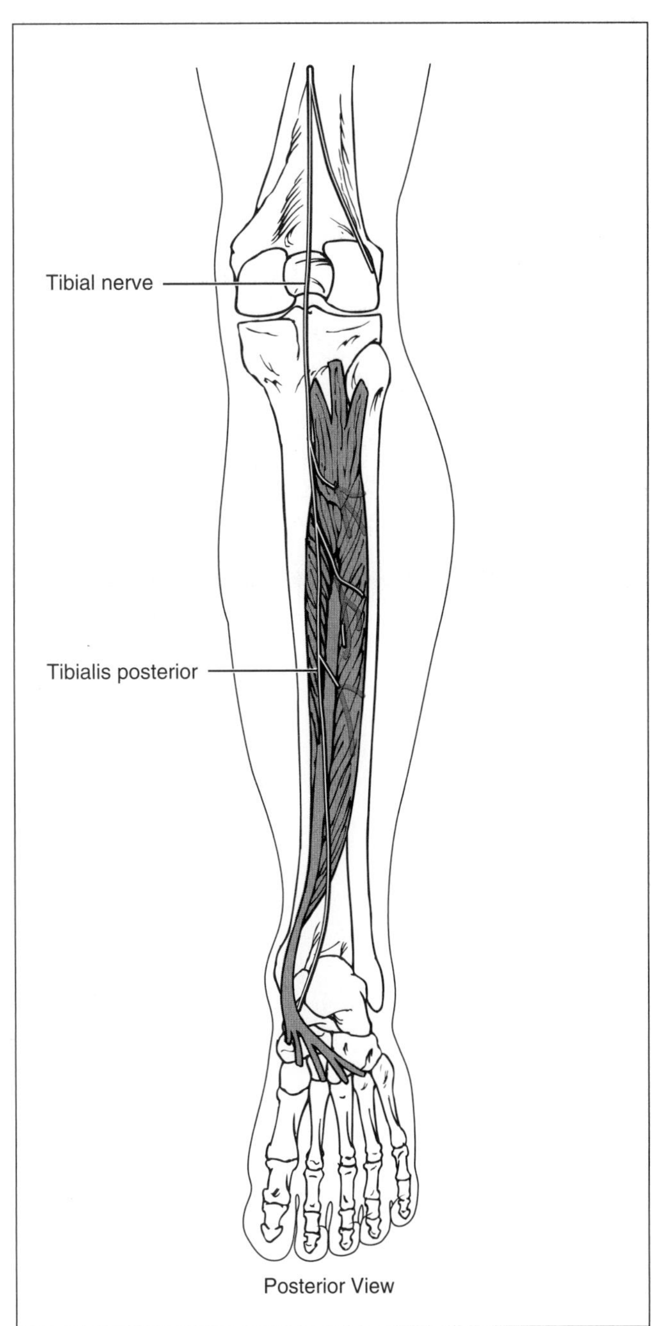

	ATTACHMENTS	NERVE SUPPLY	FUNCTION
Tibialis posterior	Origin: Posterior aspect of the interosseous membrane, posterior surface of the body of the tibia, proximal ⅔ of the medial surface of the fibula Insertion: Tuberosity of the navicular bone, cuboid bone, all three cuneiform bones, bases of metatarsals 2–4	Peripheral nerve: Tibial Nerve root: L5, S1	Inversion of the foot at the subtalar joint, plantar flexion of the foot at the ankle

Gravity-Resisted Test (Grades 5, 4, and 3)

Patient position: Side lying on side to be tested, with ankle slightly plantar flexed, foot extended beyond edge of table (Fig. 4-92).

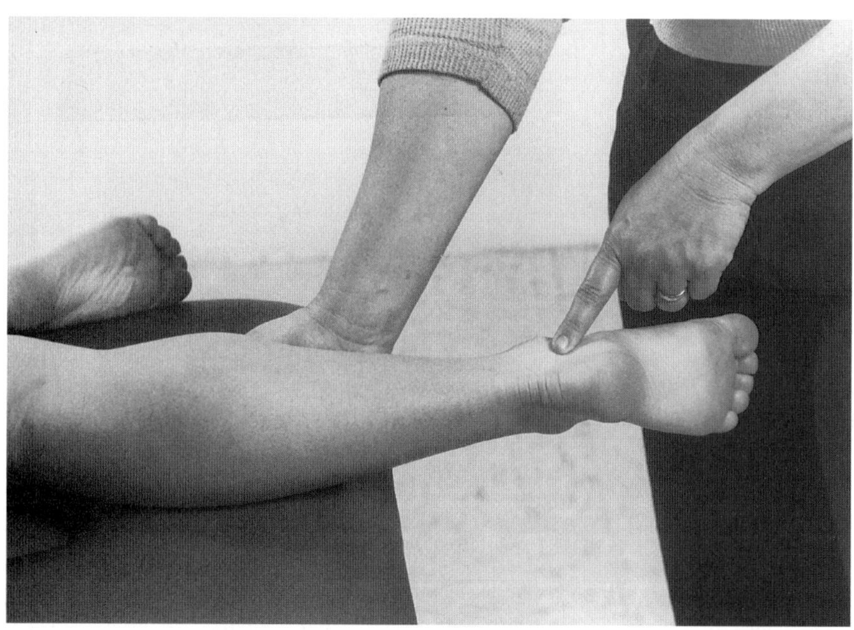

Fig. 4-92.

Stabilization/palpation: Stabilize over anteromedial aspect of tibia. With opposite hand, palpate tibialis posterior directly distal and posterior to medial malleolus (Fig. 4-92).

Examiner action: While instructing patient in motion desired, invert patient's foot through full available ROM. Return limb to starting position. Performing passive movement allows determination of patient's available ROM and shows patient exact motion desired.

Patient action:

Patient inverts subtalar joint through full available ROM (toes should remain relaxed or extended during movement). Examiner stabilizes tibia and palpates tibialis posterior during patient's active movement (Fig. 4-93).

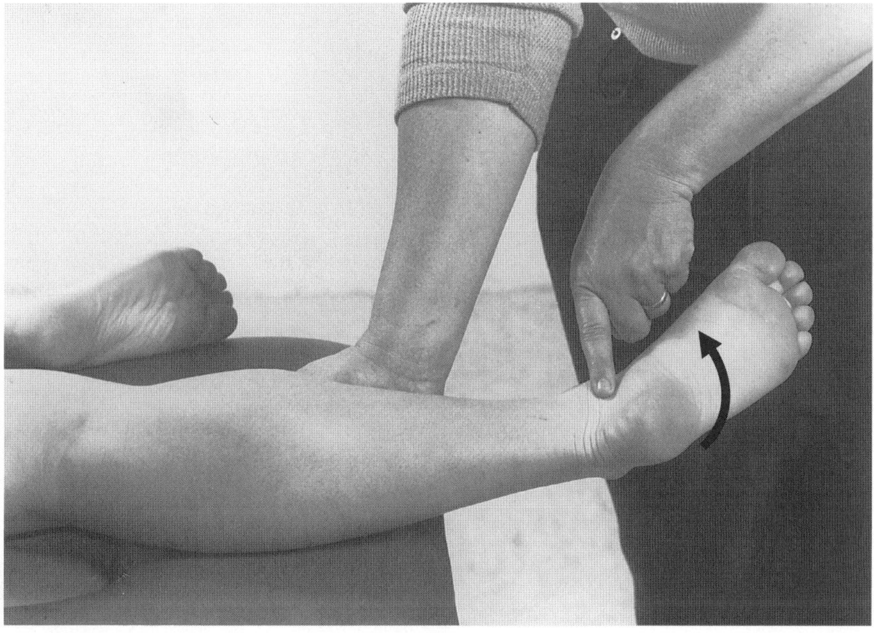

Fig. 4-93. Arrow indicates direction of movement.

Resistance:

Apply resistance over medial aspect of foot in direction of eversion. Palpating hand is moved to foot to apply resistance (Fig. 4-94).

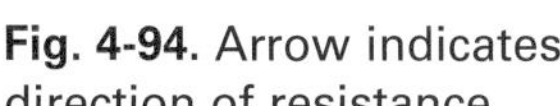

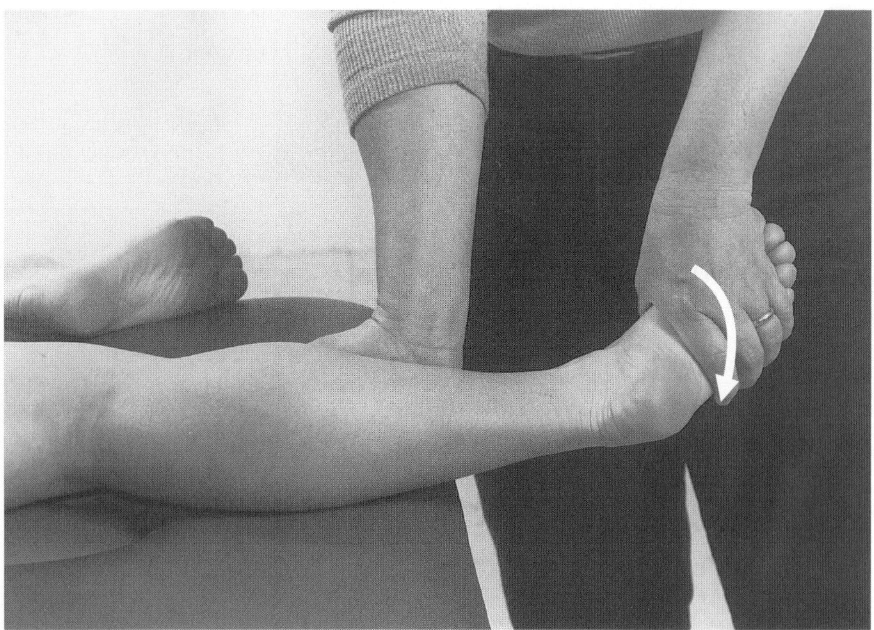

Fig. 4-94. Arrow indicates direction of resistance.

Gravity-Eliminated Test (Grades Below 3)

Patient position: Supine with lower extremities extended, ankle of test limb in slight plantar flexion, foot extended beyond edge of table (Fig. 4-95; starting position of ankle not shown).

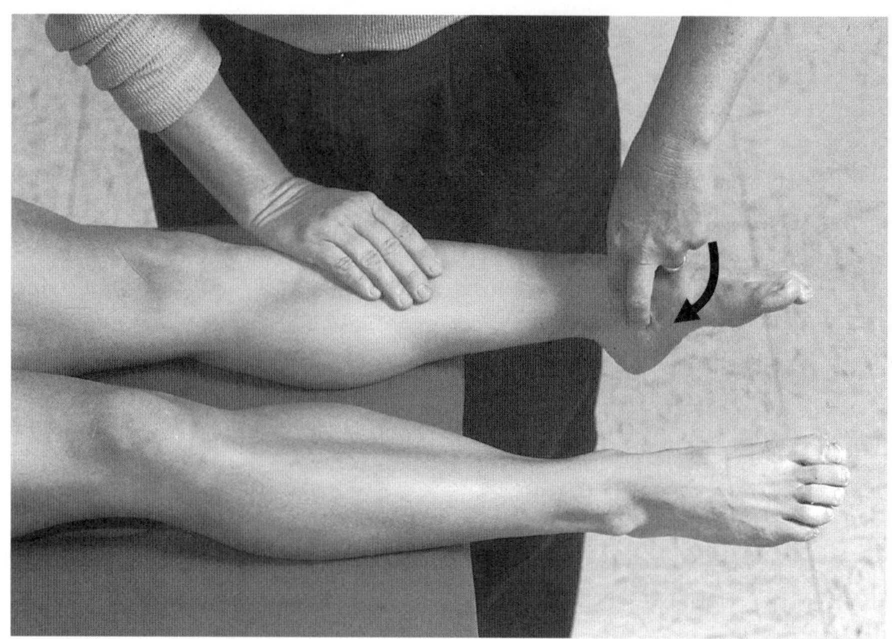

Fig. 4-95. Arrow indicates direction of movement.

Stabilization/palpation: As in gravity-resisted test (Fig. 4-95).

Examiner action: As in gravity-resisted test.

Patient action: Patient inverts subtalar joint through full available ROM (toes should remain relaxed or extended during movement). Examiner stabilizes tibia and palpates tibialis posterior during patient's active movement (Fig. 4-95).

COMMON SUBSTITUTIONS

1. Long toe flexors: Substitution by long toe flexors results in flexion of toes during inversion movement. Care should be taken to keep toes relaxed or extended during movement.
2. Tibialis anterior: Substitution by tibialis anterior results in dorsiflexion of ankle during subtalar inversion. Care should be taken to prevent dorsiflexion during test for tibialis posterior.

■ SUBTALAR EVERSION

PERONEUS LONGUS AND BREVIS (Figs. 4-96 and 4-97)

Fig. 4-96.

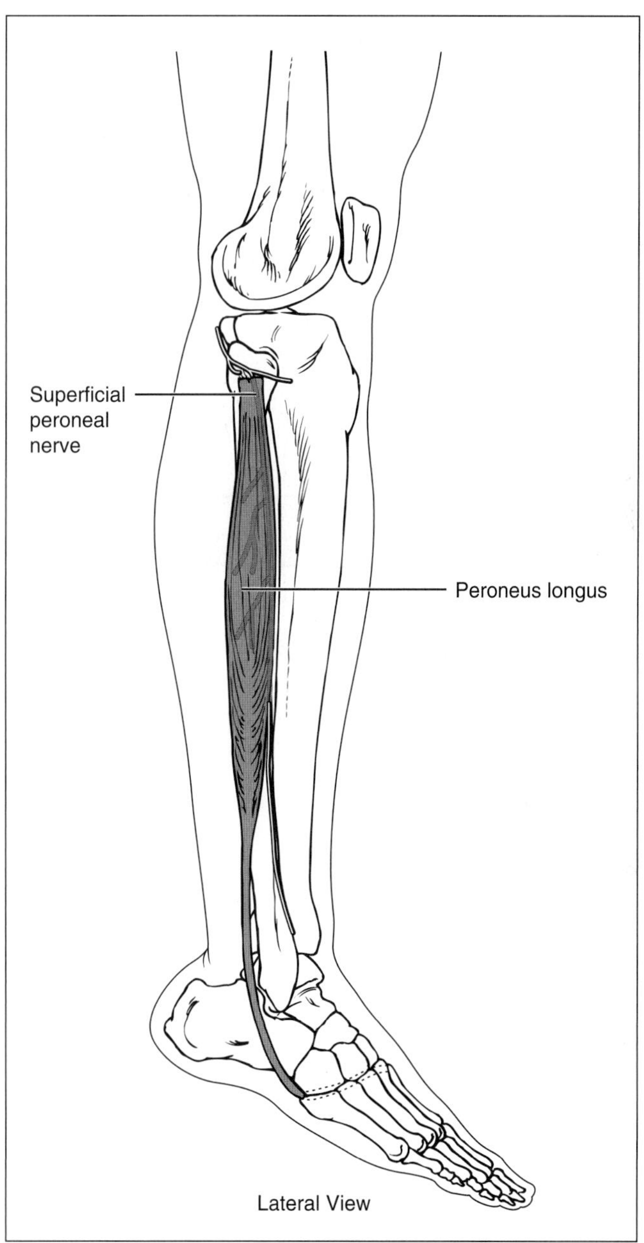

Fig. 4-97.

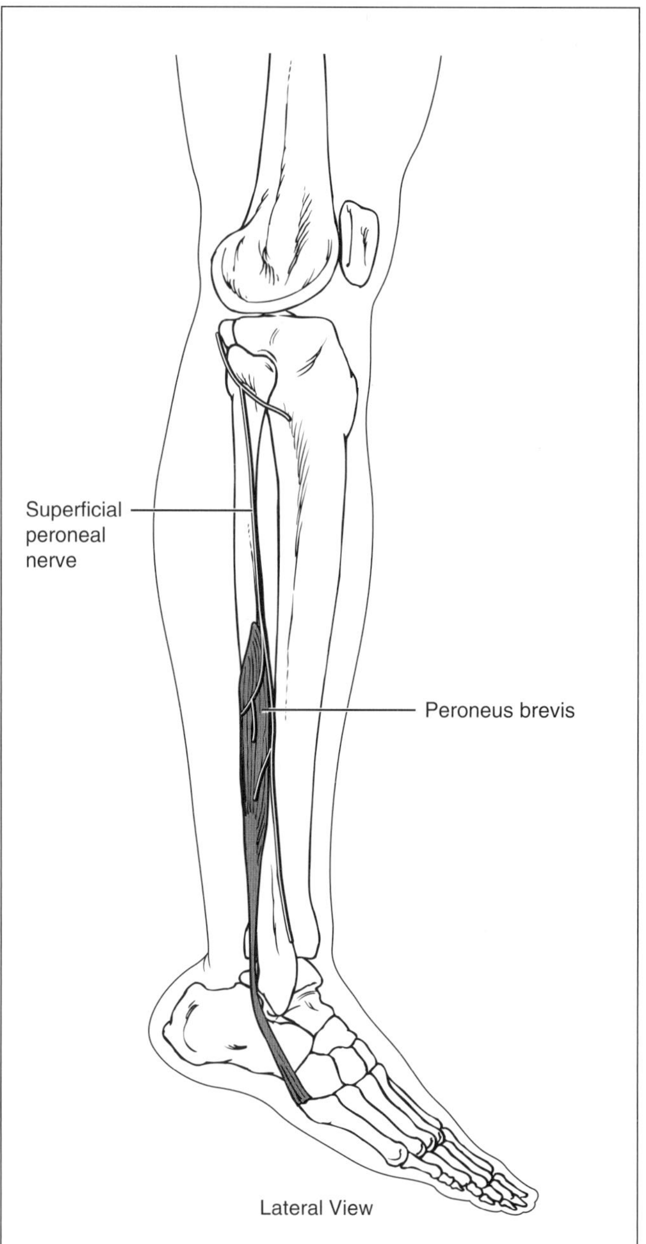

	ATTACHMENTS	NERVE SUPPLY	FUNCTION
Peroneus longus	Origin: Head and upper ⅔ of the lateral surface of the fibula Insertion: Base of the 1st metatarsal, lateral aspect of the medial cuneiform	Peripheral nerve: Superficial peroneal nerve Nerve root: L4, L5, S1	Eversion of the foot at the subtalar joint; weak plantar flexor of the foot at the ankle
Peroneus brevis	Origin: Distal ⅔ of the lateral surface of the fibula Insertion: Tuberosity of the 5th metatarsal	Peripheral nerve: Superficial peroneal nerve Nerve root: L4, L5, S1	Eversion of the foot at the subtalar joint; weak plantar flexor of the foot at the ankle

Gravity-Resisted Test (Grades 5, 4, and 3)

Patient position: Side-lying with limb to be tested uppermost, ankle neutral, foot extended beyond edge of table (Fig. 4-98).

Fig. 4-98.

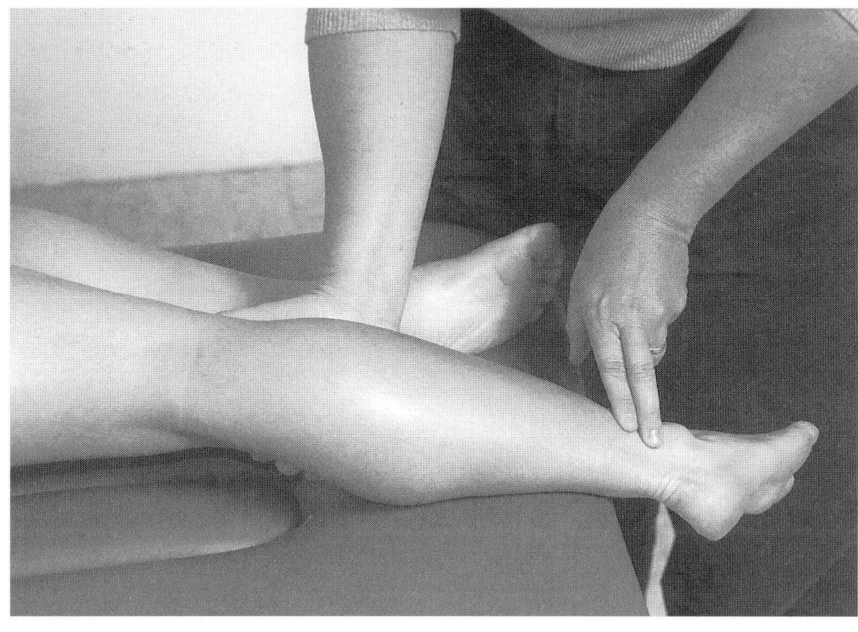

Stabilization/palpation: Stabilize medial aspect of distal leg. With opposite hand, palpate tendons of peroneus longus and brevis just posterior to lateral malleolus (peroneus brevis tendon is just posterior to malleolus and peroneus longus tendon is just posterior to brevis). Two tendons also can be distinguished as they pass above (brevis) and below (longus) peroneal tubercle (Fig. 4-98).

Examiner action: While instructing patient in motion desired, evert patient's foot through full available ROM. Return limb to starting position. Performing passive movement allows determination of patient's available ROM and shows patient exact motion desired.

Patient action: Patient everts subtalar joint through full available ROM. Examiner stabilizes distal leg and palpates ankle evertoers during patient's active movement (Fig. 4-99).

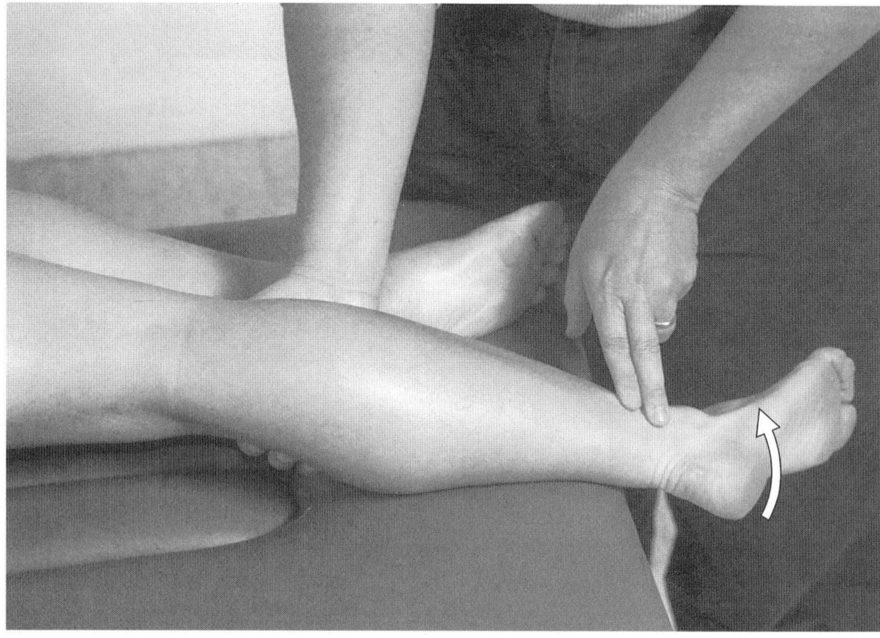

Fig. 4-99. Arrow indicates direction of movement.

Resistance: Apply resistance against lateral border and plantar surface of foot in direction of inversion. Palpating hand is moved to foot to apply resistance (Fig. 4-100).

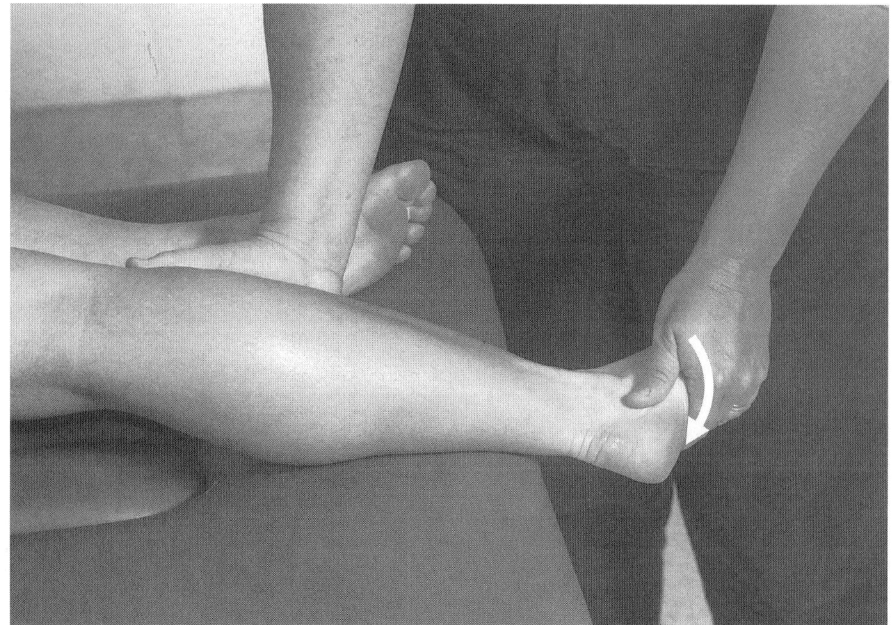

Fig. 4-100. Arrow indicates direction of resistance.

To test only peroneus longus:

Resistance is applied on plantar surface of head of first metatarsal in direction of inversion (Fig. 4-101).

Fig. 4-101.

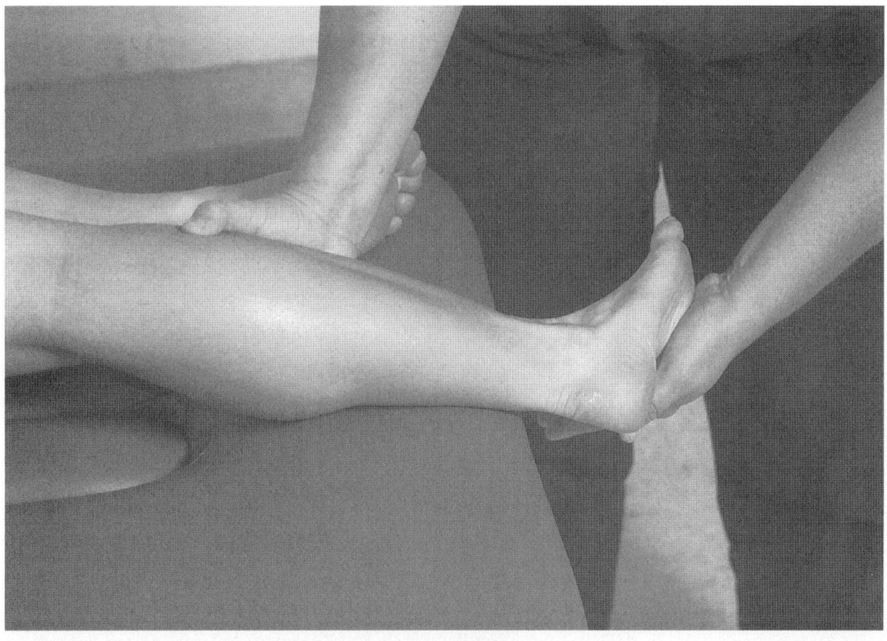

To test only peroneus brevis:

Resistance is applied on lateral border of foot along shaft of fifth metatarsal in direction of inversion (Fig. 4-102).

Fig. 4-102. Arrow indicates direction of resistance.

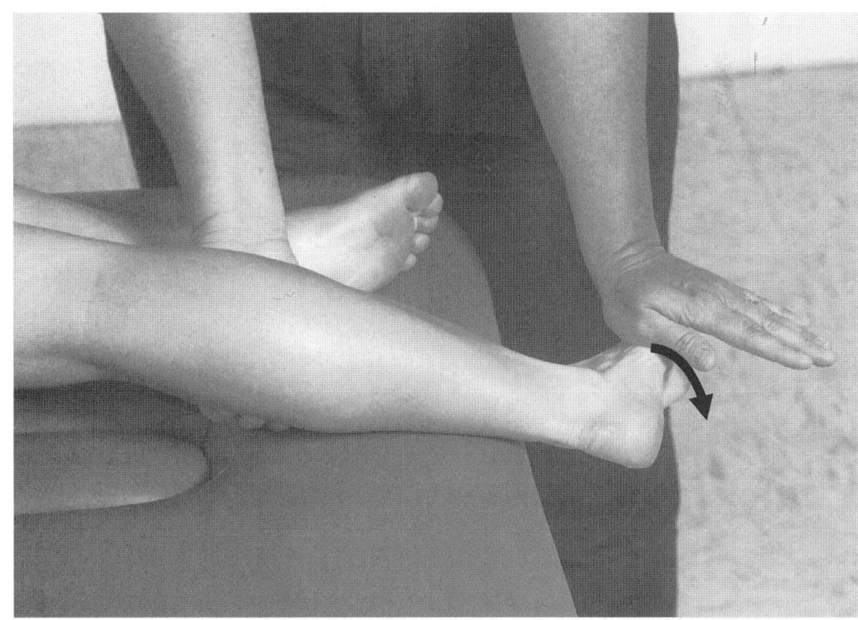

Gravity-Eliminated Test (Grades Below 3)

For patients unable to move completely through available ROM against gravity.

Patient position: Supine with lower extremities extended, ankle of test limb in neutral position, foot extended beyond edge of table.

Stabilization/palpation: As in gravity-resisted test (Fig. 4-103).

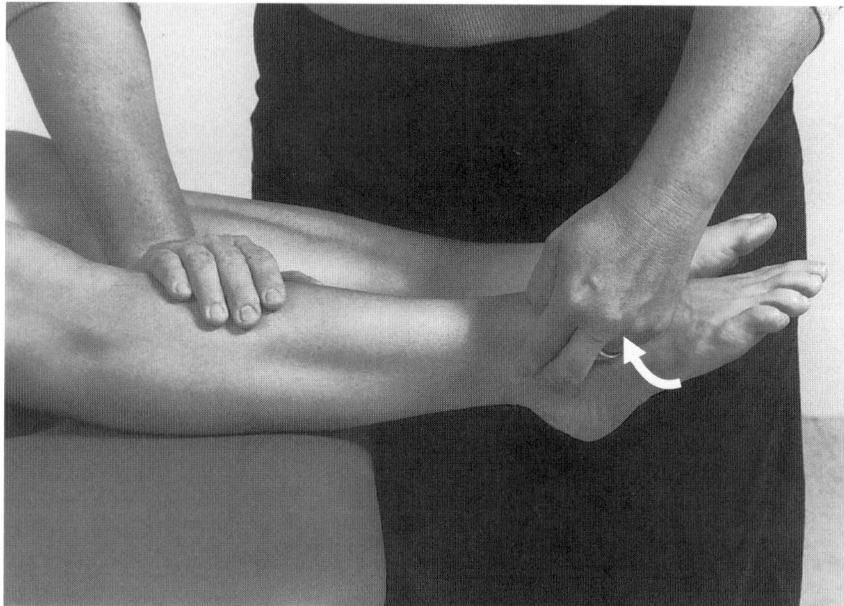

Fig. 4-103. Arrow indicates direction of movement.

Examiner action: As in gravity-resisted test.

Patient action: Patient everts subtalar joint through full available ROM. Examiner stabilizes distal leg and palpates ankle evertors during patient's active movement (Fig. 4-103).

CLINICAL COMMENT: SUBTALAR EVERTOR MUSCLES AND S1 NEUROLOGIC ASSESSMENT

The evertors of the subtalar joint (peroneus longus and brevis) are key muscles for examining the integrity of the S1 spinal nerve or neurologic segment of the spinal cord. Complete assessment of the S1 neurologic level includes:

Strength assessment of:
Gluteus maximus (pp. 265-267)
Gastrocnemius (pp. 317-321)
Soleus (pp. 317-321)
Peroneus longus and brevis (pp. 339-342)

Reflex testing of:
Achilles reflex (p. 551)

Sensory testing of:
Skin over plantar surface of foot and little toe (S1 dermatome; pp. 528-532)

■ METATARSOPHALANGEAL FLEXION

LUMBRICALS, FLEXOR HALLUCIS BREVIS (Fig. 4-104)

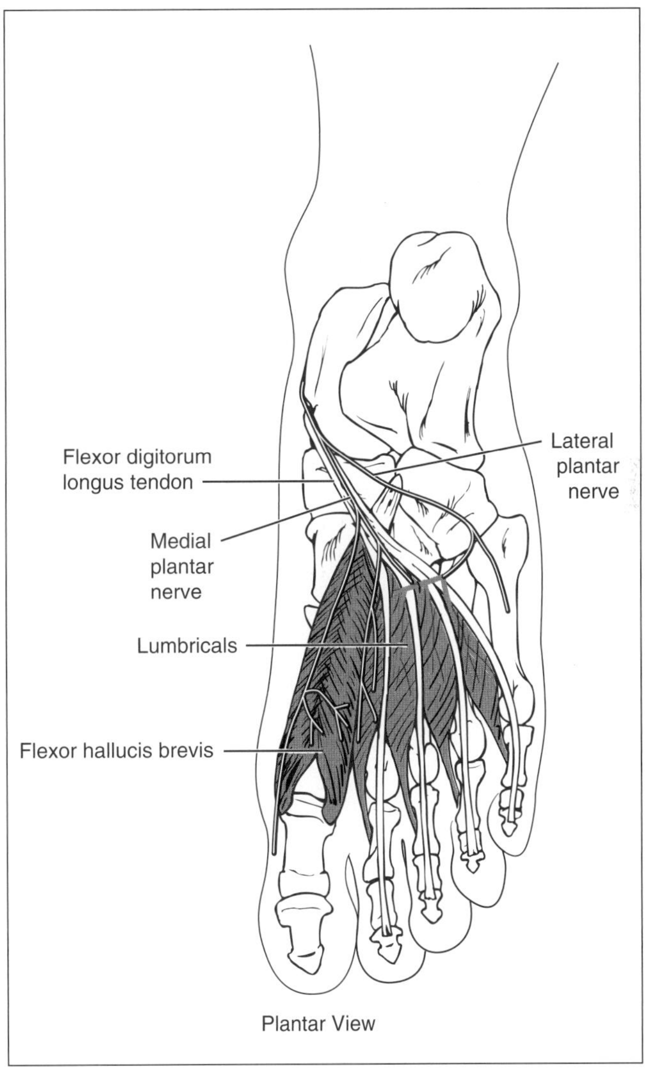

Fig. 4-104.

	ATTACHMENTS	NERVE SUPPLY	FUNCTION
Lumbricals	Origin: Tendons of the flexor digitorum longus Insertion: Tendons of the extensor digitorum longus	Peripheral nerve: Medial plantar (1st lumbrical) and lateral plantar (lumbricals 2–4) nerves Nerve root: L5, S1 (1st lumbrical), S2, S3	Flexion at the MTP joints and extension at the IP joints of the lateral four toes
Flexor hallucis brevis	Origin: Plantar surface of the cuboid and lateral cuneiform bones Insertion: Base of the proximal phalanx of the great toe	Peripheral nerve: Medial plantar nerve Nerve root: L5, S1	Flexion at the MTP joint of the great toe

Grades 5 and 4

Patient position: Supine or seated with ankle neutral. If patient is seated, patient's foot rests on examiner's thigh (Fig. 4-105).

Fig. 4-105.

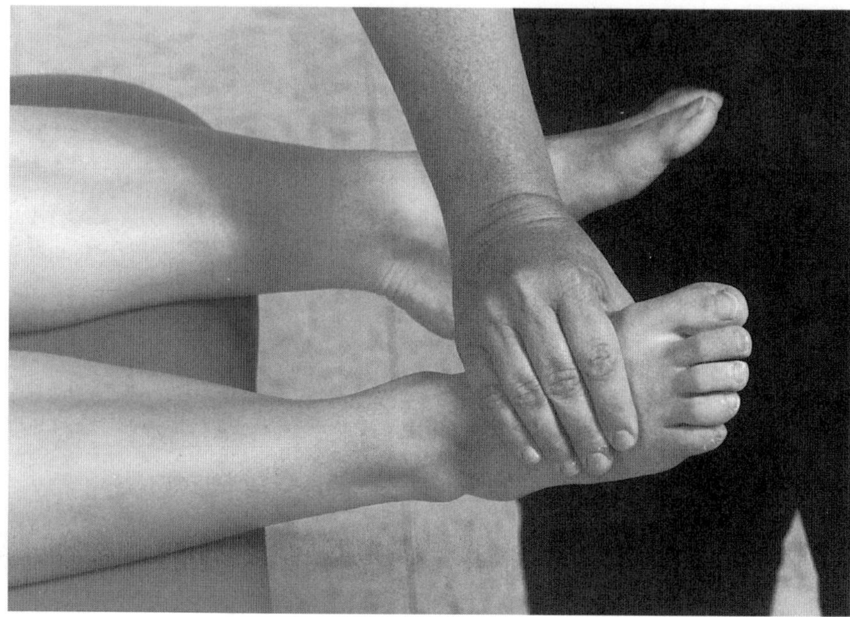

Stabilization/palpation: Stabilize metatarsals. Lumbricals and flexor hallucis brevis are too deep to palpate (Fig. 4-105).

Examiner action: While instructing patient in motion desired, flex patient's metatarsophalangeal (MTP) joints, keeping interphalangeal (IP) joints straight. Return limb to starting position. Performing passive movement allows determination of patient's available ROM and shows patient exact motion desired.

Patient action:

Patient flexes all five toes at MTP joints and attempts to keep IP joints extended. Examiner stabilizes metatarsals during patient's active movement (Fig. 4-106).

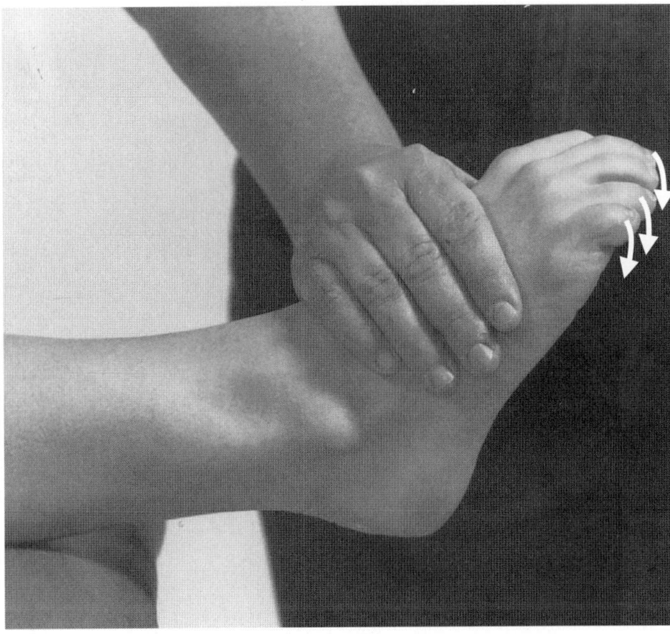

Fig. 4-106. Arrows indicate direction of movement.

Resistance:

Apply resistance with nonstabilizing hand in direction of MTP extension. Resistance is applied over plantar surface of proximal phalanx of first toe for flexor hallucis brevis (Fig. 4-107) and lateral four toes for lumbricals (Fig. 4-108).

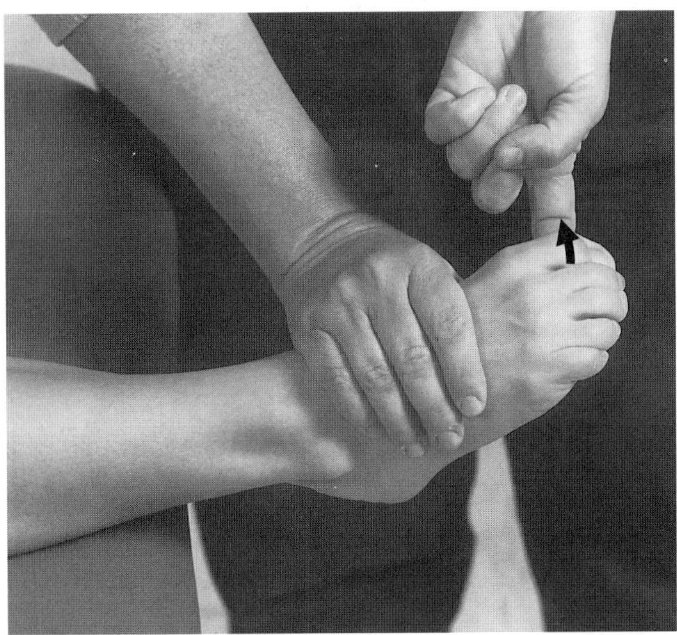

Fig. 4-107. Arrow indicates direction of resistance.

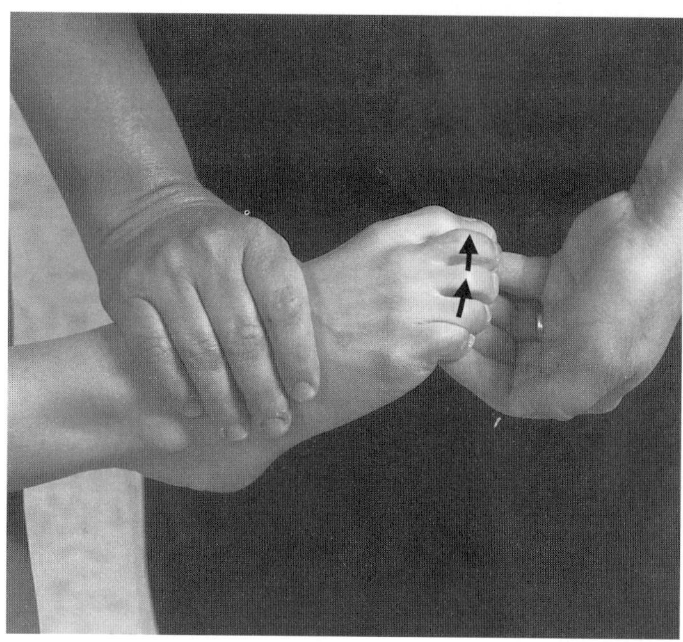

Fig. 4-108. Arrows indicate direction of resistance.

Grades 3 and Below

There is no separate test for these muscles for grades below 3. Grading is altered as follows to accommodate lack of a gravity-eliminated position.

For grade 3: Patient flexes joint through full ROM without resistance.

For grade 2: Patient flexes joint through partial ROM.

Grades 1 and 0 are difficult to distinguish because lumbricals and flexor hallucis brevis are not palpable.

■ INTERPHALANGEAL FLEXION OF TOES

FLEXOR DIGITORUM LONGUS AND BREVIS AND FLEXOR HALLUCIS LONGUS (Figs. 4-109 and 4-110)

Fig. 4-109.

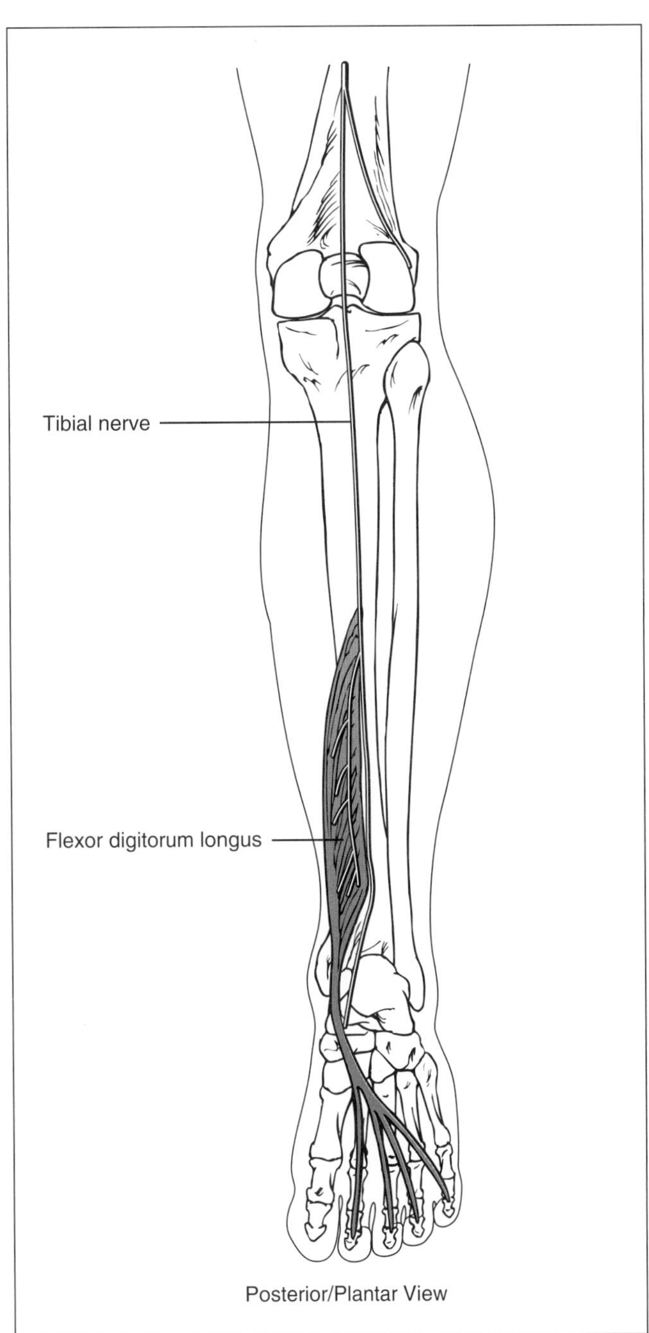

Fig. 4-110.

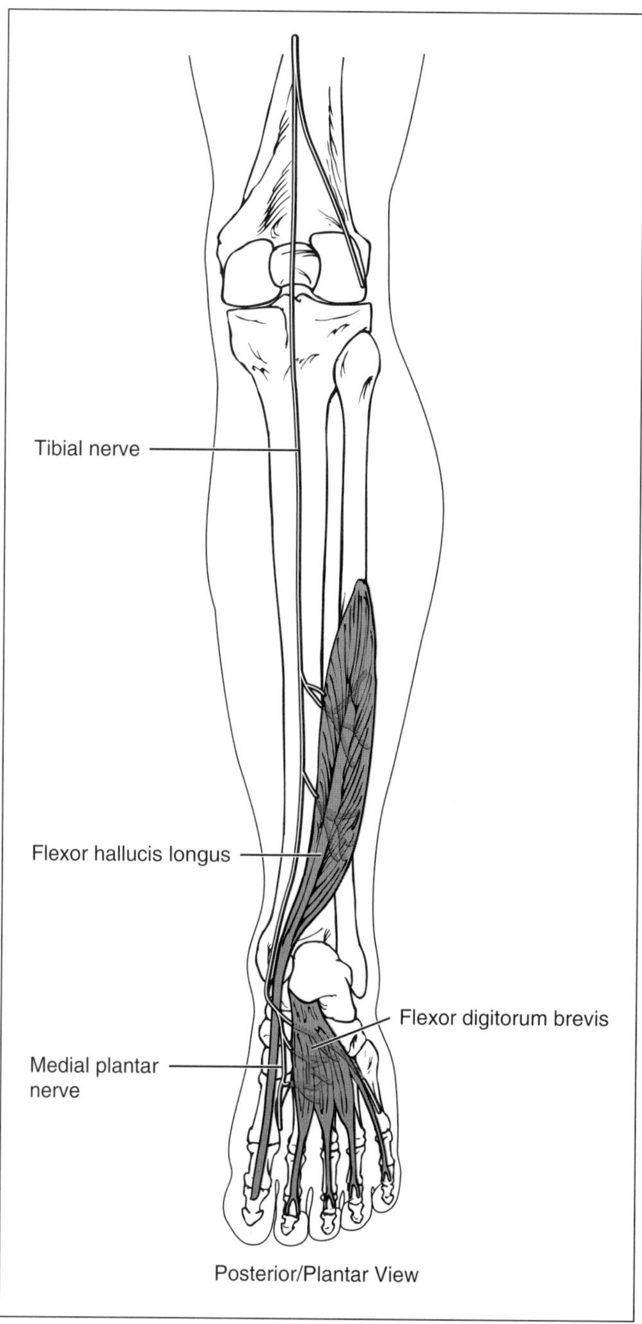
Tibial nerve
Flexor hallucis longus
Flexor digitorum brevis
Medial plantar nerve
Posterior/Plantar View

	ATTACHMENTS	NERVE SUPPLY	FUNCTION
Flexor digitorum longus	Origin: Posterior aspect of the body of the tibia Insertion: Base of the distal phalanges of toes 2–5	Peripheral nerve: Tibial nerve Nerve root: L5, S1	Flexion at the distal and proximal IP joints of the lateral four toes
Flexor digitorum brevis	Origin: Tuberosity of the calcaneus, plantar aponeurosis Insertion: Sides of the middle phalanges of toes 2–5	Peripheral nerve: Medial plantar nerve Nerve root: L5, S1	Flexion at the proximal IP joints of the lateral four toes
Flexor hallucis longus	Origin: Posterior aspect of the body of the fibula, interosseous membrane Insertion: Base of the distal phalanx of the great toe	Peripheral nerve: Tibial nerve Nerve root: L5, S1, S2	Flexion at the IP joint of the great toe

Grades 5 and 4

Patient position: Supine or seated with ankle neutral. If patient is seated, patient's foot rests on examiner's thigh (Fig. 4-111).

Fig. 4-111.

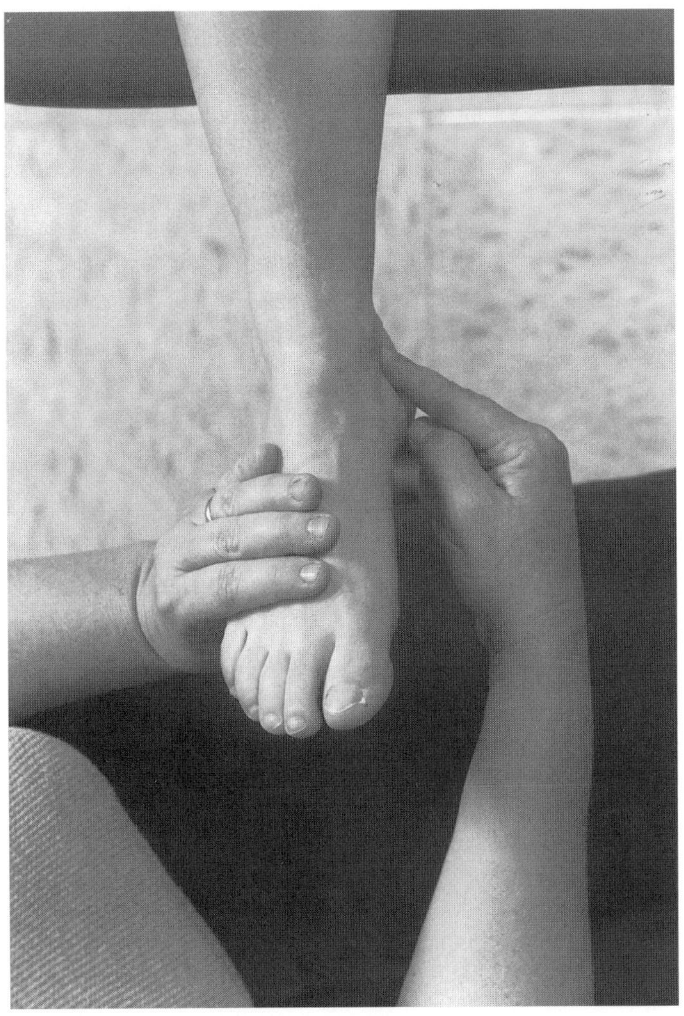

Stabilization/palpation: Stabilize proximal phalanges of lateral four toes for flexor digitorum longus and brevis (Fig. 4-112) and of great toe for flexor hallucis longus (Fig. 4-113). Palpate tendons of flexor digitorum longus and flexor hallucis longus posterior to medial malleolus between malleolus and sustentaculum tali (tendon of flexor digitorum longus is anterior to tendon of flexor hallucis longus; Figs. 4-111 and 4-113).

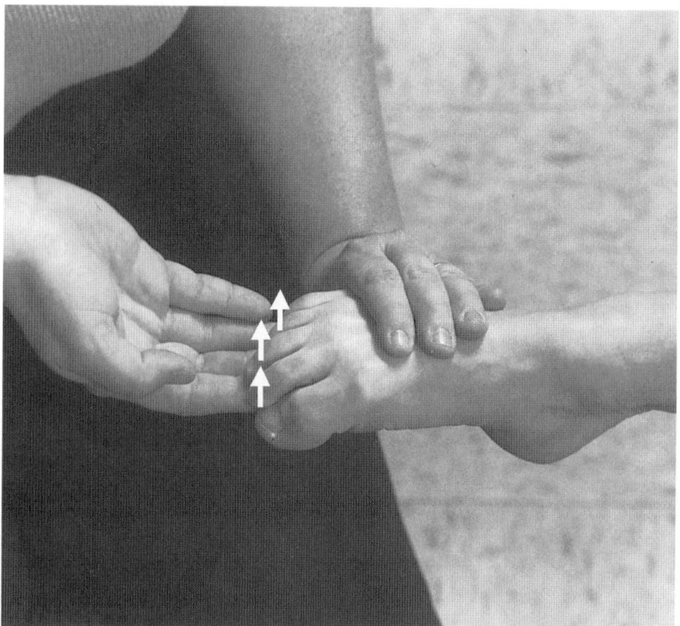

Fig. 4-112. Test for flexor digitorum longus and brevis; arrows indicate direction of resistance.

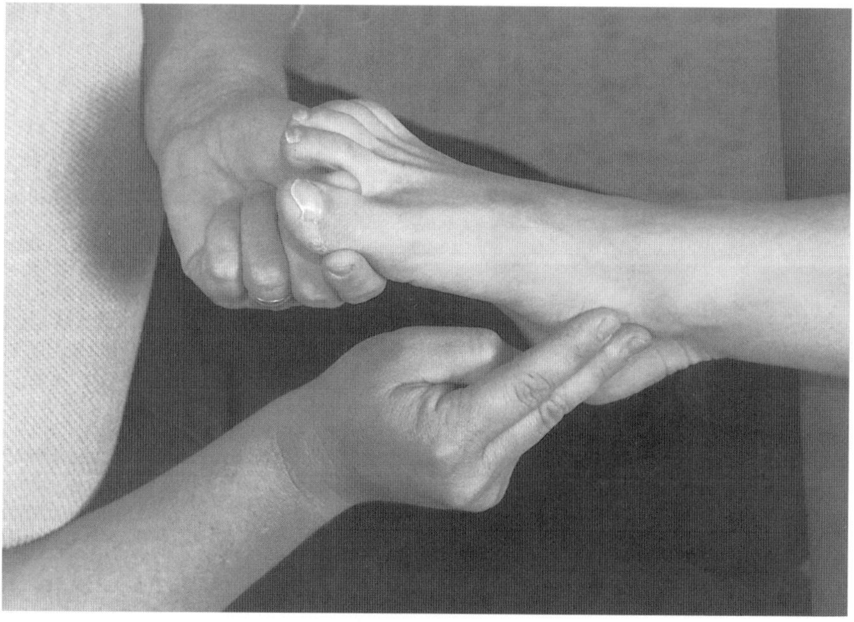

Fig. 4-113.

Examiner action: While instructing patient in motion desired, flex IP joints of patient's toes through full available ROM. Return limb to starting position. Performing passive movement allows determination of patient's available ROM and shows patient exact motion desired.

Patient action:

Patient flexes IP joints of lateral four toes (flexor digitorum longus and brevis; see Fig. 4-112) and great toe (flexor hallucis longus; Fig. 4-114) through full available ROM. Examiner stabilizes proximal phalanges and palpates long toe flexors during patient's active movement.

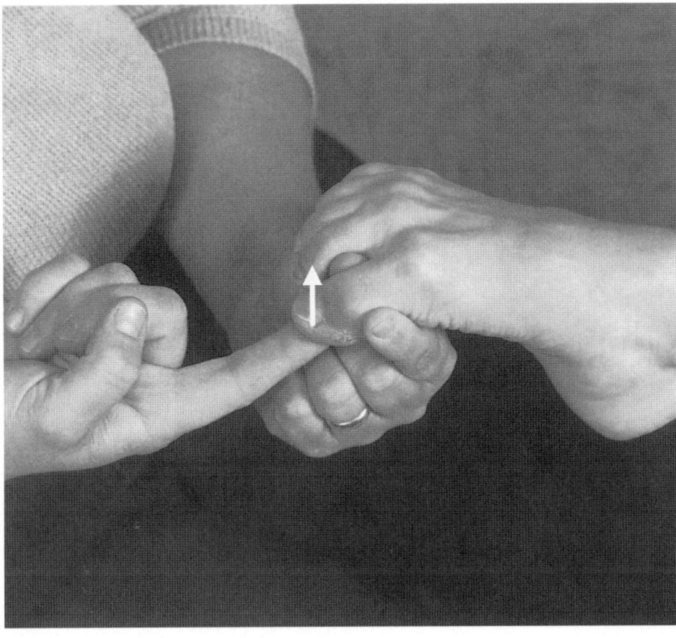

Fig. 4-114. Test for flexor hallucis longus; arrow indicates direction of resistance.

Resistance:

Apply resistance against middle and distal phalanges of lateral four toes for flexor digitorum longus and brevis (see Fig. 4-112) and against distal phalanx of great toe for flexor hallucis longus (Fig. 4-114). Palpating hand is moved to toes to apply resistance.

Grades 3 and Below

There is no separate test for these muscles for grades below 3. Grading is altered as follows to accommodate lack of a gravity-eliminated position.

For grade 3: Patient flexes joint through full ROM without resistance.

For grade 2: Patient flexes joint through partial ROM.

For grade 1: No motion, but a palpable contraction is present. Palpation occurs as described earlier (see Figs. 4-111 and 4-113).

For grade 0: No motion or contraction is present.

■ METATARSOPHALANGEAL EXTENSION

EXTENSOR DIGITORUM LONGUS AND BREVIS (Figs. 4-115 and 4-116)

Fig. 4-115.

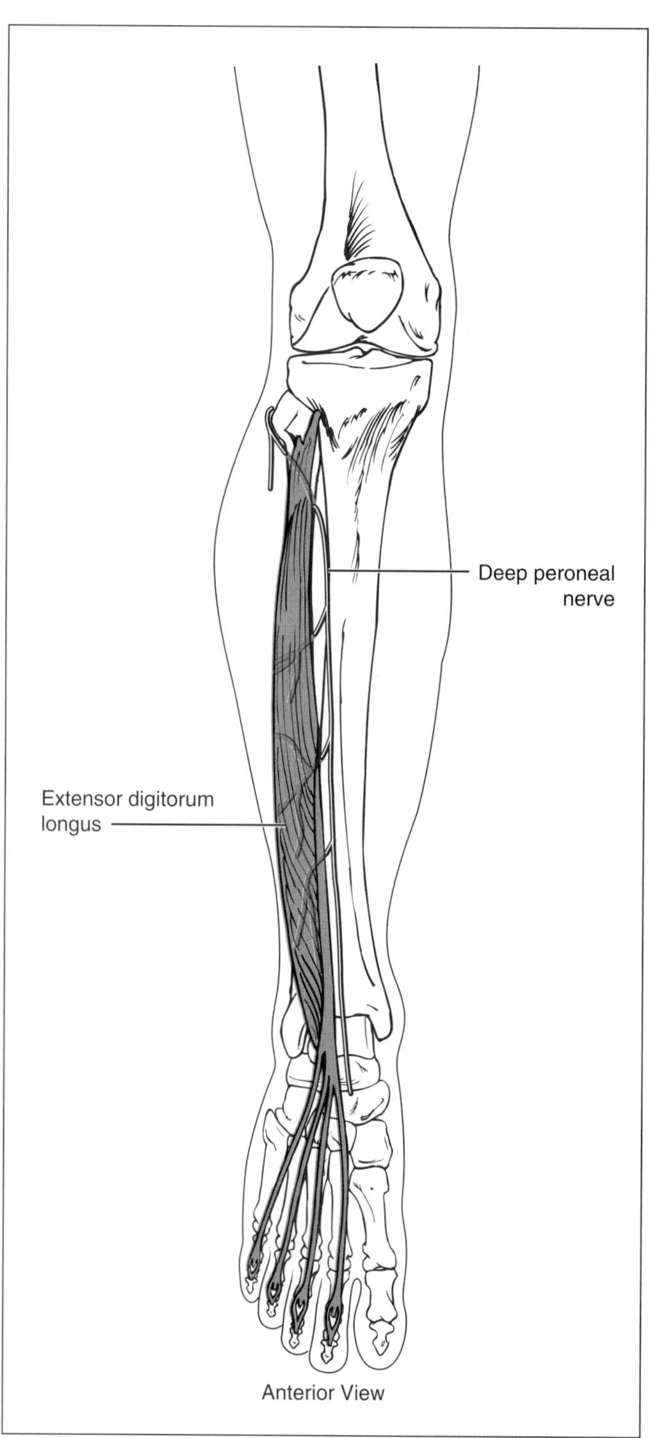

Fig. 4-116.

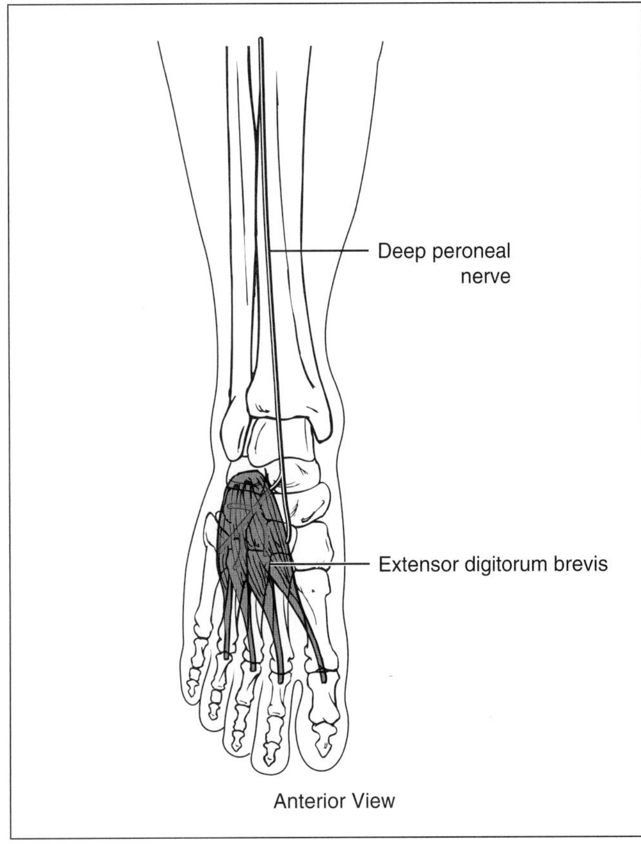

	ATTACHMENTS	NERVE SUPPLY	FUNCTION
Extensor digitorum longus	Origin: Lateral tibial condyle, anterior surface of the body of the fibula, interosseous membrane Insertion: Dorsum of the middle and distal phalanges of toes 2–5	Peripheral nerve: Deep peroneal nerve Nerve root: L4, L5, S1	Extension at the MTP joints of the lateral four toes
Extensor digitorum brevis	Origin: Superior surface of the calcaneus, lateral talocalcaneal ligament, inferior extensor retinaculum Insertion: Dorsal surface of the base of the proximal phalanx of the great toe, lateral aspect of the extensor digitorum longus tendons of toes 2–4	Peripheral nerve: Deep peroneal nerve Nerve root: L5, S1	Extension at the MTP joint of the great toe and toes 2–4

Grades 5 and 4

Patient position: Supine or seated with ankle neutral. If patient is seated, patient's foot rests on examiner's thigh (Fig. 4-117).

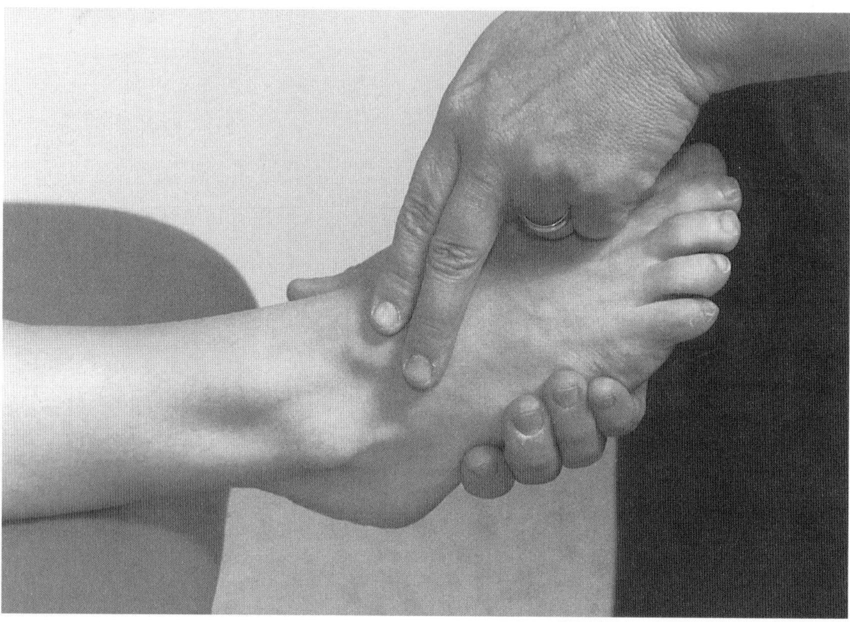

Fig. 4-117.

Stabilization/palpation: Stabilize metatarsals. Palpate extensor digitorum brevis and longus tendons on dorsolateral (brevis) and dorsal (longus) aspects of foot (Fig. 4-117).

Examiner action: While instructing patient in motion desired, extend MTP joints of patient's toes through full available ROM. Return limb to starting position. Performing passive movement allows determination of patient's available ROM and shows patient exact motion desired.

Patient action:

Patient extends all five toes at MTP joints through full available ROM. Examiner stabilizes metatarsals and palpates toe extensors during patient's active movement (Fig. 4-118).

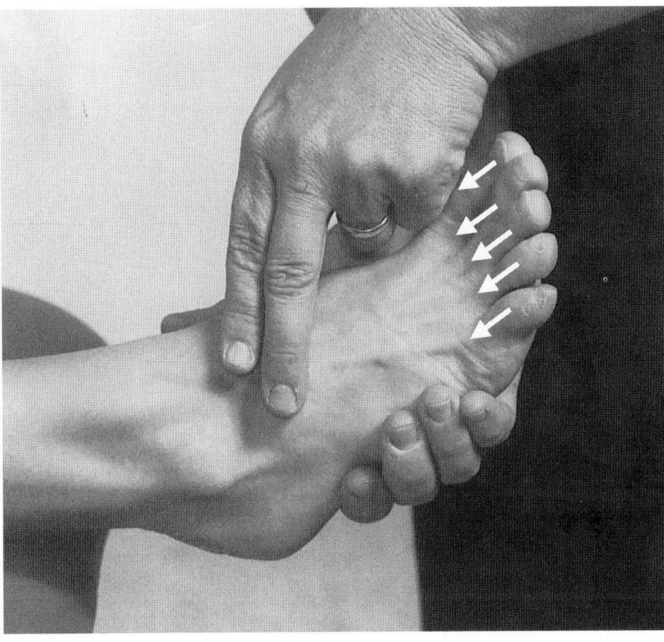

Fig. 4-118. Arrows indicate direction of movement.

Resistance:

Apply resistance over dorsum of proximal phalanx of first (Fig. 4-119) and lateral four (Fig. 4-120) toes in direction of MTP flexion. Palpating hand is moved to toes to apply resistance.

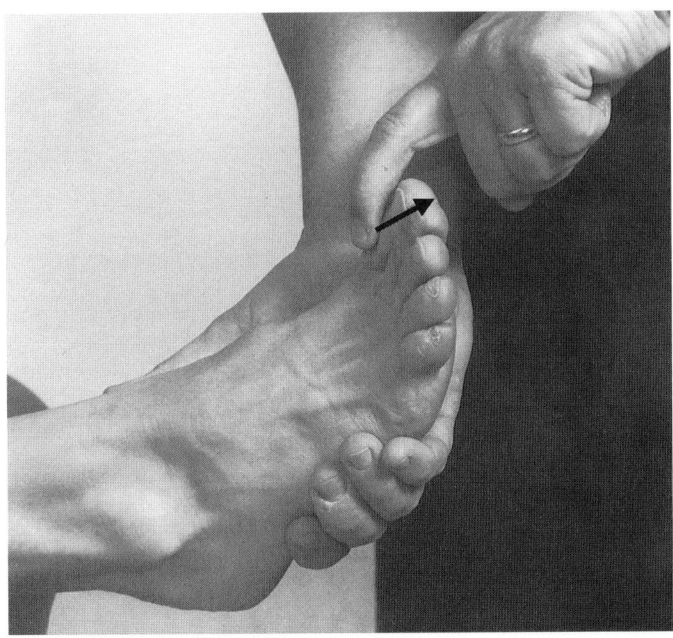

Fig. 4-119. Arrow indicates direction of resistance.

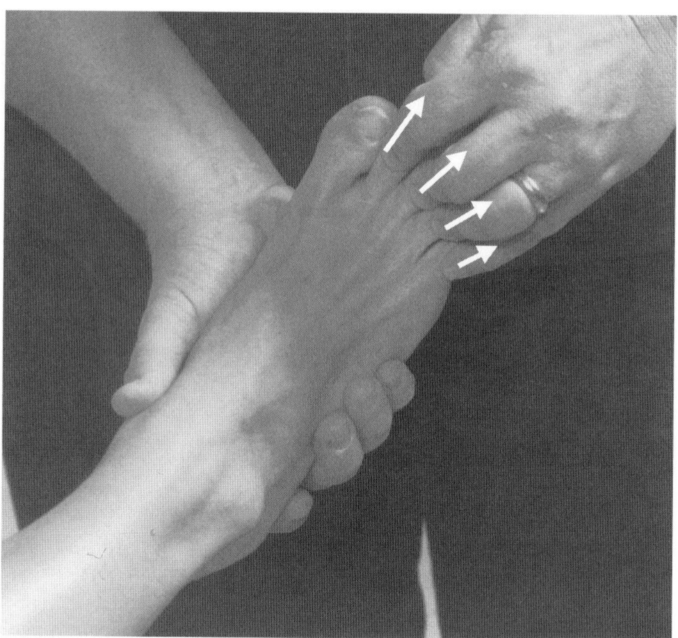

Fig. 4-120. Arrows indicate direction of resistance.

Grades 3 and Below

There is no separate test for these muscles for grades below 3. Grading is altered as follows to accommodate lack of a gravity-eliminated position.

For grade 3: Patient extends joint through full ROM without resistance.

For grade 2: Patient extends joint through partial ROM.

For grade 1: No motion, but a palpable contraction is present. Palpation occurs as described earlier (see Fig. 4-117).

For grade 0: No motion or contraction is present.

CLINICAL COMMENT: LONG TOE EXTENSOR MUSCLES AND L5 NEUROLOGIC ASSESSMENT

The long toe extensor muscles (extensor hallucis longus, extensor digitorum longus) are key muscles for examining the integrity of the L5 spinal nerve or neurologic segment of the spinal cord. Complete assessment of the L5 neurologic level includes:

Strength assessment of:
Extensor hallucis longus (pp. 358-360)
Extensor digitorum longus (pp. 354-356)
Hip abductors (pp. 274-276)

Sensory testing of:
Skin over the lateral side of the leg and dorsum of the foot (L5 dermatome; pp. 528-532)

■ INTERPHALANGEAL EXTENSION (GREAT TOE)

EXTENSOR HALLUCIS LONGUS (Fig. 4-121)

Fig. 4-121.

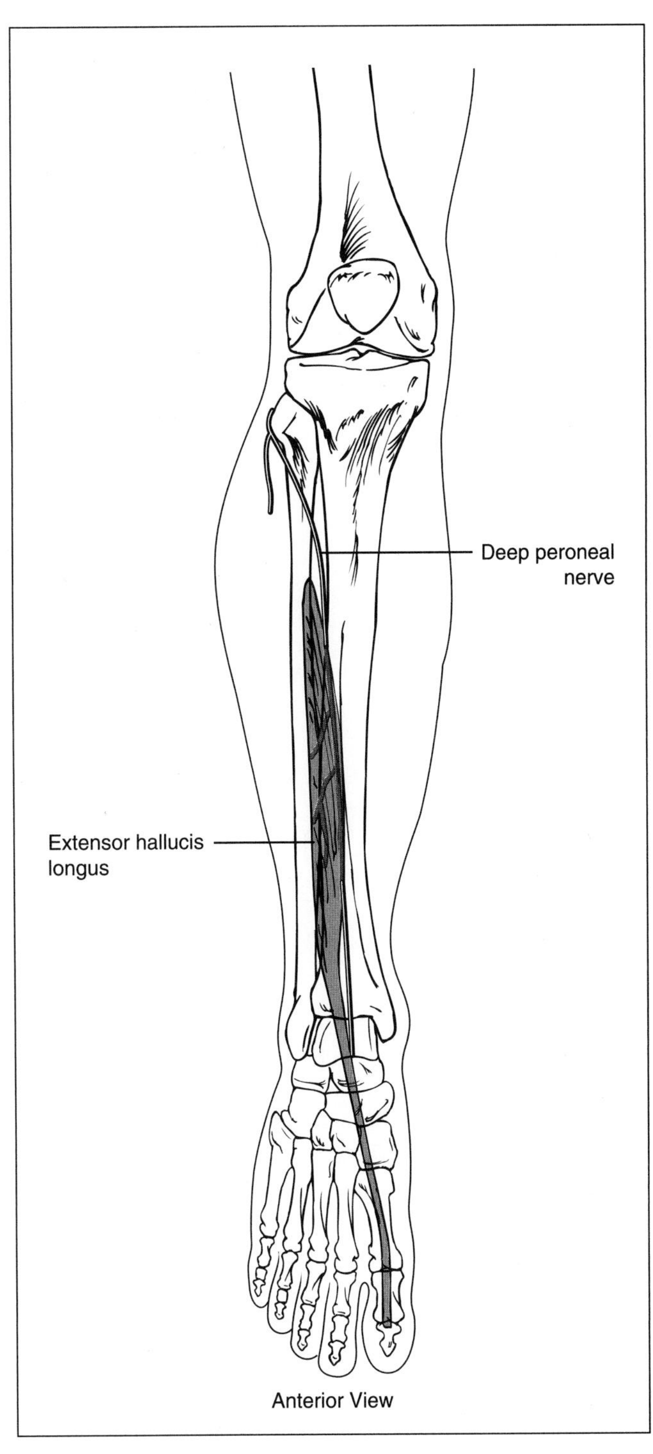

	ATTACHMENTS	NERVE SUPPLY	FUNCTION
Extensor hallucis longus	Origin: Medial surface of the body of the fibula, interosseous membrane Insertion: Base of the distal phalanx of the great toe	Peripheral nerve: Deep peroneal nerve Nerve root: L4, L5, S1	Extension at the IP joint of the great toe

Grades 5 and 4

Patient position:

Supine or seated with ankle neutral. If patient is seated, patient's foot rests on examiner's thigh (Fig. 4-122).

Fig. 4-122.

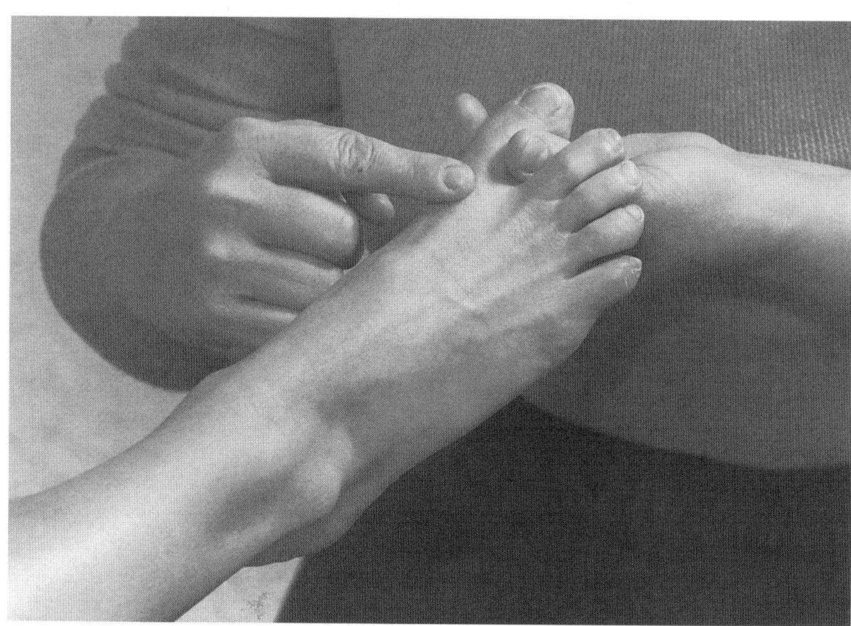

Stabilization/palpation:

Stabilize proximal phalanx of great toe. With opposite hand, palpate tendon of extensor hallucis longus along dorsomedial aspect of foot (Fig. 4-122).

Examiner action:

While instructing patient in motion desired, extend IP joint of patient's great toe through full available ROM. Return limb to starting position. Performing passive movement allows determination of patient's available ROM and shows patient exact motion desired.

Patient action:

Patient extends great toe at IP joint through full available ROM. Examiner stabilizes proximal phalanx of great toe and palpates extensor hallucis longus tendon during patient's active movement (Fig. 4-123).

Fig. 4-123. Arrow indicates direction of movement.

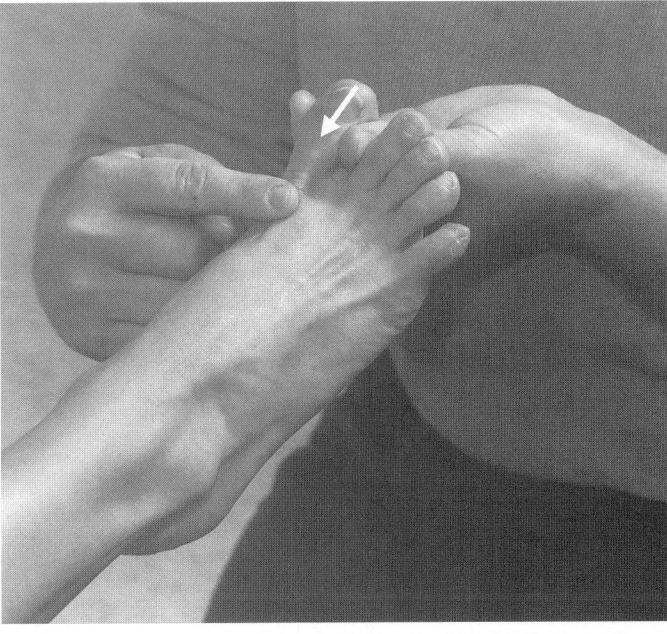

Resistance:

Apply resistance on dorsum of distal phalanx of great toe in direction of IP flexion. Palpating hand is moved to distal phalanx to apply resistance (Fig. 4-124).

Fig. 4-124. Arrow indicates direction of resistance.

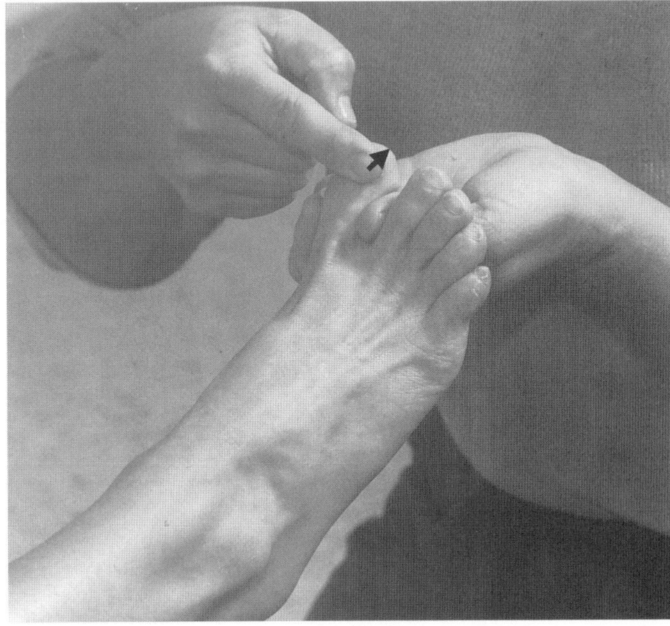

Grades 3 and Below

There is no separate test for this muscle for grades below 3. Grading is altered as follows to accommodate lack of a gravity-eliminated position.

For grade 3: Patient extends joint through full ROM without resistance.

For grade 2: Patient extends joint through partial ROM.

For grade 1: No motion, but a palpable contraction is present. Palpation occurs as described earlier (see Fig. 4-122).

For grade 0: No motion or contraction is present.

CASE 4-1 SPINAL CORD INJURY (CONTINUED FROM CASE 2-1; CHAPTER 2)

Questions 1 through 3 were answered regarding this case in Chapter 2. Answer questions 4 through 6 regarding your examination of this patient. Note: This case is continued in Chapter 8: Techniques of the Sensory Examination.

Mr. Q is a 17-year-old male who suffered a fracture of the sixth cervical vertebra during a motor vehicle accident. Due to compression of the spinal cord by the fracture fragments, he sustained an incomplete spinal cord injury at a C7 neurologic level. His fracture site has been completely stabilized, and he has been admitted to the rehabilitation unit at 3 months post injury due to multiple medical complications that delayed his transfer to rehab. As a result of prolonged hospitalization, Mr. Q is unable to tolerate an upright position. You are planning your initial examination in which you must determine his level of motor and sensory functioning.

1. Given that this patient's injury is at the C7 spinal level, which muscles would you expect to be free from motor weakness?
2. How would you need to alter the following muscle tests to accommodate for the patient's inability to maintain an upright position?
   a. Biceps brachii—gravity resisted
   b. Middle deltoid—gravity resisted
   c. Extensor carpi radialis longus and brevis—gravity resisted
   d. Upper trapezius—gravity resisted
   e. Pectoralis major—gravity eliminated
3. How would you alter your documentation to accommodate the changes in patient positioning described in your answer to question number 2?

During a screening examination of Mr. Q's lower extremity function, you observe that Mr. Q has active lower extremity movement that you believe is of sufficient strength in some muscle groups to allow movement against gravity.

4. How would you alter the following lower extremity muscle tests to accommodate for the patient's inability to maintain an upright position?
   a. Rectus femoris—gravity resisted
   b. Tibialis anterior—gravity resisted
   c. Gastroc/soleus—gravity resisted
   d. Medial hip rotators—gravity resisted
5. How would you alter your documentation to accommodate the changes in patient positioning described in your answers to question number 4?
6. How could you organize your muscle tests to minimize changes in patient positioning during the session?

CASE 4-2 PERIPHERAL NERVE INJURY

Mr. H is a 19-year-old college football player who suffered a peroneal nerve injury following a blow to the lateral side of the right knee from a defensive player's helmet during Saturday evening's game. The patient presents with foot drop and sensory loss in the lower extremity. No fracture occurred during the injury, but there is extensive bruising and swelling involving the lateral side of the knee and proximal calf.

Answer the following questions regarding your examination of this patient (you may want to refer to an anatomy text to assist with your answers). Note: This case is continued in Chapter 8: Techniques of the Sensory Examination.

1. Describe the anatomy and course of the common peroneal nerve.
2. Why would the peroneal nerve have been injured as a result of the incident described in the case?
3. What muscle in the thigh is innervated by the common peroneal nerve?
4. What are the motor branches of the common peroneal nerve in the leg? What muscles does each branch innervate?
5. How would you test strength of each of the muscles listed in your answer to question number 4?
6. Explain the mechanism of foot drop in this patient.
7. What other muscles might demonstrate weakness in this patient? What functional losses would you expect as a result of such weakness?

CASE 4-3 LUMBOSACRAL STRAIN

Questions 1 through 4 were answered regarding this case in Chapter 3. Answer questions 5 through 7 regarding your examination of this patient.

Ms. R is a 16-year-old high-school volleyball player who has complaints of left-sided lumbosacral pain following an intensive weekend volleyball tournament. During volleyball participation, the patient engages in forceful movements involving trunk rotation combined with flexion or extension. Pain is present during activity and with sitting. The patient has excessive hamstring length secondary to a 12-year history of dance (ballet and jazz) and slightly tight quadriceps bilaterally. An essential part of your examination is a strength assessment of the trunk stabilizers.

1. What muscles are stabilizers of the lumbar spine? Provide the action(s) of each muscle listed in your answer.
2. How do the abdominal muscles assist in stabilization of the spine and pelvis?
3. Which abdominal muscles produce forceful rotation of the trunk to the left? Which muscles of the spine assist in this motion?
4. How is strength assessment of the trunk stabilizers accomplished? Contrast methods described in this text with those found in texts aimed at musculoskeletal assessment. Which methods would be most appropriate for this patient? Why?

Following a more thorough examination of Ms. R, you begin to suspect that integral to her lumbosacral pain is an underlying pelvic instability. In an effort to confirm this suspicion, you perform a strength assessment of muscles providing pelvic stabilization. Answer the following questions regarding your examination of this patient (you may want to refer to a kinesiologic textbook to assist with your answers).

5. What lower extremity muscles have an attachment on the pelvis?
6. For each of the muscles listed in the answer to question number 5, provide its action *on the pelvis*.
7. What effect, if any, do you think Ms. R's hamstring length would have on the strength of her hamstring muscles? Provide a rationale for your answer based on muscle mechanics.

References

1. Basmajian JV, DeLuca CJ. *Muscles Alive: Their Function Revealed by Electromyography,* 5th ed. Baltimore: Williams & Wilkins, 1985.
2. Furlani J, Bérzin F, Vitti M. Electromyographic study of the gluteus maximus muscle. *Electromyogr Clin Neurophysiol* 1974;14:377–388.
3. Smith LK, Weiss EL, Lehmkuhl LD. *Brunnstrom's Clinical Kinesiology,* 5th ed. Philadelphia: FA Davis, 1996.
4. Daniels L, Worthingham C. *Muscle Testing: Techniques of Manual Examination,* 5th ed. Philadelphia: WB Saunders, 1986.
5. Kendall FP, McCreary EK, Provance PG. *Muscles: Testing and Function,* 4th ed. Baltimore: Williams & Wilkins, 1993.
6. Lunsford BR, Perry J. The standing heel-rise test for ankle plantar flexion: criterion for normal. *Phys Ther* 1995;75:694–698.
7. Hislop HJ, Montgomery J. *Daniel's and Worthingham's Muscle Testing: Techniques of Manual Examination,* 6th ed. Philadelphia: WB Saunders, 1995.

Bibliography

American Spinal Injury Association. *International Standards for Neurological Classification of Spinal Cord Injury*. Revised, 2002. Chicago: ASIA, 2002.

Andersson E, Oddsson L, Grundstrom H, et al. The role of the psoas and iliacus muscles for stability and movement of the lumbar spine, pelvis and hip. *Scand J Med Sci Sports* 1995;5:10–16.

Basmajian JV, Lovejoy JF. Function of the popliteus muscles in man. *J Bone Joint Surg* 1971;53A:557–562.

Clarkson HM. *Musculoskeletal Assessment: Joint Range of Motion and Manual Muscle Strength,* 2nd ed. Philadelphia: Lippincott, Williams & Wilkins, 2000.

Clemente CD. *Gray's Anatomy, 30th American ed*. Philadelphia: Lea & Febiger, 1985.

Cresswell AG, Loscher WN, Thorstensson A. Influence of gastrocnemius muscle length on triceps surae torque development and electromyographic activity in man. *Exp Brain Res* 1995;105:283–290.

Devinsky O, Feldmann E. *Examination of the Cranial and Peripheral Nerves*. New York: Churchill Livingstone, 1988.

Dostal WF, Soderberg GL, Andrews JG. Actions of hip muscles. *Phys Ther* 1986;66:351–359.

Fischer FJ, Houtz SJ. Evaluation of the function of the gluteus maximus muscle. *Am J Phys Med* 1968;47:182–191.

Fisher NM, Pendergast DR, Calkins EC. Maximal isometric torque of knee extension as a function of muscle length in subjects of advancing age. *Phys Med Rehabil* 1990;71:896–899.

Florence JM, Pandya S, King WM, et al. Intrarater reliability of manual muscle test (Medical Research Council scale) grades in Duchenne's muscular dystrophy. *Phys Ther* 1992;72:115–126.

Frese E, Brown M, Norton BJ. Clinical reliability of manual muscle testing: middle trapezius and gluteus medius muscles. *Phys Ther* 1987;67:1072–1076.

Gravel D, Richards CL, Filion M. Angle dependency in strength measurements of the ankle plantar flexors. *Eur J Appl Physiol* 1990;61:182–187.

Hart DL, Stobbe TJ, Till CW, et al. Effect of trunk stabilization on quadriceps femoris muscle torque. *Phys Ther* 1984;64:1375–1380.

Hoppenfeld S. *Physical Examination of the Spine and Extremities*. New York: Appleton-Century-Crofts, 1976.

Inman VT. Functional aspects of the abductor muscles of the hip. *J Bone Joint Surg* 1947;29A:607–619.

Jarvis DK. Relative strength of the hip rotator muscle groups. *Phys Ther Rev* 1952;32:500–503.

Keagy RD, Brumlik J, Bergan JJ. Direct electromyography of the psoas major muscle in man. *J Bone Joint Surg* 1966;40A:817–832.

Lindsay DM, Maitland ME, Lowe RC, et al. Comparison of isokinetic internal and external hip rotation torques using different testing positions. *J Orthop Phys Ther* 1992;16:43–50.

Mendler HM. Effect of stabilization on maximum isometric knee extensor force. *Phys Ther* 1967;47:375–379.

Murray MP, Baldwin JM, Gardner GM, et al. Maximum isometric knee flexor and extensor muscle contractions. *Phys Ther* 1977;57:637–643.

Neumann DA, Soderberg GL, Cook TM. Electromyographic analysis of hip abductor musculature in healthy right-handed persons. *Phys Ther* 1989;69:431–440.

Olson VL, Smidt GL, Johnston RC. The maximum torque generated by the eccentric, isometric, and concentric contractions of the hip abductor muscles. *Phys Ther* 1972;52:149–157.

Pare EB, Stern JT, Schwartz JM. Functional differentiation within the tensor fasciae latae. *J Bone Joint Surg* 1981;63A:1457–1471.

Reider B. *The Orthopaedic Physical Examination*. Philadelphia: WB Saunders, 1999.

Signorile JF, Applegate B, Duque M, et al. Selective recruitment of the triceps surae muscles with changes in knee angle. *J Strength Cond Res* 2002;16:433–439.

Skyrme AD, Cahill DJ, Marsh HP, et al. Psoas major and its controversial rotational action. *Clin Anat* 1999;12:264–265.

Wadsworth CT, Krishnan R, Sear M, et al. Intrarater reliability of manual muscle testing and hand-held dynametric muscle testing. *Phys Ther* 1987;67:1342–1347.

Wintz MM. Variations in current manual muscle testing. *Phys Ther Rev* 1959;39:466–475.

5

TECHNIQUES of FUNCTIONAL MUSCLE TESTING

Reta J. Zabel, PhD, PT, GCS

Maturation and aging are associated with many physiologic and physical changes.[11] Spirduso[26] described the maturation process as physical development and decline in cardiovascular and pulmonary function, muscle strength and endurance, and motor control, coordination, and skill. This chapter focuses on assessment of muscle strength and endurance from the perspective of function; however, the reader should be reminded of the complexity of physical maturation and the impact on functional performance.

Although the physiologic phenomenon of muscle aging is not fully understood, the result is a decrease in muscle strength and power evidenced by differing degrees of muscle weakness and functional loss.[9] Researchers have determined that an inability to complete motor tasks is frequently associated with muscle weakness.[6,16,21,28] Furthermore, muscle weakness may be the primary factor in the movement deficits associated with disorders like muscular dystrophy and may be a secondary factor in disorders that limit, alter, or prevent usual movement; for example, rheumatoid arthritis, cerebrovascular accident, or musculoskeletal trauma.

The likelihood of strength changes in these disorders is accepted as is the need to test muscle strength. However, the traditional techniques used for quantification of strength are assessed in linear movements involving single muscle groups and may be inadequate as indicators of functional performance.[15] Brown et al.[4] proposed that strength and function are best assessed by performance of a specific task that combines key muscle groups. Bohannon[2] suggested that many of the objective methods of strength testing may be limited by factors such as the strength of the tester, extremity stabilization, and expensive equipment requirement. Amundsen[1] recommended a logical sequence for more effectively assessing the muscle strength component of functional movement. He proposed that activities of daily living (ADLs) be assessed first, followed by functional strength tests, and finally performance of appropriate manual muscle tests.

Tests of ADLs and instrumental activities of daily living (IADLs) assist the clinician in identifying motor dysfunction that limits the individual's ability to function in the home and community. Most of the tools provide a gross overview of the patient's ability to function in areas of mobility, cognition, self-care, and community interaction. Examples include the KATZ ADL Index,[14] Barthel Index,[18] and Instrumental Activities of Daily Living Index.[8,17] These tests provide information on functional status but fail to provide specific information on the limitations of motor performance.

Performing a more detailed examination of movement using functional strength testing is recommended following assessment of ADLs.[1] Functional strength tests examine the capacity of synergistic muscle groups to generate a force output adequate to complete a specific task. Synergistic muscle groups may be flexors, extensors, and rotators acting as a unit to accomplish the motor goal. For example, rising from sitting includes hip flexors and extensors, knee flexors and extensors, and ankle plantar flexors. An appropriate functional strength test should involve assessment of all of these muscle groups. Therefore, assessment of chair rise would be useful in determination of the functional strength of these muscles.

Because functional strength testing involves more patient-specific task performance, the issues of standardization, validity, reliability, and normative performance scores should be considered. Test standardization exists for few functional strength tests; however, when available, standardization will be included with the test description. Nonetheless, even with attempts at standardization, procedural differences exist in the literature. For example, for the repeated chair rise, chair height ranges from 43 to 44.5 cm[5,24] and position in chair differs from forward on chair seat to back against back of chair.[13,22,28] In addition, scoring differences are present in the literature ranging from counting the number of repetitions completed in a specified amount of time (time range, 10 to 30 seconds[2,12]) or recording time required to complete a predetermined number of repetitions (one, three, five, or 10 repetitions).[5,10,23,28]

Validity, the ability of a test to measure what it was intended to measure, is a very important aspect to consider in selection of functional strength tests. An accepted means for determination of test validity is to examine how well the measurement correlates with other valid measures of strength. For example, the chair rise test was correlated with isokinetic measures of knee extensor and knee flexor strength and was found to be moderately correlated (0.77) for both men and women.[13] Bohannon[3] reported construct validity (r = 0.578-0.702) between manual muscle testing, handheld dynamometry, and sit-to-stand test. Likewise, Eriksrud and Bohannon[7] found significant correlations (r = 0.652-0.708) for sit-to-stand without use of hands and knee extension force.

Reliability or consistency of a measure has been reported by many researchers. Reliability may be determined by using a test-retest model where the test is repeated on different days, usually 2 to 5 days apart, and scores between the days are correlated.[22] A reliability of 0.80 (high correlation) is acceptable reliability for a measure.[20] For the chair rise test, test-retest reliability has been reported by several investigators with values ranging from 0.88 to 0.89, which is acceptable by the aforementioned standard.[13,19]

Normative performance scores are important to compare performance scores with the expected score of similar individuals performing the same task. Given the heterogeneity of functional performance, establishment of normative values has proven to be challenging for most researchers. Therefore, the examiner should review the latest research on normative values. At the least, the examiner should determine an individual's performance baseline to support comparison over time. When possible, normative scores have been developed by testing large numbers of people in a selected population, and summarization scores have been organized into descriptive categories. Rikli and Jones[22] reported normative data for the chair rise test in 7183 adults using percentile tables and age categories. Using this method, the investigators found that the normal range for the number of successful chair rises completed in 30 seconds was 12 to 17 for women and 14 to 19 for men aged 60 to 64. Therefore a score falling below 12 for women or 14 repetitions for men would be considered below normal, and scores above 17 (women) and 19 (men) would be above normal for individuals in this age category. Amundsen[1] proposed ranking functional strength tests on the basis of patient status as a way of standardizing the test results. Therefore the level of performance may be ranked using this suggested ordinal scoring 0 through 5 as follows:

0 = Unable
1 = Able but severely limited (requires set up, physical assistance, or dysfunctional amount of time)
2 = Able but moderately involved (requires same as for score of 1 except to a lesser degree)
3 = Able but mildly involved (same as score of 2 except to a lesser degree)
4 = Able but slowed
5 = Able

This ranking would allow comparison of an individual's performance over time rather than a comparison with normative scores. For example for a score of 5 on a low-level test, the individual would be expected to have adequate functional strength whereas a score of 1 on the same test would be indicative of a limitation in functional strength. The ordinal ranking system is based on inferences by Amundsen[1] and Guralnik et al.[10] and, although presented here, requires further testing. Additionally, the examiner should be aware that the above ranking is clinically applicable and useful for individual patients/clients but that further epidemiologic data are needed to establish normative scores and a more standard ranking system. As with muscle testing in pediatrics, the examiner is encouraged to establish intrarater reliability for the functional strength tests and interrater reliability where the test will be assessed by more than one examiner.

In functional muscle testing, the tester should consider that functional motor performance (ability to perform motor tasks essential to fulfill one's desires and role in life) is multifactorial. Performance involves more than muscle strength and power and requires complex interactions of the musculoskeletal, neuromuscular, cardiopulmonary, and integumentary systems as well as motor skill.[7] Functional motor performance is demonstrated in performance of ADLs like bathing, toileting, dressing, and feeding oneself.[14] Further functional performance incorporates IADLs like community mobility, recreation and socialization, and shopping.[17] For efficient, safe, functional motor performance to take place successfully, three factors should be considered—individual factors, task factors, and environmental factors.

Individual factors include cognition; muscle strength; smooth, pain-free range-of-motion (ROM); endurance; and power adequate for successful completion of the task. Task factors are related to the dynamics of the task itself and whether the task is simple (i.e., coming from sit to stand) or complex (walking). Environmental factors are associated with the context within which the task is performed and the constraints placed upon the individual and the task by the environment. Some examples of environmental factors are height of chairs, curbs, or stairs; carpet or tile; stable surface or moving surface; and carrying a load or unloaded. These factors will affect the individual's ability to complete the task and must be considered when examining functional motor performance.

Because the emphasis of this chapter is on functional strength testing (an individual factor), the tester will be asked to assume that the other individual factors such as cognitive ability have been taken into account. Recommendations for controlling the environmental factors will be included within the test description under equipment.

IMPORTANT DEFINITIONS

1. Function—performance that supports physical, social, psychological well-being and meaningful living and is determined to be essential by the individual

2. Strength-force output capacity—maximum force or tension generated by a single muscle or related muscle groups[2]
3. Functional strength—capacity to generate a force output adequate to complete a specific task[1]

Upper Body Tests

The upper body is functionally divided into components of extremities and upper trunk/head. The trunk is involved largely in postural control in static and dynamic activities requiring shifts of the body's mass within the base of support.[25] The upper extremities are involved in light load activities, reaching, and "bringing to" types of tasks.[27] These tasks require combinations of extension, flexion, and rotation with object manipulation.

The trunk acts to hold the body in position as in maintenance of upright posture in relation to gravity. The trunk musculature also is important in maintaining equilibrium during transitional movements involving changes of body position. The head is important as an initiator or leader of movement. The primary goal of head movement is to keep the head in a vertical position with the eyes close to horizontal such that the eyes can participate in motor planning and organization of movement in relation to the external environment. To evaluate functional strength of the head and trunk, activities should include translations of the body mass forward, backward, laterally, and diagonally in relation to the base of support. Tests of functional strength of the head and trunk should incorporate both tonic (holding) and phasic (moving) aspects in forward, backward, lateral, and diagonal. These directions require extension, flexion, and rotational strength.

Tests used to evaluate functional strength of the upper body should include all aspects of these movements. The tests described in this section are sweep curl, sitting up lift, sitting down lift, diagonal up lift (standing), diagonal down lift (standing), long sit—head, prone roll—head, and supine to side roll—head.

Lower Body Tests

The lower body is functionally comprised of the lower trunk/pelvis and the lower extremities. The lower trunk/pelvis is involved in postural control in static and dynamic activities, acting during shifts of the body's mass within the base of support. Lower extremities are involved in heavy load activities like sit to stand, walking, or double-/single-limb stance.[27] These types of tasks involve hip, knee, and ankle movements of flexion, extension, and rotation in reciprocal patterns using open-chain and closed-chain (weight-bearing) positions. To evaluate functional strength the tests used should include all of these movements in single-limb and double-limb activities. The tests included in this section are repeated chair rise, step test, stair climb, side-step stair climb, sitting leg cross, lateral hip scoot, hip hike, forward stepping, and backward stepping.

Gross Body Tests

The tests in this section assess upper trunk and head, which includes the shoulder girdle and the upper thoracic trunk segment, and the lower trunk, which includes the low back and pelvis. The tests to assess gross body functional strength are floor sit, floor rise, and supine to side sit.

■ UPPER BODY TESTS

SWEEP CURL

Assessment of functional strength of elbow flexors and shoulder musculature (pectoralis major, subscapularis, latissimus dorsi, teres major).

Functional Strength (Grades 5 and 4)

Equipment: Straight wooden chair with a seat height of 43 to 44 cm placed against a wall; barbell weights of 0.45 kg, 1.35 kg, and 2.25 kg.

Constraints: Shoulder pain, ROM deficits, grip strength deficit, sitting balance deficit, or cognitive deficits that would limit understanding of instruction.

Patient position: Sitting in middle of chair with back approximately 10 cm from back of chair and feet flat on floor slightly posterior of knee joint. Hips should be at 90°, shoulders level, and head upright. Begin test with patient holding a 2.25-kg weight in hand on the side being tested with the elbow extended, palm facing forward, and arm at side (Fig. 5-1).

Fig. 5-1.

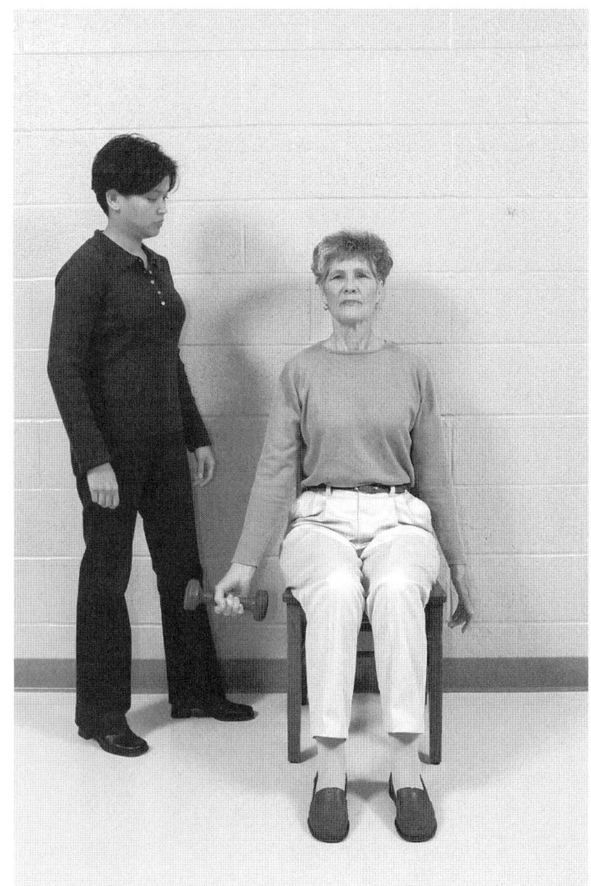

Examiner position: At side being tested and far enough away to allow free movement of the sweep motion (Fig. 5-1).

Examiner action: Instruct patient as follows: "When I say to, I want you to bend your elbow to bring the barbell to touch your opposite shoulder and then bring the barbell back to your side. During the movement, keep your elbow close to your side. Repeat the task five times." As you describe the task, demonstrate one complete movement.

Examiner command: "Now bend your elbow and touch your opposite shoulder. Repeat the action five times."

Patient action: Patient will flex elbow to touch the barbell to the opposite shoulder and then extend the elbow to bring the arm back to the side (Figs. 5-2, 5-3, and 5-4).

Repeat test with the other arm.

SCORING RECOMMENDATIONS

For grade 5: Patient completes five repetitions without difficulty.

For grade 4: Patient completes four repetitions.

Note: Document the amount of weight used in the test.

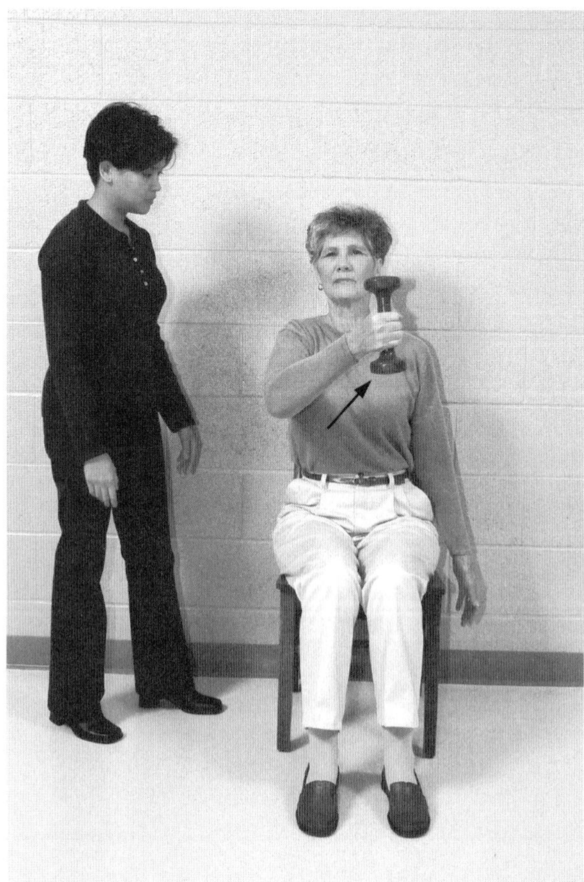

Fig. 5-2. Arrow indicates direction of movement.

Fig. 5-3.

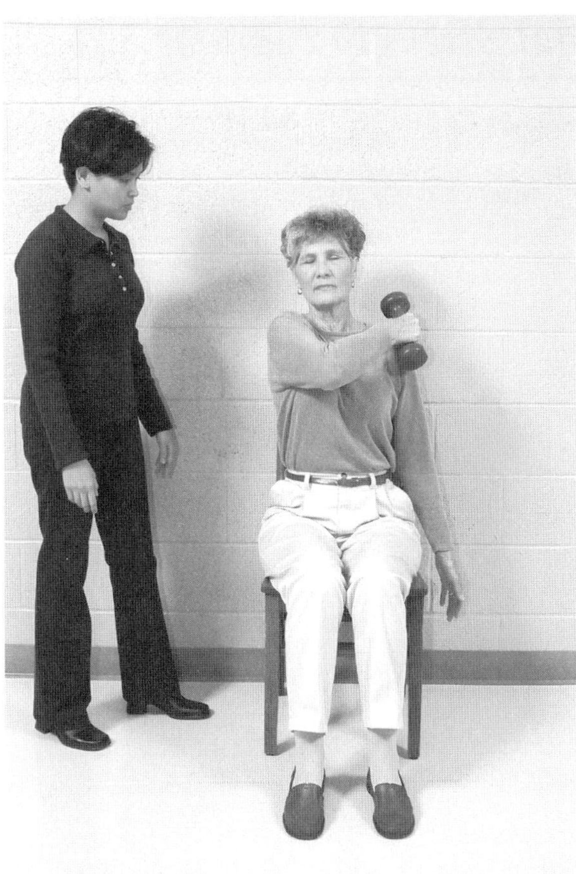

Fig. 5-4. Arrow indicates direction of movement.

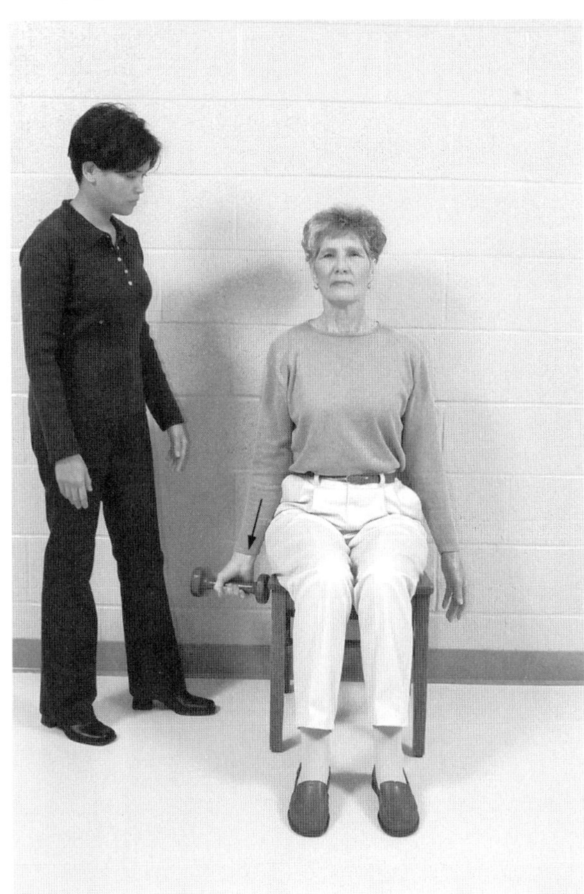

Functional Strength (Grades 3 and Below)

For grade 3: Patient completes five repetitions using the 0.45-kg barbell. If the patient is unable to complete the five repetitions, refer to instructions for grade 2.

For grade 2: Patient completes less than five repetitions, but is able to initiate the movement through partial range without allowing the arm to drop back to the side.

For grade 1: Examiner palpates a contraction of the biceps and shoulder muscles.

For grade 0: No contraction is observed or palpated by the examiner.

SITTING UP LIFT

Assessment of functional strength of upper trunk extensors, shoulder flexors, and scapular rotators.

Functional Strength (Grades 5, 4, and 3)

Equipment: Straight wooden chair with a seat height of 43 to 44 cm and a can or 15-cm square wooden block held by examiner at patient's arm length in front and center of the patient.

Constraints: Shoulder pain, ROM deficits, grip strength deficit, sitting balance deficit, or cognitive deficits that would limit understanding of instruction.

Patient position: Sitting in middle of chair with back approximately 10 cm from back of chair and feet flat on floor slightly posterior of knee joint. Hips should be at 90°, shoulders level, and head upright. Begin test with patient's hands resting on the thighs (Fig. 5-5).

Examiner position: To side close enough to position the block in front and center of the patient and to prevent a loss of balance in the forward direction (Fig. 5-5).

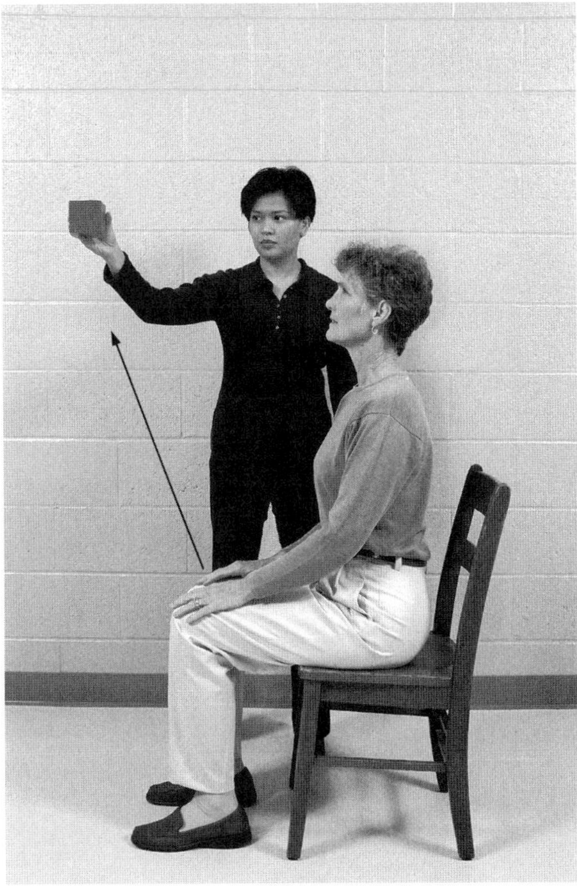

Fig. 5-5. Arrow indicates direction of movement.

Examiner action: Instruct patient as follows: "When I say to, I want you to reach up with both hands to take the block from me. After you have taken the block, hold it with both hands and place it in your lap. I will ask you to repeat the task five times, ending with the block in your lap each time." As you describe the task, demonstrate the movement to the patient.

Examiner command: "Now, reach up and take the block with both hands and place it in your lap." At the end of each repetition, retrieve the block from the patient and repeat the command.

Patient action: Patient will bring arms forward and up with elbows extended while the trunk extends to take the block from the examiner and then will return to a neutral posture with the elbows slightly flexed and the object held in both hands (Figs. 5-6, 5-7, and 5-8).

SCORING RECOMMENDATIONS

For grade 5: Patient completes five repetitions without difficulty.

For grade 4: Patient completes four repetitions but movement uncoordinated.

For grade 3: Patient completes three of the five repetitions but requires added time and movement is poorly controlled.

Functional Strength (Below Grade 3)

For grade 2: Patient is able to initiate the movement through partial range without allowing the arms to drop back to the thighs.

For grade 1: Examiner palpates a contraction of the biceps and shoulder muscles.

For grade 0: No contraction is observed or palpated by the examiner.

Fig. 5-6.

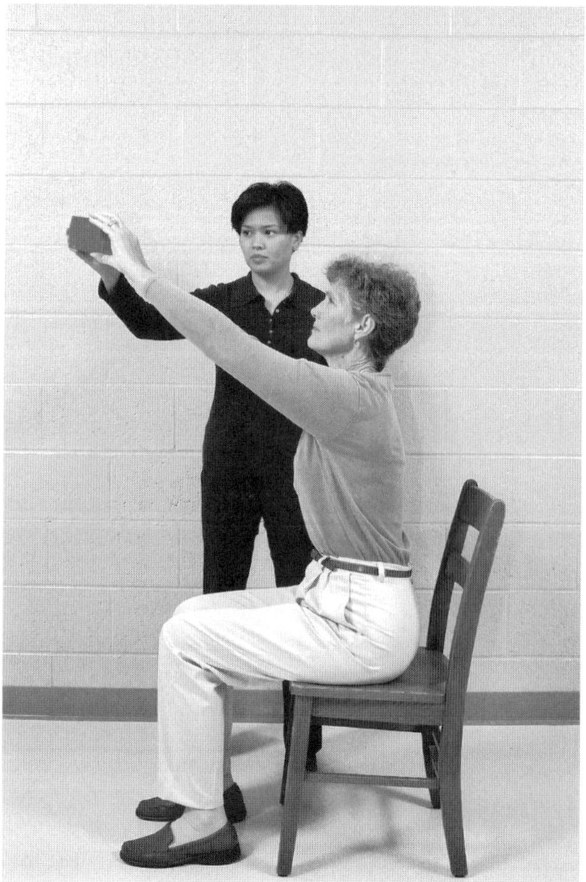

Fig. 5-7.

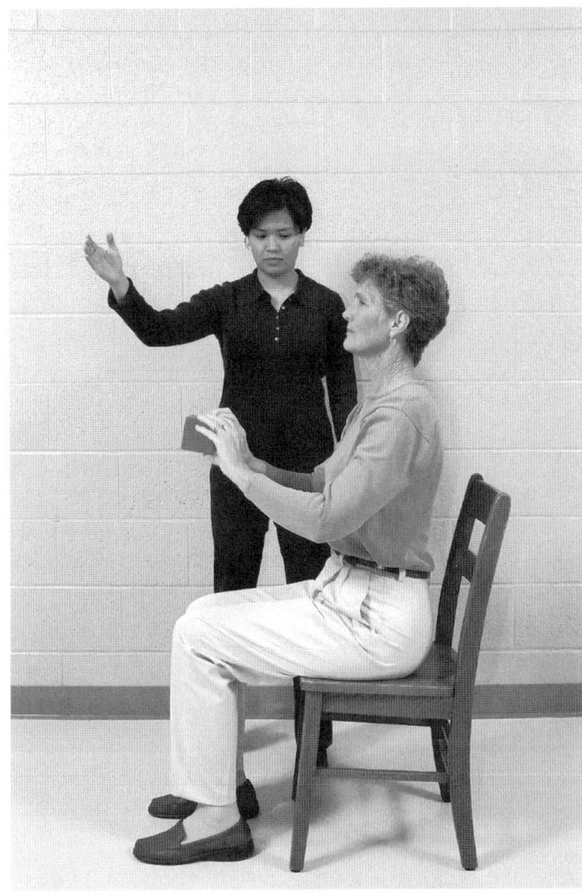

Fig. 5-8.

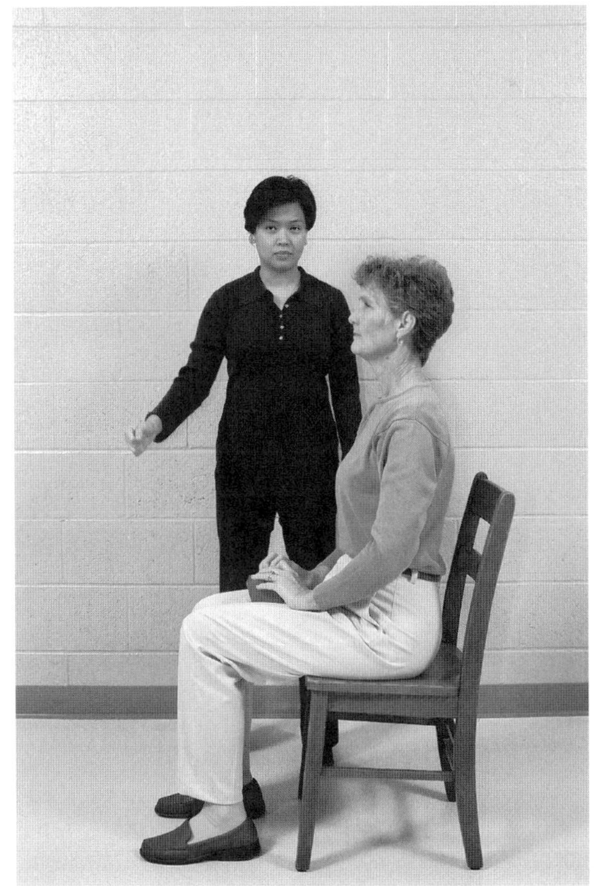

SITTING DOWN LIFT

Assessment of functional strength of upper trunk flexors (down movement) and extensors (movement back to upright).

Functional Strength (Grades 5, 4, and 3)

Equipment: Straight wooden chair with a seat height of 43 to 44 cm and a 15-cm square wooden block or can of sufficient size that the patient can comfortably grasp with both hands.

Constraints: Shoulder pain, ROM deficits, grip strength deficit, sitting balance deficit, or cognitive deficits that would limit understanding of instruction.

Patient position: Sitting in middle of chair with back approximately 10 cm from back of chair and feet flat on floor slightly posterior of knee joint. Hips should be at 90°, shoulders level, and head upright. Begin test with patient's hands resting in the lap holding the block with both hands (Fig. 5-9).

Examiner position: To side, close enough to prevent a loss of balance in the forward direction.

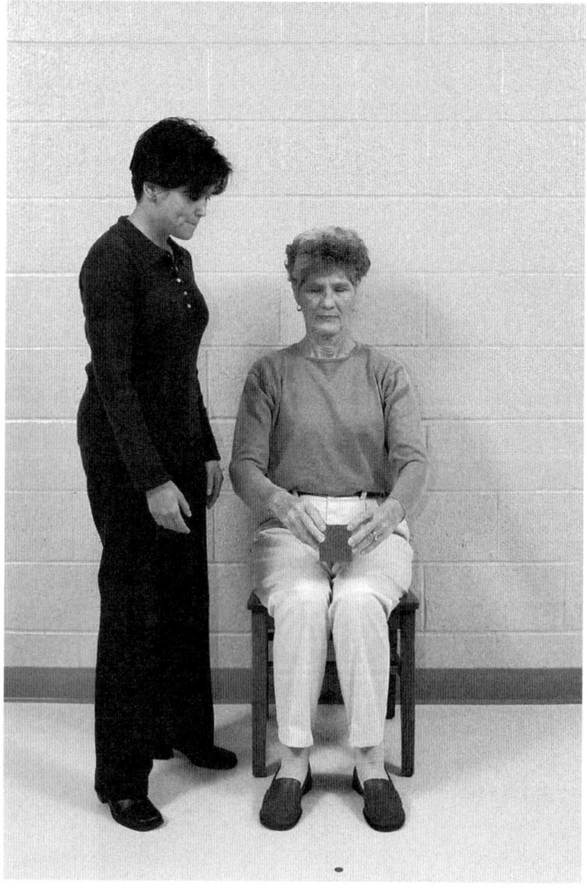

Fig. 5-9.

Examiner action: Instruct patient as follows: "When I say to, I want you to reach down with both hands to place the block on the floor in front of you. After you have placed the block on the floor, return to sitting upright with your hands on your thighs. I will ask you to repeat the task five times, ending with the block on the floor each time." As you describe the task, demonstrate the movement to the patient.

Examiner command: "Now, take the block with both hands and place it on the floor in front of you and leave it there." At the end of each repetition, retrieve the block from the floor, return it to the patient, and repeat the command.

Patient action: Patient will bring arms forward and down with elbows extended while the trunk flexes to place block on the floor in front of the feet. The patient will extend the trunk to return to a neutral posture with hands resting on thighs (Figs. 5-10, 5-11, and 5-12).

Fig. 5-10.

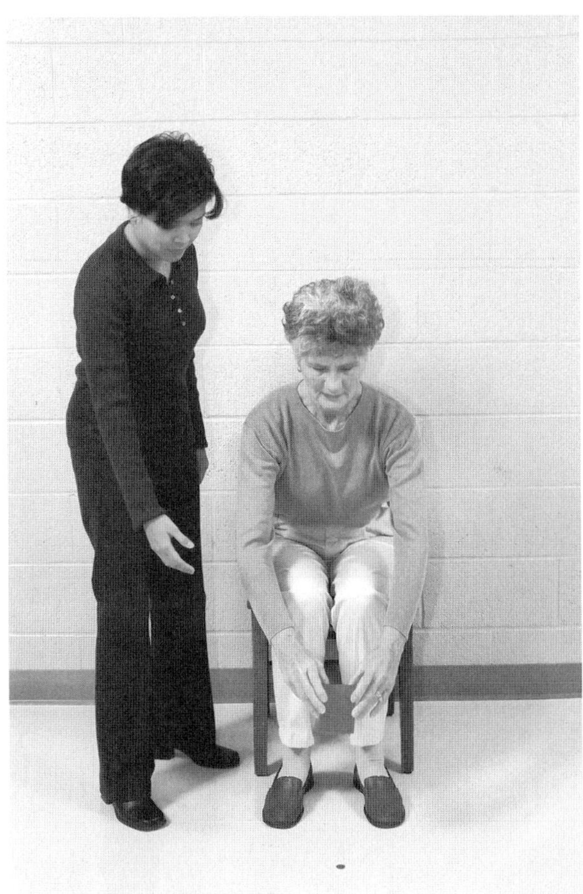

Fig. 5-11.

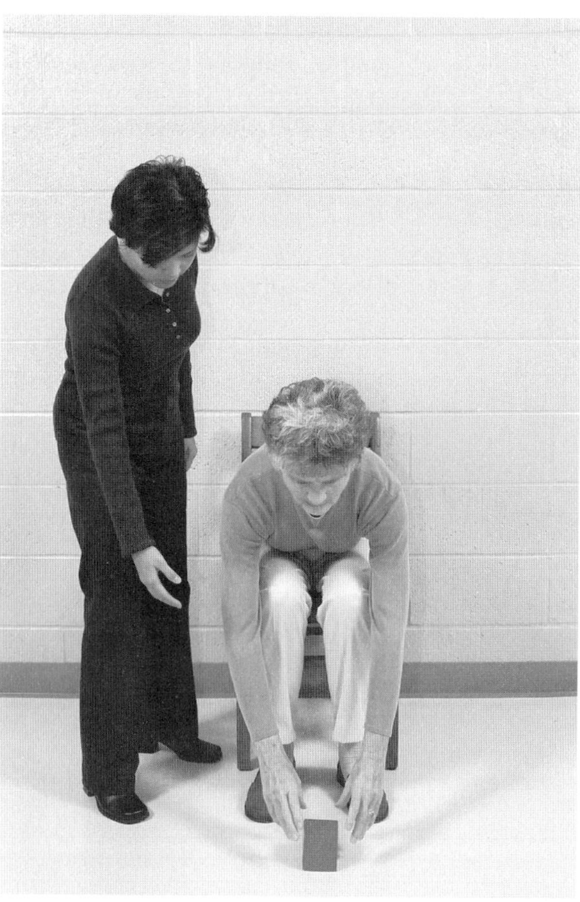

Fig. 5-12.

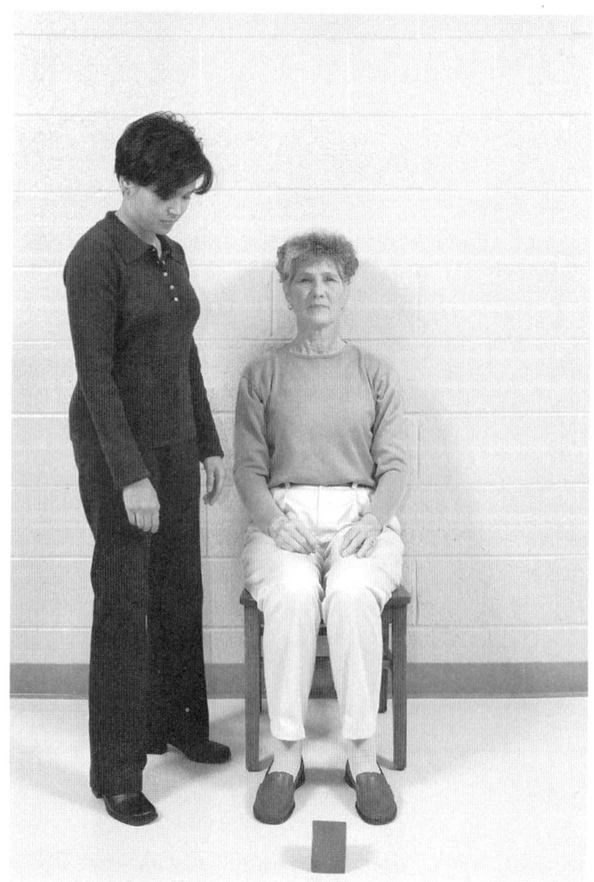

SCORING RECOMMENDATIONS

For grade 5: Patient completes five repetitions without difficulty.

For grade 4: Patient completes four repetitions but movement uncoordinated.

For grade 3: Patient completes three of the five repetitions but requires added time and movement is poorly controlled.

Functional Strength (Below Grade 3)

For grade 2: Patient is able to initiate the movement through partial range without dropping the object or losing balance.

For grade 1: Examiner observes movement in forward direction but patient unable to initiate placement of the block without loss of balance.

For grade 1: No contraction is observed or palpated by the examiner.

DIAGONAL UP LIFT

Assessment of concentric and eccentric functional strength of trunk, shoulder abductors and flexors, and scapular rotators

Functional Strength (All Grades)

Equipment: Standard wooden chair with seat height of 43 to 44 cm placed next to a shelf approximately 168 cm high and 0.45-kg, 1.35-kg, and 2.25-kg weights. Mark shelf and chair with "X" using colorful tape or sticky labels to provide a visual target and standardization of placement from time to time. The marker should be placed to provide a diagonal-reach pattern, for example if the patient is reaching with the right arm, the marker should be placed on the left side of the chair seat.

Constraints: Pain, ROM limitations, balance deficits, and cognitive deficits that would limit understanding of instruction.

Patient position: Standing close to and facing the chair with arms at sides.

Begin with right arm close to shelf. Trunk is upright with head forward and pelvis is level without rotation. Feet are shoulder width apart.

Examiner position: In back of patient with hands on each side of pelvis to prevent loss of balance (Fig. 5-13).

Fig. 5-13.

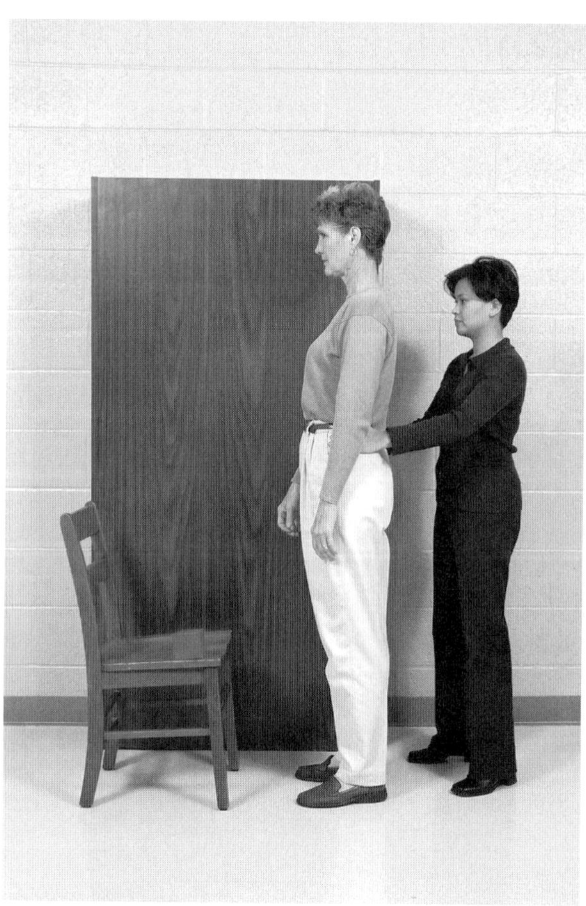

Examiner action: Instruct patient as follows: "When I say for you to, reach forward and across with the right arm to grasp weight and lift upward to place on marked area on the shelf." Start with the 2.25-kg weight. Place the weight on the marker as previously indicated. As you describe the task, demonstrate the movement to the patient (Figs. 5-14 and 5-15).

Examiner command: "Now reach with your right hand to pick up the weight and place it on the shelf and leave it there."

Fig. 5-14.

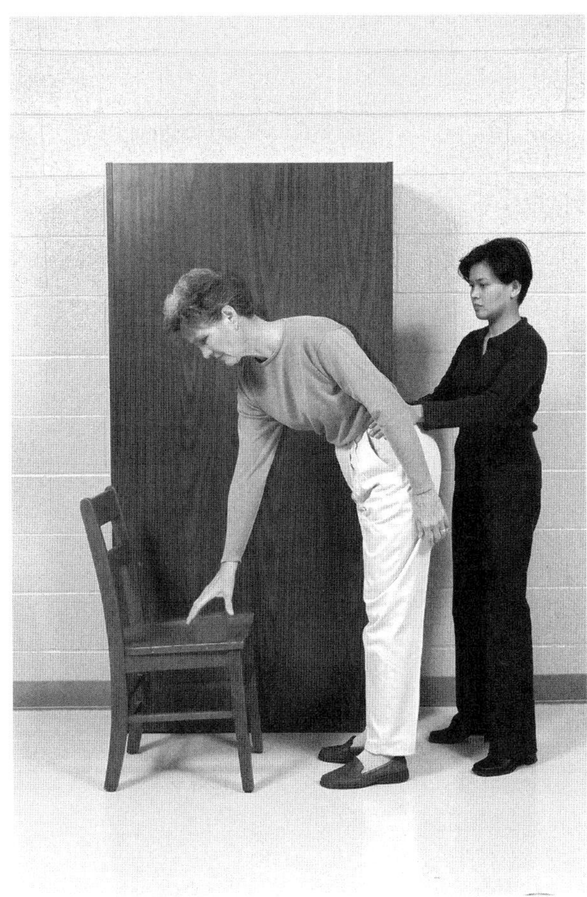

Fig. 5-15. Arrow indicates direction of movement.

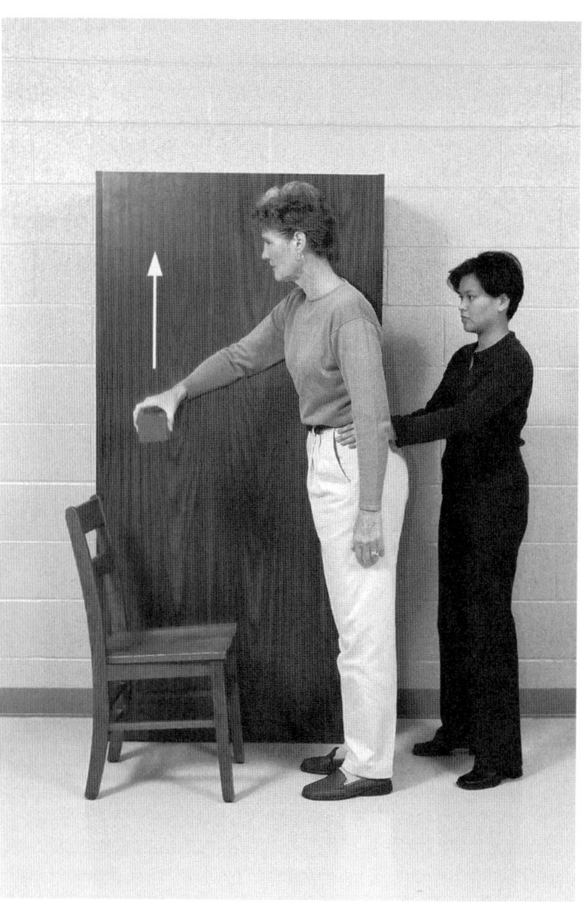

Patient action: Patient will flex and slightly rotate the trunk while the arm is adducted to retrieve the weight then will abduct and flex the shoulder and extend the trunk to place the weight on the shelf. Slight knee flexion and extension may also occur depending on the patient's height (Fig. 5-16).

Repeat the task changing the chair position such that the patient is now reaching forward and across with the left arm.

SCORING RECOMMENDATIONS

For grade 5: Patient completes lift of 2.25 kg without difficulty.

For grade 4: Patient completes lift of 1.35 kg but movement jerky and slowed.

For grade 3: Patient completes more than one-half lift of 0.45 kg but with added time, and movement is poorly controlled.

For grade 2: Patient completes less than one half of the lift test against gravity (no weight).

For grade 1: Patient is unable to complete task; slight contraction is palpated or observed.

For grade 0: Patient is unable to complete task; no contraction is palpated or observed.

Fig. 5-16.

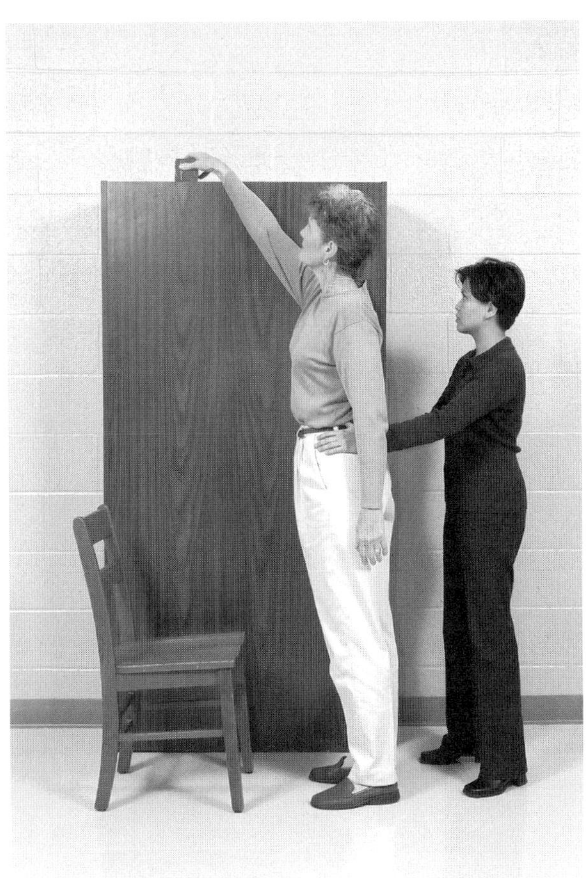

DIAGONAL DOWN LIFT

Assessment of concentric and eccentric functional strength of the trunk, shoulder flexors, horizontal adductors, and scapular rotators.

Functional Strength (Grades 5, 4, and 3)

Equipment: Standard wooden chair with seat height of 43 to 44 cm placed next to a shelf approximately 168 cm high and 0.45-kg, 1.35-kg, and 2.25-kg weights. Mark shelf and chair with "X" using colorful tape or sticky labels to provide a visual target and standardization of placement from time to time. The marker should be placed to provide a diagonal reach pattern, for example if the patient is reaching with the right arm, the marker should be placed on the left side of the chair seat. The marker should be placed on the shelf slightly forward of the patient such that they will be required to reach forward and up to the target.

Constraints: Pain, ROM limitations, balance deficits, and cognitive deficits that would limit understanding of instruction.

Patient position: Standing close to and facing the chair with arms at side.

Begin with right arm close to shelf. Trunk is upright with head forward and pelvis level without rotation. Feet are shoulder width apart (Fig. 5-17).

Fig. 5-17.

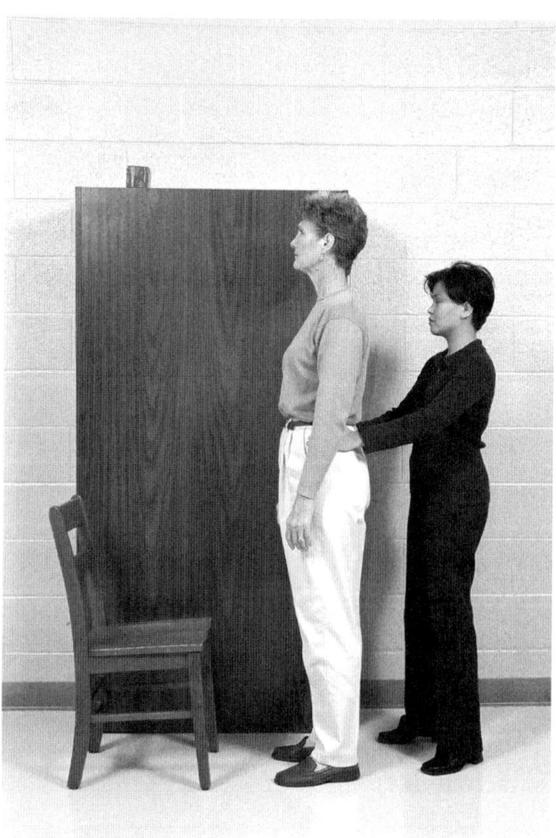

Examiner position: In back of patient with hands on each side of pelvis to prevent loss of balance (Fig. 5-18).

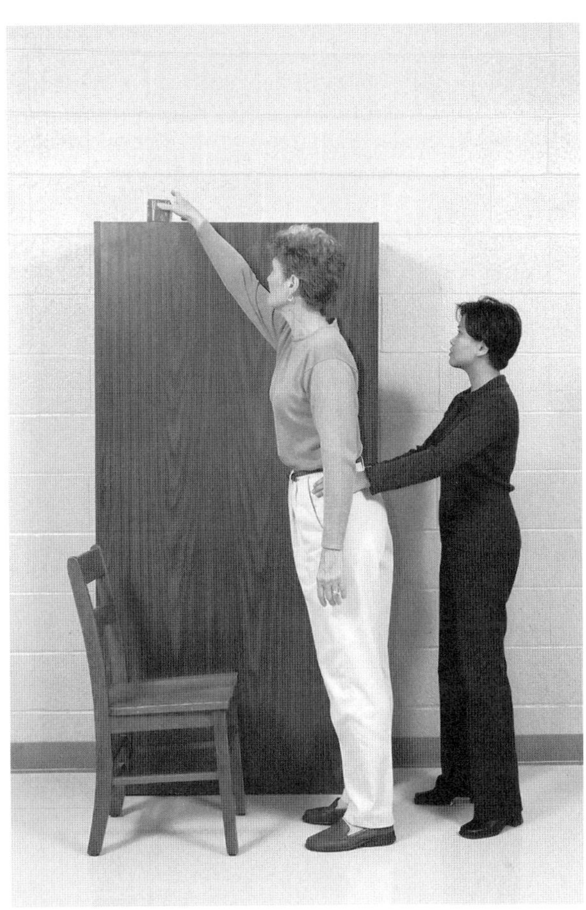

Fig. 5-18.

Examiner action:

Instruct patient as follows: "When I say for you to, reach forward and up with the right arm to grasp the weight on the shelf and bring it down and across to place it on marked area on the chair." Start with the 2.25-kg weight. Place the weight on the marker on the shelf as previously indicated. As you describe the task, demonstrate the movement to the patient.

Examiner command:

"Now reach with your right hand to pick up the weight and place it on the marker on the chair and leave it there." (Fig. 5-19).

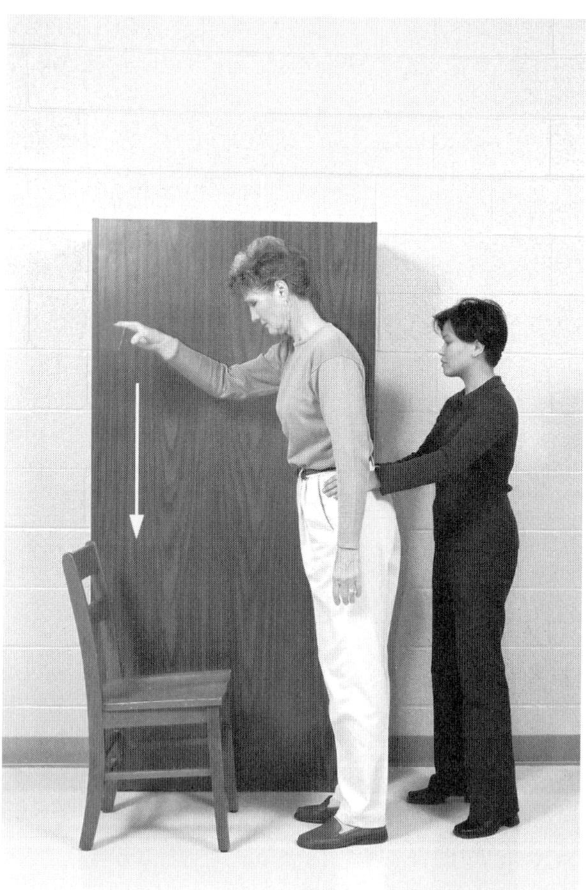

Fig. 5-19. Arrow indicates direction of movement.

Patient action: Patient will extend the trunk while the shoulder is abducted and flexed to retrieve the weight and then will adduct and extend shoulder with slight trunk flexion and rotation to place the weight on the chair. Slight knee flexion and extension also may occur depending on the patient's height (Fig. 5-20).

Fig. 5-20.

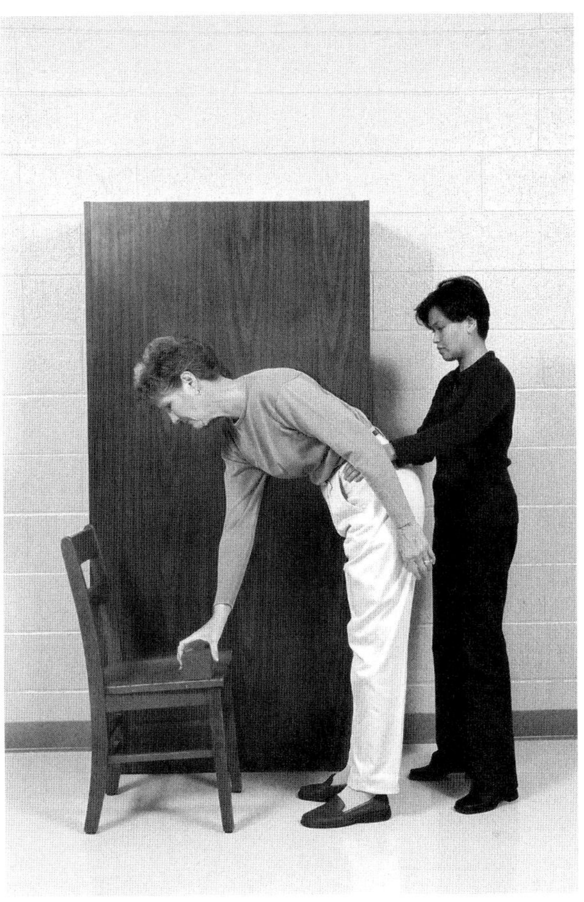

Repeat the task changing the chair position such that the patient is now reaching forward and across with the left arm.

SCORING RECOMMENDATIONS

For grade 5: Patient completes test with 2.25 kg without difficulty.

For grade 4: Patient completes test with 1.35 kg but movement jerky and with decreased speed.

For grade 3: Patient completes more than one half of the test with 0.45 kg but with poorly controlled downward movement.

Functional Strength (Grades Below 3)

SCORING RECOMMENDATIONS

For grade 2: Examiner passively moves patient's arm to reach position and releases; patient's arm falls back to side.

For grade 1 and 0: Test not recommended.

LONG SIT

Assessment of concentric and isometric neck flexors

Functional Strength (All Grades)

Equipment: Wall mat or firm surface (a firm bed or sofa if in patient's home) of adequate width and length to permit completion of task and two towel rolls.

Constraints: Pain, abdominal strength deficit, sitting trunk balance deficit, limitations in ROM (trunk and lower extremities), and cognitive deficits that limit understanding of instruction.

Patient position: Supine with the arms at the sides and the hands resting on each side of the pelvis. Knees and hips are extended and feet are slightly apart. If needed, pressure may be relieved from lower back using a small towel roll under each knee (Fig. 5-21).

Examiner position: At the side of the mat or surface toward the head and in position to observe the movement and prevent the head or trunk from falling backward too rapidly. Examiner position will change slightly with a weight shift from one foot to the other to remain in the recommended position as the patient moves through the task (Figs. 5-22, 5-23, and 5-24).

Examiner action: Instruct patient as follows: "When I ask you to, I want you to sit straight up as far as you comfortably can with your legs out in front of you. You may use your arms as needed to complete the task. You will be asked to complete the task five times." As you describe the task, passively assist the patient to attain the long sit position and return to the starting position. This passive action allows assessment of adequate trunk and lower extremity flexibility and strength.

Fig. 5-21.

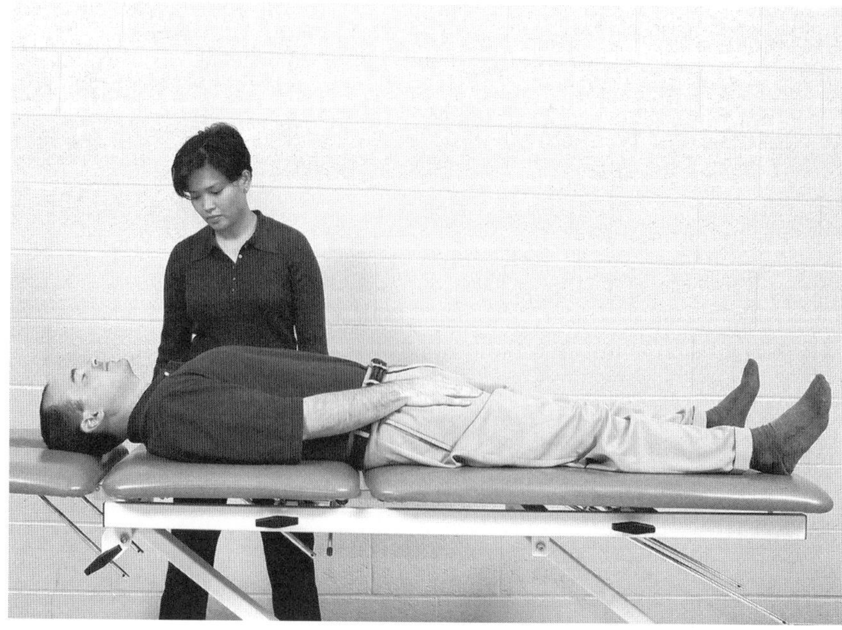

Fig. 5-22.

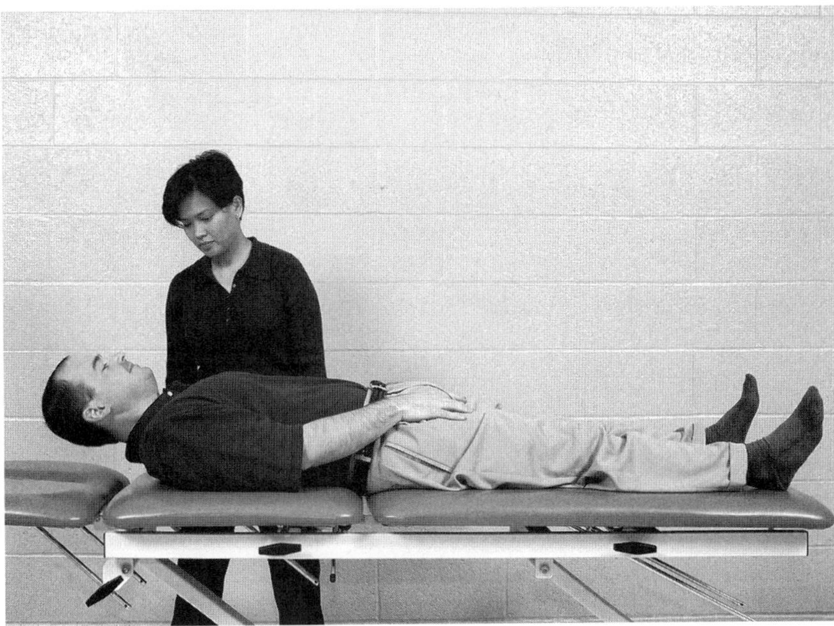

Fig. 5-23.

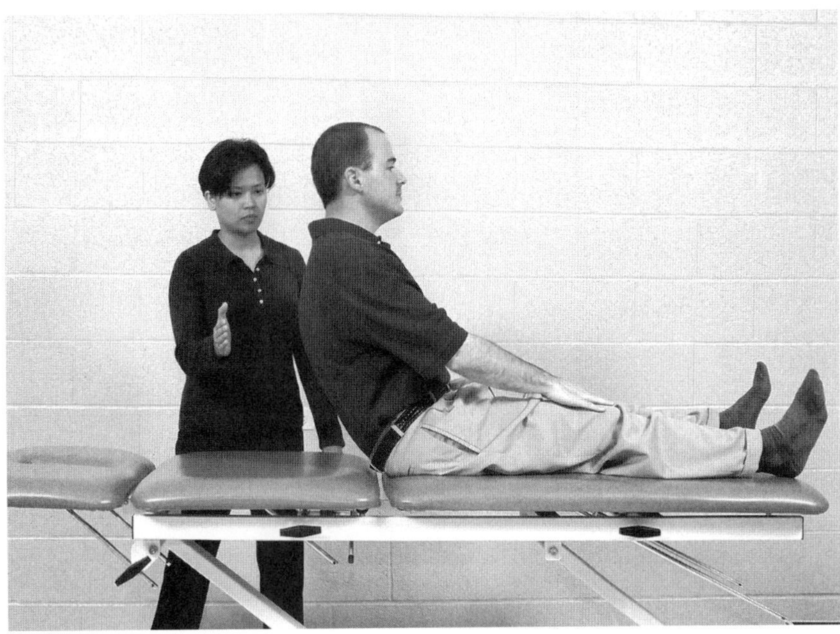

Examiner command: "Now sit up and hold your head upright."

Patient action: Patient assumes long sitting from supine while maintaining head in line with or anterior to the shoulders. The movement will begin with a chin tuck and flexion of the neck, and then the head will lift from the surface followed by trunk and hip flexion. The head will remain in varied degree of flexion until the trunk attains upright position with hips at 90°.*

*If abdominal strength is limited, the test may be altered by asking the patient to come to approximately 75% of a full upright sitting position and then return to the supine position. This change will still allow assessment of the neck flexors through most of the long sit movement. Document any alterations or changes in the test protocol.

Fig. 5-24.

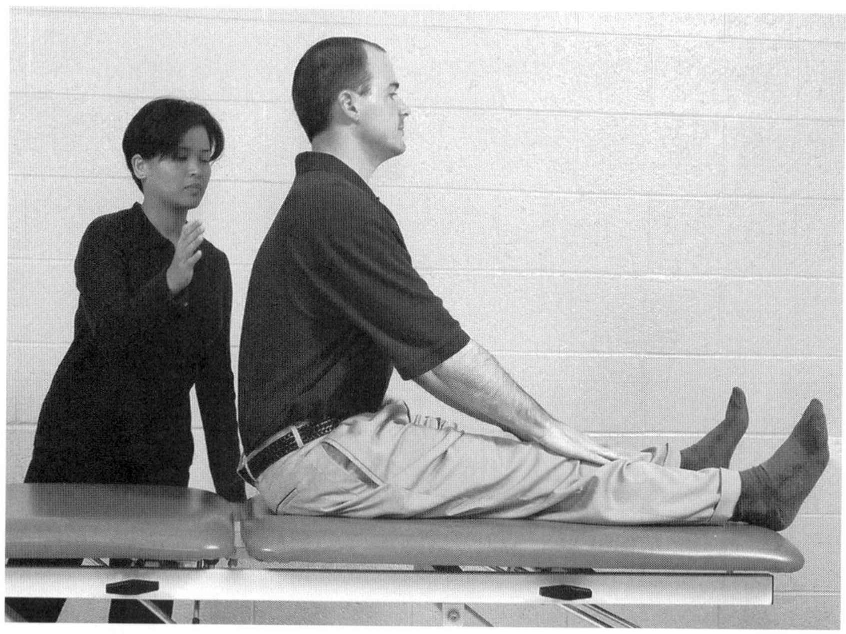

SCORING RECOMMENDATIONS

For grade 5:	Patient is able to initiate and maintain neck flexion through five repetitions of the movement.
For grade 4:	Patient is able to initiate and maintain neck flexion through three repetitions of the movement.
For grade 3:	Patient is able to initiate and maintain neck flexion through one repetition of the movement.
For grade 2:	Patient is able to lift head from surface but is unable to maintain through test range against gravity.
For grade 1:	Contraction is observed or palpated but patient is unable to lift head from surface.
For grade 0:	No movement or contraction occurs; patient's head remains supported by the surface.

PRONE ROLL

Assessment of concentric and isometric functional strength of neck extensors

Functional Strength (All Grades)

Equipment: Wall mat or firm surface (a firm bed or sofa if in patient's home) of adequate width and length to permit completion of task.

Constraints: Pain, abdominal strength deficit, sitting trunk balance deficit, limitations in ROM (trunk and upper extremities), discomfort in prone position, and cognitive deficits that limit understanding of instruction.

Patient position: Prone in slight neck flexion with forehead resting on the surface. The shoulders are abducted to 90° and the elbows flexed approximately 90 to 100° (Fig. 5-25).

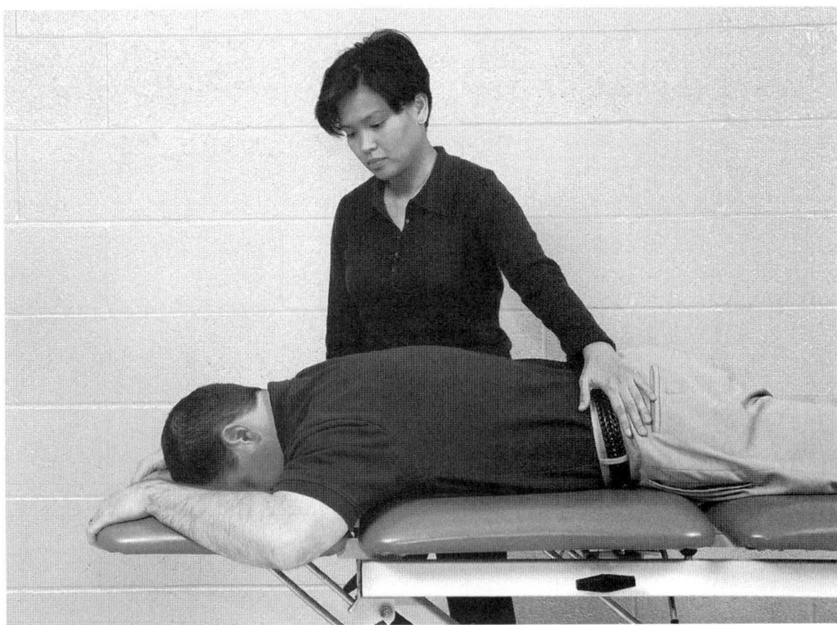

Fig. 5-25.

Examiner position: At the side of the mat or surface toward the head and positioned to observe the movement, prevent the head from falling too rapidly, and for safety during the patient's roll. Examiner position will change slightly with a weight shift from one foot to the other to remain in the recommended position as the patient moves through the task. Examiner may place a hand on the pelvis to guide the rolling movement (Fig. 5-26).

Examiner action: Instruct patient as follows: "When I ask you to, I want you to lift your head and roll over to your side using your arms for support as needed. You may roll to either the right or left as you prefer. I will ask you to repeat the movement five times." As you describe the task, passively move the patient through the task and return patient to the starting position.

Examiner command: "Now lift your head and roll to your side, and then I will assist you to return to the prone starting position."

Fig. 5-26.

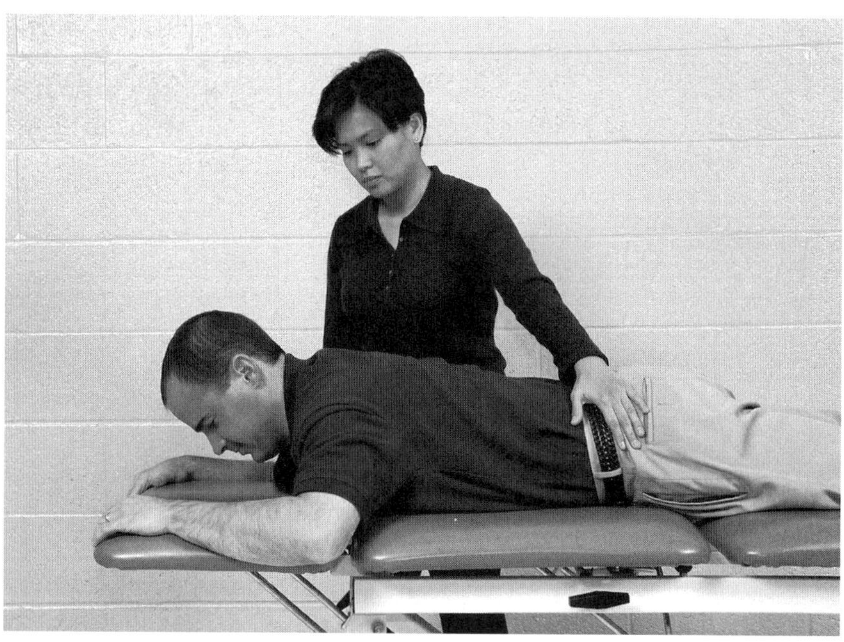

Patient action: Patient extends the head and neck while pushing up with arms to roll to the preferred side. Patient should move head and neck into extension, then to neutral at side-lying position (Fig. 5-27).

Fig. 5-27.

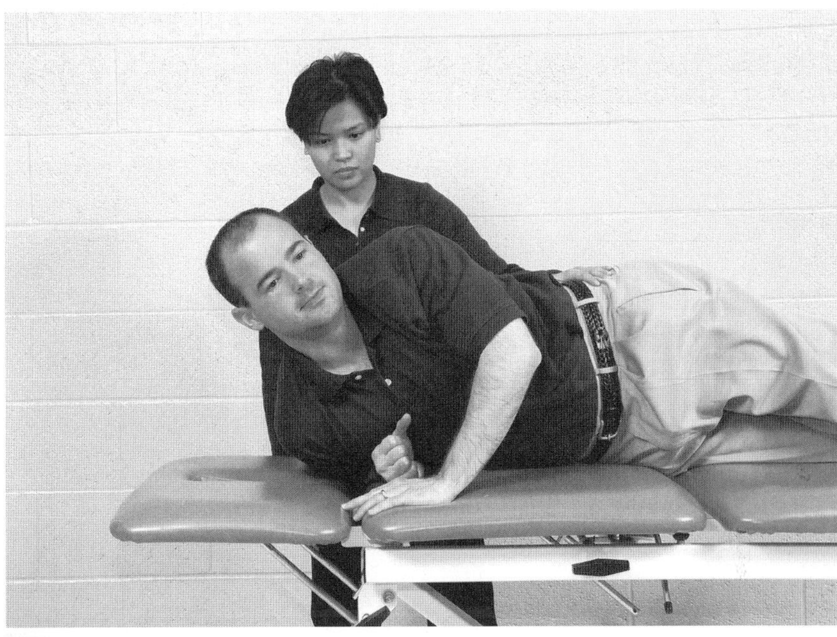

SCORING RECOMMENDATIONS

For grade 5: Patient is able to initiate and maintain neck flexion through five repetitions of the movement.

For grade 4: Patient is able to initiate and maintain neck flexion through three repetitions of the movement.

For grade 3: Patient is able to initiate and maintain neck flexion through one repetition of the movement.*

For grade 2: Patient is able to lift head from surface but is unable to maintain through test range against gravity.

For grade 1: Contraction is observed or palpated but the patient is unable to lift head.

For grade 0: No movement or contraction occurs; the head remains supported by the surface.

*If strength is limited, the test may be altered by asking the patient to come to approximately 75% of a side-lying position and then return to the prone position. This change will still allow assessment of neck extension through most of the prone roll movement. Document any alterations or changes in the test protocol.

SUPINE TO SIDE ROLL

Assessment of functional strength neck rotators

Functional Strength (All Grades)

Equipment: Mat or firm surface large enough to permit rolling from supine to side-lying position in either direction.

Constraints: Pain, abdominal strength deficit, trunk balance deficit, limitations in ROM (trunk and upper extremities), and cognitive deficits that limit understanding of instruction.

Patient position: Supine with head turned away from the side being tested. The shoulders are abducted to 90°, and the dorsal aspects of the forearms are resting on the table. The lower extremities are fully extended (Fig. 5-28).

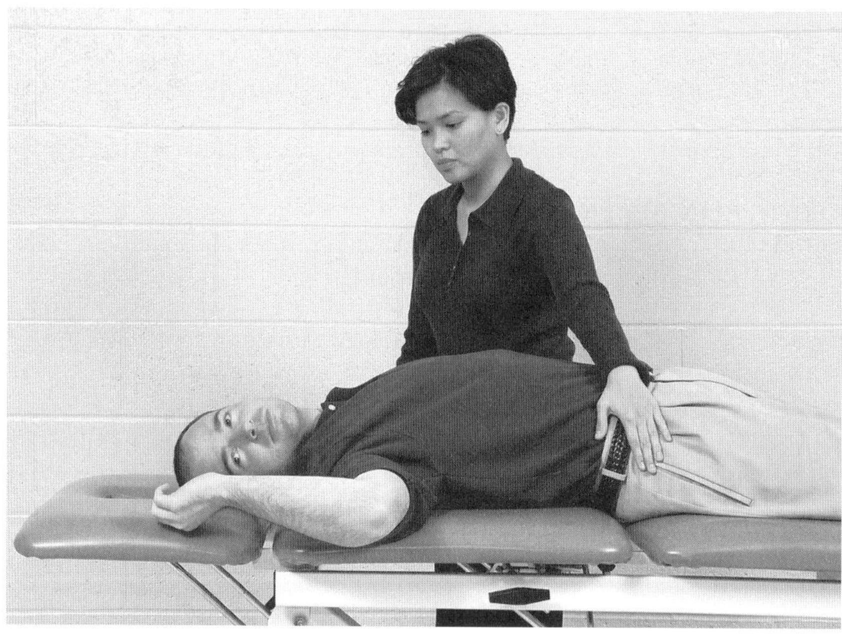

Fig. 5-28.

Examiner position: On the side of the mat toward which the patient is rolling near the head and in such a position to observe the movement and to provide safety during the patient's roll. Examiner position will change slightly with a weight shift from one foot to the other to remain in the recommended position as the patient moves through the task. Examiner may place a hand on the opposite side of the pelvis to guide the rolling movement (Fig. 5-29).

Examiner action: Instruct patient as follows: "When I say to, I want you to turn your head toward the opposite side and roll over onto that side. For example, if you are looking to your left, I want you to turn your head toward the right and roll onto your right side. I will ask you to repeat the task five times." As you describe the task, passively rotate the patient's head away from then toward the side being tested. Once the movement has been demonstrated, return the patient to the starting position.

Examiner command: "Now, turn your head and roll onto your right side and then back."

Fig. 5-29.

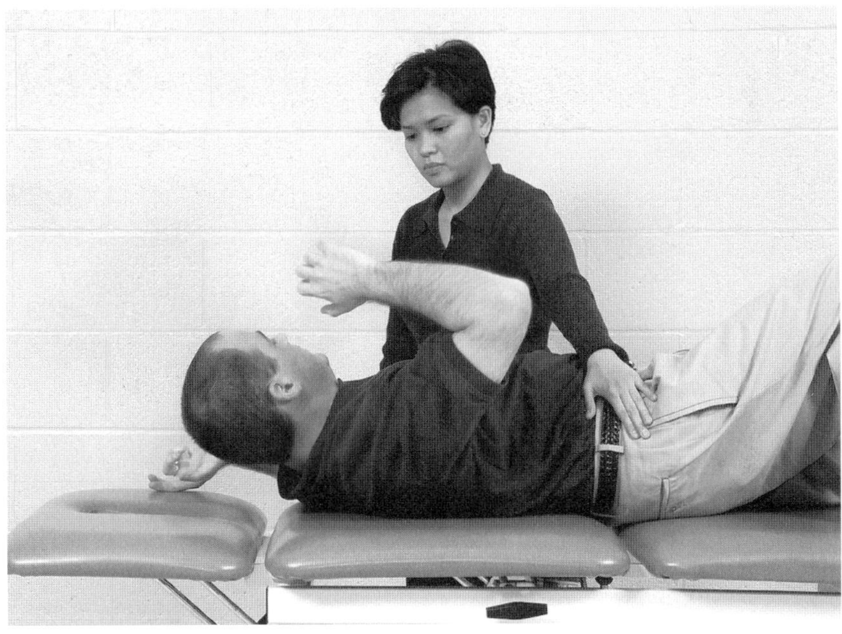

Patient action:

Patient will laterally rotate the neck and turn to look in the direction of the roll while assuming a side-lying position on the side being tested (Figs. 5-30 and 5-31).

Test should be repeated with rolling to the left.

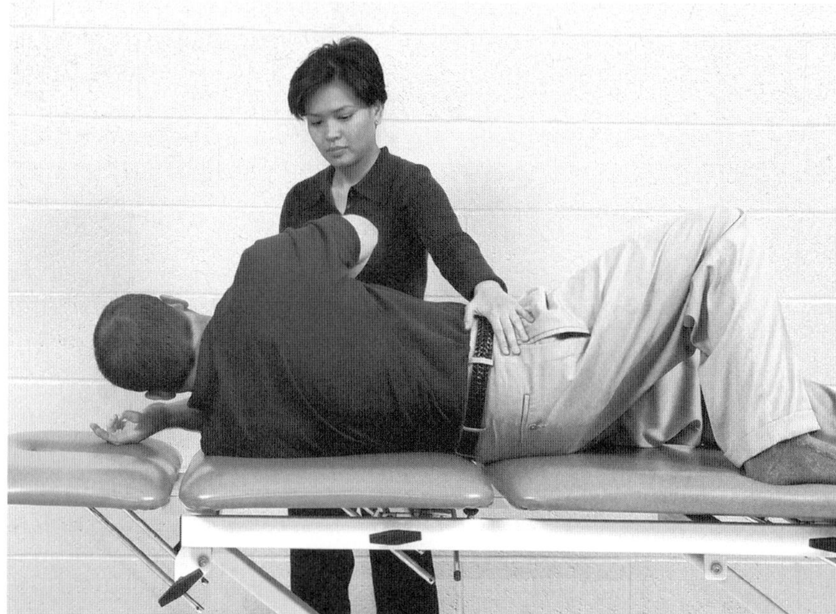

Fig. 5-30.

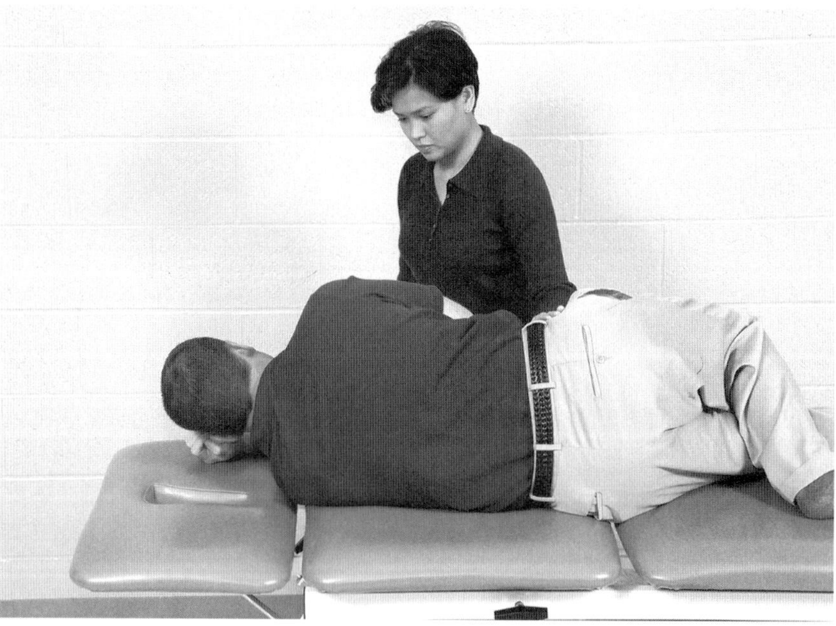

Fig. 5-31.

SCORING RECOMMENDATIONS

For grade 5: Patient is able to complete five repetitions.

For grade 4: Patient is able to complete three repetitions.

For grade 3: Patient is able to complete one repetition.

For grade 2: Patient is able to complete less than one half of the roll against gravity.

For grade 1: Contraction is observed or palpated but the patient is unable to initiate the roll.

For grade 0: No movement or contraction occurs; the patient remains supine.

■ LOWER BODY TESTS

REPEATED CHAIR RISE

Assessment of functional strength of knee extensors and gross lower body muscle groups[21]

Functional Strength (All Grades)

Equipment: Straight wooden chair with a seat height of 43 to 44 cm placed against the wall for stability and a standard stopwatch.

Constraints: Pain, ROM deficits, sitting balance deficit, or cognitive deficits that would limit understanding of instruction.

Patient position: Sitting in middle of chair with back approximately 10 cm from back of chair and feet flat on floor slightly posterior to knee joint. Hips should be at 90°, shoulders level, and head and trunk upright. Begin test with patient's arms crossed at the wrists and across the chest (Fig. 5-32).

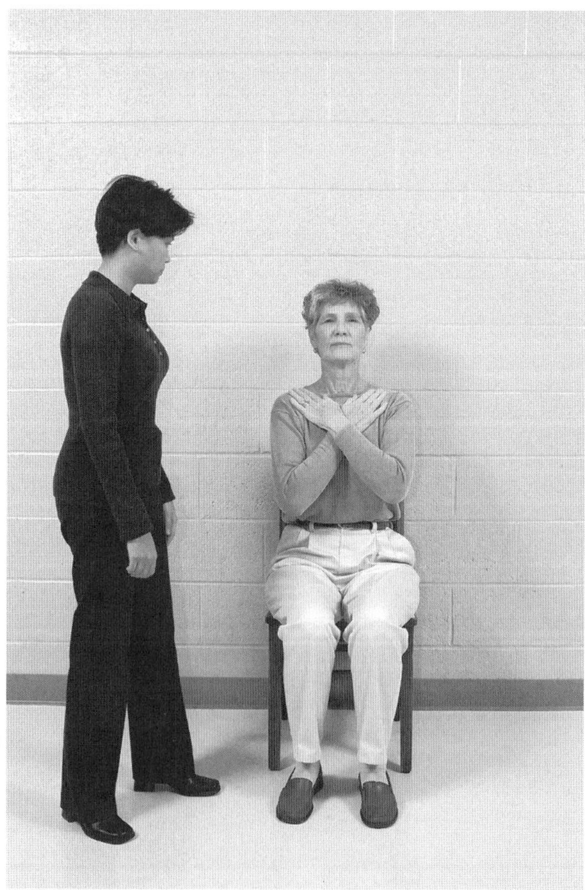

Fig. 5-32.

Examiner position: To the side near enough to observe lift off from the chair seat and to prevent a loss of balance in the forward direction or a fall back into the chair.

Examiner action: Instruct the patient as follows: "When I say to, I want you to rise from the chair without using your arms, come to full standing, and then sit back into the chair. I want you to repeat the sit to full stand and back to sit as many times as you can in 30 seconds without stopping. I will give you a chance to try the task once before beginning the test." As you describe the task, demonstrate and allow the patient to perform one repetition of the task. If the patient is able to perform the task without using the arms, begin the test by timing the patient from the start command for 30 seconds and counting the number of successful rises. As suggested by Rikli and Jones,[22] if the patient is more than halfway to full standing at the end of the 30 seconds, count as a full stand.

Examiner command: "Now, you may start."

Patient action: Patient will perform the sit-to-stand maneuver for 30 seconds (Figs. 5-33 and 5-34).

SCORING RECOMMENDATIONS

The score is the total number of successfully completed rises in 30 seconds.

This score may be used to establish a baseline or compare with the normative values published by Jones and Rikli.[13]

Fig. 5-33.

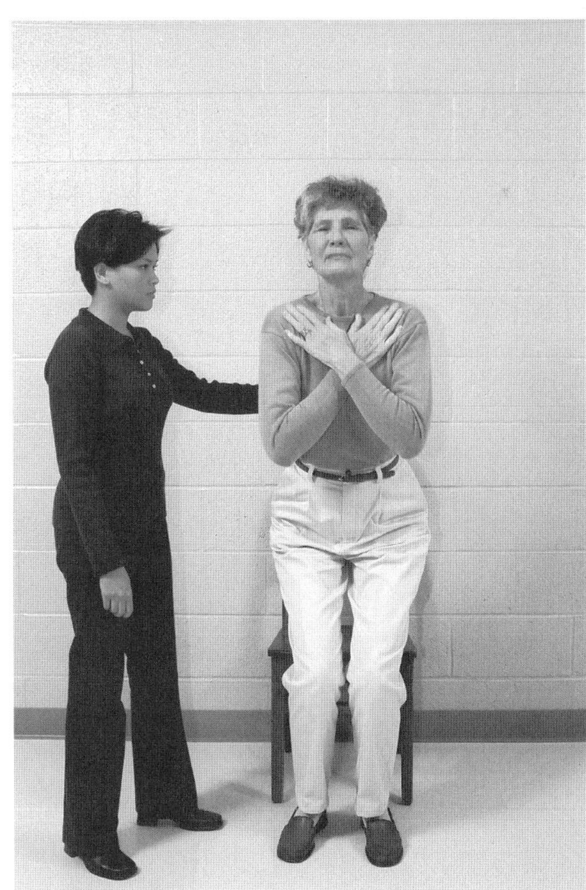

Fig. 5-34.

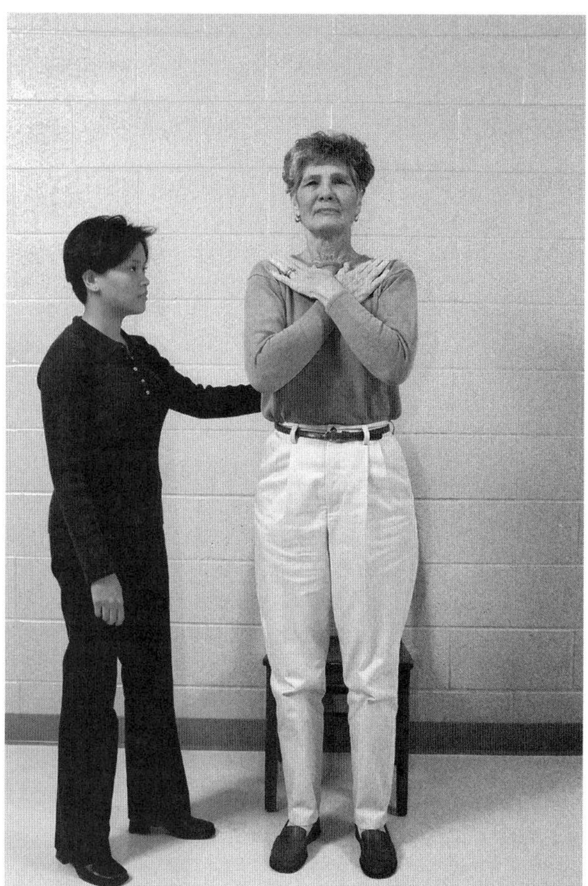

STEP TEST

Assessment of functional strength of gross lower body muscle groups.

Functional Strength (Grades 5, 4, 3, and 2)

Equipment: Step approximately 10 to 15 cm high placed on nonskid surface with "X" markers for foot placement.

Constraints: Pain, ROM deficits, balance deficit, or cognitive deficits that would limit understanding of instruction.

Patient position: Standing in double-limb stance facing the step with feet approximately shoulder-width apart (Fig. 5-35).

Examiner position: To the side or back of the patient near enough to prevent a loss of balance, but without touching the patient or restricting the stepping movement.

Examiner action: Instruct the patient as follows: "When I say to, I want you to bring your foot up to place your entire foot on the "X" on the step and then bring your foot back to the floor. Now step up with the other foot and back to the floor. I want you to repeat this sequence five times. You will be allowed to practice one time before the test begins." As you describe the task, demonstrate the task to the patient and allow them to practice one complete sequence to check for proper understanding of stepping task.

Fig. 5-35.

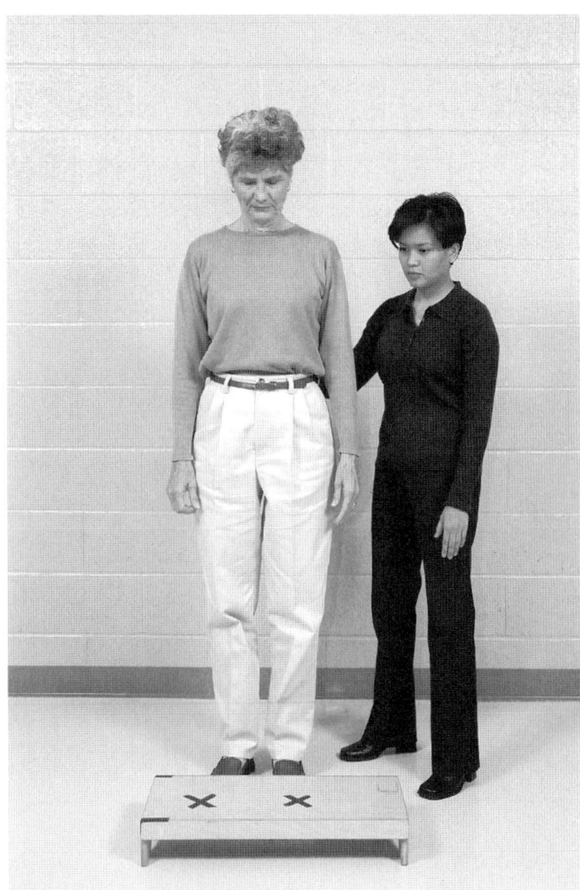

Examiner command: "Now, begin stepping up and back five times with each foot beginning with the right foot first."

Patient action: Patient will shift weight to left limb and step up with the right foot to place the entire foot on the marker and then return to initial double-limb stance position (Figs. 5-36 and 5-37).

The action should be repeated with the left limb involving a weight shift to the right limb.

Fig. 5-36.

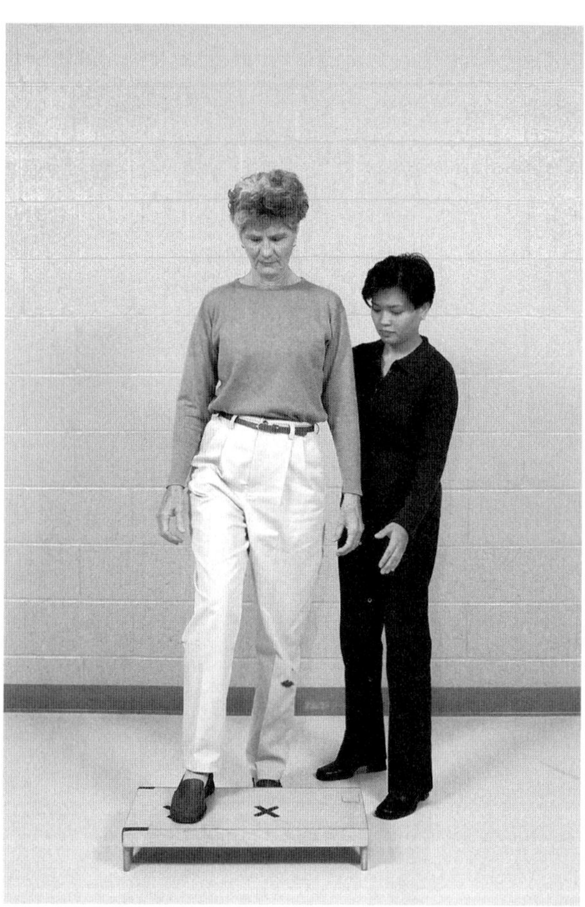

Fig. 5-37.

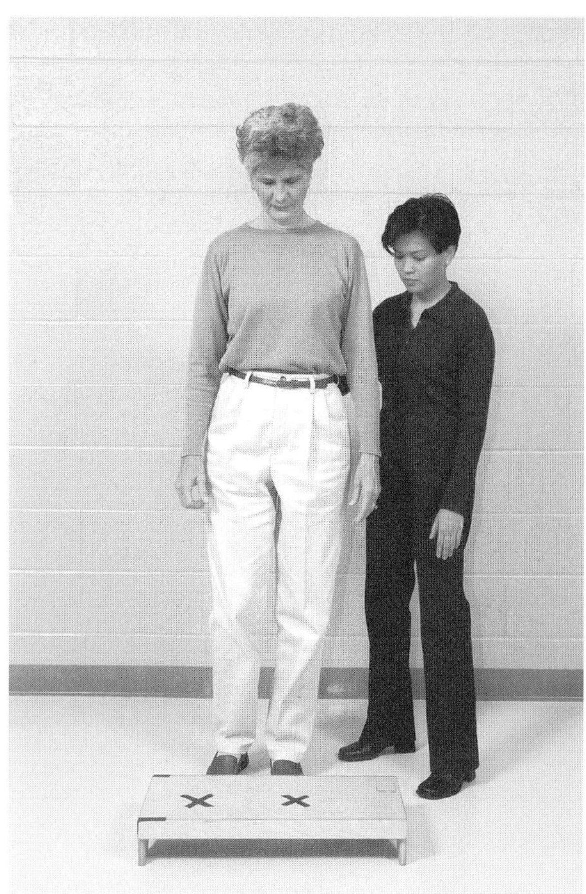

SCORING RECOMMENDATIONS

For grade 5: Patient completes the task without difficulty.

For grade 4: Patient completes task but movement may be slowed.

For grade 3: Patient completes task but movement is slow and more labored.

For grade 2: Patient initiates movement but is unable to complete task safely and requires moderate assistance to prevent fall.*

*Refer to Functional Strength (Grade 2 and Below).

Functional Strength (Grade 2 and Below)

Equipment: Standard mat or plinth, pillow, and two towel rolls.

Patient position: Supine on the mat with the head supported on a pillow and a towel roll under each knee.

Examiner position: Standing beside the mat near the patient's lower extremity (Fig. 5-38).

Examiner action: Instruct the patient as follows: "When I say to, I want you to bend your knee and slide your foot up to place it flat on the mat and then straighten your knee by sliding your foot down to return to your initial position. Then bend and straighten your other knee to place your other foot flat on the mat. I want you to repeat this sequence five times." As you describe the task, move the patient's limb passively through the described movement.

Fig. 5-38.

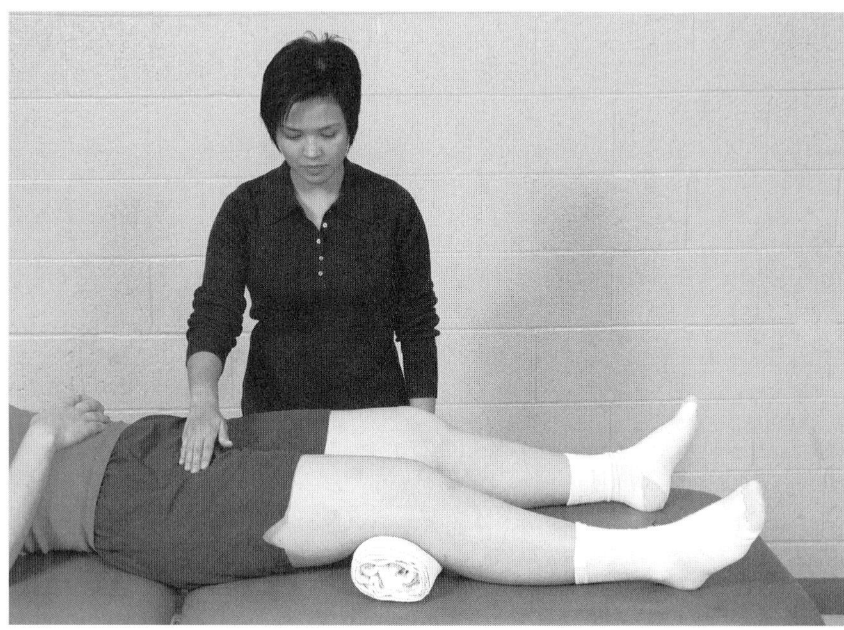

Examiner command: "Now, begin bending and straightening your knees alternately, repeating five times with each leg beginning with your right leg" (Fig. 5-39).

Fig. 5-39.

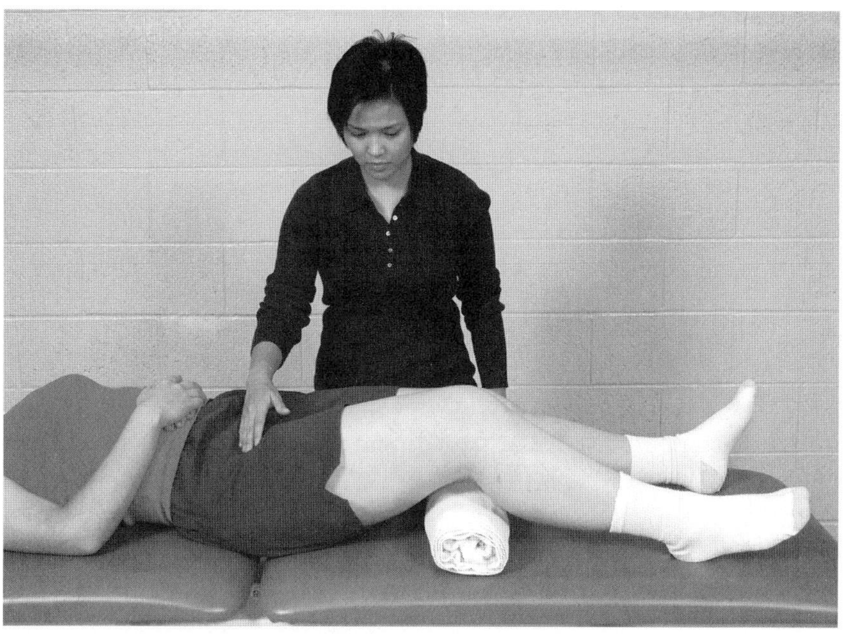

SCORING RECOMMENDATIONS

For grade 2: Patient bends knee to place the foot flat on mat surface at least three of five attempts on each limb.

For grade 1: Examiner observes and palpates a contraction of hip and knee flexors.

For grade 0: No contraction is observed or palpated by the examiner.

STAIR CLIMBING

Assessment of functional concentric strength of lower extremities

Functional Strength (Grades 4 and 5)

Equipment: At least three steps of standard (15 cm) height.

Constraints: Pain, ROM limitations, balance deficits, limitations in control of momentum, and cognitive deficits that would limit understanding of instruction.

Patient position: Standing facing the stairs with toes 5 to 8 cm from first step. The trunk and head is upright. Hands may be on handrails.

Examiner position: Examiner is to the side and behind the patient during ascent and in front of the patient during descent. The examiner is near enough to prevent a loss of balance without touching the patient or hindering the patient's movement (Fig. 5-40).

Examiner action: Instruct the patient as follows: "When I say to, climb up as many of the steps as you can, turn around, and go back down the steps to the floor. You may use the handrails as you need to for safety. I will be behind you going up and in front of you going down." As you describe the test, demonstrate the completed test (Figs. 5-41 and 5-42).

Examiner command: "Now, climb up and down the steps."

Patient action: Patient will shift weight slightly backward and laterally to the down limb as the up limb rises to the first step. The patient will shift weight forward and diagonal to place weight on the up limb as the down limb begins to flex at the hip and knee to move toward stepping to next step. The sequence is then repeated cyclically in a step over step pattern.

Fig. 5-40.

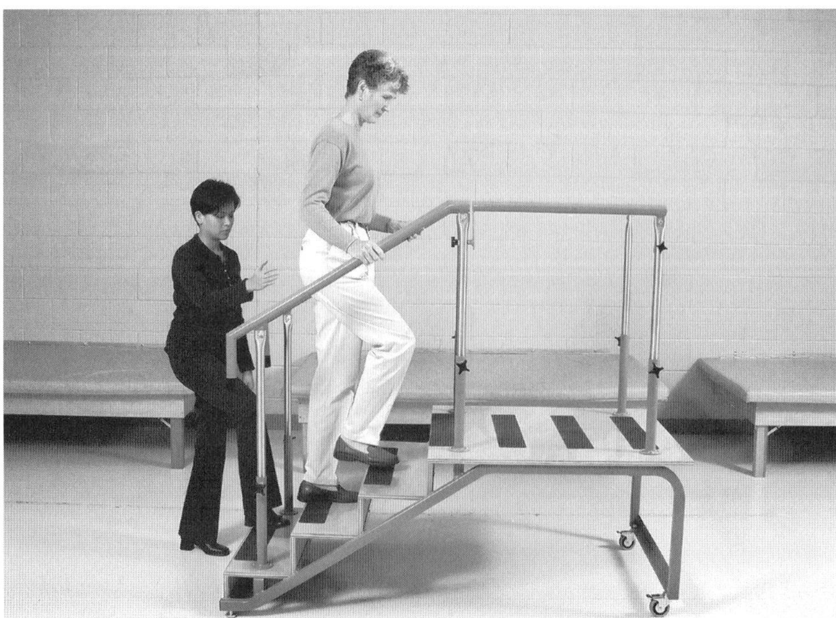

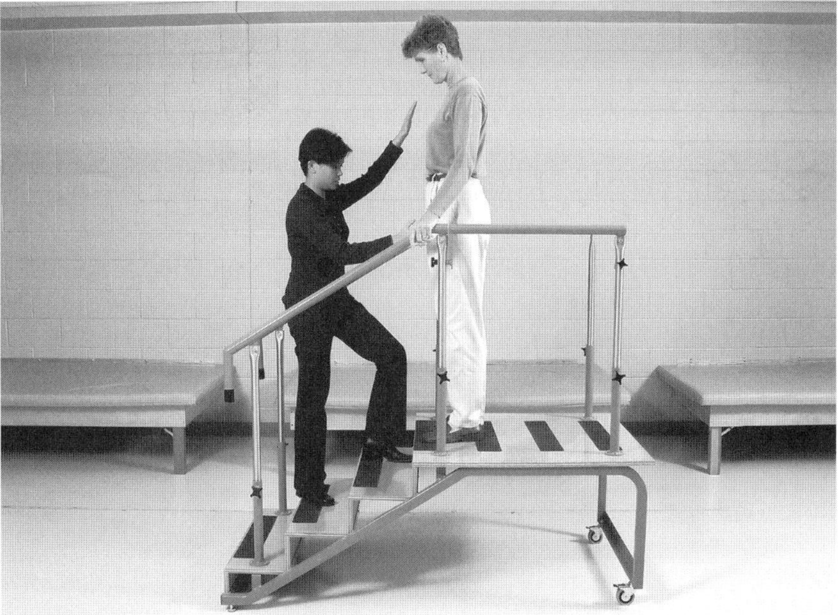

Fig. 5-41.

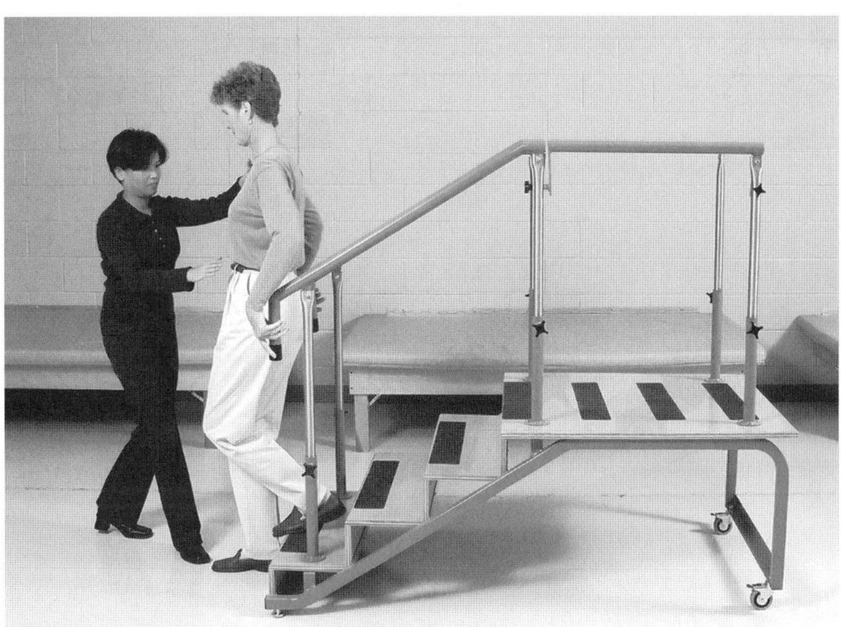

Fig. 5-42.

SCORING RECOMMENDATIONS

For grade 5: Patient ascends and descends at least 3 steps without difficulty.

For grade 4: Patient ascends and descends at least 3 steps but is slower and hesitant.

Functional Strength (Grades 3 and Below)

For grade 3: Same as grades 4 and 5 except movement will be slow and more labored with increased dependence on handrails.

For grade 2: Patient will be able to initiate movement but be unable to complete task for cyclical stepping.

For grades 1 and 0: If uncompensated by assistive device, physical assistance, or one limb grade 3 or higher, stair climb test is **not recommended.**

SIDE STEP STAIR CLIMB

Assessment of functional concentric strength of hip abductors

Functional Strength (Grades 5 and 4)

Equipment: At least three steps of standard height (15 cm).

Constraints: Pain, ROM limitations, balance deficits, limitations in control of momentum, and cognitive deficits that would limit understanding of instruction.

Patient position: Standing parallel with first step. Feet are side by side; trunk and head is upright. Arms are at side or hands are placed on handrail or wall (Fig. 5-43).

Examiner position: Examiner is to the side and behind the patient during ascent and descent. The examiner is near enough to prevent a loss of balance without touching the patient or hindering the patient's movement (Fig. 5-43).

Fig. 5-43.

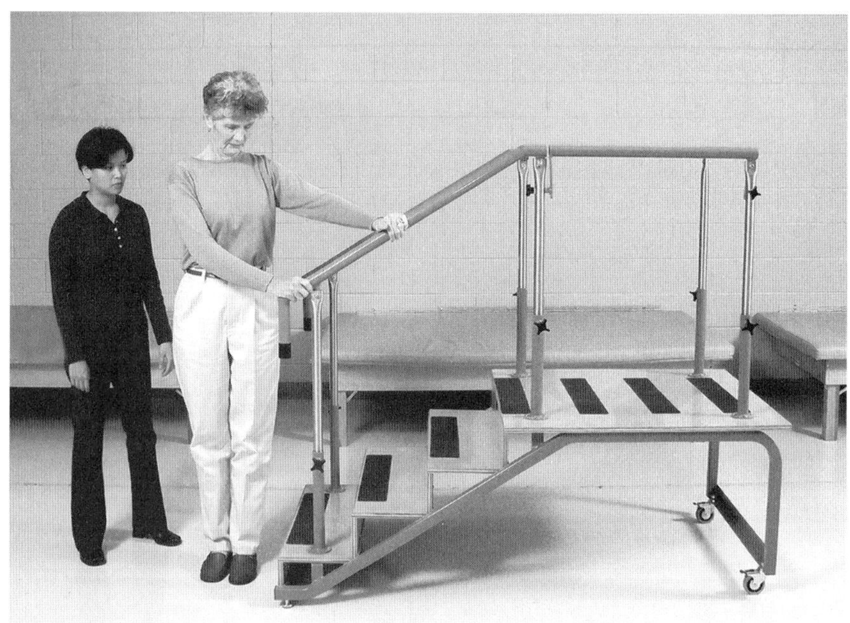

Examiner action: Instruct the patient as follows: "When I say to, step sideways up as many steps as you can safely ascend and then change your position and come down the steps sideways. You may use the handrails if you need them. I want you to stay upright and facing sideways during the test." As you describe the test, demonstrate by ascending and descending the steps sideways (Figs. 5-44 and 5-45).

Examiner command: "Now, climb up and down the steps sideways."

Patient action: Patient will shift weight laterally to down limb as the up limb rises sideways to the first step. The patient should keep the toes forward and the trunk should not be rotated or flexed.

Repeat test leading with the other limb.

Fig. 5-44.

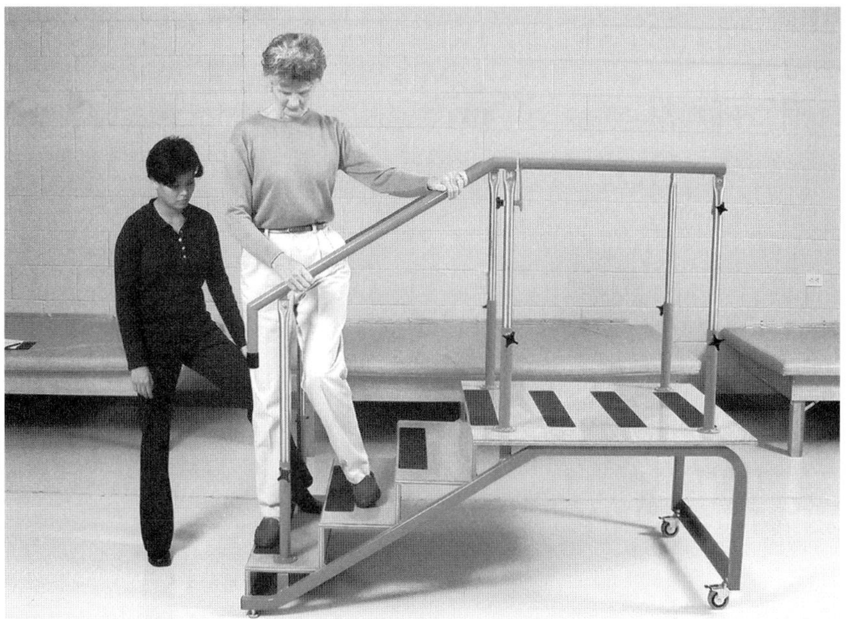

Fig. 5-45.

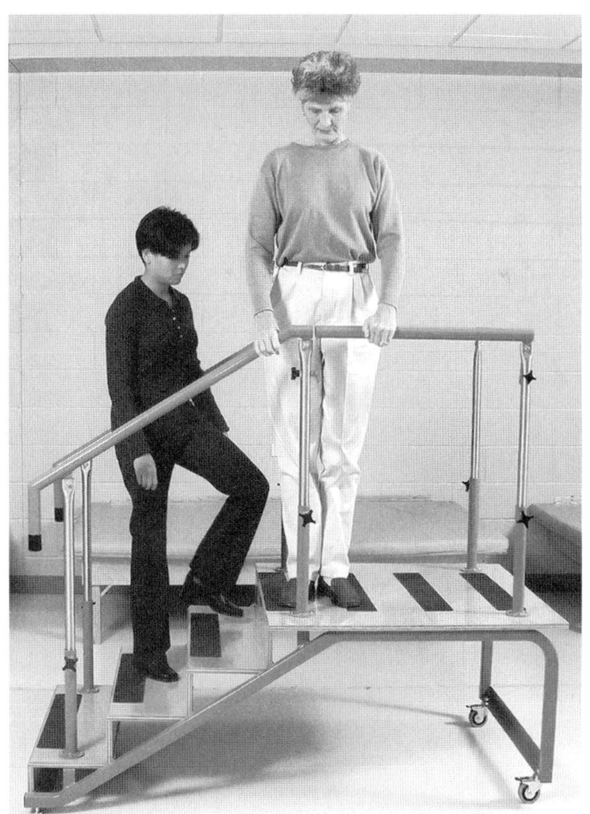

SCORING RECOMMENDATIONS

For grade 5: Patient ascends and descends at least 3 steps without difficulty.

For grade 4: Patient ascends and descends at least 3 steps but is slower and hesitant.

Functional Strength (Grades 3 and Below)

SCORING RECOMMENDATIONS

For grade 3: Same as grades 4 and 5 except movement will be slow and more labored.

For grade 2: Patient will be able to initiate movement but be unable to complete task for repeated stepping.

For grades 1 and 0: If uncompensated by assistive device, physical assistance, or one limb grade 3 or higher, side-step stair climb test is **not recommended.**

SITTING LEG CROSS

Assessment of functional strength of lower trunk flexors

Functional Strength (All Grades)

Equipment: Straight wooden chair (seat height of 43-44 cm) placed against a wall.

Constraints: Pain, balance deficit, limitations in ROM (trunk and extremities), and cognitive deficits that limit understanding of instruction.

Patient position: Seated in middle and at least 10 cm from back of chair with trunk upright and shoulders in line with hips, feet hip width apart and flat on floor. Knees and hips flexed 90°. Hands are resting on sides of chair to provide trunk stabilization (Fig. 5-46).

Examiner position: To the side near enough to prevent a loss of balance.

Examiner action: Instruct the patient as follows: "When I say to, I want you to cross your right leg over your left leg at the knee. I want you to repeat the task five times without stopping." As you describe the task, passively demonstrate the sequence of the movement and return the patient to the starting position.

Examiner command: "Now cross your legs with your right knee over your left and then return to the starting position. Repeat the movement five times without stopping."

Fig. 5-46.

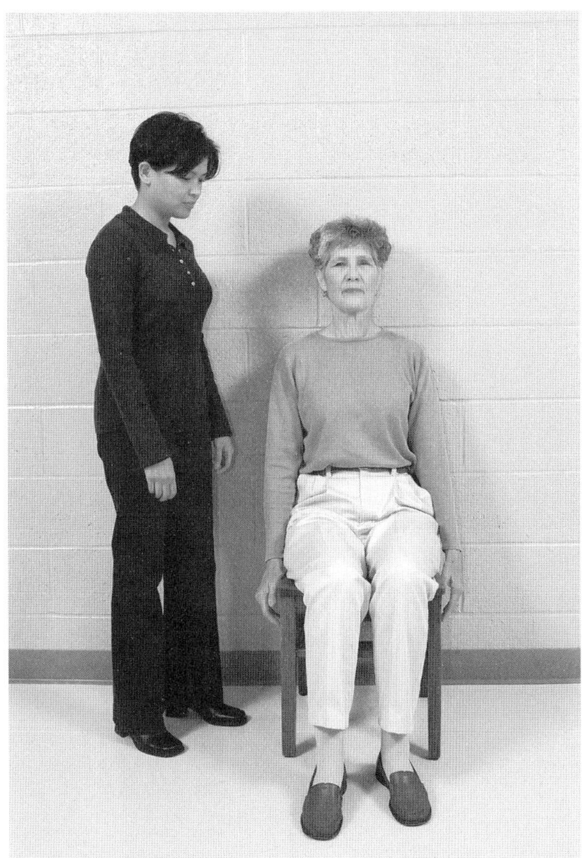

Patient action:

Patient will posteriorly tilt pelvis, flex right hip, and place the right knee over the left knee (Figs. 5-46, 5-47, and 5-48).

Test should be repeated with left leg crossing over right.

Fig. 5-47.

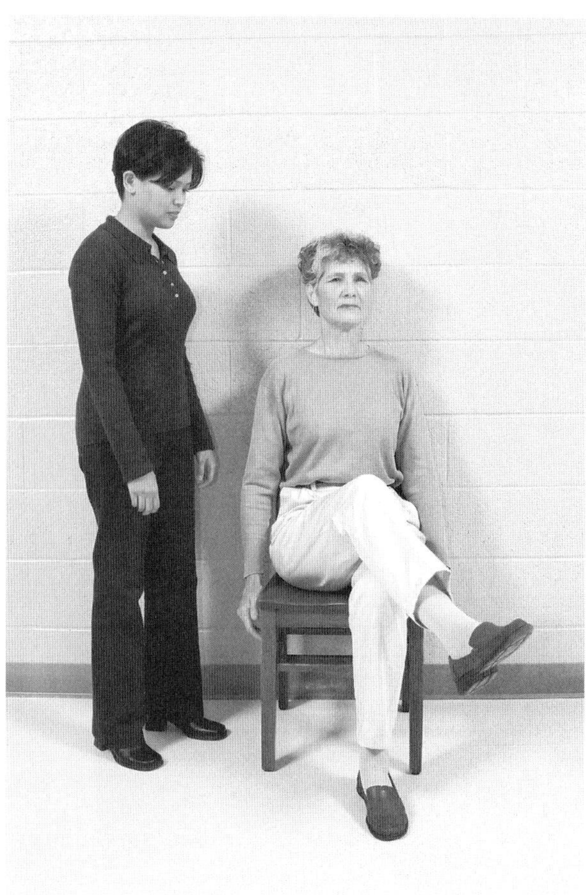

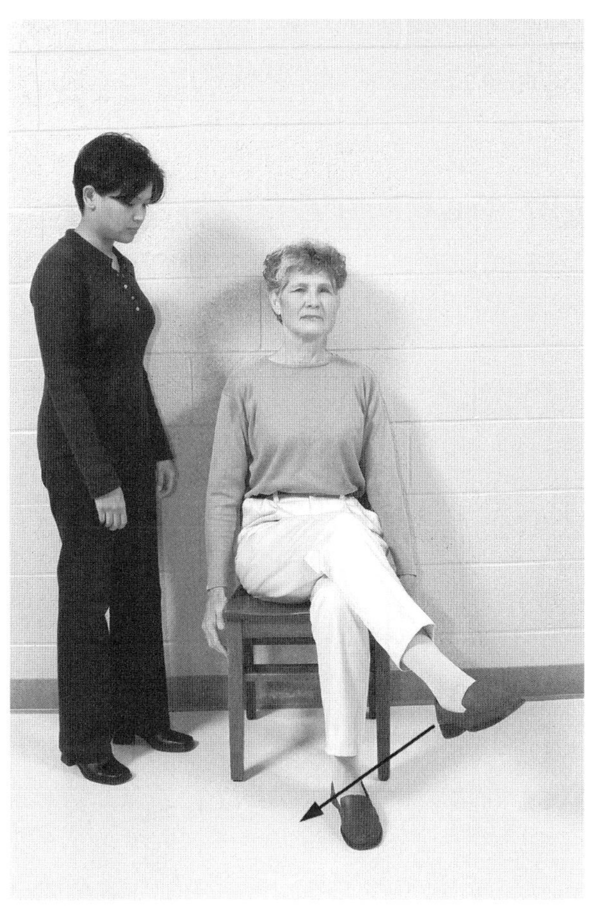

Fig. 5-48. Arrow indicates direction of movement.

SCORING RECOMMENDATIONS

For grade 5: Patient is able to complete five repetitions.

For grade 4: Patient is able to complete three repetitions.

For grade 3: Patient is able to complete one repetition.

For grade 2: Patient is able to complete less than one half of the movement against gravity.

For grade 1: Contraction is observed or palpated by the examiner but the patient is unable to initiate lifting foot from floor.

For grade 0: No movement or contraction occurs.

LATERAL HIP SCOOT

Assessment of functional strength of lower trunk rotators

Functional Strength (All Grades)

Equipment: Straight wooden chair (seat height of 43-44 cm) placed against a wall.

Constraints: Pain, balance deficit, limitations in ROM (trunk and extremities), and cognitive deficits that limit understanding of instruction.

Patient position: Seated in middle of chair with back against chair with trunk upright and shoulders in line with hips, feet hip width apart and flat on floor. Knees and hips are flexed 90°. Hands are hanging loosely at sides (Fig. 5-49).

Fig. 5-49.

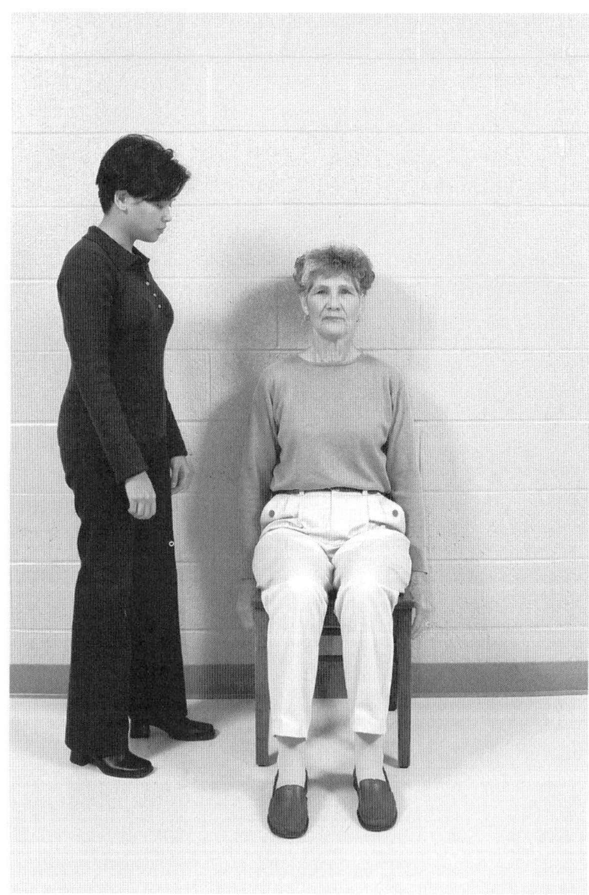

Examiner position: To the side near enough to observe movement and prevent a loss of balance (Fig. 5-50).

Examiner action: Instruct patient as follows: "When I say to, I want you to scoot one hip at a time to the front of the chair and then scoot back one hip at a time to the back of the chair. You may begin with either hip." As you describe the task, demonstrate.

Examiner command: "Now scoot to the front of the chair one hip at a time." Once achieved say, "Now scoot back in chair one hip at a time."

Patient action: Patient will weight shift to unweight the forward moving hip, moving one hip forward and then repeating weight shift and movement until forward in chair. Similar movements will occur when moving in reverse. Lower trunk will remain aligned in the frontal plane (Fig. 5-51).

Fig. 5-50.

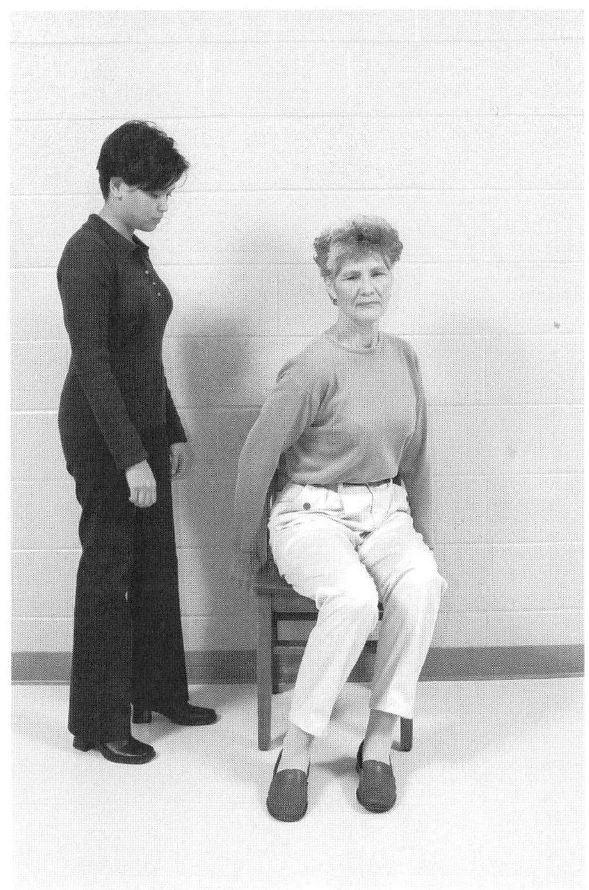

Fig. 5-51.

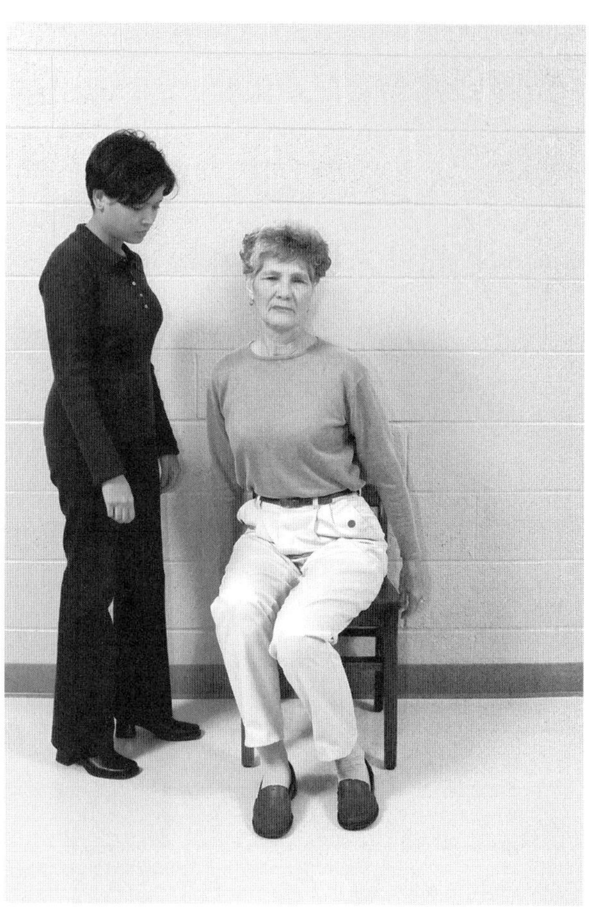

SCORING RECOMMENDATIONS

For grade 5: Patient is able to complete forward and backward movement.

For grade 4: Patient is able to complete forward and backward movement but is slowed.

For grade 3: Patient is able to complete forward and backward movement but with excessive trunk lean to utilize momentum.

For grade 2: Patient is able to complete less than one half of the forward task.

For grade 1: Contraction is observed or palpated by the examiner but the patient is unable to initiate movement.

For grade 0: No movement or contraction occurs.

HIP HIKE

Assessment of functional strength of ipsilateral lower trunk, lateral flexors, and contralateral hip abductors

Functional Strength (Grades 5, 4, and 3)

Equipment: Low stool (height, 8-10 cm) placed on nonskid surface and beside a support surface (plinth or wall).

Constraints: Pain, balance deficits, limitations in ROM (trunk and extremities), and cognitive deficits that limit understanding of instruction.

Patient position: Standing on low stool with the side being tested in non–weight-bearing so that the contralateral stance limb is supporting the body weight. The pelvis is level in the horizontal plane. The patient may place a hand on the support surface for stability as needed (Fig. 5-52).

Examiner position: Examiner is to the side and back of patient in close proximity of patient in case of loss of balance.

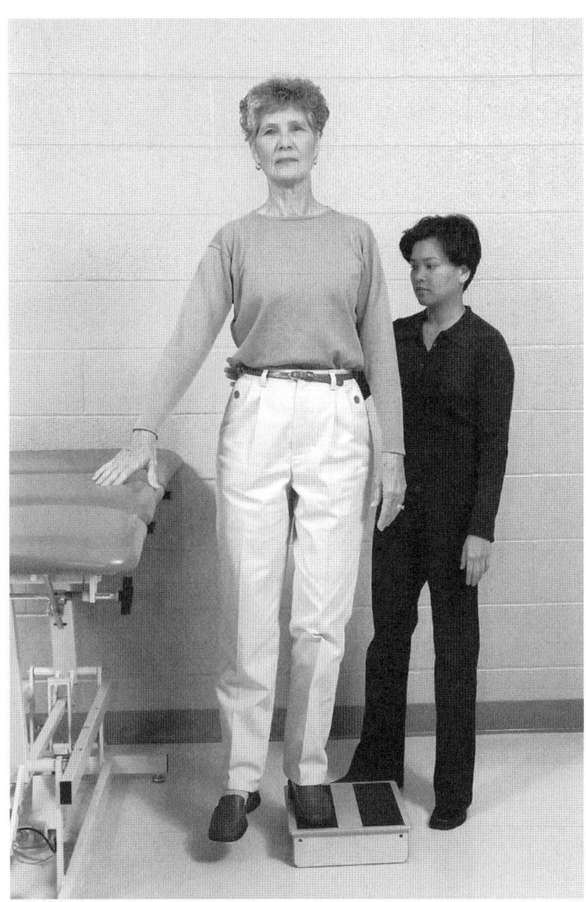

Fig. 5-52.

Examiner action: Instruct patient as follows: "When I say to, I want you to bring your right hip up toward your right shoulder. Do not rotate your hips from their position. I want you to repeat the task five times." As you describe the test, demonstrate.

Examiner command: "Now, bring your hip up toward your shoulder and back down five times."

Patient action: Patient will laterally flex the right trunk bringing the iliac crest upward while maintaining trunk upright. Pelvis will tilt in the frontal plane (Fig. 5-53).

Test should be repeated on the left side.

Fig. 5-53.

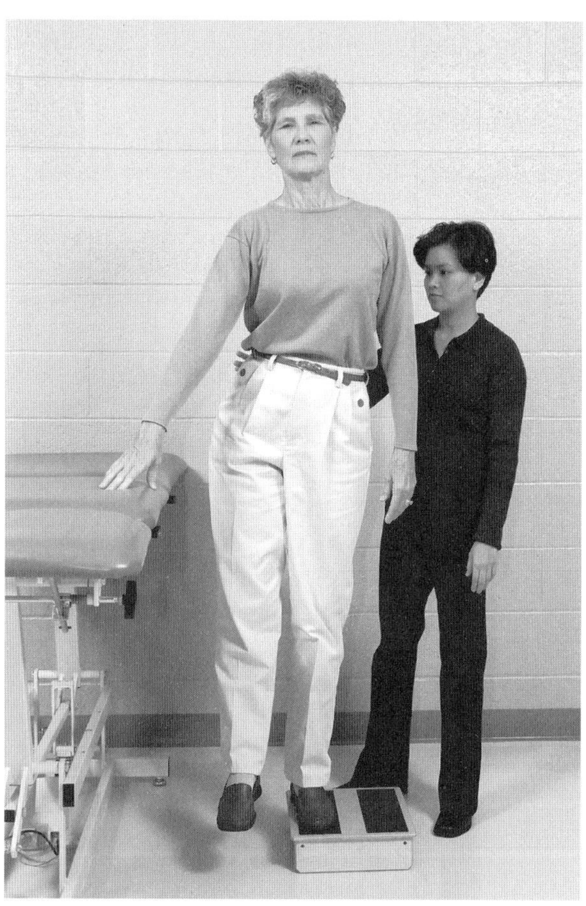

SCORING RECOMMENDATIONS

For grade 5: Patient is able to complete five repetitions.

For grade 4: Patient is able to complete three repetitions.

For grade 3: Patient is able to maintain the pelvis level but is unable to laterally flex the trunk

Functional Strength (Grades Below 3)

Patient position: Standing facing a wall with feet approximately 15 to 20 cm from wall and shoulder-width apart. The pelvis is level in the horizontal plane. The patient's hands are placed on the wall for stability as needed.

Examiner position: Examiner is to the side and back of patient in close proximity to patient in case of loss of balance.

Examiner action: Instruct patient as follows: "When I say to, I want you to bring your right hip up toward your right shoulder. Do not rotate your hips from their position." As you describe the test, demonstrate.

Patient action: Patient will attempt to laterally flex the right trunk.

Test should be repeated on the left side.

SCORING RECOMMENDATIONS

For grade 2: Patient is able to initiate lateral trunk flexion, but unable to clear foot from floor (heel may come up).

For grade 1: Contraction is observed or palpated by the examiner but the patient is unable to initiate lifting foot from floor.

For grade 0: No movement or contraction occurs.

FORWARD STEPPING

Assessment of functional strength, lower extremities

Functional Strength (All Grades)

Equipment: Obstacle-free level walking area 3 m in length and stopwatch.

Constraints: Pain, balance deficits, sensory deficits, limitations in ROM (trunk and extremities), and cognitive deficits that limit understanding of instruction.

Patient position: Standing at one end of the 3-m course.

Examiner position: To the side and back of patient, near enough to prevent a fall or loss of balance. The examiner will need to move along the 3-m course with the patient (Figs. 5-54 and 5-55).

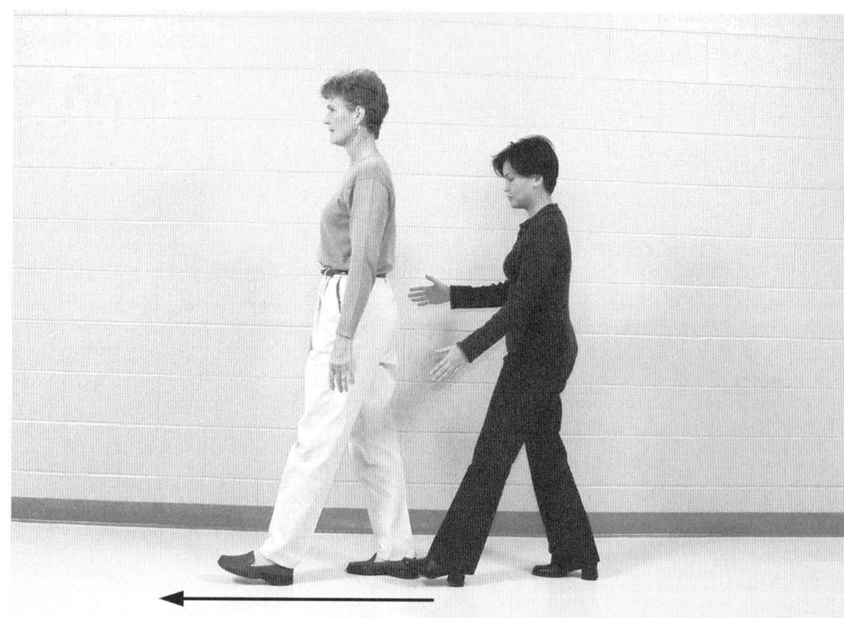

Fig. 5-54. Arrow indicates direction of movement.

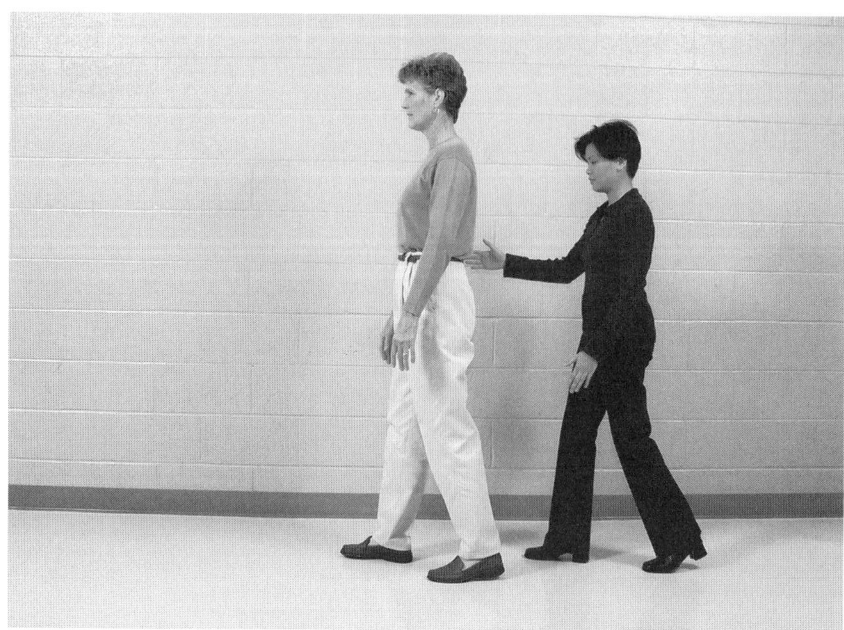

Fig. 5-55.

Examiner action: Instruct patient as follows: "When I say to, I want you to walk forward to the end of the course, turn around, and come back to the starting point." As you describe the task, allow the patient to practice and return to the starting position.

Examiner command: "Now begin."

Patient action: Patient will walk forward, turn, and walk back.

SCORING RECOMMENDATIONS

Timing should begin on the "begin" command and stop when the patient returns to the original position. Time should be rounded to the nearest tenth of a second. Although some comparison values for gait speed have been published,[10,22] lack of standardization limits applicability to a broad population. Therefore the timed value may be used to establish a more quantitative baseline and as a monitor for progression or decline.

For grade 5: Patient is able to complete 3-m course in forward-stepping direction.

For grade 4: Patient is able to complete 3-m course in forward-stepping direction but is slowed.

For grade 3: Patient is able to complete 3-m course in forward-stepping direction but is slowed, inconsistent in steps, and hesitant in stepping.

For grade 2: Patient is able to complete less than one half of the 3-m course without assistance.

For grade 1: Contraction is observed or palpated by the examiner but the patient is unable to safely initiate forward stepping of the swing limb.

For grade 0: No movement or contraction occurs in advancing limb.

BACKWARD STEPPING

Assessment of functional strength of lower trunk extensors

Functional Strength (All Grades)

Equipment: Obstacle-free level walking area 3 m in length and two cone course markers.

Constraints: Pain, balance deficits, sensory deficits, limitations in ROM (trunk and extremities), and cognitive deficits that limit understanding of instruction.

Patient position: Standing at one end of the marked course with back to the course (or facing outward). Standing in appropriate postural alignment, hips and knees vertically aligned, feet hip width apart.

Examiner position: To the side and back of patient, near enough to prevent a fall or loss of balance. The examiner will need to move along the 3 m course with the patient.

Examiner action: Instruct patient as follows: "When I say to, I want you to step backward to the end of walking course, which is 3 m. You may start stepping with either foot." Examiner should remain close to patient at all times during the test in case of loss of balance. As you describe the stepping task, demonstrate the movement to the patient and return to the starting position (Fig. 5-56).

Fig. 5-56.

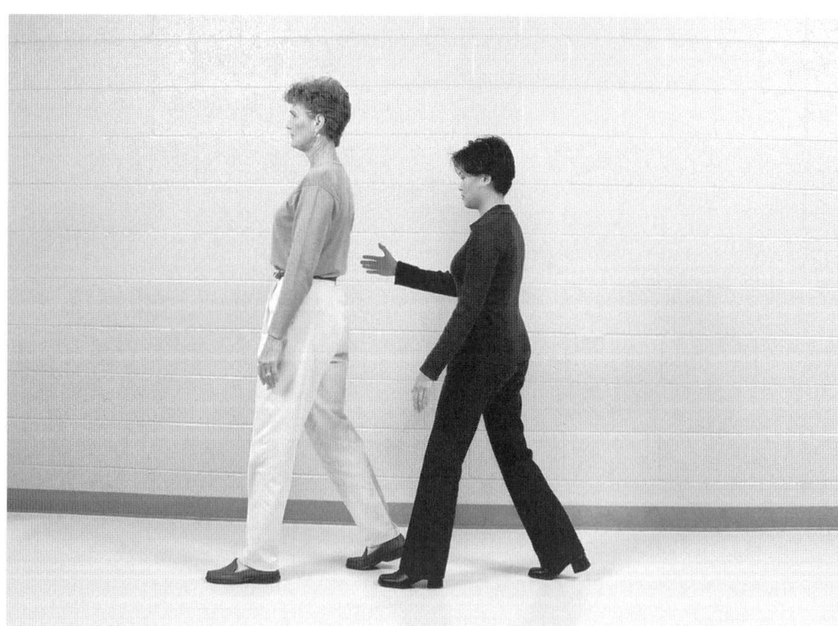

Examiner command: "Now begin stepping backward until I tell you to stop."

Patient action: Patient will shift weight to stance limb, anteriorly tilt pelvis, flex knee then extend stepping limb, and swing limb backward landing in a toe-to-heel loading pattern (Fig. 5-57).

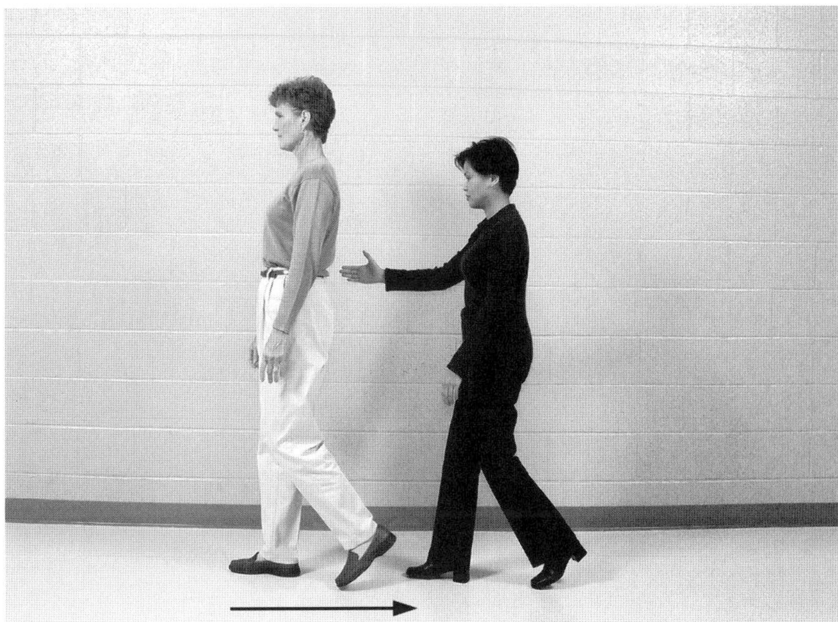

Fig. 5-57. Arrow indicates direction of movement.

SCORING RECOMMENDATIONS

For grade 5: Patient is able to complete 3-m course in backward-stepping direction.

For grade 4: Patient is able to complete 3-m course in backward-stepping direction but is slowed.

For grade 3: Patient is able to complete 3-m course in backward-stepping direction but is slowed, inconsistent in steps, and hesitant in stepping.

For grade 2: Patient is able to complete less than one half of the 3-m course without assistance.

For grade 1: Contraction is observed or palpated by the examiner but the patient is unable to safely initiate backward stepping.

For grade 0: No movement or contraction occurs.

■ GROSS BODY MOVEMENTS

FLOOR SIT

Assessment of functional strength of gross upper and lower body muscle groups.

Functional Strength (All Grades)

Equipment: Straight wooden chair with a seat height of 43 to 44 cm placed against the wall for stability and a floor mat or pad.

Constraints: Pain, ROM deficits, sitting balance deficit, or cognitive deficits that would limit understanding of instruction.

Patient position: Sitting in middle of chair with back against back of the chair and feet flat on floor slightly posterior to knee joint. Hips should be at 90°, shoulders level, and head and trunk upright. Begin test with patient's arms at each side or resting on sides of chair (Fig. 5-58).

Examiner position: To the side near enough to prevent a loss of balance in the forward direction. The examiner should shift position as patient moves in order to remain in close proximity to prevent a fall as patient moves from chair to the floor (Fig. 5-59).

Examiner action: Instruct patient as follows: "When I say to, I want you to come forward and down to sit on the floor. You may get down to the floor in any safe way you choose. Once on the floor, remain there for the next test, the floor rise." As you describe the task, demonstrate the task to the patient.

Examiner command: "Now, move to the floor."

Fig. 5-58.

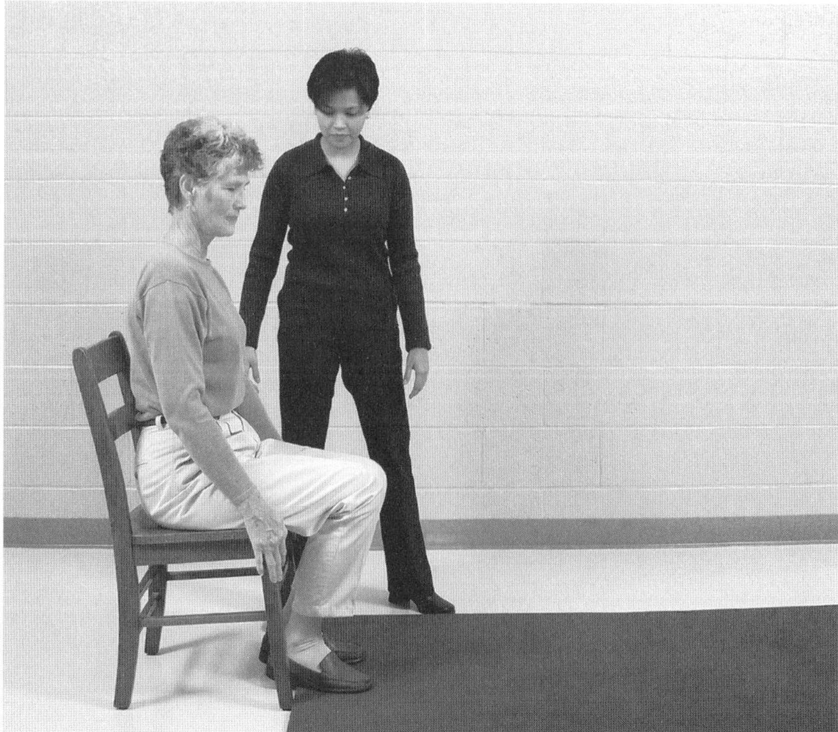

Fig. 5-59.

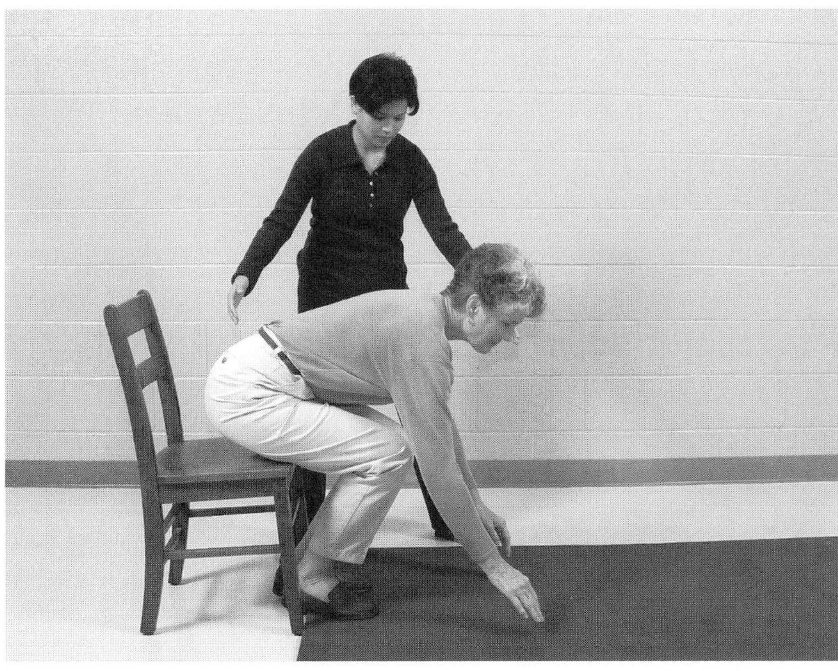

Patient action: Patient will move forward in the chair and lower themselves to sit on the floor (Figs. 5-60 and 5-61).

Fig. 5-60.

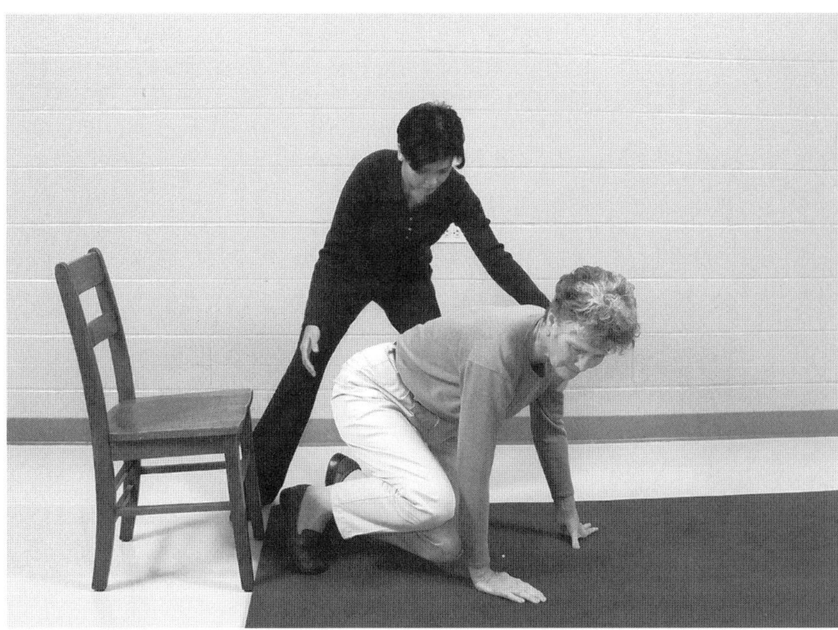

Fig. 5-61.

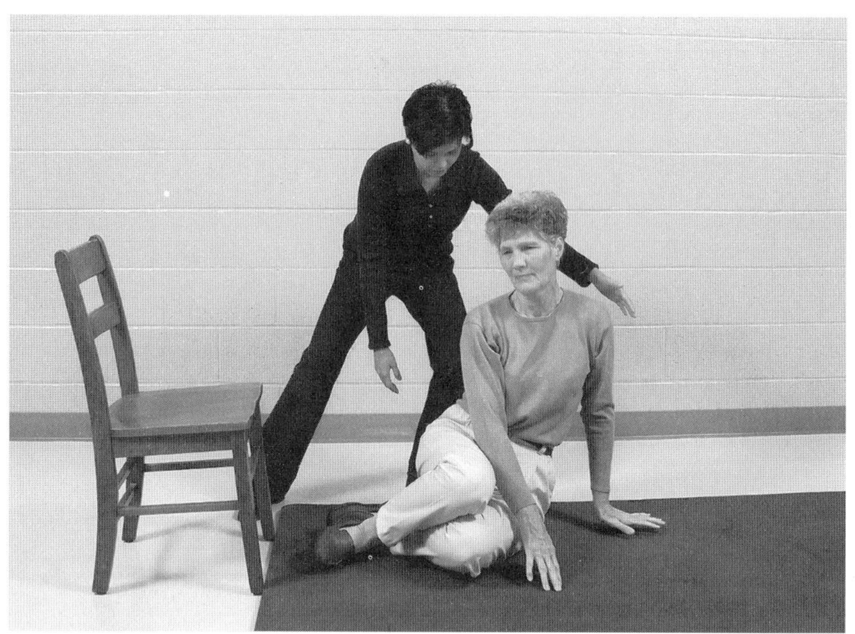

SCORING RECOMMENDATIONS

For grade 5: Patient completes the task safely without loss of balance.

For grade 4: Patient completes task but movement is labored and less controlled.

For grade 3: Patient completes task but uses chair for support until sitting on floor.

For grade 2: Patient initiates movement but is unable to complete task safely and requires assistance to prevent fall.

For grade 1: Patient is unable to safely complete the task beyond forward movement in chair.

For grade 0: Patient is deemed unsafe to attempt task.

Note: The floor sit test should be followed by the floor rise test. Refer to following.

FLOOR RISE

Assessment of whole body movement and functional strength of upper and lower extremities in complex rotational patterns

Functional Strength (Grades 5, 4, and 3)

Equipment: Straight wooden chair with a seat height of 43 to 44 cm placed against the wall for stability and a floor mat or pad.

Constraints: Pain, ROM deficits, sitting balance deficits, or cognitive deficits that would limit understanding of instruction.

Patient position: Sitting on the floor mat. Begin test with patient's arms in a supporting position at the side (Fig. 5-62).

Examiner position: To the side or back of the patient near enough to prevent a loss of balance during the rise to the chair. The examiner should shift position as patient moves in order to remain in close proximity to prevent a fall as patient moves from floor and back to chair (Fig. 5-63).

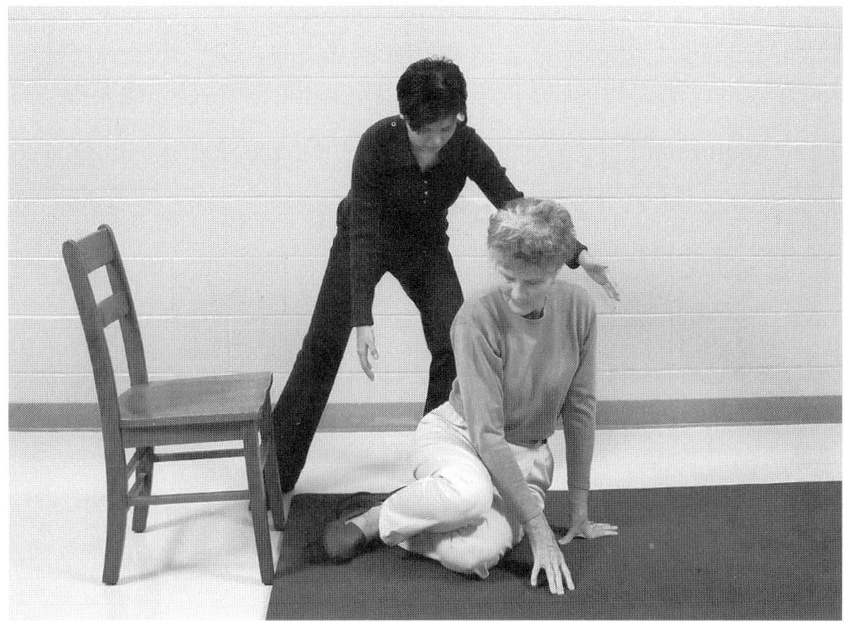

Fig. 5-62.

Fig. 5-63.

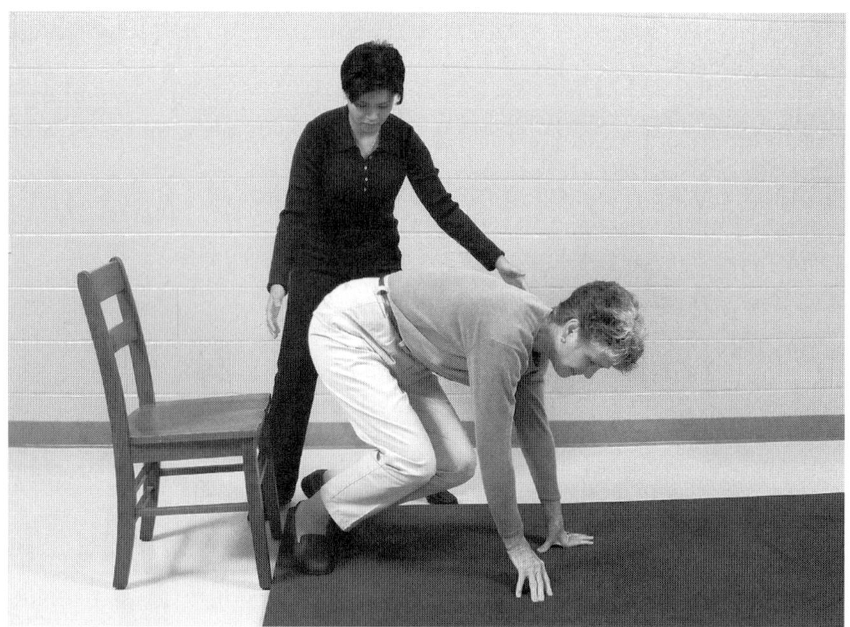

Examiner action:

Instruct patient as follows: "When I say to, I want you to rise from the floor and get into the chair. You may get up from the floor in any safe way you choose. Once in the chair, please scoot to the back of the chair." As you describe the task, demonstrate the task to the patient.

Examiner command: "Now, rise from the floor and get into the chair."

Patient action: Patient will shift position to rise from the floor and rotate to get into the chair (Figs. 5-64 and 5-65).

Fig. 5-64.

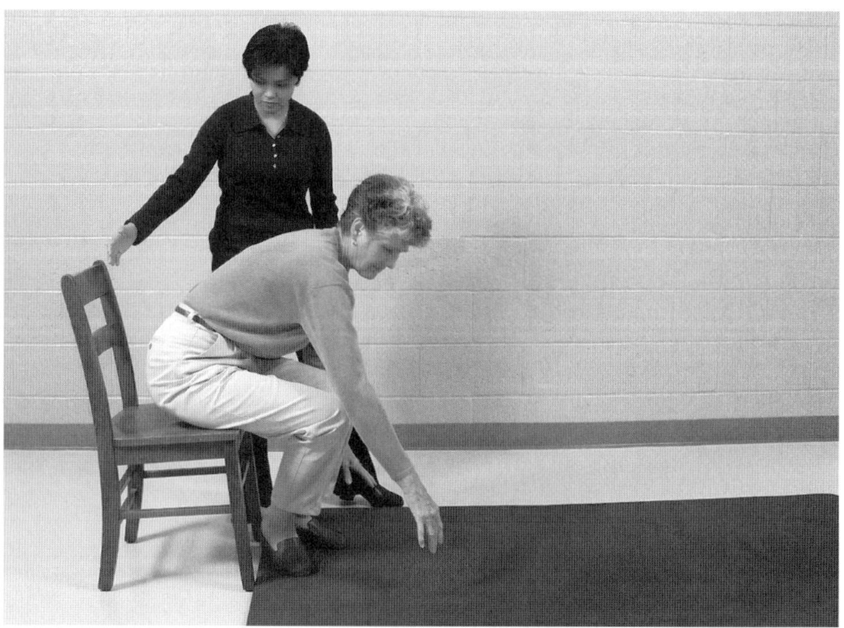

Fig. 5-65.

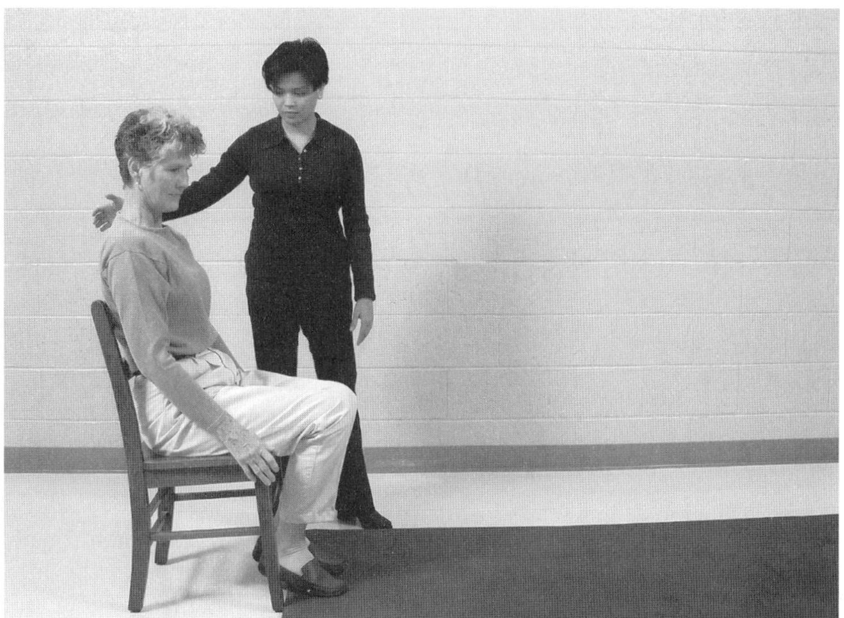

SCORING RECOMMENDATIONS

For grade 5: Patient completes the task safely without loss of balance.

For grade 4: Patient completes the task but movement is labored and less controlled.

For grade 3: Patient completes the task but pushes down on chair to rise from floor.

Functional Strength (Grades Below 3)

The following grades will require maximal assistance to place patient into chair and are considered unnecessary except in circumstances involving assessment of caregiving needs and training:

For grade 2: Patient initiates movement but is unable to complete task safely and requires moderate assistance to prevent fall.

For grade 1: Patient is unable to safely complete the task beyond minimal movement toward chair and requires maximal assistance for completion of task.

For grade 0: Patient requires maximal assistance for completion of task.

SUPINE TO SIDE-SIT

Assessment of functional strength of whole body transitional movement against gravity

Functional Strength (All Grades)

Equipment: Mat or firm surface large enough to permit rolling from supine to side sitting in either direction.

Constraints: Pain, abdominal strength deficit, balance deficit, limitations in ROM (trunk and extremities), and cognitive deficits that limit understanding of instruction.

Patient position: Supine with arms resting at the side, elbows fully extended, and with palm in pronation. The lower extremities are fully extended (Fig. 5-66).

Examiner position: On the side of the mat toward which the patient is moving near the head and in such a position to both observe the movement and for safety during the patient's transition to sitting. Examiner position will change slightly with a weight shift from one foot to the other in order to remain in the recommended position as the patient moves through the task. Examiner may place a hand near but not touching the patient's back during the movement for safety.

Examiner action: Instruct patient as follows: "When I say to, I want you to bring your left arm over, push up with your right arm, and sit up to your right. You may use your arms for assist and support as needed. I want you to repeat the task five times. I will assist you back to the starting position after each movement." As you describe the task, passively move the patient through the sequence of movements and return them to supine (Fig. 5-67).

Examiner command: "Now sit up to your right and stay there."

Fig. 5-66.

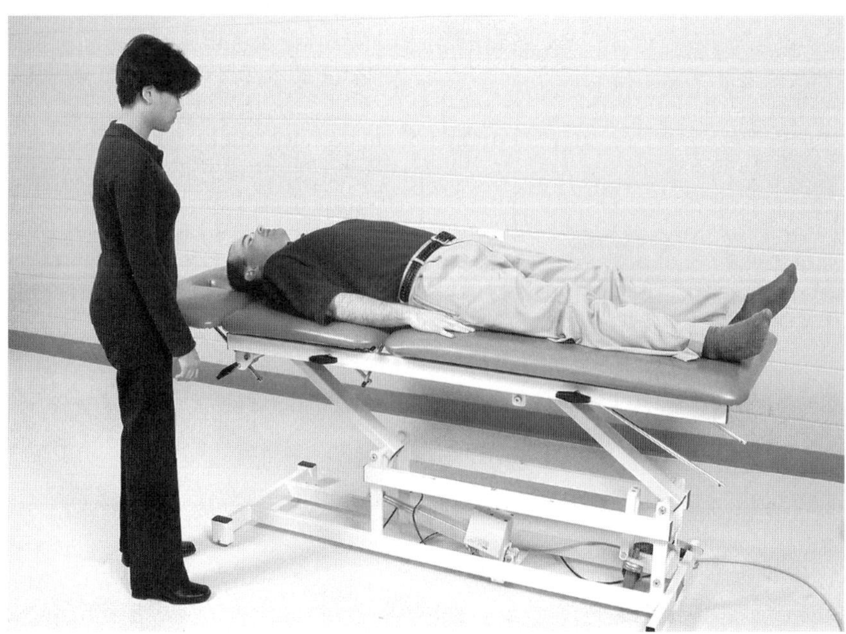

Fig. 5-67.

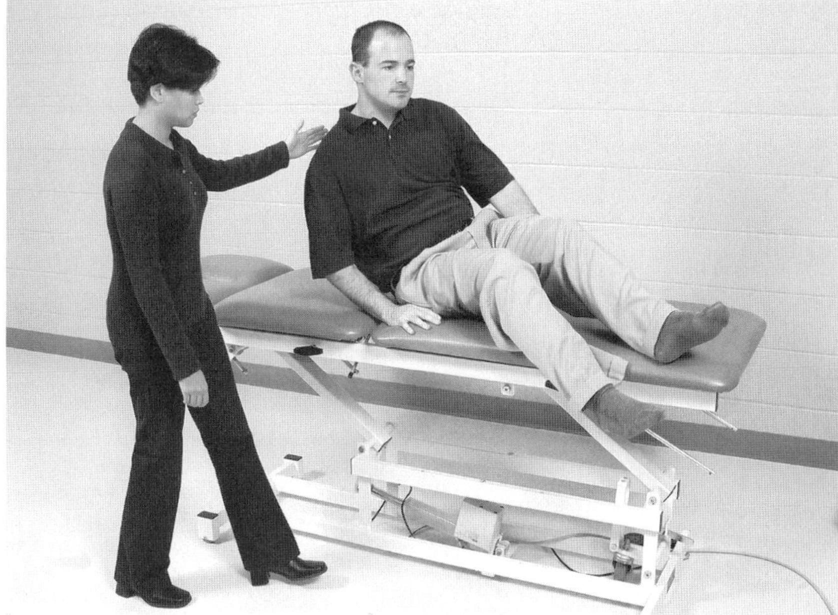

Patient action: Patient will bring left arm across body, flex right elbow, and rotate upper body to the right, ending the task by redistributing weight onto each hip and extended arms (Fig. 5-68).

Test should be repeated with sitting up to the left.

Fig. 5-68.

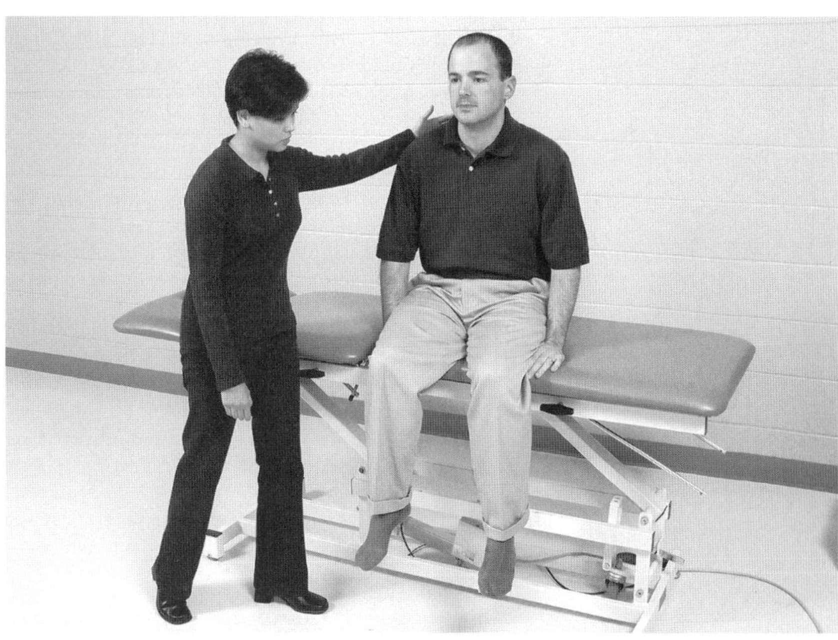

SCORING RECOMMENDATIONS

For grade 5: Patient is able to complete five repetitions.

For grade 4: Patient is able to complete three repetitions.

For grade 3: Patient is able to complete one repetition.

For grade 2: Patient is able to complete less than one half of the movement against gravity.

For grade 1: Contraction is observed or palpated by the examiner but the patient is unable to initiate roll.

For grade 0: No movement or contraction occurs; the patient remains supine.

References

1. Amundsen LR. *Muscle Strength Testing. Instrumented and Non-instrumented Systems.* New York: Churchill Livingstone, 1990.
2. Bohannon RW. Sit to stand test for measuring performance of lower extremity muscles. *Percept Mot Skills* 1995;80:163–166.
3. Bohannon RW. Alternatives for measuring knee extension strength of the elderly at home. *Clin Rehab* 1998;12:434–440.
4. Brown M, Sinacore DR, Host HH. The relationship of strength to function in the older adult. *J Geront A Biol Sci Med Sci* 1995;50A:55–59.
5. Csuka M, McCarty DJ. Simple method for measurement of lower extremity muscle strength. *Am J Med* 1985;78–81.
6. Dancewicz TM, Krebs DE, McGibbon CA. Lower-limb extensor power and lifting characteristics in disabled elders. *J Rehab Res Dev* 2003;40:337.
7. Eriksrud O, Bohannon RW. Relationship of knee extension force to independence in sit-to-stand performance in patients receiving acute rehabilitation. *Phys Ther* 2003;83:544.
8. Fisher AG. The assessment of IADL motor skills: an application of the many faceted Rasch analysis. *Am J Occup Ther* 1993;47:319–329.
9. Frontera WR, Hughes VA, Lutz KJ, et al. A cross-sectional study of muscle strength and mass in 45- to 78-yr-old men and women. *J Appl Physiol* 1991;71:644–650.
10. Guralnik JM, Ferrucci L, Pieper CF, et al. Lower extremity function and subsequent disability: Consistency across studies, predictive models, and value of gait speed alone compared with the short physical performance battery. *J Geront A Biol Sci Med Sci* 2000;55A:M221–M231.
11. Hyatt RH, Whitelaw MN, Bhat A, et al. Association of muscle strength with functional status of elderly people. *Age Ageing* 1990;19:330–336.
12. Jones CJ, Rikli RE. Development and validation of a functional fitness test for community-residing older adults. *Res Q Exer Sports* 1999;7:129–161.
13. Jones CJ, Rikli RE, Bean WC. A 30-s chair stand test as a measure of lower body strength in community-residing older adults. *J Phys Act Ageing* 1999;70:113–119.
14. Katz S, et al. Studies of illness in the aged: the index of ADL—a standard measure of biologic and psychosocial function. *JAMA* 1963;185:914–919.
15. Knutzen KM, Brilla L, Caine D, et al. Absolute vs. relative machine strength as predictors of function in older adults. *J Strength Cond Res* 2002;16:628–640.
16. Landers KA, Hunter GR, Wetzstein CJ, et al. The interrelationship among muscle mass, strength, and the ability to perform physical tasks of daily living in younger and older women. *J Geron A Biol Sci Med Sci* 2001;56A:B443–B448.
17. Lawton MP. The functional assessment of elderly people. *J Am Geriatr Soc* 1971;19:465–481.
18. Mahoney FI, Barthel DW. Functional evaluation: the Barthel Index. *Md State Med J* 1965;14:61–65.
19. Newcomer KL, Krag HE, Mahowalk ML. Validity and reliability of the timed-stands test for patients with rheumatoid arthritis and other chronic diseases. *J Rheumatology* 1993;20:21–27.
20. Portney LG, Watkins MP. *Foundations of Clinical Research: Applications to Practice,* 2nd ed. Upper Saddle River, NJ: Prentice Hall, 2000.
21. Rantanen T, Guralnik JM, Izmirlian G, et al. Association of muscle strength with maximum walking speed in disabled older women. *Am J Phys Med Rehabil* 1999;77:299–305.
22. Rikli RE, Jones CJ. Functional fitness normative scores for community-residing older adults ages 60-94. *J Aging Phys Act* 1999;7:162–181.
23. Schiller BC, Casas YG, DeSouza CA, et al. Age-related declines in knee extensor strength and physical performance in healthy Hispanic and Caucasian women. *J Geront A Biol Sci Med Sci* 2000;55A:B563–B570.
24. Schot PK, Knutzen KM, Poole SM, et al. Sit-to-stand performance of older adults following strength training. *Res Q Exer Sport* 2003;74:1–8.
25. Shumway-Cook A, Woollacott MH. *Motor Control Theory and Practical Applications,* 2nd ed. Hagerstown, MD: Lippincott, Williams & Wilkins. 2000.
26. Spirduso WW. *Physical Dimension of Aging.* Champaign, IL: Human Kinetics, 1994.
27. Stockmeyer SA. An interpretation of the approach of Rood to the treatment of neuromuscular dysfunction. *Am J Phys Med* 1967;46:900–956.
28. Suzuki T, Bean JF, Fielding RA. Muscle power of the ankle flexors predicts functional performance in community-dwelling older women. *JAGS* 2001;49:1161–1167.

6

TECHNIQUES of PEDIATRIC MUSCLE TESTING

Venita Lovelace-Chandler, PhD, PT, PCS

Johnson[17] wrote an article to assist physicians in examining infants and small children suspected of having muscle weakness. He noted the need to present a relatively simple routine for such an examination, and he gave the three steps of palpation, examination for muscle tightness, and demonstration of muscle function as the appropriate routine. Johnson[17] stated that the only requirements for the examiner were a working knowledge of functional anatomy and acquaintance with the motor development of infants. He suggested that knowledge of functional anatomy was easily obtained by a review of an anatomy textbook, and an understanding of motor development was attained by observation of infants and familiarity with developmental scales. Although Johnson[17] was correct that a routine was not clearly available in existing literature, he underestimated the knowledge and skills involved in applying functional anatomy and principles of normal development to the assessment of the quantity and quality of muscle force exhibited by infants and young children.

In 1960, Schenck and Tomberlin wrote "Hints for Manual Muscle Testing of Infants" (while employed at the University of Texas Medical Branch) for use in teaching muscle testing to physical therapy students. Those "hints" suggested techniques for assessing the strength of individual muscles, and in some cases, muscle groups, for children from newborn to 5 years of age. Developmental reflexes were used to elicit most of the responses for children in the newborn to the 6- or 7-month range. From the sixth or seventh month to approximately 1 year, muscle strength was assessed by stimulating a voluntary movement without particular regard for gravity. From approximately 1 to 5 years of age, strength was assessed by stimulating a voluntary response against gravity. The authors advocated the use of the hints only in instances when voluntary or play activities would not elicit the desired muscle contraction according to criteria established for adult testing, and the hints have not been subjected to testing for reliability and validity. Donohoe and Bleakney[10] stated that palpation, observation of movement against gravity, and gross motor function are used to ascertain muscle grades in children.

Connolly[8] prepared a guide to muscle testing of functional movements using primarily the developmental activities listed in the Peabody developmental motor scales and activity cards developed by Folio and Fewell.[11] Connolly noted that therapists must have knowledge of normal movement in children and familiarity with motor milestones and performance in functional activities to perform muscle strength testing. Turman and Van Vranken[31] provided a guide for muscle testing of infants, toddlers, and preschool children that is designed to be compatible with multiple developmental assessments. Such developmental activities and assessments may not be appropriate for all populations of children. Smith, Danoff, and Parks[27] used the Peabody developmental motor scales to evaluate gross and fine motor skills in 143 children who had human immunodeficiency virus (HIV) infection. They found that children with HIV who were younger than 5 years performed below the levels of children who were not diagnosed with HIV. The group averages for children with HIV for 1.5 years of living with the infection were 1 to 1.5 standard deviations below the mean of a healthy reference population.

Other authors have studied strength or strength changes in atypically developing children using functional activities as well as other methods for measuring strength. Using children with cerebral palsy, Blundell et al.[5] measured lower limb muscle strength with dynamometry and the lateral step-up test. Functional performance was measured by the motor assessment scale (sit-to-stand), minimum chair height test, timed 10-m test, and 2-minute walk test. The authors found that children aged 4 to 8 years were able to demonstrate strength and functional performance with these methods. Muscle strength of adolescents with cerebral palsy was measured with a handheld dynamometer by Darrah et al.[9] in a study to evaluate a community fitness program.

Pitetti and Yarmer[23] compared children on isometric strength of knee flexion and extension and combined leg and back strength at the ages 8 to 18 years with and without mental retardation. Children without mental retardation were significantly stronger than their same-gender peers for all strength measurements. Stemmons Mercer and Lewis[28] compared 17 children with Down syndrome between the ages of 7 and 15 years with a peer group. A handheld dynamometer was used to measure hip abductor and knee extensor muscle strength. The children with Down syndrome had lower mean peak values than the comparison group, and the authors concluded that anthropometric characteristics and physical activity could be significant predictors of peak torque production.

Svien[29] compared children aged 7 to 10 years who were born 5 to 10 weeks preterm with control subjects and found that the preterm children exhibited impairments in muscular strength and endurance at school age. However, the impairments did not interfere with reported involvement in physical activity or sports. Barlett and Kneale Fanning[4] found that infants born preterm preferred play positions of sitting and supine, with the prone position being the least favored by infants. The authors concluded that infants who spend more time in sitting and supine positions have less opportunity for gross motor exploration.

Lieberman and McHugh[21] found that sighted children performed significantly better on a health-related fitness test than children with visual impairments. Chapman[7] studied the effect of movement context on the frequency and quality of spontaneous leg movements of infants with spina bifida and peers. A specially designed infant seat elicited more movements from both groups than did placement in other movement contexts.

Knutson et al.[18] and Krefting[19] have reported that cultural influences affect behavior. Abbott et al.[1] failed to find statistically significant correlations between home environment and infant motor development, but their observations suggested that stimulating home environments are associated with higher infant motor developmental scores. This chapter uses developmental activities for determining muscle strength, but examiners are encouraged to consider impairments or pathologies when making clinical decisions. For the purposes of muscle testing, examiners should consider that the current medical emphasis on supine positioning for sleep to reduce the incidence of sudden infant death syndrome may reduce an infant's ability to develop muscle strength in the prone position. Examiners need to include a parent/caregiver interview with attention to culture and home environment to determine the possible prior movement experiences of the child.

During the first year of life, children are striving to obtain motor control against gravity. During this period, the child exhibits varied reflexive and functional movements. Between 1 and 5 years of age, children continue the use of these movements in a variety of ways against gravity. Muscle testing below the age of 5 years is challenging and may not offer a true, implying reliable, muscle test.[7,9,11] Several authors have suggested that strength in children can be quantified beginning at approximately 6 years of age,[7,11,13] and most studies of strength have been conducted with older children.[21,23,29,31]

In one study of young children, Romero[24] described the development of trunk flexor muscle strength of 3-, 4-, 5-, and 6-year-old children using a reliable methodology that she indicated could be replicated in a clinical setting. She found that mean muscle grades increased with age; the greatest gain was between the ages of 4 and 5 years. Although the mean muscle grades were significantly different at each age, the author hypothesized that improvement in coordination may have been a greater factor than the child's ability to exert greater muscular force at the older ages further supporting the concept that assessing muscle strength in children is difficult.

Barrett and Harrison[3] compared 6-year-old children with 22-year-old adults in an effort to examine whether muscle function changes from childhood to adulthood could be accounted for by growth related changes in muscle size. They used a specific scaling technique, and their results suggested that muscle volume accounted for the differences in power measurements of children and adults. The findings supported the concept that muscle function is relatively unchanged from 6 years to adulthood (defined in their study as 22-years-old).

Gajdosik and Gajdosik[12] suggested that isokinetic systems can be used with children large enough to fit the components and that further modification of components could be accomplished. These authors further noted that handheld dynamometers may be able to offer precise measurements in children, and Hinderer and Hinderer[13] suggested using handheld instruments in conjunction with manual muscle testing. Sloan[26] summarized articles that used handheld dynamometers to quantify muscle strength in children with particular regard to reliability and validity. She found seven articles published between 1983 and 1992. The ages of children ranged from 5 to 21 years of age and included typically as well as atypically developing children. Sloan concluded that stabilization was essential to reliability of the handheld dynamometer and that children presented unique concerns in maintaining stabilization. Sloan's review should be helpful to examiners considering the use of handheld dynamometers for determining strength in children. The use of dynamometers in children younger than 3.5 years of age has not been reported in the literature.[2] Photographs and instructions for performing muscle tests in children using the handheld dynamometer are provided for selected muscle groups of the upper and lower extremities on the DVD accompanying this text. Regardless of the method used, Gajdosik and Gajdosik[12] caution that standardization of testing procedures and awareness of the influence of such factors as spasticity on assessing muscle strength should improve the reliability of strength testing in children.

When assessing children younger than 6 years, Connolly[8] observed that adult grading scales could be used with minor changes in the operational definitions or that grading could be accomplished by characterizing the weakness as minimal, mild, moderate, or severe. Hinderer et al.[14] reviewed manual muscle testing literature for children, particularly related to children with myelodysplasia, and recommended using the full manual muscle test scale regardless of age. These authors concluded that manual muscle testing in infancy is useful in providing information for prognosis and treatment planning. However, they noted that manual muscle testing is not a method of choice for assessing changes in strength over time.

Examiners may need to measure hand strength in children as the preschool age range is the range at which hand problems are usually corrected. Readers are directed to a review article by Innes[15] in which handgrip strength testing is reviewed and an extensive reference list is available. Lee-Volkov et al.[20] were able to establish normative data for grip and pinch strength for 3- to 5-year-olds. They also obtained normative values for dexterity using the functional dexterity test, but they found low correlation values suggesting that dexterity values are not correlated with grip or pinch strength. The authors were surprised that the factors governing dexterity and strength were independent and that a child could be strong but the strength did not necessarily translate into fine motor control.

Although challenges in accurate muscle testing for the 1- to 5-year range continue, this chapter focuses on strength development against gravity during the first year of life using hints for individual muscle testing and developmental activities that provide information on muscle groups. One or more test positions are offered for functional movements. Notes are provided when other activities might allow observation of the movement. Palpation may be accomplished using the techniques described for adult manual muscle testing in the other chapters of this text. Asymmetry between the two sides of the body for any grade is reason for concern during the first year of life.[15] Evidence of hand preference would be inappropriate during the first year, as are differences in strength between the upper and lower extremities or between the distal and proximal components of the extremities. Feeding difficulties may be a sign of weakness, and facial and eye movements should be examined for normal appearance.

Examiners are encouraged to establish intratester reliability, and if necessary, intertester reliability when using the suggestions in this chapter or any other source. Parents may share not only cultural and environmental perspectives but also motivational strategies, but the use of parents must be considered when analyzing reliability.

Mental state is very important, and the infant needs to be alert or crying.[13,24] Unhappy infants are likely to exhibit more spontaneous movements, which can be an advantage in manual muscle testing. Spontaneous movements may be suppressed if the infant is handled,[13] but tickling the infant or passively positioning an infant in an awkward position may elicit a spontaneous movement.[24] However, as indicated in the chapters in this text relating to adult testing, passively taking the infant through the movement allows determination of the infant's available range of motion (ROM).

Examiners need to continue to seek methods for accurate muscle strength testing for young children. Certainly, examiners can note if no response can be elicited, and a normal response might be defined as no apparent deficit in the quantity and quality of movement considering age level. Clinical judgment may be the only tool available currently for combining palpation and observation of functional movements with such factors as spasticity, cognition, attention, and cultural experiences when assessing muscle strength in children at levels between zero and normal.

■ HEAD MOVEMENTS

NECK EXTENSION

Gravity-Resisted Tests (Grades 5, 4, and 3)

PRONE

Infant position: Prone with the arms placed to allow forearm support.

Examiner action: Offer an auditory or visual stimulus such as calling the infant's name or using a musical toy.

Infant action: Birth to 3 months: The infant lifts the head. The newborn may free the face by turning the head[5,10] or may bob the head (Fig. 6-1). A small roll may be used to provide support under the arms (Fig. 6-2). By 3 months, the infant is actively extending the head past 45°.[10]

4 to 6 months: The infant lifts the head to at least 90° and maintains the position.[5]

7 to 9 months: The infant lifts the head past 90°.[5]

Resistance: For grade 5 or 4, gently press down on the back of the infant's head while continuing the auditory or visual stimulus.

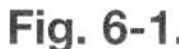

Fig. 6-1.

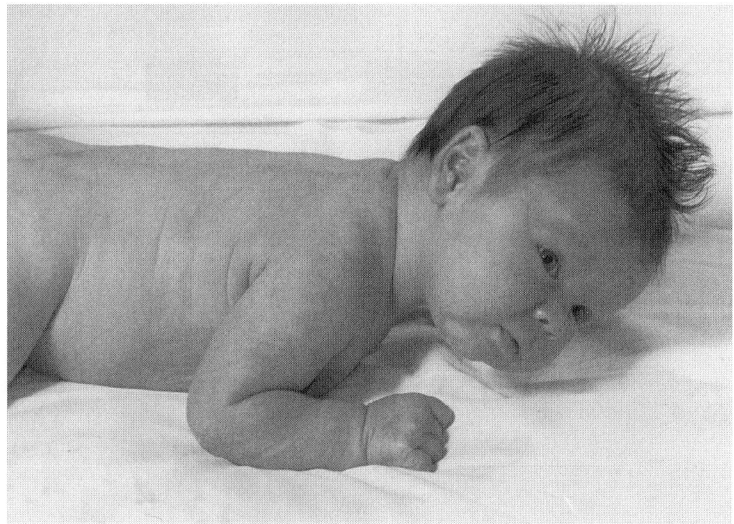

Fig. 6-2.

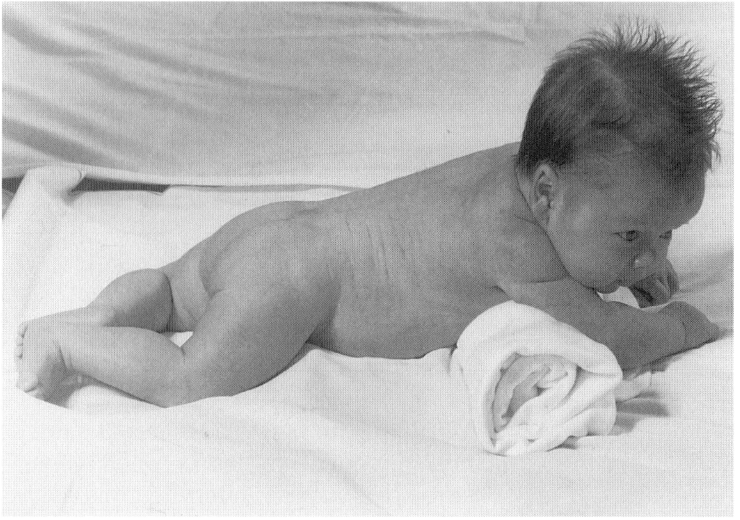

HORIZONTAL SUSPENSION

Infant position: Held horizontally in space with the examiner's hands supporting the infant under the chest and abdomen.

Examiner action: Offer an auditory or visual stimulus such as calling the infant's name or using a musical toy.

Infant action: Birth to 3 months: The infant lifts the head in line with the body. The newborn may hold the head upright only momentarily or may bob the head (Fig. 6-3). By 3 months, the infant holds the head steady and may lift it beyond the plane of the body.

4 to 6 months: The infant lifts the head to 90° or higher and maintains the position (Fig. 6-4).

Resistance: For grades 5 or 4, gently press down on the back of the infant's head while continuing the auditory or visual stimulus.

Fig. 6-3.

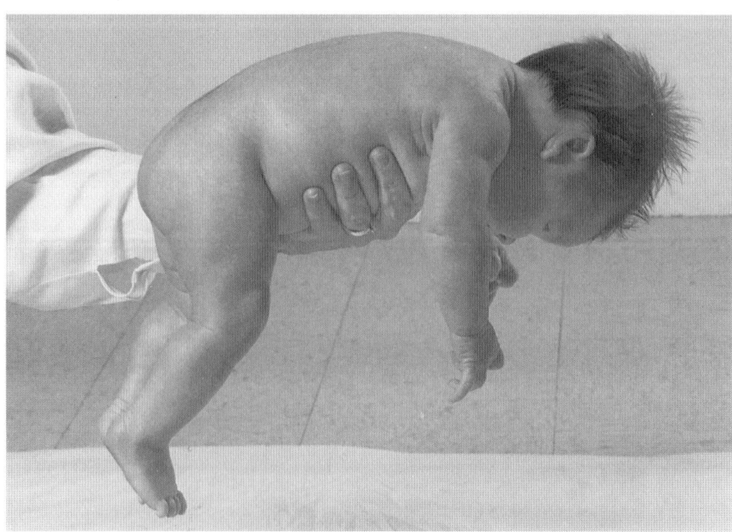

Fig. 6-4.

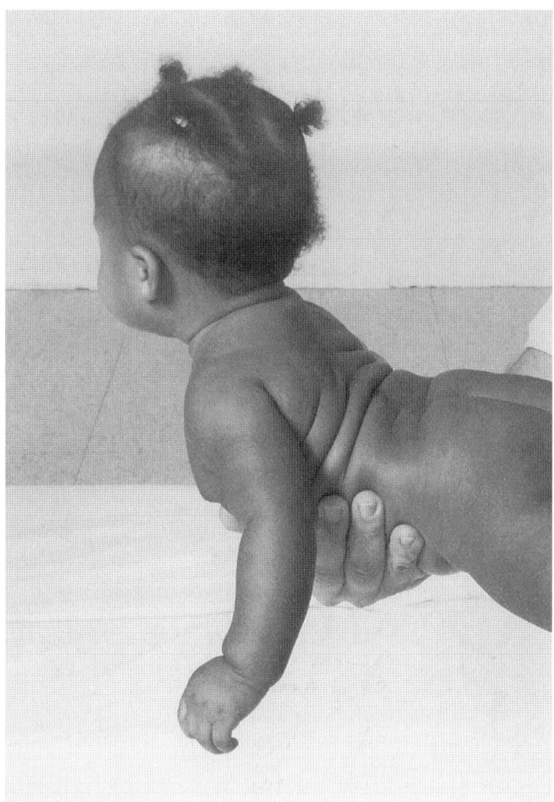

Grades Below 3

Grade 2: The infant extends the head through partial ROM. The examiner must consider the expected range for various ages.

Grades 1 and 0: With the infant prone and the face down, stroke the posterior neck muscles and observe for any contraction, or lift the head slightly off the surface and palpate for a contraction of the posterior neck muscles as the head is allowed to drop 5° into the examiner's hand.

NECK FLEXION (FORWARD)

Gravity-Resisted Test (Grades 5, 4, and 3)

Infant position: Supine with the examiner's hands grasping the infant's wrists and hands.

Examiner action: Pull the infant into a sitting position while offering an auditory or visual stimulus such as calling the infant's name.

Infant action: Birth to 3 months: The infant's head will lag behind the body (Fig. 6-5) until a sitting position is attained. The infant holds the head upright momentarily when sitting (Fig. 6-6).

4 to 5 months: The infant tucks the chin and keeps the head in line with the body.

6 to 7 months: The infant brings the head forward of the line of the body (Fig. 6-7).

Fig. 6-5.

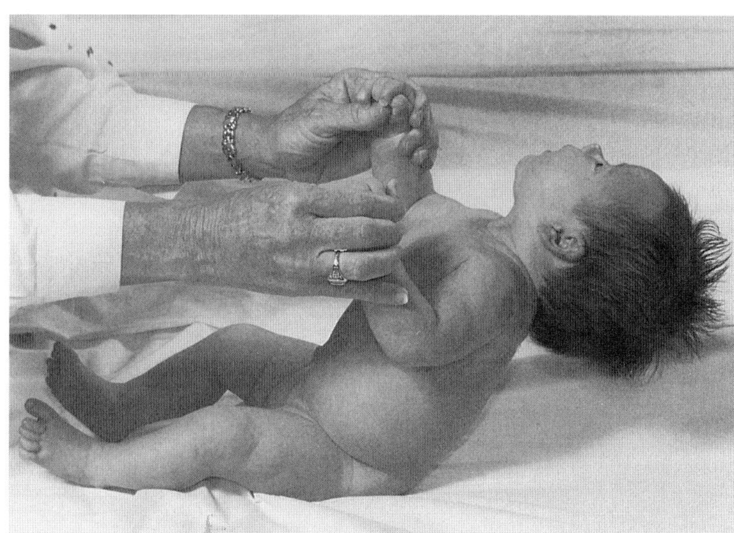

Fig. 6-6.

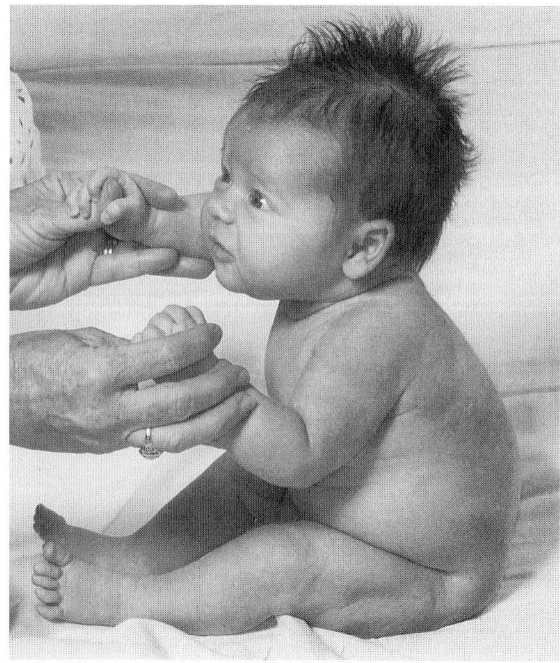

Fig. 6-7.

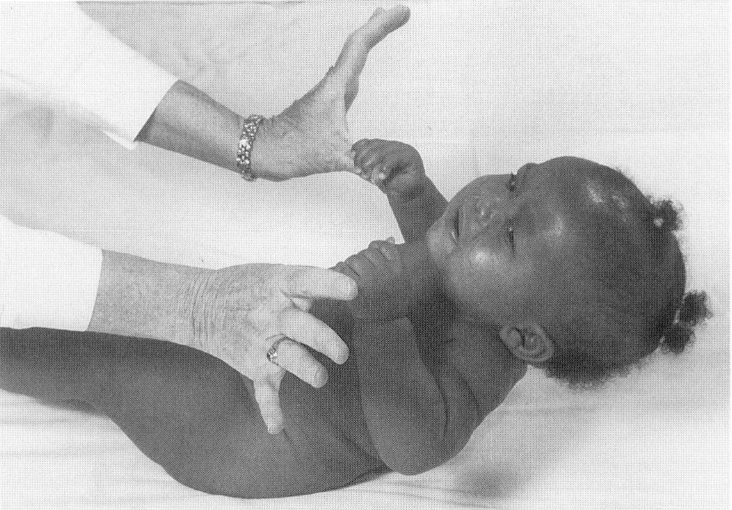

Note: Infants placed in a reclining seat will bring the head forward off the surface beginning at age 4 months. Infants placed supine but not given the stimulus of pulling on the wrists and hands are able to lift the head off the surface at 6 months of age.

Resistance: For grades 5 and 4, gently press backward on the infant's forehead while continuing the auditory or visual stimulus. The examiner may be able to hold both of the infant's arms with one hand and apply resistance with the other hand, or resistance may be applied by an assistant.

Grades Below 3

Grade 2: The infant flexes the head through partial ROM. It may be difficult to determine before 6 months when full range can be expected from a supine position.

Grades 1 and 0: With the infant supine, lift the head slightly off the surface and palpate for a contraction of the anterior neck muscles as the head is allowed to drop 5° into the examiner's hand.

NECK FLEXION (LATERAL)

Gravity-Resisted Test (Grades 5, 4, and 3)

This vertical position may be used to test neck flexion (forward) or neck extension by tilting the infant forward or backward or to assess cocontraction of neck flexors and extensors as shown in Fig. 6-8.

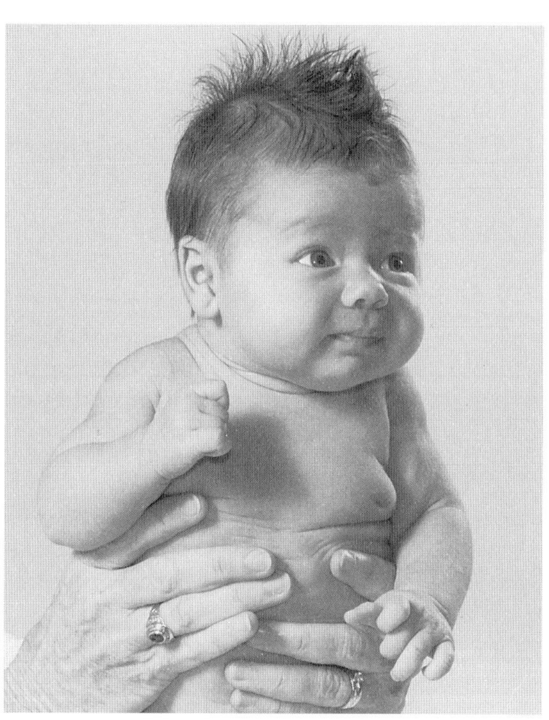

Fig. 6-8.

Infant position: Held vertically with the examiner's hands around the trunk and without support for the head.

Examiner action: Tilt the infant laterally 5° to 10° (or a greater distance for older infants) while offering an auditory or visual stimulus such as calling the infant's name or using a musical toy.

Infant action: Birth to 3 months: The infant keeps the head from falling sideways (Fig. 6-9).

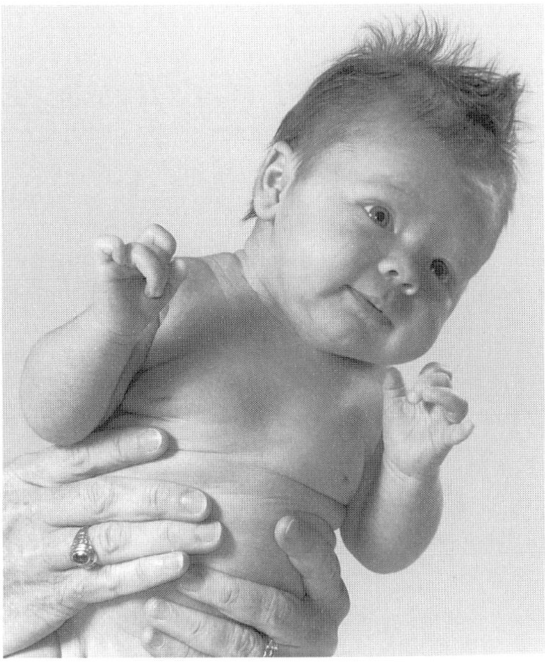

Fig. 6-9.

4 months: The infant corrects the head so that the face is vertical.

Resistance: Grades 5 and 4, push on the side of the head laterally in the direction of the tilt. An assistant is needed to apply resistance while the examiner maintains support around the trunk.

Grades Below 3

Grade 2: The infant laterally flexes the head through partial ROM. It may be difficult to determine before age 4 months, when full range is expected.

Grades 1 and 0: With the infant in a side lying position, lift the head slightly off the surface and palpate for a contraction of the lateral neck muscles as the head is allowed to drop 5° into the examiner's hand.

■ TRUNK MOVEMENTS

TRUNK FLEXION

Gravity-Resisted Test (Grades 5, 4, and 3)

PULLED-TO-SIT

Infant position: Supine with the examiner's hands grasping the infant's wrists and hands.

Examiner action: Pull the infant into a sitting position while offering an auditory or visual stimulus such as calling the infant's name or using a musical toy.

Infant action: Birth to 3 months: The abdominals do not participate during the first 2 months. Beginning at about 3 months, the abdominals and hip flexors become active and provide stability to the thorax.[5]

4 to 6 months: The abdominals assist in bringing the body forward. If the cervical vertebral stabilizers and abdominals are active, the sternocleidomastoid will flex the head. If the cervical vertebral stabilizers and abdominals are inactive, the sternocleidomastoid will extend the head during pulled-to-sit. The hips and knees will flex (Fig. 6-10).[5]

7 to 12 months: The abdominals contract to bring the infant forward. The hips flex and the knees extend, elongating the hamstrings and bringing the infant into a sitting position (Fig. 6-11).[5]

Fig. 6-10.

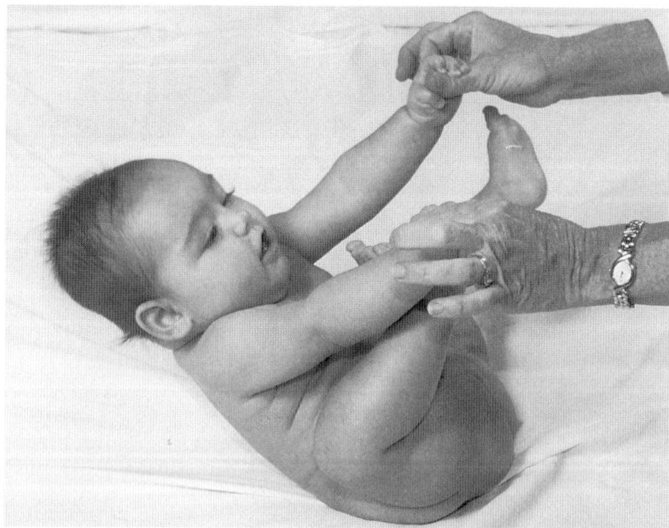

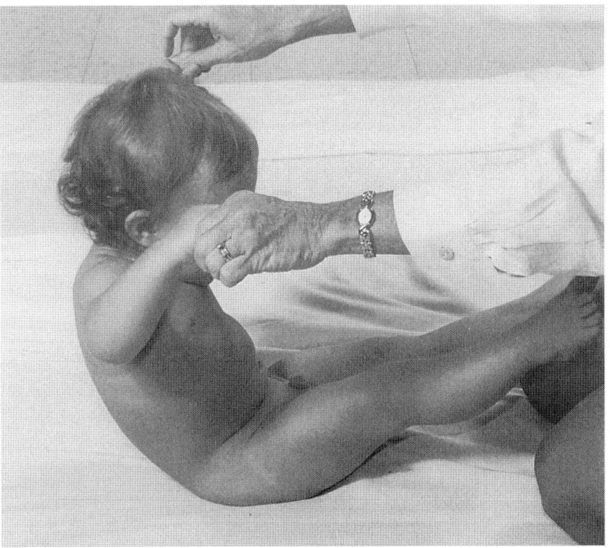

Fig. 6-11.

Resistance: Grades 5 and 4, gently push backward on the infant's chest while maintaining an auditory or visual stimulus. An assistant is needed to apply resistance while the examiner grasps the wrists and hands.

Grades Below 3

PULLED-TO-SIT

Grade 2: The infant is unable to assist through the full ROM to achieve sitting or the hips do not flex through the full range.

Grades 1 and 0: With the infant supine, grasp both of the infant's wrists in one hand. Pull the infant into a sitting position while palpating for abdominal contractions, or lift the infant's head and shoulders off the surface and palpate for a contraction while the trunk is allowed to drop 5 to 10° into the examiner's arm.

Gravity-Resisted Test (Grades 5, 4, and 3)

SUPINE

Infant position: Supine.

Examiner action: Observe for spontaneous lifting of the hips and feet. If no movement occurs, bend the child's knees and bring the feet toward the head.[10] For the older infant, use verbal encouragement and say, "Get your feet."

Infant action: Term to 3 months: The infant spontaneously lifts the legs off the surface and may alternate kicking and flexing the hips and knees.

4 to 6 months: The infant will lift the pelvis and bring the feet to the mouth for play (Fig. 6-12).[10]

Fig. 6-12.

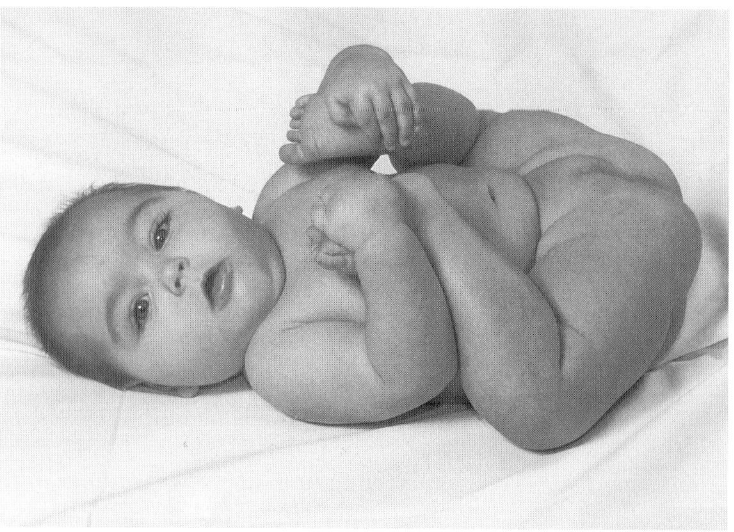

7 to 9 months: The infant lifts the pelvis, and the legs are held straight upright. The arms come to the feet for play. The abdominal muscles are very active, but minimal spinal flexion occurs.[5]

Resistance: Grades 5 and 4, gently push downward on the infant's legs.

Grades Below 3

SUPINE

Grade 2: The infant is unable to bring the legs and pelvis through the full ROM or the infant is unable to hold the legs and pelvis up when the legs are placed in flexion by the examiner.

Grades 1 and 0: Hold the legs up and let them drop 10° into the examiner's arm while palpating the lower abdominals for a contraction.

TRUNK EXTENSION

Gravity-Resisted Test (Grades 5, 4, and 3)

Infant position: Held horizontally in space with the examiner's hands supporting the infant under the chest and abdomen.

Examiner action: Offer an auditory stimulus such as calling the infant's name or a visual stimulus such as the caregiver's face.

Infant action: 4 to 6 months: The infant lifts the head and upper trunk into extension above the plane of the rest of the body. The legs are in line with the body (Fig. 6-13).

Fig. 6-13.

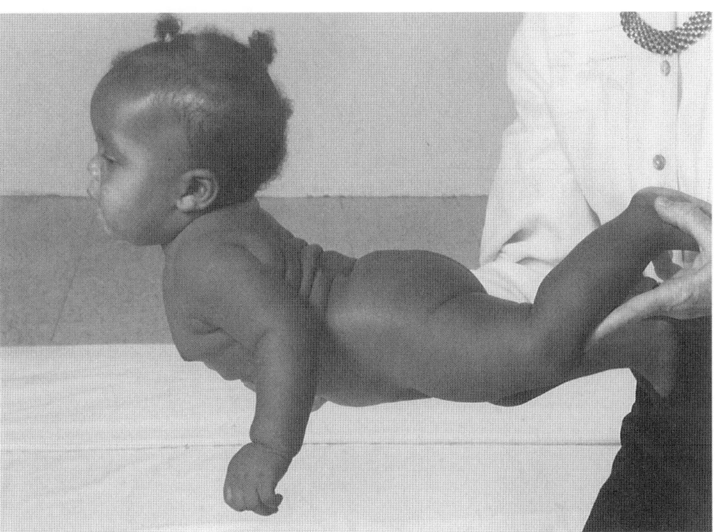

Note: Trunk extension may be noted in a 5-month-old infant who balances on the stomach and rocks (Fig. 6-14).

Fig. 6-14.

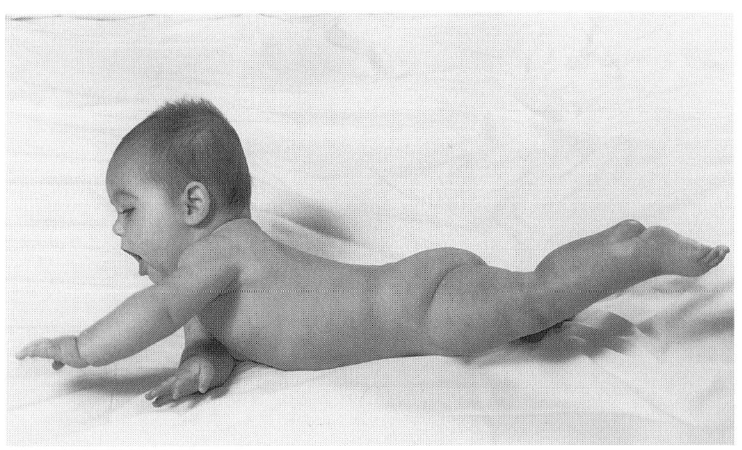

7 to 9 months: The infant lifts the entire trunk into extension, and the legs extend above the plane of the trunk.

Resistance: Gently press down on the infant's upper or lower trunk while continuing the auditory or visual stimulus and support under the abdomen.

Grades Below 3

Grade 2: The infant extends the trunk through a partial ROM.

Grade 1 or 0: With the infant prone, stroke the upper trunk and observe for any contraction. Lift the lower extremities and pelvis off the surface and palpate for contractions of the buttocks as the legs are lowered a short distance.

TRUNK EXTENSION AND FLEXION

Gravity-Resisted Tests (Grades 5, 4, and 3)

SITTING

Infant position: Sitting.

Examiner action: Offer an auditory or visual stimulus such as calling the infant's name or using a musical toy.

Infant action: 6 months: At 6 months, the infant has sufficient abdominal (and back extensor) activity in the sagittal (flexion and extension) plane to sit independently for at least 1 minute.[10] The baby lacks sufficient trunk activity in the transverse and frontal planes and will fall frequently with weight shifts into those directions (Fig. 6-15).[5]

Fig. 6-15.

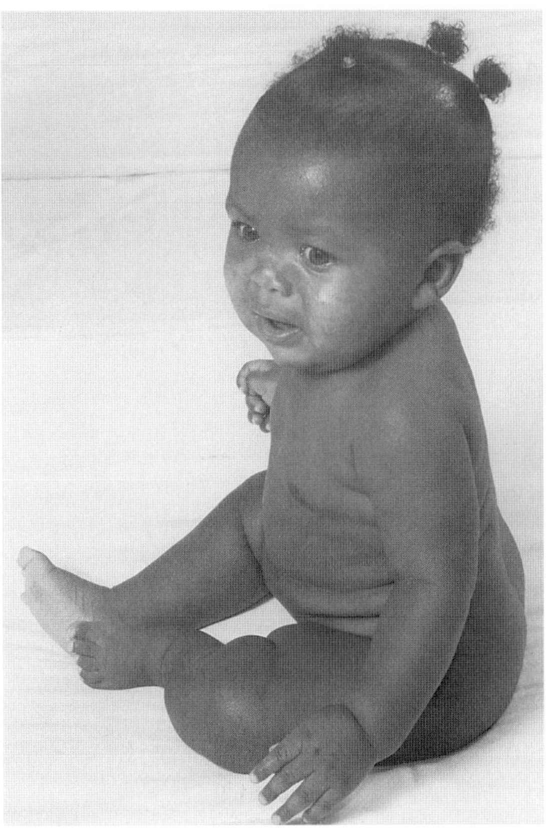

7 to 9 months: Abdominal (and pelvic) control in flexion and extension is very active. The infant sits independently and is able to adjust to weight shifts that occur as a result of head and arm movements.[5] The pelvis can be maintained in a neutral position.[7]

Resistance: Grades 5 and 4, gently push the infant backward or forward at 6 months. From 7 months on, the infant can respond to resistance applied in all planes. The resistance is minimal during the seventh month and can be increased as full control is obtained at 9 months.

Grades Below 3

Grade 2: The infant sits with a posterior tilt.

Grades 1 and 0: Support the infant in sitting and palpate for contractions of the abdominals and trunk extensors.

Gravity-Resisted Test (Grades 5, 4, and 3)

QUADRUPED

Infant position: On hands and knees.

Examiner action: Offer an auditory or visual stimulus to maintain interest.

Infant action: 6 months: The infant has sufficient strength to hold the hands and knees position, but some lordosis may be present.

7 to 9 months: The infant can hold the position for lengthy periods and can even creep without lumbar lordosis (Fig. 6-16).[5]

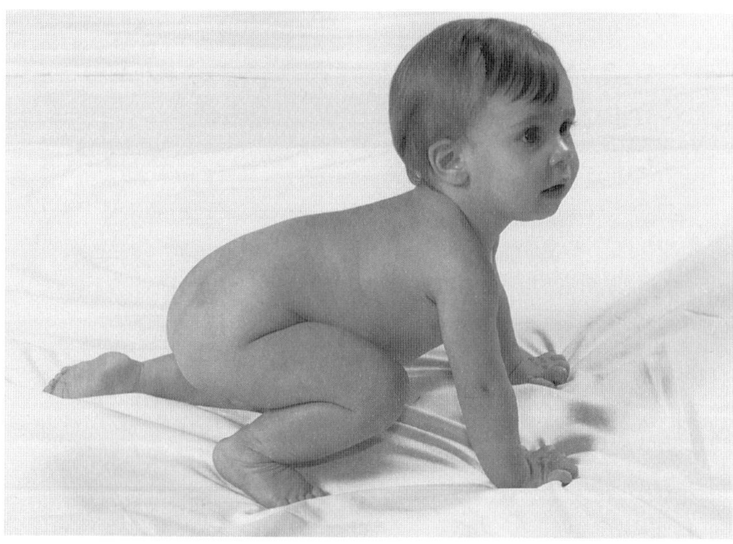

Fig. 6-16.

Resistance: Grades 5 and 4, gently push up or down on the trunk.

Grades Below 3

QUADRUPED

Grade 2: The infant maintains a quadruped position with an excessive lordosis.

Grade 1: The infant holds the position only momentarily and with lordosis.

TRUNK ROTATION

Gravity-Resisted Test (Grades 5, 4, and 3)

SUPINE

Infant position: Supine.

Examiner action: Use an auditory or visual stimulus above and to the side of the infant's head.

Infant action: 4 months: The infant rolls from a supine to a side lying position using a flexed posture with both hips and knees flexed (some infants may roll to side lying position through the use of excessive head and neck extension).[5]

Fig. 6-17.

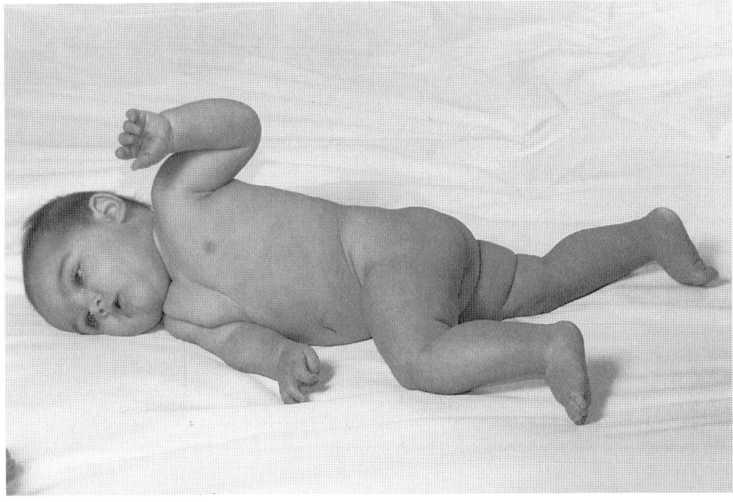

5 months: The infant rolls from a supine to a side lying position using trunk rotation and separation of the legs (Fig. 6-17).[7]

6 months: The infant rolls from a supine to a prone position using trunk rotation (Fig. 6-18).[5]

Fig. 6-18.

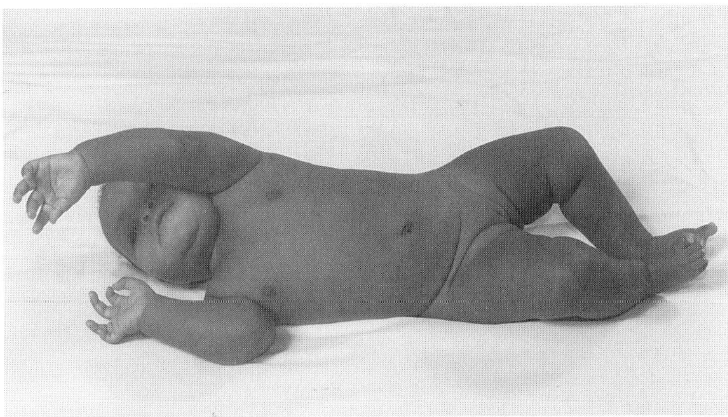

8 to 9 months: The infant rolls from a supine to a prone position using counterrotation: The shoulder rotates in one direction, and the hip rotates in the other direction.[5]

Note: The infant demonstrates head and trunk lateral flexion during the transition from a side lying position into a prone position (Fig. 6-19).

Fig. 6-19.

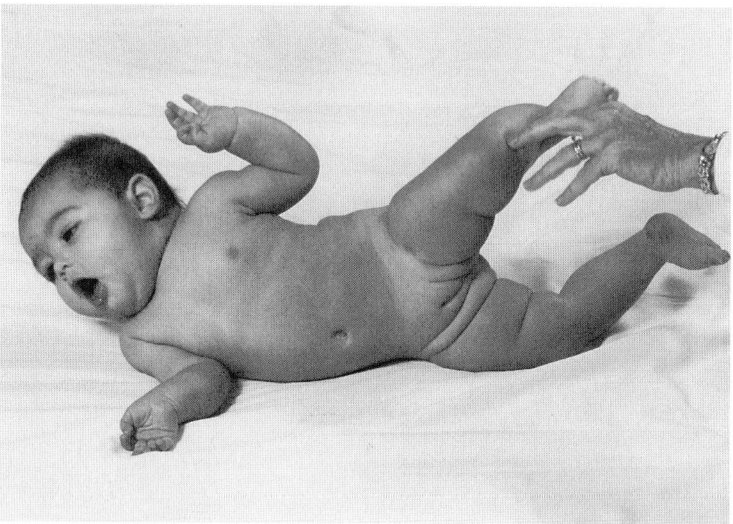

Resistance: Grades 5 and 4, gently push the infant back into a supine position by applying pressure at the shoulder or the pelvis.

Grades Below 3

SUPINE

Grade 2: The infant maintains a side lying position when placed there.

Grade 1: The infant attempts to maintain a side lying position when placed there.

Gravity-Resisted Test (Grades 5, 4, and 3)

ROTATION INTO SITTING

Infant position: Prone.

Examiner action: Use a toy at the child's side to attract attention.[10]

Infant action: 7 to 9 months: The infant shifts weight laterally and places the unweighted lower extremity on the floor with hip flexion abduction and external rotation. The head and trunk show lateral flexion. The infant actively externally rotates the weight-bearing hip to pull the pelvis and trunk backward to sit (Fig. 6-20).

Fig. 6-20.

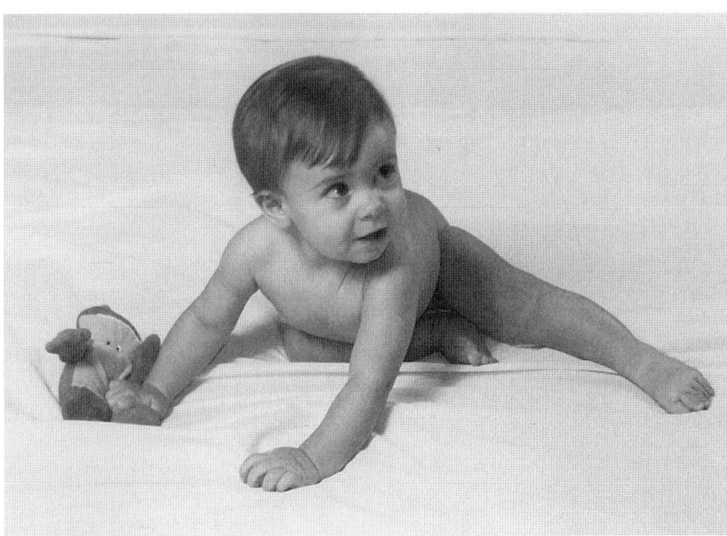

Resistance: Grades 5 and 4, gently push the infant toward a prone position.

Grades Below 3

Grade 2: The infant moves through a partial ROM in an attempt to assume a sitting position.

Grade 1: The infant attempts to rotate the trunk up from a prone position.

■ UPPER EXTREMITY MOVEMENTS

SHOULDER FLEXION

Gravity-Resisted Test (Grades 5, 4, and 3)

SUPINE: OPTION I

Infant position: Supine with the examiner offering a toy overhead.

Examiner action: Encourage the infant to reach for the toy.

Infant action: 6 months: The infant reaches overhead using shoulder flexion and elbow extension (Fig. 6-21).

Fig. 6-21.

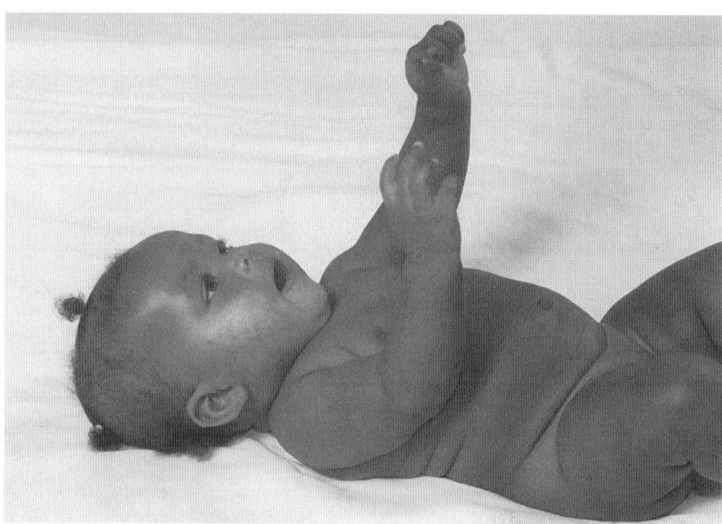

Resistance: Grades 5 and 4, gently push the arms down toward the surface and into shoulder extension.

Grades Below 3

Grade 2: The infant is unable to bring the arms into full 90° of shoulder flexion.

Grade 1: Observe any attempts to lift the arms.

Gravity-Resisted Test (Grades 5, 4, and 3)

SUPINE: OPTION II

Infant position: Supine with the examiner's hands offered to the infant.

Examiner action: Encourage the infant to pull into a sitting position.

Infant action: 6 months: The infant reaches for the examiner's hands using shoulder flexion, adduction, and elbow extension and pulls into a sitting position with shoulder and elbow flexion (Fig. 6-7).

Resistance: Grades 5 and 4, an assistant can apply resistance downward into extension as the infant reaches for or holds the examiner's hands.

Grades Below 3

Grade 2: The infant will exhibit only a partial ROM for shoulder flexion to 90°.

Grade 1: The examiner palpates for efforts of the infant to flex the shoulder.

Gravity-Resisted Test (Grades 5, 4, and 3)

SITTING

Infant position: Sitting.

Examiner action: Hold an object above the child's head.

Infant action: 6 months: The infant reaches for the toy with shoulder flexion and elbow extension (Fig. 6-22).

Fig. 6-22.

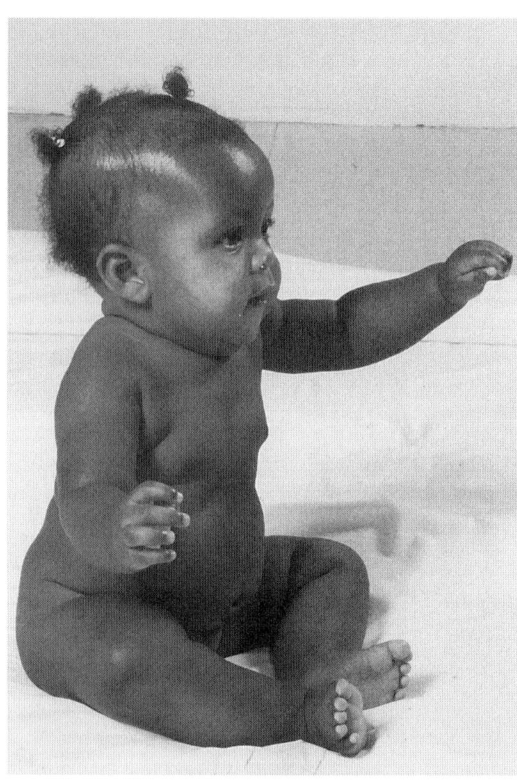

11 months: Able to reach overhead for the last 20° of shoulder flexion.[7]

Resistance: Grades 5 and 4, gently push down on the arms as the infant reaches for the toy.

Grades Below 3

Grade 2: The infant will exhibit only a partial ROM for shoulder flexion to 90°.

Grade 1: The examiner palpates for efforts of the infant to flex the shoulder.

ELBOW EXTENSION

Gravity-Resisted Test (Grades 5, 4, and 3)

PRONE

Infant position: Prone with the arms forward to allow support.

Examiner action: Offer an auditory or visual stimulus such as calling the infant's name or using a toy.

Infant action: Birth to 3 months: The infant shows an increasing ability to push up on the arms and to prop up on the elbows (Fig. 6-1).[5]

6 months: The infant pushes up on fully extended arms (Fig. 6-23).

Fig. 6-23.

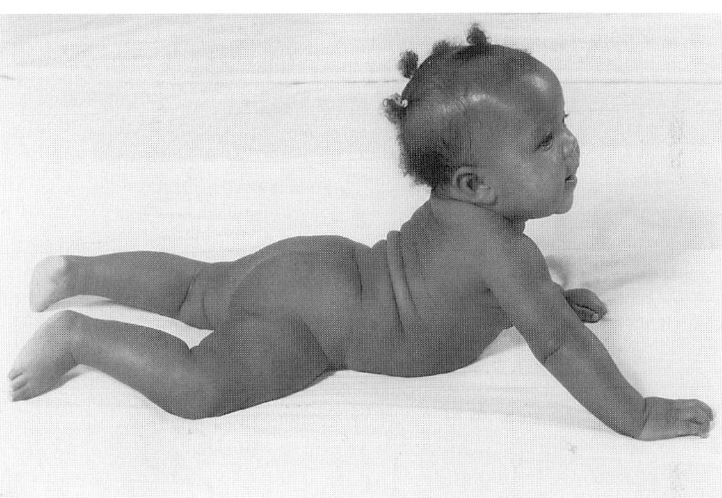

Resistance: Grades 5 and 4, push gently on the shoulder girdle with consideration for the amount of elbow extension that should be present. Also, the arms could be gently pushed into elbow flexion.

Grades Below 3

Grade 2: The infant will be unable to move through the expected range of elbow extension. The infant could be placed on propped arms to determine if the infant can hold momentarily.

Grade 1: The examiner should palpate for efforts at extension.

Gravity-Resisted Test (Grades 5, 4, and 3)

SITTING

Infant position: Sitting.

Examiner action, option I: While holding the infant's elbows extended, place the infant's arms forward in propping position and temporarily remove support from the elbows.

Infant action: 4 months: The infant momentarily props up with elbow extension.[5]

Examiner action, option II: Gently push the infant to the side (7 months) or backward (9 to 12 months).

Infant action: 7 months: The infant will demonstrate protection to the side with elbow extension and shoulder abduction (Fig. 6-24).

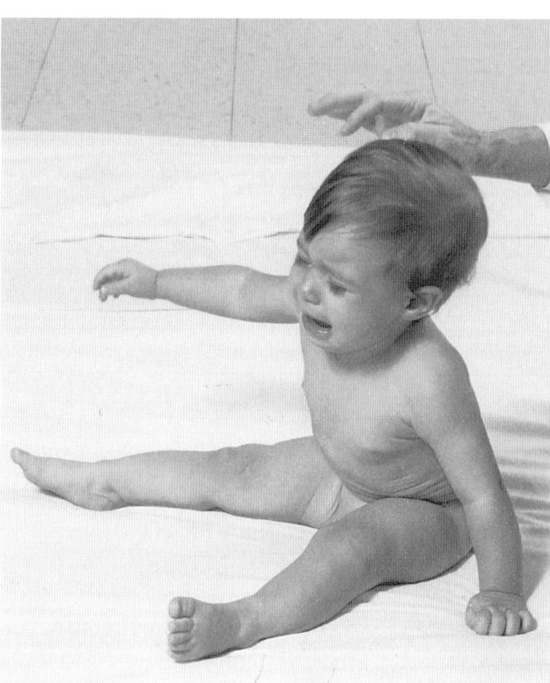

Fig. 6-24.

9 to 12 months: The infant will demonstrate protection backward (unilaterally or bilaterally) (Fig. 6-25).

Note: A downward parachute reaction may also be used to obtain elbow extension. The wrist, fingers, head, and upper trunk will also extend (Fig. 6-26).

Fig. 6-25.

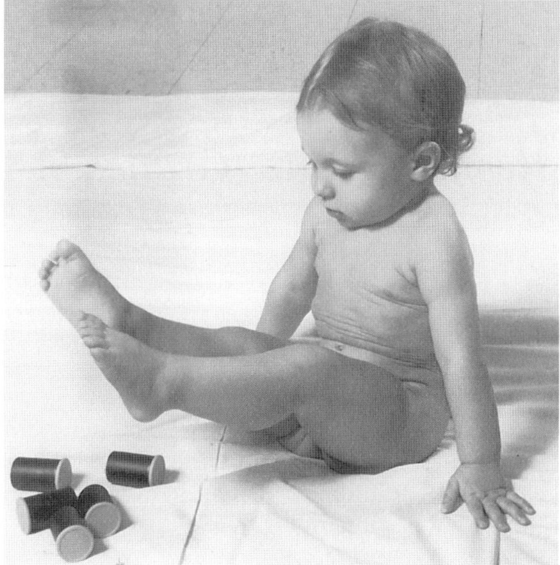

Fig. 6-26.

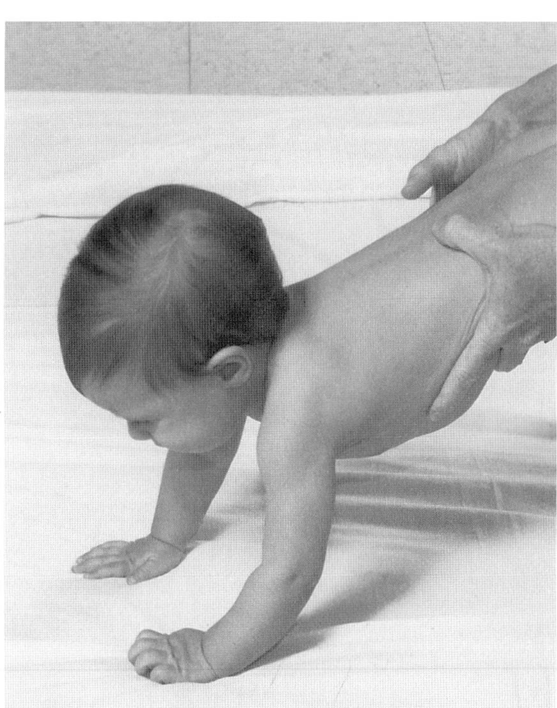

Resistance: These movements are done with speed for protection, and resistance is awkward to apply. The task is made more difficult for the infant by increasing the speed of the stimulus sideways, backward, or downward.

Grades Below 3

Grade 2: The infant will not be able to hold the protected position or may only move through a partial ROM.

Grade 1: The examiner observes or palpates for efforts at protection.

■ LOWER EXTREMITY MOVEMENTS

HIP AND KNEE FLEXION

Gravity-Resisted Tests (Grades 5, 4, and 3)

SUPINE

Infant position: Supine.

Examiner action: Observe spontaneous movements. Tickle or stroke the feet to encourage movement.

Infant action: Birth to 3 months: The newborn holds the hips and knees in flexion with the feet resting on the surface and the knees and thighs remaining in the air.[5] By 3 months, active, symmetric, reciprocal kicking occurs (seen in 6-month-old infant; Fig. 6-27).

Fig. 6-27.

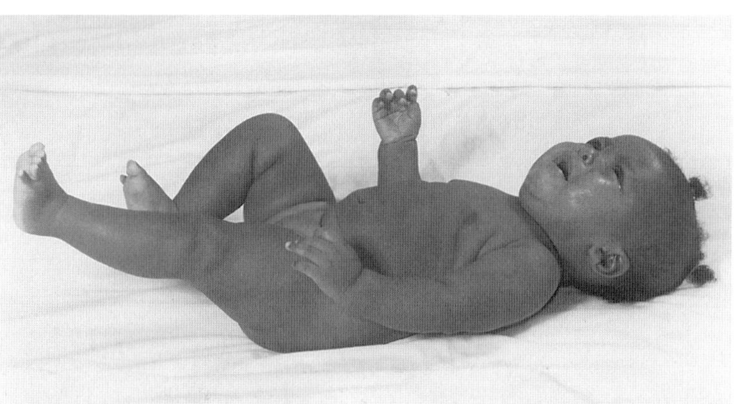

4 to 6 months: The infant flexes the hips and knees and brings the feet to the mouth for play (Fig. 6-28).[10]

Fig. 6-28.

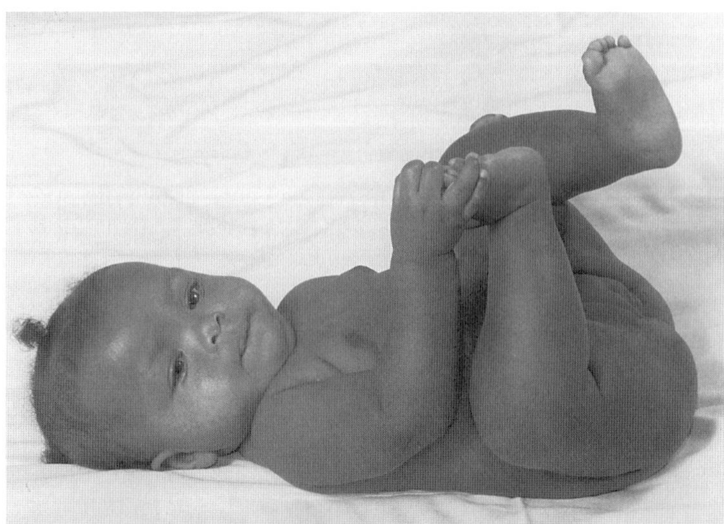

7 to 9 months: The infant moves in and out of hip and knee flexion when in transition from a prone to a sitting position and from a sitting to a prone position (Fig. 6-29).

Fig. 6-29.

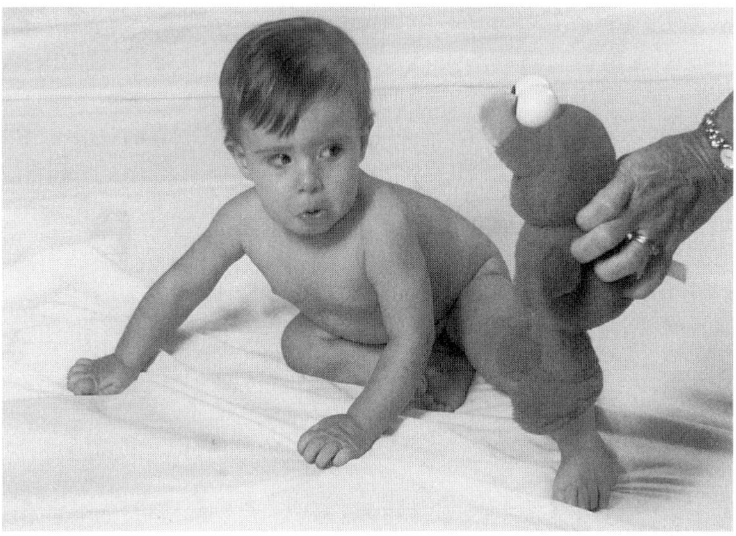

12 months: The infant kneels (low kneeling) with hip and knee flexion and hips aligned under the shoulders (Fig. 6-30).

Fig. 6-30.

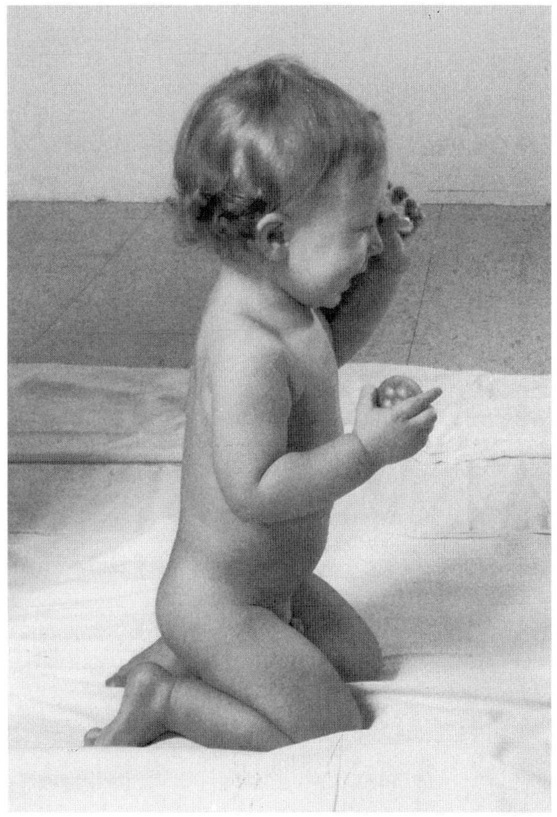

PRONE

Infant position: Prone.

Examiner action: Observe spontaneous movements. Tickle or stroke the feet to encourage movement, or lift up on the pelvis.

Infant action: Birth to 3 months: The infant pulls the hip and knee into flexion (Fig. 6-31).

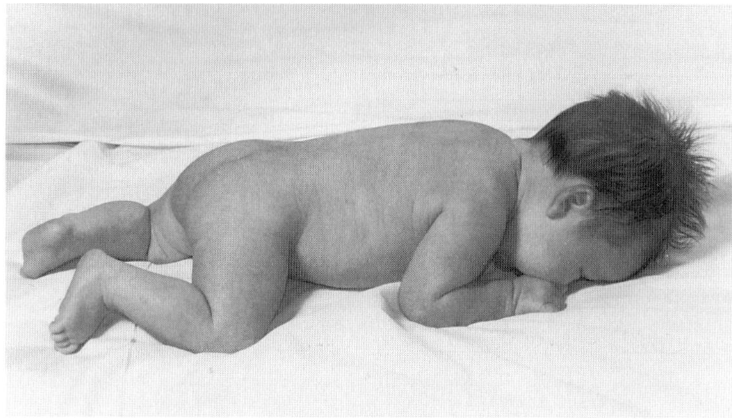

Fig. 6-31.

4 to 6 months: The infant maintains the quadruped position.

7 to 10 months: The infant creeps and may keep one knee up with the foot placed flat on the surface (Fig. 6-32).

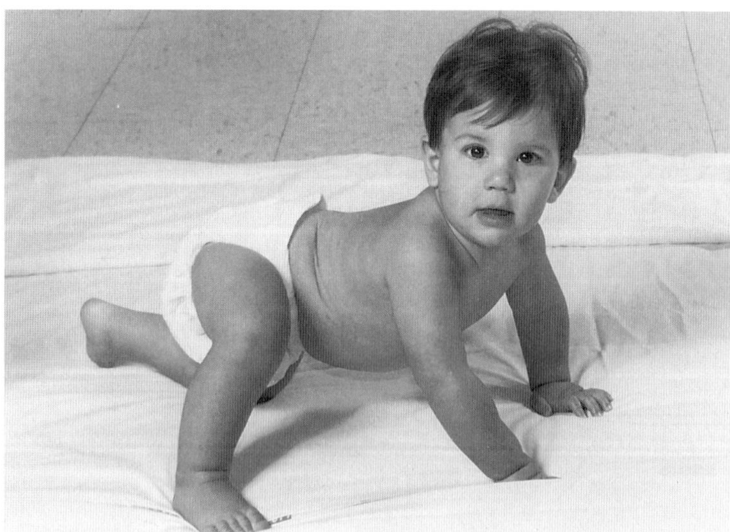

Fig. 6-32.

10 to 12 months: The infant pulls into standing by flexing the hip and knee and then abducting the flexed leg (Figs. 6-33 and 6-34).

Fig. 6-33.

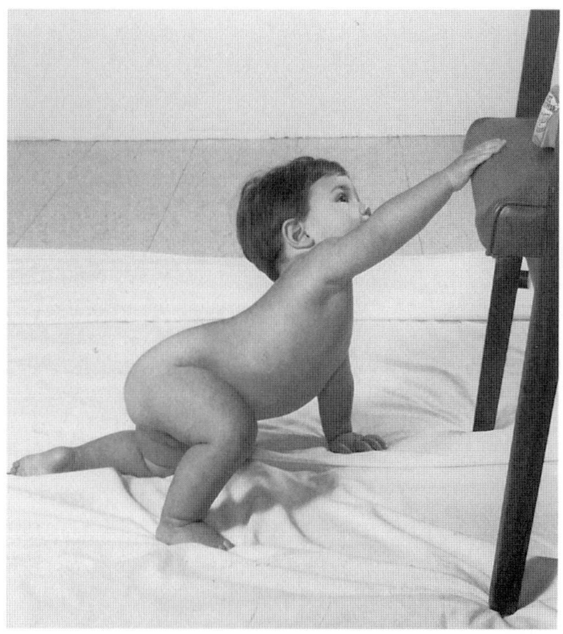

Fig. 6-34.

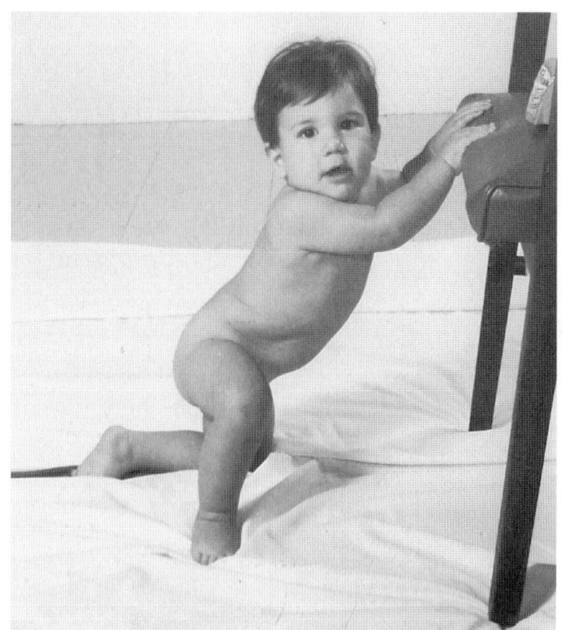

12 months: The infant demonstrates hip and knee flexion in one leg when stepping and maintaining hip and knee extension on the weight-bearing leg (Fig. 6-35).

Fig. 6-35.

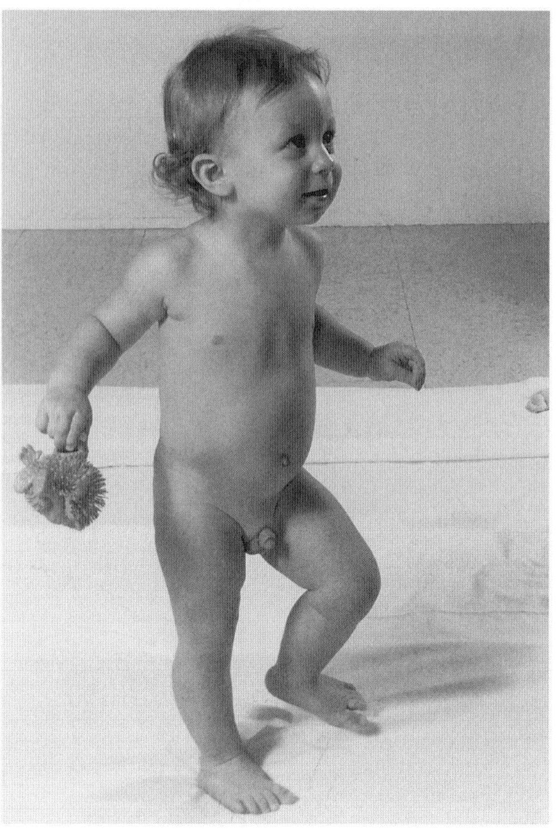

Resistance: Grades 5 and 4, apply resistance to hip and knee flexion in the various positions and movements appropriate for the age of the infant.

Grades Below 3

Grade 2: The infant exhibits only partial hip and knee flexion in the various positions and movements.

Grade 1: The examiner palpates or observes for attempts at contractions of the hip and knee flexors.

HIP AND KNEE EXTENSION

Gravity-Resisted Test (Grades 5, 4, and 3)

PRONE

Infant position: Prone or in horizontal suspension with the examiner's hands supporting the infant under the chest and abdomen.

Examiner action: Observe spontaneous movements or tickle or stroke the lower back or legs to encourage movement.

Infant action: 4 to 6 months: The infant extends the legs off the surface.[10] At 5 months, the infant rocks in a prone position (Fig. 6-19).[5]

7 to 9 months: The infant extends the legs during horizontal suspension.

12 months: The infant kneels (high kneeling) with hips extended and knees flexed and with the hips aligned under the shoulders.

Resistance: Grades 5 and 4, gently push downward on the extended leg or attempt to flex the leg.

Grades Below 3

PRONE

Grade 2: The infant exhibits only partial hip and knee extension in the various positions and movements.

Grade 1: The examiner palpates or observes for attempts at contractions of hip and knee extensors.

Gravity-Resisted Test

STANDING

Infant position: Standing independently.

Examiner action: Place an object on the floor and attract the infant's attention to the object.

Infant action: 12 months: The infant squats to pick up the object and returns to standing without falling (Fig. 6-36).

Fig. 6-36.

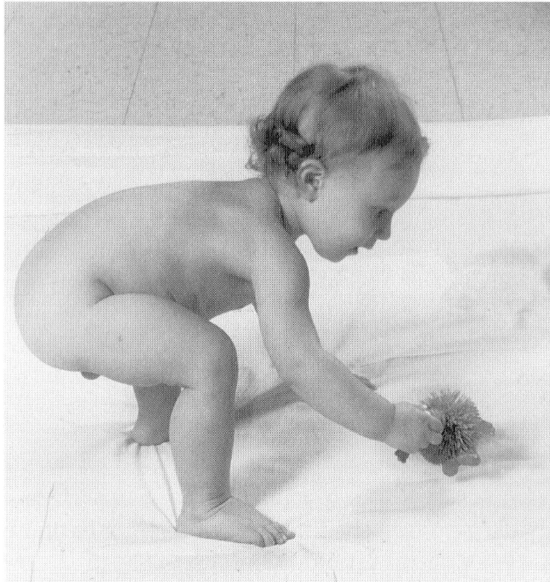

Note: The infant may exhibit combinations of hip and knee flexion and extension during plantar grade or bear walking. The infant may walk on the hands and feet with the knees extended (Fig. 6-37) or may keep the pelvis lower and walk on the hands and feet with the knees more flexed (Fig. 6-38).

Fig. 6-37.

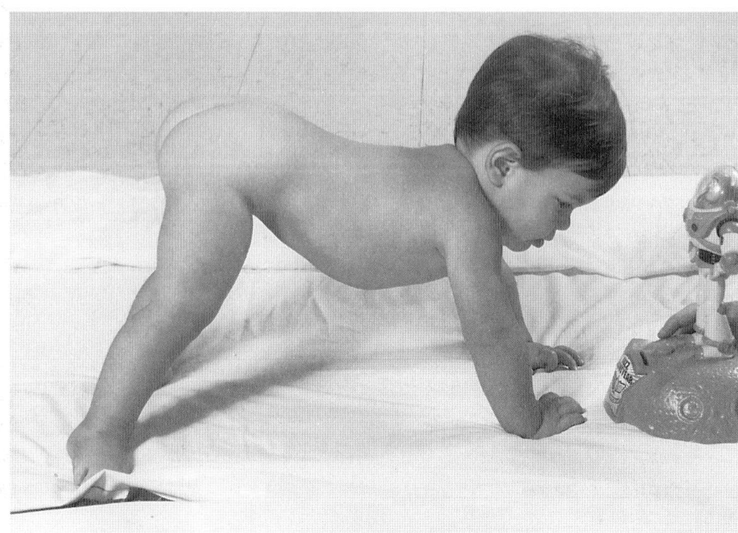

Fig. 6-38.

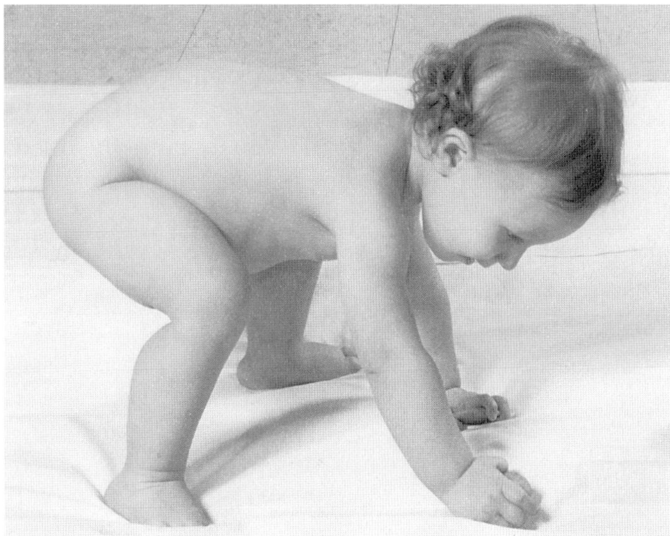

Gravity-Resisted Test (Grades 5, 4, and 3)

INDEPENDENT STANDING

Infant position: Supported in standing progressing to independent standing.

Examiner action: Provide support in standing or protect the infant who is standing with self-support or independently.

Infant action: Birth to 3 months: The infant takes some weight and extends the legs. The flexor tone results in a semiextended knee, and the hips remain flexed and behind the shoulders. The feet are close together, but the knees bow apart (Fig. 6-39).[5]

Fig. 6-39.

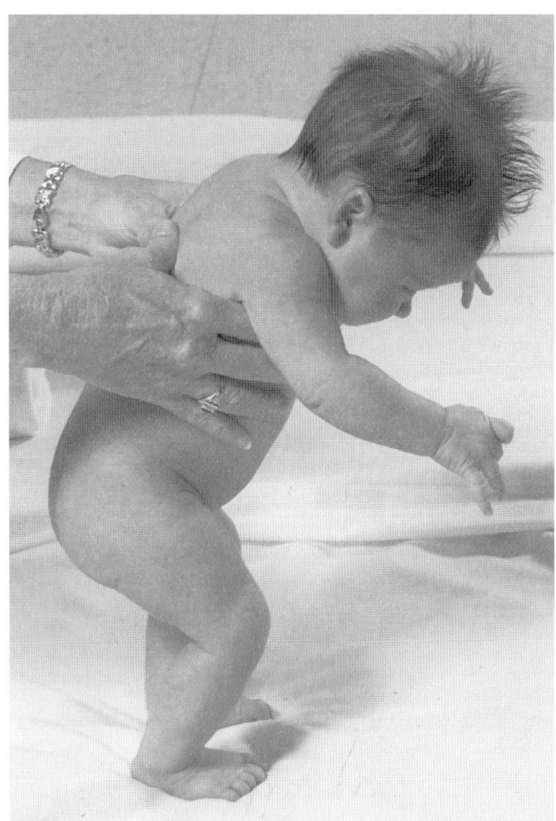

4 to 5 months: The infant takes almost the full weight with strong knee extension, but releases the extension and often collapses into flexion with attempts at practicing knee flexion.[5]

6 months: The infant takes the full weight on the legs and may stand momentarily without support. The hip extensors are not fully active (Fig. 6-40).[5]

Fig. 6-40.

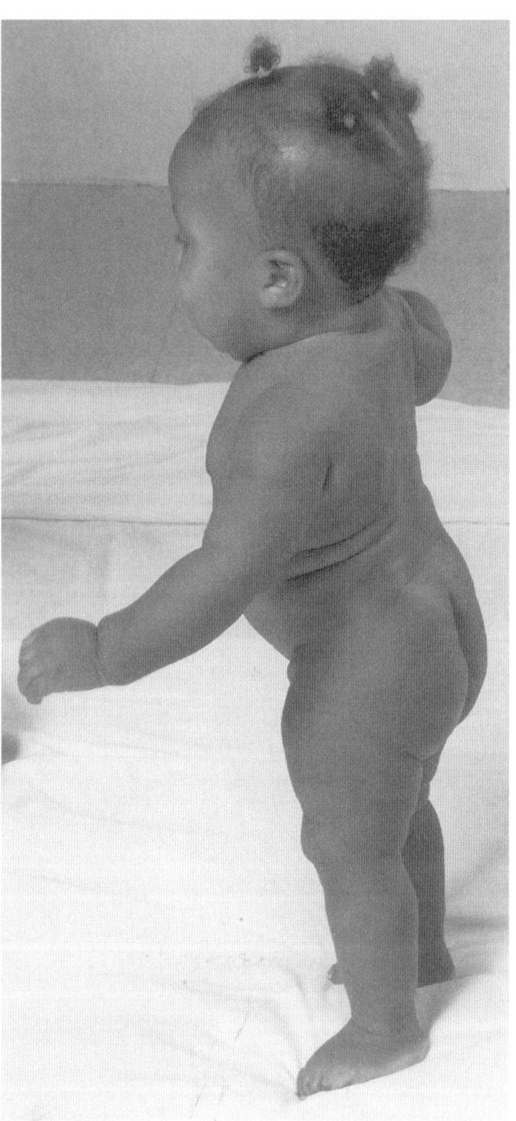

9 months: The infant takes the full weight but uses the hands on furniture to stabilize.[5] Infants who have been standing with self-support for a short time often exhibit strong ankle plantar flexion (Fig. 6-41).

Fig. 6-41.

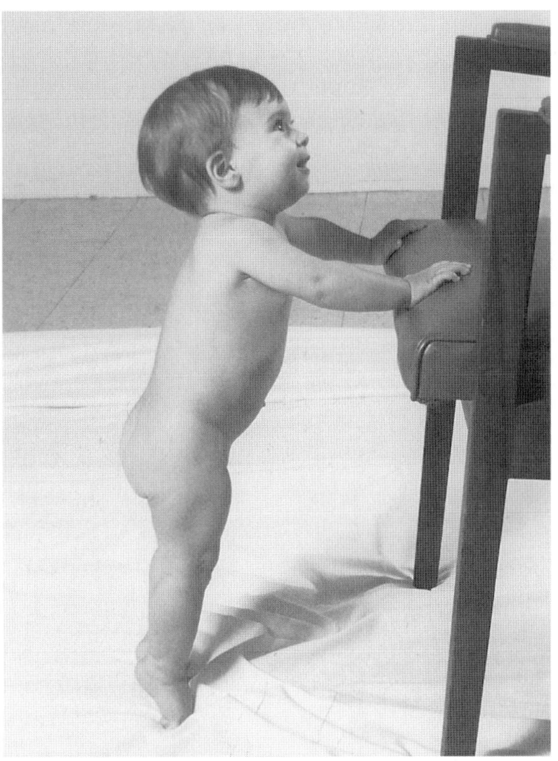

10 months: The infant practices rotation in standing, with the trunk and pelvis rotating over the face and side and causing external rotation of that leg.[5] The infant may still stand with ankle plantar flexion, but the lower extremities are more flexible (Fig. 6-42).

Fig. 6-42.

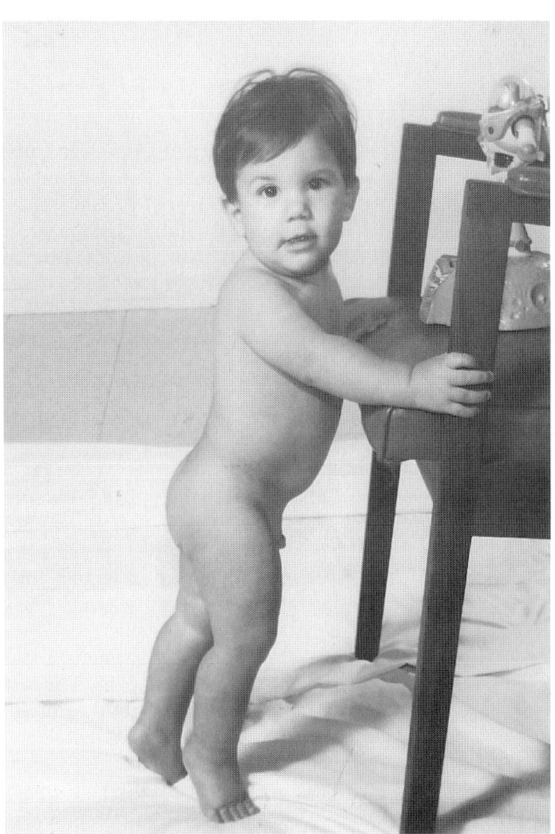

12 months: The infant stands without external support. Wide abduction is used for a stable base of support.[5] The arms often exhibit scapular adduction for upper trunk stability. The feet are placed flat on the surface (Fig. 6-43).

Fig. 6-43.

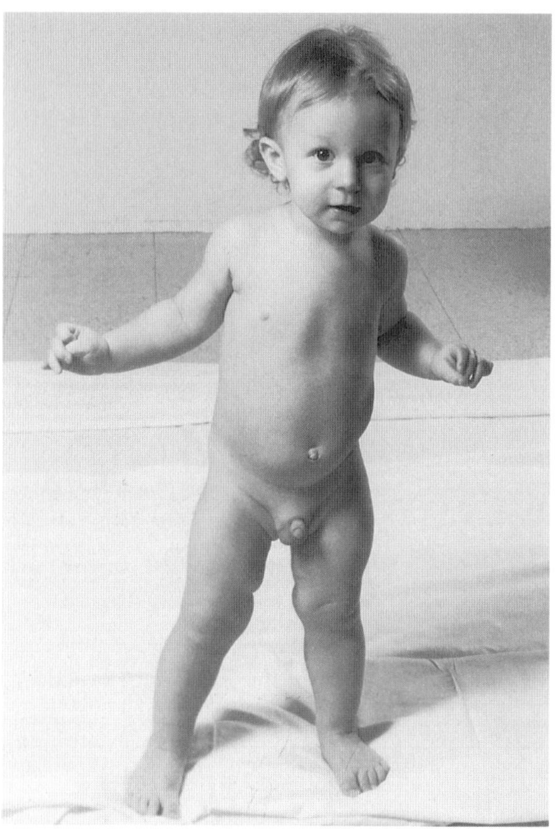

References

1. Abbott AL, Bartlett DJ, Kneale Fanning JE, et al. Infant motor development and aspects of the home environment. *Pediatr Phys Ther* 2000;12:62–67.
2. Backman E, Odenrick P, Henriksson KG, et al. Isometric muscle force and anthropometric values in normal children aged between 3.5 and 15 years. *Scand J Rehab Med* 1989; 21:105–114.
3. Barrett U, Harrison D. Comparing muscle function of children and adults: effects of scaling for muscle size. *Pediatr Exer Sci* 2002;14:369–376.
4. Bartlett DJ, Kneale Fanning JE. Relationships of equipment use and play positions to motor development at eight months corrected age of infants born preterm. *Pediatr Phys Ther* 2003; 15:8–15.
5. Blundell SW, Shepherd RB, Dean CM, et al. Functional strength training in cerebral palsy: a pilot study of a group circuit training class for children aged 4-8 years. *Clin Rehab* 2003; 17:48–57.
6. Bly L. *Motor Skills Acquisition in the First Year: An Illustrated Guide to Normal Development*. Tucson, AZ: Therapy Skill Builders, 1994.
7. Chapman D. Context effects on the spontaneous leg movements of infants with spina bifida. *Pediatr Phys Ther* 2002;14:62–73.
8. Connolly B. Testing in infants and children. In: Hislop HJ, Montgomery J, eds. *Daniels and Worthingham's Muscle Testing: Techniques of Manual Examination*, 6th ed. Philadelphia: WB Saunders, 1995, 235–260.
9. Darrah J, Wessel J, Nearingberg P, et al. Evaluation of a community fitness program for adolescents with cerebral palsy. *Pediatr Phys Ther* 1999;11:18–23.
10. Donohoe M, Bleakney DA. Arthrogryposis multiplex congenital. In: Campbell SK, ed. *Physical Therapy in Children*, 2nd ed. Philadelphia: WB Saunders, 2000:261–277.
11. Folio M, Fewell RR. *Peabody Developmental Motor Scales and Activity Cards*. Allen, TX: DLM Teachings Resources, 1983.

12. Gajdosik CG, Gajdosik RL. Musculoskeletal development adaptation. In: Campbell SK, ed. *Physical Therapy in Children*, 2nd ed. Philadelphia: WB Saunders, 2000:105–126.
13. Hinderer KA, Hinderer SR. Muscle strength development and assessment in children and adolescents. In: Harms-Ringdahl K, ed. *International Perspectives in Physical Therapy, Vol. 6: Muscle Strength*. London: Churchill Livingstone, 1993:93–140.
14. Hinderer KA, Hinderer SR, Shurtleff DB. Myelodysplasia. In: Campbell SK, ed. *Physical Therapy in Children*, 2nd ed. Philadelphia, WB Saunders, 2000;571–619.
15. Innes E. Handgrip strength testing: a review of the literature. *Aust Occup Ther J* 1999; 46:120–140.
16. Jacobson RD. Approach to the child with weakness or clumsiness. *Pediatr Clin North Am* 1998;45:145–168.
17. Johnson EW. Examination for muscle weakness in infants and small children. *JAMA* 1958;8:1306–1313
18. Knutson LM, Leavitt RL, Sarton KR. Race, ethnicity and other factors influencing children's health and disability: implications for pediatric physical therapists. *Pediatr Phys Ther* 1995;7:175–183.
19. Krefting L. The culture concept in the everyday practice of occupational and physical therapy. *Phys Occup Ther Pediatr* 1991;11:1–16
20. Lee-Volkov PM, Aaron DH, Eladoumikdachi F, et al. Measuring normal hand dexterity values in normal 3-, 4-, and 5-year-old children and their relationship with grip and pinch strength. J Hand Ther 2003; 16:22–28.
21. Lieberman LJ, McHugh E. Health-related fitness of children who are visually impaired. *J Visual Impair Blind* 2001;95:272–287.
22. Merlini L, Dell'Accio D, Granata C. Reliability of dynamic strength knee muscle testing in children. *J Orthop Sports Phys Ther* 1995;22:73–76.
23. Pitetti KH, Yarmer DA. Lower body strength of children and adolescents with and without mild mental retardation: a comparison. *Adapted Phys Act Q* 2002;19:68–81.
24. Romero PW. Trunk flexor muscle strength in healthy children 3 to 6 years old. *Pediatr Phys Ther* 1990;2:3–9.
25. Schneider JW, Gabriel KL. Congenital spinal cord injury. In: Humphrey DA, ed. *Neurological Rehabilitation*, 2nd ed. St. Louis: CV Mosby, 1990:397–389.
26. Sloan C. Review of the reliability and validity of myometry with children. *Phys Occup Ther Pediatr* 2002;22:79–93.
27. Smith MR, Danoff JV, Parks RA. Motor skill development of children with HIV infection measured with the Peabody Developmental Motor Scales. *Pediatr Phys Ther* 2002;14:74–84.
28. Stemmons Mercer V, Lewis CL. Hip abductor and knee extensor muscle strength of children with and without Down syndrome. *Pediatr Phys Ther* 2001;13:18–26.
29. Svien LR. Health-related fitness of seven- to 10-year-old children with histories of preterm birth. *Pediatr Phys Ther* 2003;15:74–83.
30. Tabin GC, Gregg JR, Bonci T. Predictive leg strength values in immediately prepubescent and postpubescent athletes. *Am J Sports Med* 1985;13:387–389.
31. Turman JE, Van Vranken T. Testing of infants, toddlers, and preschool children. In: Hislop HJ, Montgomery J, eds. *Daniels and Worthingham's Muscle Testing: Techniques of Manual Examination*, 7th ed. Philadelphia: WB Saunders, 2002, 253–288.
32. Weltman A, Tippet S. Measurements of isokinetic strength in prepuberal males. *J Orthop Sports Phys Ther* 1998;9:345–351.

7

HANDHELD DYNAMOMETRY for MUSCLE TESTING

Gary L. Soderberg, PhD, PT, FAPTA

The advent of technology, combined with data showing poor reproducibility of manual techniques and the need for more objective measures of human performance, has led to the development of various devices to measure force created by human segments, primarily during isometric conditions. The devices produced to make the desired force measurements are of small to moderate size and capable of accurately measuring relatively large forces when adequate stabilization and other technical considerations are taken into account. This chapter provides a brief historical overview of the development of handheld dynamometry (HHD) and presents the advantages, limitations, and clinical utility of the measurements. Considerations associated with the reliability, validity, and desirability of replacing force measurements with torque are discussed, and the chapter concludes with a presentation of representative values for samples of normal and patient populations.

HISTORY

In a review article about the two earliest dynamometers used to assess human muscle strength, Pearn states that the first dynamometer was developed in 1763 by Graham and Desaguliers.[115] The first study reporting the use of HHD was published in 1916, when Lovett and Martin[96] described the use of a spring balance system for muscle testing. These authors emphasized the importance of assigning quantitative values to muscle "strength" to measure progress and regression. Their system measured from 1 oz to 100 lb in their testing of 22 upper extremity muscles. They are considered by most to be the first to use what we consider today as the break test.[96] Thirty-three years later another device, the myometer, was designed, asserting that "no batteries, electronic amplifiers, or other electrical or mechanical connections for its operation" were required. For these measurements, three dynamometers were developed that were capable of recording either 0 to 5, 0 to 15, or 0 to 60 lb. Newman[111] asserted that strengths over 60 lb did not need to be measured with a gauge. Then, in the mid 1950s, two articles were published that dealt with measurements in children.[11,119]

Progress toward using HHDs continued to be slow, including two articles in the 1960s[56,83] and only four publications in the 1970s,[66,80,109,115] one being a review article focusing on two "early" dynamometers.[115] However, in the decade of the 1980s, numerous other articles were published in which some type of handheld dynamometer was used for measurements of human performance in both the normal and pathologic state.[1,2,5,7,13-17,19,21,24,27,28,31,34,35,58,69,82,100,102,113,127,135,145,146,149,152] Sixteen other articles, commonly authored, use data derived from measurements on patients with hemiparesis.[18,20,22,23,25,26,28-30,32,33,35,37,38,41,43] Obviously, during this time several different products had been introduced, primarily for use in the clinical setting.[80,112] In addition to the standard spring scale and electromechanical dynamometers, the suggestion has been made that the sphygmomanometer can be used for similar measurements.[71,76,84,124] There are many limitations associated with the use of this device, and continued use has not recently occurred.

Many of the published works have focused on the establishment of the reliability of the instrument where specific muscle groups are tested on a limited group of subjects with a relatively small age range. The literature expanded rather remarkably in the 1990s, as reported by Bohannon in 1998[51] and 2001.[53] In his latter report, he noted that electronic databases yielded 347 articles published through December 2000 in which handheld dynamometry has been used. Articles have now appeared in a broad scope of journals, requiring the type of comprehensive review of the literature included in the formulation and presentation in this chapter. Review articles also exist but are located in sources difficult to find.[40,134] As more HHDs become available to the clinician, more information will likely be readily available.

GENERAL UTILITY

Advantages

Handheld dynamometry has become useful in the clinical setting for a number of reasons, not the least of which are the technologic advances that have facilitated the development of devices that can be used with ease and with a wide range of applications. Use has now included a variety of patients, examples of which are muscular dystrophy[67,78,130,131] spinal muscular atrophy,[62,108] arthritis,[74,147] neuropathic weakness,[72,73,87,88,94] thyroid dysfunction,[64] Down syndrome,[107,110] spinal cord injury,[100,114] renal transplant candidates,[47] the elderly,[45,85] varied musculoskeletal conditions,[91,101,121,126,136,152] lower motor neuron syndromes,[116] and patients who have experienced a stroke. Special applications have also been made for the assessment of spasticity,[55,60,98] reflex-mediated changes,[92,99] for assessing "tone,"[110] and for studying the passive compliance of calf muscles as a result of the application of casting.[65] In this specific application, the examiner applies a force to the joint of interest, usually the ankle, and evaluates the effect of the motion and/or the resulting force or torque. In general, the special application of the HHD in these studies has shown high levels of reliability when force values or torque measures are assessed.[55,92,98]

Also to be considered are the measurement constraints associated with the use of manual muscle testing (MMT). For example, for the two highest grades of the MMT system, the grading is rather insensitive to differences in the ability of the body to generate torque at a joint. In one reported case, up to a 25% difference was not discriminated by the MMT. Children who had suffered from poliomyelitis had 50% deficits that were given grades of 5/5.[12] In general, the higher the torque that the patient can generate, the more difficult it will be for the clinician to distinguish differences. Furthermore, some investigators have established an overlap among different MMT values, a factor that may lead to the poor reliability for MMT at the higher grades.[2,17,70,153] Noreau and Vachon[114] have noted that "the MMT method does not seem to be sufficiently sensitive to assess muscle strength, at least for grade 4 and higher and to detect small or moderate increases of strength over the course of rehabilitation." Duyff et al.[64]

also state that HHD is "more sensitive for the detection of weakness." However, in testing 43 ambulatory patients with chronic osteoarthritis Hayes and Falconer[74] noted that HHD was questionable for weak patients even though differences were noted between HHD and MMT measurements. A more complete discussion of the reliability and validity issues associated with MMT is contained in the work of Hinderer and Hinderer.[77]

Bohannon[17] has reported that MMT values for knee extensors in patients were 69% of normal but using dynamometry these resulting values were only 48% of normal; this highlights the magnitude of the differences that can exist between the two measurement systems. In addition, as pointed out by Resnick et al.[122] in 1981 (citing a Beasley exhibit at the American Congress of Rehabilitation Medicine in 1961), different muscles require different percentages of their maximal capacity to move the respective limb segment against gravity. For example 2% of the elbow flexor muscles' capacity is used when flexing the elbow against gravity, the hip abductors require 24%, and the knee requires less than 10%.[122] Thus it is neither logical nor sound to give the muscles similar grades of 3/5 if they cannot move the segment through the range of motion against gravity. Because many of these limitations are implicit to the ordinal scale of measurement used in MMT,[3,59,83,112,128,138] more quantifiable measures, like the data yielded from the HHD, are appropriately recommended.

Limitations

Although HHDs are a convenient, portable, noninvasive, relatively quick, easy, and inexpensive way to objectively measure forces exerted as humans attempt to move, they are not without some limitations, both technical and practical. Some of the technical limitations are inherent to the design of the system. For example, in the modified sphygmomanometers, which some will not include in the HHD category, there are limitations in the upper limit of the measured force, approximately 30 kg of force (kgf), and nonlinearity at the higher end of the scale.[43]

Relative to the spring-gauge type of dynamometers, limitations exist in the upper range of possible force values. The range is determined by the specific characteristics of the dynamometer but care should be taken to establish this limit and the linearity of the system throughout the range.[34] In general the most reliable types of HHDs are those that are electromechanical in nature. They will typically have the capability of recording higher force values while maintaining linearity. The constraint is that the clinician has to ensure that the power supply is available and at the correct level required for operation.[34,137,139]

Practical limitations of HHD testing include at least some of those for which all testing applies. Subjects, both healthy and patient types, must be capable of understanding instructions. Hyperactive individuals and those with mental retardation may preclude testing, although Surberg has reported the successful testing of a group with IQs ranging from 36 to 69.[148] Also, those with disorders that preclude the generation of maximum tension may provide a limitation. Patients with cerebral palsy provide an example of this case. However, although maximum force may not be generated, the maximum effort may be readily quantified. These data may be helpful in serial evaluations or in special cases, such as in the quantification of spasticity.[55] Further, in cases where maximum cannot be generated as a result of pain or for reasons of injury exacerbation, maximum testing may be precluded. However, some cases of patients with or recovering from diseases have been documented[13,14,19,67,95,122] with dynamometry data. The very young, particularly those younger than

5 years,[62] may be difficult to test. However, some data do exist that show that HHD is applicable for those as young as 3.5 years of age.[7]

Probably the biggest limitation of the HHD is that the clinician perceives that he or she is not able to provide an adequate resistive force; thus, the contraction is not isometric and the reading is not valid. The upper limit of force that can be resisted is dependent on the age, strength, experience, and stabilizing abilities of the clinician doing the testing. Research has shown, however, that experience is not a factor but that strength of the examiner can make a difference.[44,155] Beck et al.[10] state that HHD can provide data at a precision level similar to maximal voluntary isometric contraction (MVIC) up to 20 kgf. The author of this chapter, however, believes there is no real upper limit of patient's strength that can be tested, given that the appropriate test procedures detailed later are used. Clinicians must ensure test validity by making sure that the patient is performing to his or her maximum, that shortening or lengthening (concentric and eccentric contractions, respectively) are not occurring, and that as much isolation of the muscle or muscle group being tested is being achieved. All of these are similar principles as for MMT as elucidated in Chapter 1. The following two cases will clarify:

A. A patient is supine while being tested for shoulder function at 90° of abduction of the glenohumeral joint (Fig. 7-1). The patient holds the arm in this position, and as the examiner pushes to equal the force (and torque) generated by the patient, the arm moves in the direction of adduction. Allowing this motion to occur is a test of the eccentric capability of the abductors (as well as of the scapular musculature), and not a true isometric test. This can occur when testing at any joint, but those to be particularly cautious of include those where the examiner has a large mechanical advantage (such as at the shoulder because of the long length of the humerus) and when limited range of motion may allow the passive tension of the muscle to provide a resistive force; such as occurs if too much ankle dorsiflexion is allowed and the passive tension of the gastrocsoleus group is tested rather than the active component associated with plantar flexion.

B. The knee extension force is to be measured. The examiner wishes to do so at the position of 45° from complete joint extension. When positioned to do the test the patient pushes the examiner away, as the resistive force is inadequate to "match" the resistive force produced by the quadriceps muscles as the knee is extended. Several options are available, including: (a) altering the patient's position so that the muscle is placed at a shorter length, thus decreasing the force output; (b) resorting to a cable tensiometer or an isokinetic dynamometer set at zero velocity; or (c) repositioning the subject and

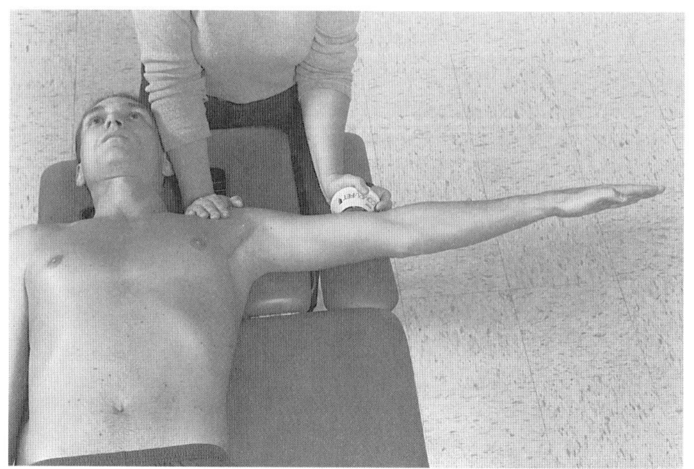

Fig. 7-1. Shoulder abduction. Resistance with a long lever arm used by therapist, increasing likelihood that muscle contraction tested will be eccentric rather than a true isometric. Note: Lever arm may be increased by moving dynamometer to wrist (not shown).

the supporting surface so that the HHD is adequately stabilized to record the force accurately. Examples include putting a second plinth directly in front of the subject to be tested, imposing the HHD between the lower leg of the subject and the second plinth, and sitting on the second plinth while the contraction is completed (Fig. 7-2). Another way to cope with this problem is to secure a strong strap around the leg of the table supporting the subject and the dynamometer (Fig. 7-3).

Resources

Availability of HHDs has improved dramatically in recent years. A list of the type of products available, the approximate cost, and the address of the

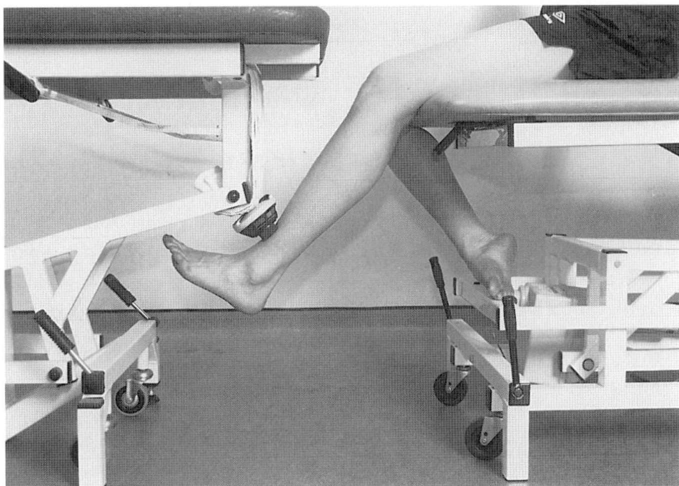

Fig. 7-2. Knee extension. Test modified to remove examiner from test because of inability of therapist to provide sufficient resistance, thus avoiding testing of a concentric contraction.

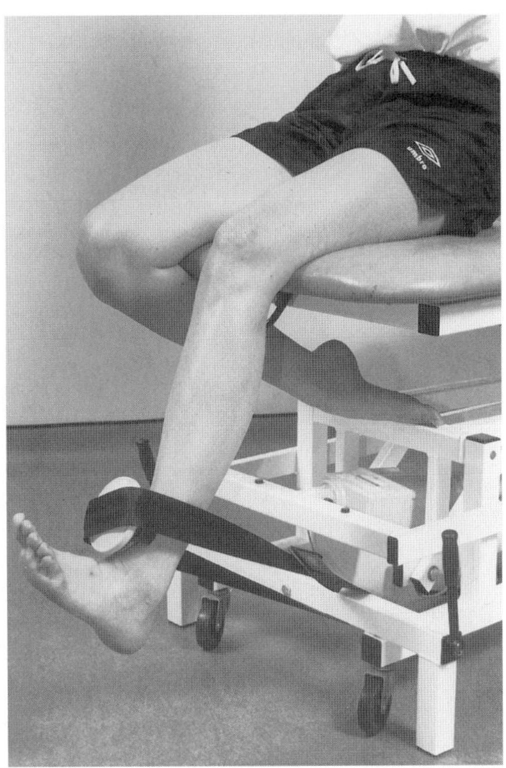

Fig. 7-3. Knee extension. Test modified differently to remove examiner from test because of inability of therapist to provide sufficient resistance, thus avoiding testing of a concentric contraction.

manufacturer is provided in Table 7-1. Further technical advances are expected to enrich the options available for clinicians and as additional reliability and other studies are published, more widespread use of the HHD is expected.

CLINICAL UTILITY

General Principles of Measurement

The rules for application of MMT also apply to any situation in which the HHD would be used. These rules are included in Chapter 1, but key points to consider with the application of HHD include the following:

Table 7-1. SOURCES FOR HAND-HELD DYNAMOMETERS

DYNAMOMETER NAME	COMPANY ADDRESS	APPROXIMATE COST
Accuforce/Ametek	Ametek, Mansfield and Green Division 8600 Somerset Dr. Largo, FL 33543	$695 and up
Baseline Push-Pull Plus Dynamometers (various others)	Best Priced Products Inc. P.O. Box 1174 White Plains, NY 10602 (800) 824-2939 www.best-pricedproducts.com	$59.00 and up
C.I.T. Hand Held Dynamometer	C.I.T. Technics BV Rijksstraatweg 384 9752 CR HAREN The Netherlands Tel.: +31 50 - 406 17 54	Unknown
Chatillon CSD 300 or 400	Chatillon Medical Products P.O. Box 35668 Greensboro, NC 27425-5668	$1,200.00 - $1,400.00
Compufet, Microfet, Ergofet	Hoggan Health Industries P.O. Box 957 12411S. 265 W. Draper, UT 84020-0957 (800) 678-7888 www.hogganhealth.com	$995.00 - $1,095.00
Jamar Grip and Pinch Gauges	Pro-Med Products 6445 Powers Ferry Road, #199 Atlanta, GA 30339 (800) 542-9297 www.promedproducts.com	$199.00 - $449.00
Lafayette Electronic Manual Muscle Tester	Pro-Med Products 6445 Powers Ferry Road, #199 Atlanta, GA 30339 (800) 542-9297 www.promedproducts.com	$795.00
Muscle Examination and Exercise Dosimeter 3000	SPARK Instruments and Academics Inc. P.O. Box 5123 Coralville, IA 52241	$445.00 and up
Penny and Giles Electronic Myometer	Penny & Giles Inc. 2716 Ocean Park Blvd., Suite 1005 Santa Monica, CA 90405 (213) 393-0014	$500.00

- Maintain consistency in test position from one test to another.[36] In some cases guidelines are available from the manufacturer of the HHD, but use good judgment because some recommendations are not well justified. Some have provided recommendations based on a specific subject population.[61,77] A standardized position for testing in your clinic is advised. Examples of test positions are provided in Figures 7-4 to 7-30.
- Ensure that the joint position is the same from test to test. Small changes can produce rather large changes in values produced because of the patient's muscle length, your position relative to the subject, and other such factors.
- Consider and account for variations in the age, sex, state of training, body mass and other factors that will influence torque.[86,141]
- Offer maximum stabilization to help ensure maximum reliability.
- Have the same therapist perform all testing, at least within a patient unless you have established intertherapist reliability with the HHD in your clinical setting. Gain experience before you begin testing patients and expect to get acceptable reliability.
- Perform a number of trials depending on how consistent (reliable) you are. No or very limited variability requires only one measurement.[42] If you are inexperienced, take the mean of two or three measurements. Ideally, perform the necessary procedures and subsequent statistics to establish that you are reliable. If you want all in your clinic to be reliable (intratherapist), you need to collect the data and do the statistics. Note: one study showed that variability within a group of novice HHD users was lower when the mean of three repeated measurements was compared with the highest of the three measures.[154]
- Test in gravity-eliminated positions whenever possible. Without eliminating the effect of gravity, there are forces (such as the segment mass of your subject) that are unaccounted for in the values you record. Avoid the problem of incorporating them in your measurement by using gravity-eliminated positions.[139] If you test in other positions recognize the implications for not accounting for gravity.
- **Apply the dynamometer at a known location. The HHD will record force at that location, and if you vary the location, you will get a different value even if the subject is generating the same force in the muscle you are testing. This is because the patient is generating a torque at the joint, but you are measuring force. To be able to compare across subjects, you need to know the distance at which your measurements were taken so you can multiply the force from the HHD times the distance to give you the torque value (torque = force × perpendicular distance of the force to the joint center). One study has reported that reliability of measurements tended to be higher when the HHD was placed at sites farther from the joint center of rotation.[105] CALCULATING THE TORQUE IS THE ONLY MEANINGFUL WAY TO COMPARE ACROSS SUBJECTS. USE THE DISTANCE.[139]**
- Apply the dynamometer perpendicularly to the segment of the patient. If you do not, the force will not be the true value. In addition, you will make it harder on yourself (i.e., you will have to apply more force as a resistance) if you do not apply the force perpendicularly. Not doing so will invalidate your measurement.[4,139] This point is just as important as the previous one.
- Ensure that the test is truly isometric, otherwise the values will be incorrect, as discussed in earlier sections of this chapter.[31,37,119]
- Apply the force for 3 to 5 seconds, although the amount of time for the actual trial is somewhat arbitrary. This duration allows for the generation of the tension and the reaching of the maximum state. Both "break" and "make" tests have been used, although there is some evidence against using the "make" type of test.[81] Intertrial time is also not specified, 20 to 30 seconds is the approximate standard.

Applicability Relative to Issues of Reliability and Validity

With the advent of any new measurement system, the focus of evaluation of the technique should be on reliability of the measures obtained.[143] This has been the case for the handheld dynamometer, in that numerous studies have evaluated a number of instruments under a variety of conditions. The differences between each of the published works lead to difficulties in generalization of the reliability of the instrument when applied to any situation, thus the following paragraphs summarize the state of knowledge regarding this matter.

Several types of reliability are important, including intrarater, interrater, and intersession comparisons. In the first case, comparisons are made within raters, as compared with the interrater situation in which comparisons are made between raters or clinicians. We would expect that the reliability, or the reproducibility of the data, would be better for the former because there are no individual differences such as stature and experience to influence the measurement. Evaluation of Tables 7-2 and 7-3 show several things. First, numerous studies have addressed the issue of reliability of HHD. The intratester (intrarater) values are relatively high and would be considered acceptable by most, within the constraints of each of the studies. Although there are differences in the values, partly due to the type of statistics used, generalization of the results indicates that intratester reliability reaches acceptable levels to be used in the clinical setting.

Evaluation of the studies in which intertester reliability has been assessed leads to the conclusion that the values are lower, in some cases unacceptable. A partial listing of studies was published by Bohannon.[52] However, because experience is a factor in reliability many of the lower values may be caused by this factor alone. Muscle tested and the relatively low number of subjects per study may also account for the values. In general, testing by a number of therapists becomes more questionable but is dependent on what is tested, the experience and strength of the clinician and other factors. It is always best to establish intertherapist reliability if the data are to be useful for purposes of reporting, either to the insurance company or to the literature.

Intersession data, shown in Table 7-4, are typically derived from a protocol that uses the same examiner(s) after a period of time has elapsed. Thus the values are high, similar as for the intratester values of Table 7-2, because the same examiner has been used. Note should be made, however, that overall a few muscles have been evaluated in a few subjects.

Another interest is the relationship of the data from the HHD in comparison with other instruments or manual techniques that measure force and/or preferably use the force value to convert to a torque. More limited work has been completed in this arena.[17,38,39,46,50,57,63,104,118,120,144,151] Only one study was located that related dynamometer values to function.[48] Considerable differences exist across studies as to the equipment used, the variables tested and the actual measurements being taken. Briefly, Bohannon[39] has shown an interinstrument correlation of 0.80 for a HHD with a Cybex II isokinetic device when the knee extensors of 20 healthy women were tested. Sullivan had similar results in healthy male subjects for the motion of shoulder external rotation.[146] Still another group established Pearson correlation coefficients of 0.72 to 0.85 between elbow and knee flexion and extension strength measurements derived by HHD versus a Lido isokinetic dynamometer.[120] Others have shown that HHD indicated weak knee extensor muscles in patients with osteoarthritis compared with manual muscle test scores of good. The Kendall tau correlation coefficient between the two measurement techniques was 0.24.[74]

Table 7-2. INTRARATER RELIABILITY STUDIES WITH HAND-HELD DYNAMOMETERS

REFERENCE	SAMPLE	STATISTIC	JOINTS TESTED	RESULT
Andrews et al (1996)[4]	156 healthy	ICC[82]	13 upper and lower extremities	.93 - .98
Bohannon (1990a)[36]	24 healthy	ICC	Elbow extension	.98
Bohannon (1990c)[39]		ICC	Knee extension	.95
Bohannon (1990e)[41]	30 neurology patients	r	18 muscle groups	.84 - .99 except shoulder & hip abduction
Bohannon (1989)[33]	stroke patients	r	Knee extension	.99 paretic and non paretic
Byl et al (1988)[58]	27 healthy	r	Deltoid and biceps	.83 - .94 deltoid .93 - .96 biceps
Riddle et al (1989)[127]	15 brain damaged patients	ICC	Knee extension	.88 - .98 paretic and non paretic
Sexton (1994)[132]	52 healthy	ICC	Hip flexion	.71 - .83
Wadsworth et al (1987)[153]	11 patients	r	5 muscle groups	.69 - .90
Stuberg and Metcalf (1988)[145]	14 healthy, 14 muscular dystrophy	r	Knee ext, hip ext, elbow flex, shoulder abduction	.74 - .99 healthy .83 - .99 patients
Hyde (1983)[82]	12 muscular dystrophy	CV	6 muscle groups	4.6 hip flexors to 15.7 hip abd
Mendall and Florence (1990)[106]	30 muscular dystrophy	r	4 muscle groups	.71 - .95 5-9 y.o. .84 - .97 9-12 .91 - 1.0 12-16
Wilkolm and Bohannon (1991)[155]	27 healthy	ICC	Shoulder ext rot, elbow flexion, knee extension	.64 - .98 inter-session; above .78 intrasession (except two)
Surberg et al (1992)[148]	10 mild-mod mentally retarded	ICC	Knee ext, elbow flexion	.97 - .99
Hsieh and Phillips (1990)[81]	30 healthy	r	Iliopsoas, pectoralis major, hip ext rot	.55 - .76 method 1 .96 - .99 method 2
Deones et al (1994)[63]	21 knee injured	ICC	Knee extension	.95 at 0 degrees .93 at 60 degrees
Rheault et al (1989)[123]	20 healthy	r	Wrist extensors and flexors	.91 extensors .85 flexors
Bäckman et al (1989)[7]	10 healthy children	CV	Elbow flexion, dorsiflexors	6% dorsiflexors 12% elbow flexors
Hayes and Falconer (1992)[74]	43 osteoarthritis patients	ICC	Knee extensors	.89 - .98
May et al (1997)[100]	25 spinal cord injured	ICC	Shoulder internal and external rotation	.89 - .96 internal .89 - .94 external
Bohannon et al (1995)[47]	110 renal transplant candidates	ICC	Knee extension	.98 - .99
Horvat et al (1994)[79]	17 moderately mentally retarded	ICC	Elbow flexion and extension	.83 - .86 extension .83 - .85 flexion
McMahon et al (1992)[105]	30 healthy young	ICC	Multiple joints	.88 shoulder abd .88 hip flexors .80 wrist extension .86 ankle dorsiflex
Mercer and Lewis (2001)[107]	17 healthy and 17 Downs syndrome	ICC	Hip abductor and knee extensor	.94 Down hip abduction, .94 healthy .89 Down knee extensor, .95 healthy

Continued

Table 7-2. INTRARATER RELIABILITY STUDIES WITH HAND-HELD DYNAMOMETERS—cont'd

REFERENCE	SAMPLE	STATISTIC	JOINTS TESTED	RESULT
Schwartz et al (1992)[129]	122 quadriplegics	Spearman r	Biceps and extensor carpi radialis (ECR)	.80 - .86 biceps one week .92 - .94 ECR
Scott et al (1982)[131]	61 muscular dystrophy	Unspecified r	Knee extension	.91
Reinking et al (1996)[121]	10 healthy	ICC	Knee extension	.92
Bohannon (1997)[49]	231 healthy	ICC	Multiple joints, dominant and non-dominant	all >.94
Bohannon (1996)[48]	13 elderly, mixed pathologies	ICC	Knee extension	.87 - .98
Bohannon and Wikholm (1992)[44]	24 healthy	ICC	Knee extension	.96 experienced .95 inexperienced
Richardson et al (1998)[125]	20 healthy older	ICC	Elbow and knee extension	.88 elbow make, .94 break .89 knee make, .95 break
Goonetilleke et al (1994)[72]	19 motor neuron disease	r	Multiple joints	>.95 or all conditions
Karner et al (1998)[85]	15 older nursing home	ICC	Ankle	.86 - .92, two motions combined
Richardson et al (1997)[126]	6 healthy	ICC	Elbow extension	.89 - .98 make .68 - .98 break
Merlini et al (2002)[108]	33 spinal muscular atrophy	ICC	Elbow flexion, knee extension/flexion, ankle dorsiflexion	.98 elbow .97 knee flexion .93 knee extension .91 ankle dorsiflexion
Leggin et al (1996)[93]	17 healthy	ICC	Shoulder abduction, internal/external rotation	.94 - .97 internal .89 - .95 external .84 - .96 abduction
Kilmer et al (1997)[87]	11 healthy, 10 neuropathy patients	ICC	Multiple joints	.89 - .97 upper extremity, .63 ankle dorsiflexors, .82 - .89 knee extensors
Hsieh and Phillips (1990)[81]	30 young healthy	r	Pectoralis major, hip flexion and external rotators	.90 - .97 pectoralis major .89 - .96 hip flexion .84 - .95 hip external rotators
Balogun et al (1998)[9]	20 healthy young	ICC	Shoulder flexors, abductors, elbow flexors and extensors	.86 - .93 shoulder abductors, .87 - .94 shoulder flexors, .80 - .85 elbow flexors, .75 - .84 elbow extensors

Table 7-3. INTERRATER RELIABILITY STUDIES WITH HAND-HELD DYNAMOMETERS

REFERENCE	SAMPLE/ #TESTORS	STATISTIC	JOINTS TESTED	RESULT
Agre (1987)[1]	8 adults/3	r	8 upper & lower extremity	.85 - .99 upper –.20 - .96 lower
Andrews et al (1996)[4]	9 healthy adults/3	ICC	8 upper & lower extremity	.51 - .95
Bäckman et al (1989)[7]	11 children/4	CV	Elbow and 3 lower extremity	8 - 11%
Bohannon and Andrews (1987)[27]	30 neurology patients/2	r	Multiple upper and lower extremity	.84 - .94; means sig different for two
Bohannon and Wikholm (1992)[44]	24 healthy	ICC	Knee extension	.95
Hyde et al (1983)[82]	14 children/3	ANOVA	Knee ext, shoulder abd	no sig difference
Kaegi et al (1998)[84]				
Kilmer et al (1997)[87]				
Rheault et al (1989)[123]	20 healthy adults/3	r	Wrist extensors and flexors	.89 - .95 exts .90 - .93 flexors
Puharic and Bohannon (1993)[117]	24 healthy	ICC	Pronation, supination of dominant, non-dominant	.90 - .95 pronation .97 - .98 supination
Sexton (1994)[132]	52 healthy/2	ICC	Hip flexion	.35 - .42
Surberg et al (1992)[148]	10 mild-mod mentally retarded	ICC	Knee extension, elbow flexion	.97 - .98 for both
Hseih and Phillips (1990)[81]	30 healthy	r	Iliopsoas, pec major, hip ext rot	.59 - .77 method 1 .95 - .96 method 2
Bohannon et al (1995)[47]	110 renal transplant candidates	ICC	Knee extension	.95 - .96
McMahon et al (1992)[105]	30 healthy young	ICC	Multiple joints	.83 shoulder abd .76 hip flexors .31 wrist extension .55 ankle dorsiflex
Richardson et al (1998)[125]	20 healthy older	ICC	Elbow and knee extension	.87 elbow make, .87 break .67 knee make, .74 break
Richardson et al (1997)[126]	6 healthy	ICC	Elbow extension	.67 make .69 break
Kwoh et al (1997)[91]	44 total hip or knee arthro-plasty	Kappa	Knee extension	.94
Kimura et al (1996)[89]	12 healthy			
Merlini et al (2002)[108]	33 spinal muscular atrophy	ICC	Elbow flexion, knee extension/flexion, ankle dorsiflexion	.98 elbow .95 knee flexion .88 knee extension .69 ankle dorsi-flexion
Leggin et al (1996)[93]	17 healthy	ICC	Shoulder abduction, internal/external rotation	.90 internal .94 external .79 abduction
Wilkolm and Bohannon (1991)[155]	27 healthy	ICC	Shoulder ext rot, elbow flexion, knee extension	.93 shoulder ext rotation .78 elbow flexion .23 knee extension
Byl et al (1988)[58]	27 healthy	r	Deltoid and biceps	.84 deltoid .66 biceps

Continued

Table 7-3. INTERRATER RELIABILITY STUDIES WITH HAND-HELD DYNAMOMETERS—cont'd

REFERENCE	SAMPLE/ #TESTORS	STATISTIC	JOINTS TESTED	RESULT
Kilmer et al (1997)[87]	11 healthy, 10 neuropathy patients	ICC	Multiple joints	.72 - .96 upper extremity, .38 ankle dorsiflexors, .53 - .84 knee extensors
Escolar et al (2001)[68]	12 ambulatory children with neuromuscular disease	ICC	Knee extension ankle dorsiflexion elbow flexion	.84 - .97 knee extensors .56 - .88 ankle dorsiflexors .93 - .98 elbow flexion
Balogun et al (1998)[9]	20 healthy young	ICC	Shoulder flexors, abductors, elbow flexors and extensors	.95 shoulder abductors, .96 shoulder flexors, .83 elbow flexors, .86 elbow extensors

Table 7-4. INTERSESSION RELIABILITY STUDIES WITH HAND-HELD DYNAMOMETRY

REFERENCE	SAMPLE	STATISTIC	JOINTS TESTED	RESULT
Bäckman et al (1989)[7]	24 children	CV	10 upper and lower extremity muscles	6 - 16 %
Bohannon (1986)[16]	30 neurologic patients	r	18 upper and lower extremity	.97 - .98
Riddle et al (1989)[127]	15 brain damaged	ICC	Numerous muscle groups	.90 - .98 paretic .31 - .93 non paretic
Stuberg and Metcalf (1988)[145]	14 healthy, 14 muscular dystrophy	r ANOVA	Eight muscle groups	.83 - .99 patients .74 - .89 healthy no sig differences
Sullivan et al (1988)[146]	14 healthy	r	Shoulder external rotation	.99
Wiles and Karni (1983)[154]	20 neuromuscular patients	median error	Knee extension	%
Boiteau et al (1995)[55]	10 children with cerebral palsy	ICC	Passive ankle dorsiflexion	.79 low velocity .90 high velocity
Hsieh and Phillips (1990)[81]	30 young healthy	r	Pectoralis major, hip flexion and external rotators	.91 - .96 pectoralis major .86 - .95 hip flexion .89 - .94 hip external rotators
Balogun et al (1998)[9]	20 healthy young	ICC	Shoulder abductors and flexors, elbow flexors and extensors	.91 - 97 shoulder abductors, .95 - .97 shoulder flexors, .86 - .94 elbow flexors, .72 - .90 elbow extensors

Deones and co-workers have also found that the HHD and isokinetic dynamometer data were significantly correlated when judged by the Pearson product moment correlation coefficient. However, the HHD did not differentiate an injured from an uninjured leg, as did the isokinetic test. Tester strength, stabilization, the lack of including the effect of gravity, and pain were all considered to have an effect.[63] Each of these factors was discussed in an earlier section of this chapter that deals with HHD principles of operation and testing. Another group also compared two HHD values with the data derived from an isokinetic dynamometer operating in an isometric mode. One of the HHD devices had significantly lower scores (mean kgf, 12.5 versus 7.5) than the other HHD, leading to differences between the lowest scoring HHD and the isometric value derived from the isokinetic device.[150] However, in this study no calibration of the HHDs was completed prior to data collection. Thus these results reflect the need to calibrate any device that is used to take a measurement, otherwise, testing for comparative purposes is not justified.

Based on the two preceding paragraphs, HHD generally appears to have concurrent validity (i.e., scores are comparable with those derived from other testing procedures). Furthermore, because the HHD is able to detect the force exerted against it as the result of contraction of muscles that create a mechanical effect the device is considered to have face validity. Predictive validity is less established, but some studies support that this type of validity also exists.[23,25,32]

VALUES

Normative

For comparison with healthy subjects, the clinician needs to have a set of normative values available. Whereas quite a number of normative values are available, they are for isokinetic, fixed, or handgrip dynamometers. However, several articles have published values for data collected with the HHD. Each is limited, however, in terms of the sample from which the data are collected. For example, Bächman et al. studied children between ages 3.5 and 15[7] and between the ages of 17 and 70.[8] Another data set includes women between the ages of 20 and 40.[15] Van der Ploeg has one of the more comprehensive sets of data from 50 female and 50 male subjects between the ages of 20 and 60.[151] However, in a number of cases, the subjects exceeded the recording capability of the dynamometer used in the study. In 1996, Andrews et al.[4] published a listing of normative values for 77 men and 70 women subjects. The range of ages tested was 50 to 79 years. Mean values and regression equations are published for 13 joint motions, eight in the upper extremities and five in the lower extremities.

As has been discussed in earlier parts of this chapter, the position of the dynamometer is critical to the value recorded. In all instances, the dynamometer should be placed perpendicular to the limb segment to which it is applied. A more important consideration is the location of the HHD from the axis around which rotation is being attempted. The articles cited in the previous paragraph contain location information, at least in a generalized form. For example, citations are typically "just proximal to" a specified anatomic location such as condyles or processes. Although using this procedure may prove adequate for values used within a patient or one particular setting, the force value alone offers no ability to make comparisons across measures. In fact, an analysis of data of Andrews versus those of van der Ploeg shows considerable discrepancies in the values, although virtually identical landmarks were used in the two studies.[4,151] For example the van der Ploeg data show that for an average age of 34.4 years, the men had a fiftieth centile score of 156 N for elbow extensors.[151] The Andrews et al.[4] data show the value for the 50-year-old group as 178 and 188 N, respectively, for the dominant and nondominant arms. In general the differences appear to be fairly large, particularly for the male groups, even if subject age, body mass, and other factors are considered. If segment lengths of subjects differed, if the HHD was placed in a slightly different location, or if the test position was different, the resultant force would be different. Thus comparison is limited. Other examples of work where dynamometer location is not exactly noted are in the works of Bohannon,[54] Merlini et al.,[108] Reinking et al.,[121] Bohannon,[48] and Mascal et al.[102] This is unfortunate because without noting the exact location the measure cannot be converted to a torque, which is the only way to allow for comparable measurements across patients, joints and studies.[140] Conversions across different units are easily made.[139]

In summary, whereas normative data have some value, a better course of action is to record the force value and multiply by the distance at which the HHD is perpendicularly placed on the segment. With this technique, the location of the HHD does not matter, as the magnitude of the force will vary as the distance changes. Thus the resulting measure is torque. (These principles are exactly the reason why the clinician chooses to place the HHD as far from the joint axis as possible, as the magnitude of force required for the resistance decreases as the distance from the joint center increases.)

Clinical Relevance

Collection of information about the ability of the patient to exert joint torque can be a valuable asset in practice. Objective, repeatable HHD measurements (except possibly for ankle motions) are a cornerstone of any quality practice, and the methods detailed in this chapter should be a valuable asset to any clinician. Data from initial assessments can be compared with data collected during repeat evaluations, thus providing information about the need for continued patient care or for indicating the need for a home exercise program. Comparison of torque data with healthy subjects can also serve as an indicator for the need for continued care. Reference values have become available as a result of a recent meta-analysis that included a large number of publications in the review process.[141] Documented changes in the ability of patients to exert torques can also be submitted to third-party payers, providing contrasts and relevant comparisons to indicate the necessity for continued patient care. There are no limitations on the number of joints, the number of motions, or the number of joint angles at which data can be derived, thus providing the capability for a comprehensive analysis of patient function.

Few studies that have used HHD have reported data as torque. However, as noted earlier in this chapter, this is the preferred practice, in spite of the fact that most studies have historically reported only force. It is noteworthy that the electromechanical dynamometers, such as the Biodex (Biodex Medical Systems, Shirley, NY) and the previously manufactured Kin-Com (Chattanooga Corporation, Chattanooga, TN), Cybex (Cybex Corporation, Ronkonkoma, NY) and Lido (Loredan Biomedical Inc., Davis, California), provide data in torque. Why persistence exists for recording only the force is perplexing. If an article in the literature provides a distance at which the HHD is placed then the torque can be calculated. However, if the location is given as "just proximal to the malleoli," there is a dependence on the length of the leg in determining the torque value. The studies that have reported data as torque while using HHD are represented in Table 7-5. In some cases only a sample of the available data is included. Full reporting on these and most other studies using all types of

Table 7-5. SUMMARY OF TORQUE VALUES FROM STUDIES USING HAND-HELD DYNAMOMETRY

REFERENCE	GENDER	AGE	N	MOVEMENT	TEST POSITION	PEAK/MEAN TORQUE (Nm)
Magnussen et al (1994)[97]	m	24	26	Shoulder internal rotation	Forearm prone, shoulder abducted 90°, elbow 90°	48
				Shoulder external rotation	Same	44
				Shoulder abduction	Sit, shoulder in "scaption" internal rotation	79
Sullivan et al (1988)[146]	m	18	26	Shoulder external rotation	Supine, shoulder abducted 90°	47
Askew et al (1987)[6]	m/f	41/45	50/50	Elbow flexion	Shoulder abducted, elbow 90°, forearm "0"	71/33
				Elbow extension	Same	41/21
				Pronation	Same	7/4
				Supination	Same	9/4
Mathiowetz et al (1985)[104]	m/f	20-24	29/26	Grip	Shoulder abducted 0°, elbow 90°	121/70
		35-39	25/24	Tip pinch	Same	18/12
		55-59	21/24	Key pinch	Same	24/16
		75+	25/25	Palmar pinch	Same	19/12
KRAMER et al (1991)[90]	f	24	20	Hip abduction	Supine, hip abducted 10°	49
	f	68	20	Hip abduction	Same	77
Mercer et al (2001)[107]	m/f	7-15	17 healthy, 17 Down syndrome	Hip abduction knee extension	Hip-supine knee-sitting	40 hip, 46 knee for Down syndrome; 70 hip, 98 knee for healthy
Kilmer et al (1997)[87]	m/f m/f	55 47-59	5/6 healthy 3/7 hereditary neuropathy	Multiple joints	Supine: shoulder flexors and abductors, elbow motions, ankle dorsiflexion seated: wrist motions and knee extensors and flexors prone: shoulder extensors	M Ctrl HN SF 62 40 SE 42 24 SIR 32 27 SER 25 20 SA 76 52 EF 52 36 EE 37 26 WF 14 8 WE 11 5 KF 77 40 KE 128 73 AD 24 6
Bohannon (1990)[38]	m/f	69	13/13 post stroke	Knee extension	Seated	50 paretic 108 non-paretic
Suomi and Collier (2003)[147]	m/f	64-68	22 osteoarthritis 8 rheumatoid	Shoulder abduction, hip abduction	Referenced to previous work	ctrl=31 shoulder abduction, 69 hip abduction
Hedengren et al (2001)[75]	m/f	107	11 juvenile chronic arthritis 14 healthy	knee extension and flexion, ankle dorsi and plantar flexion	supine for knee, sitting for ankle	KE 21 JCA Ctrl KF 28 JCA Ctrl AD 8 JCA Ctrl AP 12 JCA 11 Ctrl

Abbreviations: M=motion; Ctrl=control; HN=hereditary neuropathy; SF=shoulder flexion; SE=shoulder extension; SIR and SER=shoulder internal and external rotation; SA=shoulder abduction; EF and EE=elbow flexion and extension; WF and WE=wrist flexion and extension; KF and KE=knee extension and flexion; AD=ankle dorsiflexion; AP=ankle plantarflexion.; JCA=juvenile chronic arthritis
Note: grip, tip, key and palmar pinch values are in kilograms force

dynamometry in testing normal subjects, patients, and special populations such as athletes is available in *The Clinician's Torque Manual*.[142]

SUMMARY

Handheld dynamometry is developing as an important part of science as applied to practice. The data have relevance for determining patient function prior to, during, or as the result of intervention. Instruments have been developed to objectively measure isometric forces as joint torques are produced. Recording is usually done via manual resistance at the distal end of a segment. This force value can and should be used in the subsequent calculation of the torque produced at human joints. Studies have established a high reliability of the measures within tester and within session. Within or between therapist ratings vary from poor to strong depending on joint tested, the experience of the examiner and other factors. As more therapists use this technique to objectively measure the capabilities of their patients, the literature will continue to contain more and more data. Normative values of the derived torque values will ultimately elucidate true weaknesses and the subsequent improvements that will be produced by effective treatment.

■ SCAPULAR ELEVATION

UPPER TRAPEZIUS, LEVATOR SCAPULAE

Patient position: Prone with arms at sides and shoulder to be tested completely elevated; head should not be rotated to either side (Fig. 7-4).

Fig. 7-4.

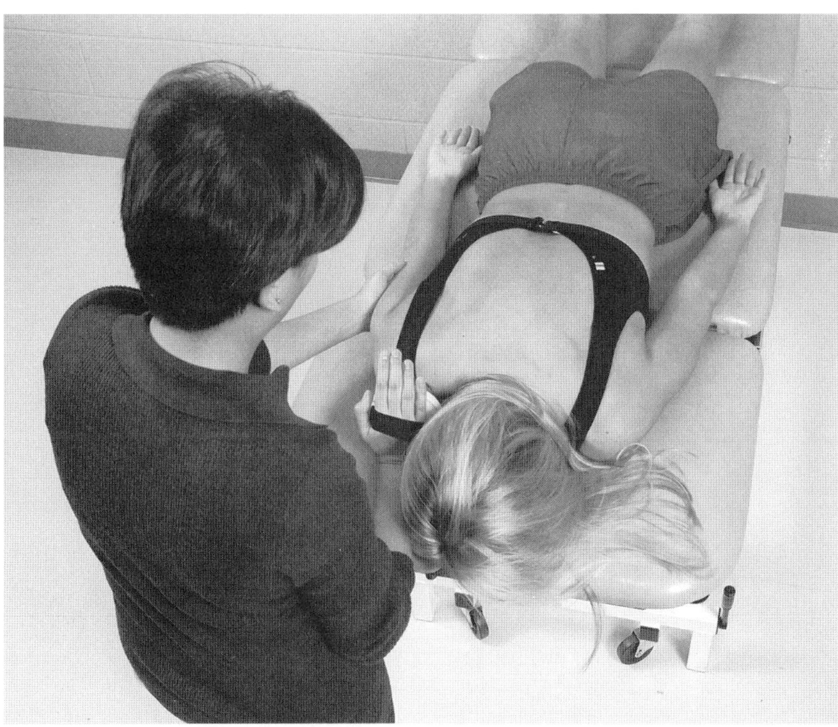

Stabilization: Stabilization is unnecessary.

Examiner command: "Hold your shoulder in that position and don't let me move it."

Dynamometer placement/resistance: Dynamometer is placed over superior aspect of acromion process of scapula. Same dynamometer placement should be used each time patient is tested so that consistency can be maintained across trials and testing sessions. Resistance is applied perpendicular to acromion in direction of scapular depression. Resistance is maintained for 3 to 5 seconds (Fig. 7-4).

■ SCAPULAR ADDUCTION

MIDDLE TRAPEZIUS

Patient position: Seated with scapula adducted and shoulder abducted to 90° and in neutral rotation, and elbow flexed. Upper extremity should be supported on a firm, smooth surface (Fig. 7-5).

Fig. 7-5.

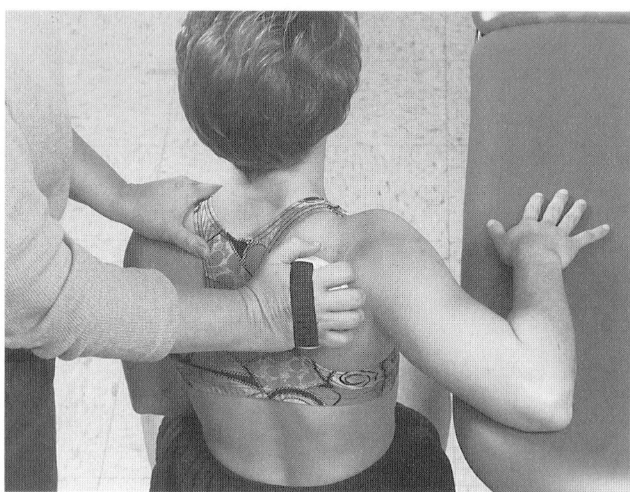

Stabilization: Over superior aspect of contralateral shoulder to prevent trunk rotation (Fig. 7-5).

Examiner command: "Hold your shoulder in that position and don't let me move it."

Dynamometer placement/resistance: Dynamometer is placed on lateral aspect of scapula near lateral border. (This location should be marked with a skin pencil and distance from thoracic spinous processes measured and recorded so that consistency can be maintained across trials and testing sessions.) Resistance is applied perpendicular to scapula in direction of scapular abduction and is held for 3 to 5 seconds (Fig. 7-5).

■ SHOULDER FLEXION

ANTERIOR DELTOID, CORACOBRACHIALIS

Patient position: Side lying with shoulder flexed 90° and in neutral rotation and elbow extended. Arm to be tested should be uppermost and supported on a smooth, flat surface (e.g. a powder board) (Fig. 7-6).

Fig. 7-6.

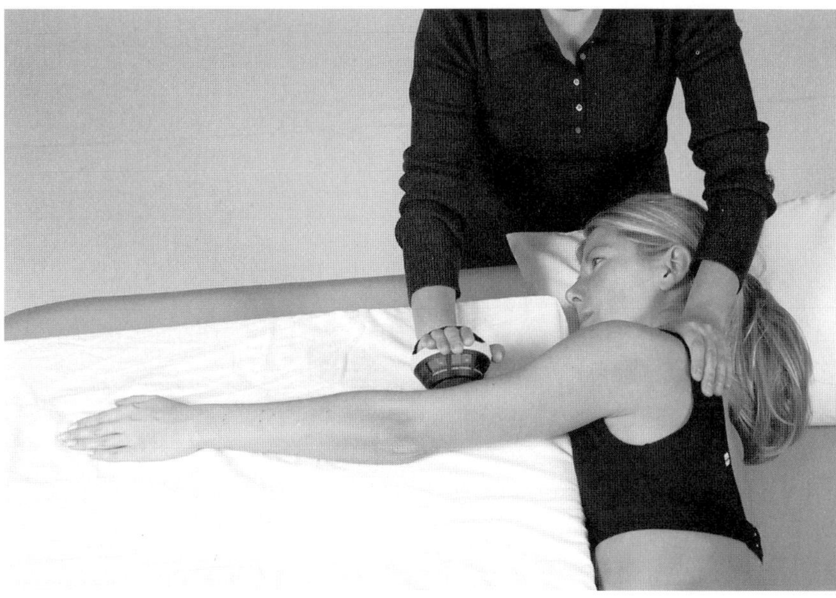

Stabilization: Over superior aspect of ipsilateral shoulder, taking care to avoid pressure over anterior fibers of deltoid (Fig. 7-6).

Examiner command: "Hold your arm in that position and don't let me move it."

Dynamometer placement/resistance: Dynamometer is placed on anterior aspect of distal humerus just proximal to elbow. (This location should be marked with a skin pencil and distance from acromion process measured and recorded so that consistency can be maintained across trials and testing sessions.) Resistance is applied perpendicular to humerus in direction of shoulder extension and is held for 3 to 5 seconds (Fig. 7-6).

■ SHOULDER EXTENSION

LATISSIMUS DORSI, TERES MAJOR, POSTERIOR DELTOID

Patient position: Side lying with shoulder extended 45° and in full medial rotation, elbow extended. Arm to be tested should be uppermost and supported on a smooth, flat surface (e.g., a powder board) (Fig. 7-7).

Fig. 7-7.

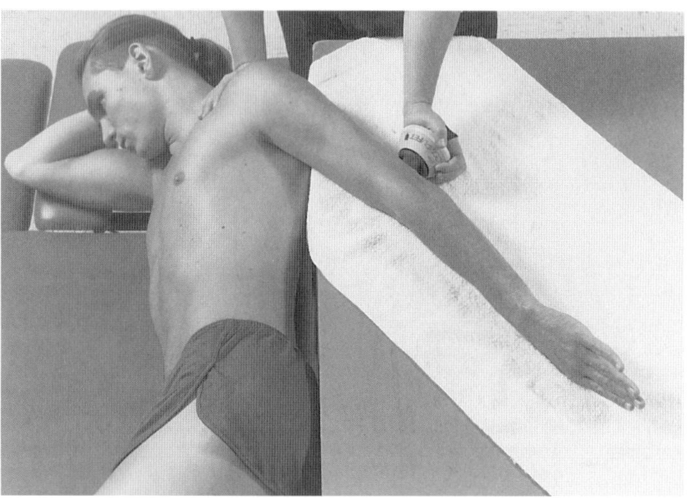

Stabilization: Over superior aspect of ipsilateral shoulder (Fig. 7-7).

Examiner action: "Hold your arm in this position and don't let me move it."

Dynamometer placement/resistance: Dynamometer is placed on dorsal aspect of distal humerus just proximal to elbow. (Location should be marked with a skin pencil and distance from olecranon process measured and recorded so that consistency can be maintained across trials and testing sessions.) Resistance is applied perpendicular to humerus in direction of shoulder flexion and is held for 3 to 5 seconds (Fig. 7-7).

■ SHOULDER ABDUCTION

MIDDLE DELTOID, SUPRASPINATUS

Patient position: Supine with shoulder abducted 90° and in neutral rotation, elbow extended (Fig. 7-8).

Fig. 7-8.

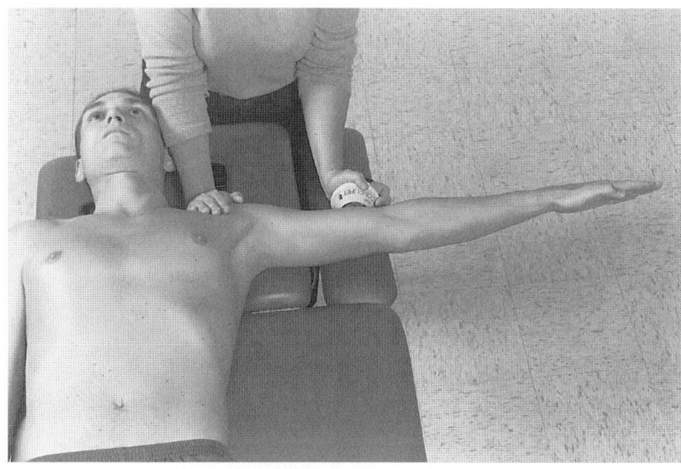

Stabilization: Over superior aspect of ipsilateral shoulder, avoiding pressure over middle deltoid (Fig. 7-8).

Examiner command: "Hold your arm in this position and don't let me move it."

Dynamometer placement/resistance: Dynamometer is placed on lateral aspect of distal humerus just proximal to elbow. (Location should be marked with a skin pencil and distance from olecranon process measured and recorded so that consistency can be maintained across trials and testing sessions.) Resistance is applied perpendicular to humerus in direction of shoulder adduction and is held for 3 to 5 seconds (Fig. 7-8).

■ SHOULDER HORIZONTAL ABDUCTION

POSTERIOR DELTOID

Patient position: Seated with shoulder abducted to 90° and in full horizontal abduction, humerus in neutral rotation, and elbow flexed to 90°. Upper extremity should be supported on a smooth, firm surface (Fig. 7-9).

Fig. 7-9.

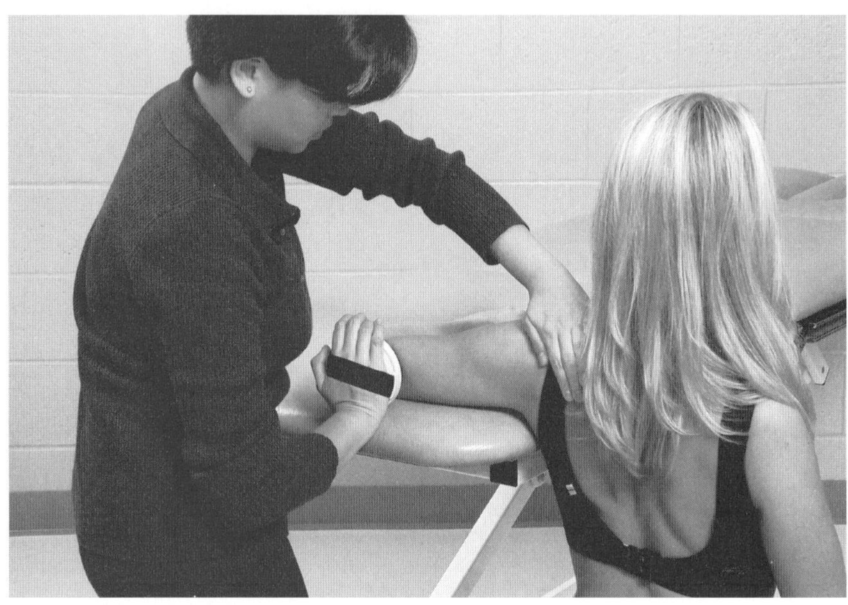

Stabilization: Over superior aspect of ipsilateral shoulder to prevent trunk rotation (Fig. 7-9).

Examiner command: "Hold your arm in this position and don't let me move it."

Dynamometer placement/resistance: Dynamometer is placed over posterior aspect of distal humerus just proximal to elbow. (Location should be marked with a skin pencil and distance from olecranon process measured and recorded so that consistency can be maintained across trials and testing sessions.) Resistance is applied perpendicular to humerus in direction of shoulder horizontal adduction and is held for 3 to 5 seconds (Fig. 7-9).

■ SHOULDER HORIZONTAL ADDUCTION

PECTORALIS MAJOR

Patient position: Seated half facing table with shoulder in 90° abduction and full horizontal adduction, elbow flexed to 90°, arm supported on table (Fig. 7-10).

Fig. 7-10.

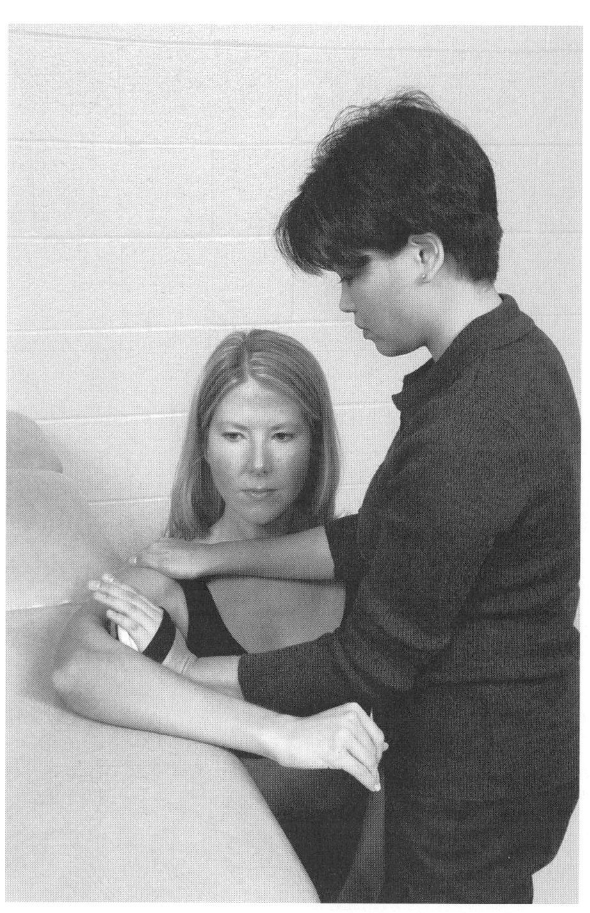

Stabilization: Over superior aspect of ipsilateral shoulder (Fig. 7-10).

Examiner command: "Hold your arm in this position and don't let me move it."

Dynamometer placement/resistance: Dynamometer is placed over anterior aspect of distal humerus just proximal to elbow. (Location should be marked with a skin pencil and distance from acromion measured and recorded so that consistency can be maintained across trials and testing sessions.) Resistance is applied perpendicular to humerus in direction of shoulder horizontal abduction and is held for 3 to 5 seconds (Fig. 7-10).

■ SHOULDER MEDIAL ROTATION

SUBSCAPULARIS, PECTORALIS MAJOR, LATISSIMUS DORSI, TERES MAJOR

Patient position: Seated with shoulder adducted and in neutral rotation, elbow flexed to 90°, forearm supported on a firm, smooth surface (Fig. 7-11).

Fig. 7-11.

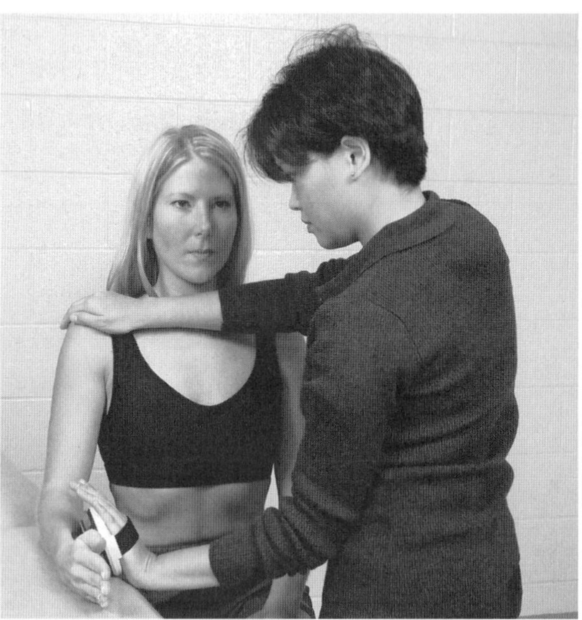

Stabilization: Over superior aspect of ipsilateral shoulder (Fig. 7-11).

Examiner command: "Hold your arm in this position and don't let me move it."

Dynamometer placement/resistance: Dynamometer is placed over anterior aspect of distal forearm just proximal to wrist. (Location should be marked with a skin pencil and perpendicular distance from radial styloid process measured and recorded so that consistency can be maintained across trials and testing sessions.) Resistance is applied perpendicular to forearm in direction of lateral rotation of shoulder and is held for 3 to 5 seconds (Fig. 7-11).

■ SHOULDER LATERAL ROTATION

INFRASPINATUS, TERES MINOR

Patient position: Seated with shoulder adducted and in neutral rotation, elbow flexed to 90°, forearm supported on a firm, smooth surface (Fig. 7-12).

Fig. 7-12.

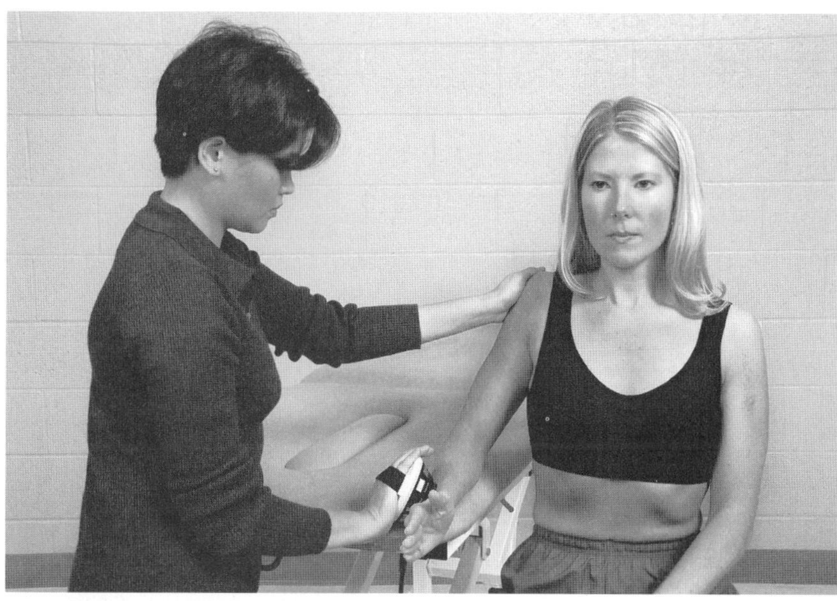

Stabilization: Over superior aspect of ipsilateral shoulder (Fig. 7-12).

Examiner command: "Hold your arm in this position and don't let me move it."

Dynamometer placement/rotation: Dynamometer is placed over dorsal aspect of distal forearm just proximal to wrist. (Location should be marked with a skin pencil and distance from olecranon process measured and recorded so that consistency can be maintained across trials and testing sessions.) Resistance is applied perpendicular to forearm in direction of medial rotation of shoulder and is held for 3 to 5 seconds (Fig. 7-12).

■ ELBOW FLEXION

BICEPS BRACHII

Patient position: Seated with arm supported on table. Shoulder is abducted to 90°, elbow flexed to 90°, forearm in full supination (Fig. 7-13).

Fig. 7-13.

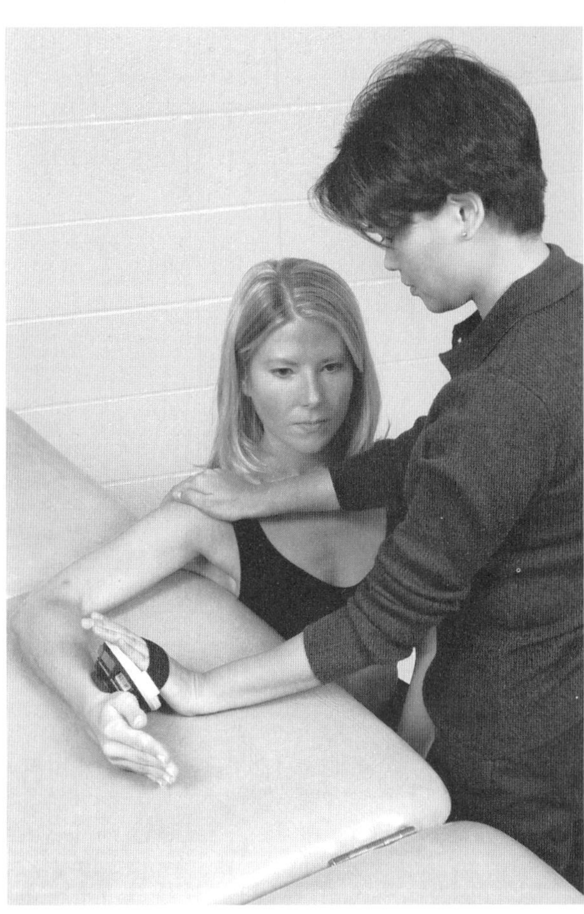

Stabilization: Over anterosuperior aspect of ipsilateral humerus, avoiding direct pressure over biceps brachii (Fig. 7-13).

Examiner command: "Hold your arm in this position and don't let me move it."

Dynamometer placement/resistance: Dynamometer is placed over ventral aspect of distal forearm just proximal to wrist. (Location should be marked with a skin pencil and perpendicular distance from radial styloid process measured and recorded so that consistency can be maintained across trials and testing sessions.) Resistance is applied perpendicular to forearm in direction of elbow extension and is held for 3 to 5 seconds (Fig. 7-13).

■ ELBOW FLEXION

BRACHIALIS

Patient position: Seated with arm supported on table. Shoulder is abducted to 90°, elbow flexed to 90°, forearm in full pronation (Fig. 7-14).

Fig. 7-14.

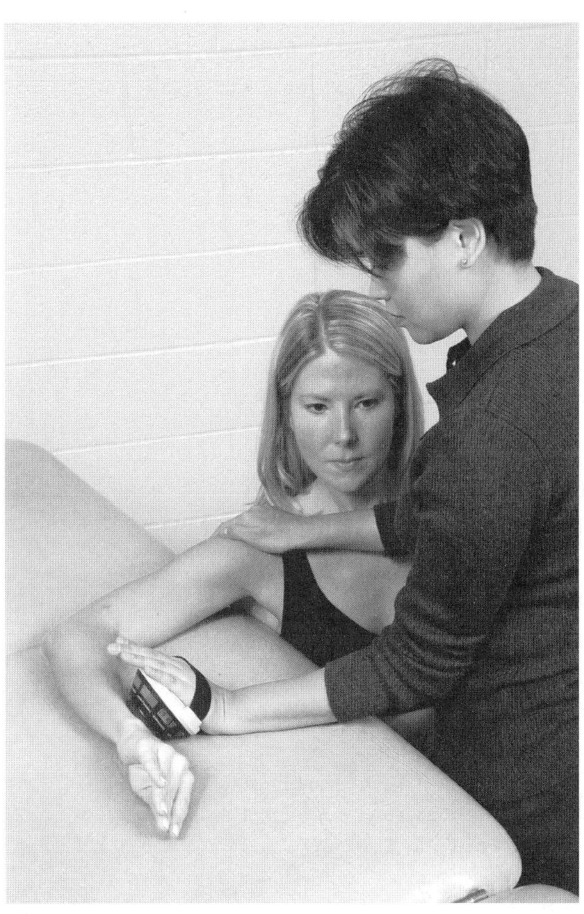

Stabilization: Over anterosuperior aspect of ipsilateral humerus (Fig. 7-14).

Examiner command: "Hold your arm in this position and don't let me move it."

Dynamometer placement/resistance: Dynamometer is placed over dorsal aspect of distal forearm just proximal to wrist. (Location should be marked with a skin pencil and perpendicular distance from radial styloid process measured and recorded so that consistency can be maintained across trials and testing sessions.) Resistance is applied perpendicular to forearm in direction of elbow extension and is held for 3 to 5 seconds (Fig. 7-14).

■ *ELBOW FLEXION*

BRACHIORADIALIS

Patient position: Seated with arm supported on table. Shoulder is abducted to 90°; elbow flexed to 90 °; and forearm in neutral rotation (Fig. 7-15).

Fig. 7-15.

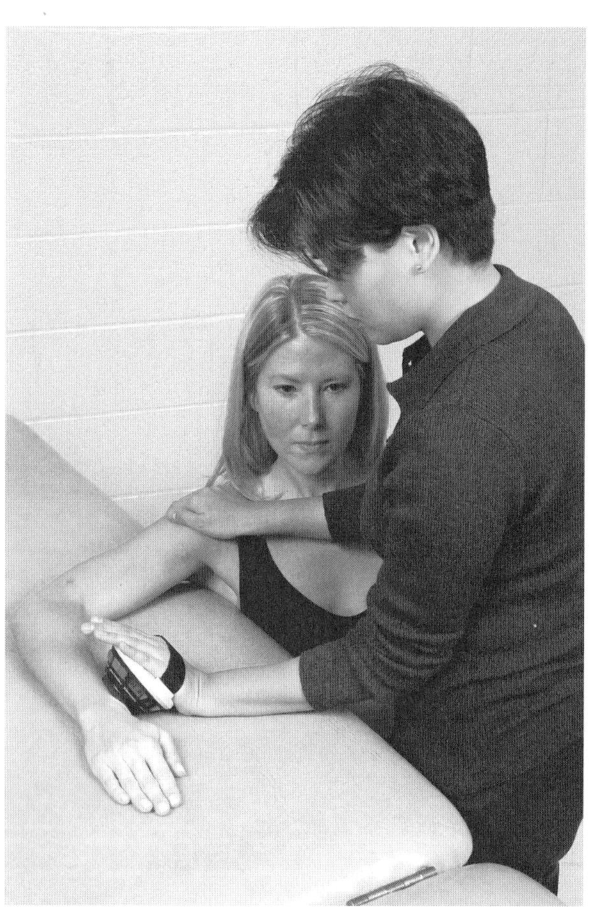

Stabilization: Over anterosuperior aspect of ipsilateral humerus (Fig. 7-15).

Examiner command: "Hold your arm in this position and don't let me move it."

Dynamometer placement/resistance: Dynamometer is placed over radial aspect of distal forearm just proximal to wrist. (Location should be marked with a skin pencil and perpendicular distance from radial styloid process measured and recorded so that consistency can be maintained across trials and testing sessions.) Resistance is applied perpendicular to forearm in direction of elbow extension and is held for 3 to 5 seconds (Fig. 7-15).

▪ *ELBOW EXTENSION*

TRICEPS BRACHII, ANCONEUS

Patient position: Seated with arm supported on table. Shoulder is abducted to 90°, elbow is 10 to 15° from full extension, forearm in supination (Fig. 7-16).

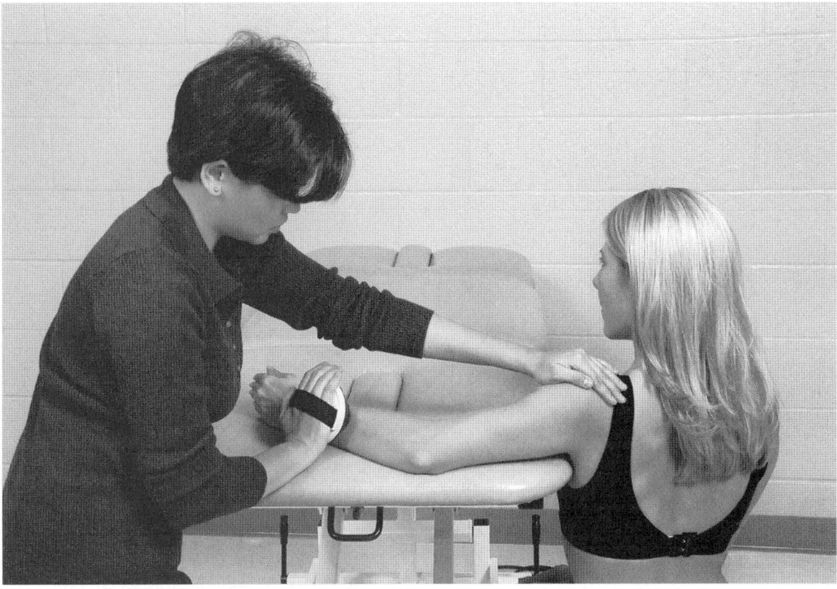

Fig. 7-16.

Stabilization: Over superior aspect of ipsilateral shoulder (Fig. 7-16).

Examiner command: "Hold your arm in this position and don't let me move it."

Dynamometer placement/resistance: Dynamometer is placed on dorsal surface of forearm just proximal to wrist. (Location should be marked with a skin pencil and distance from olecranon process measured and recorded so that consistency can be maintained across trials and testing sessions.) Resistance is applied perpendicular to forearm in direction of elbow flexion and is held for 3 to 5 seconds (Fig. 7-16).

■ WRIST FLEXION

FLEXOR CARPI RADIALIS, FLEXOR CARPI ULNARIS

Patient position: Seated with forearm in neutral rotation, wrist flexed, forearm supported on a flat surface (Fig. 7-17).

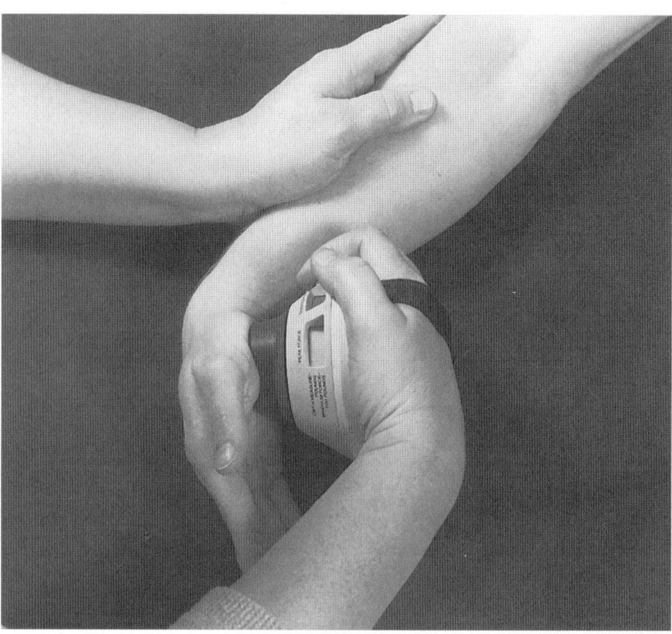

Fig. 7-17.

Stabilization: Along radial side of forearm (Fig. 7-17).

Examiner command: "Hold your wrist in this position and don't let me move it."

Dynamometer placement/resistance: Dynamometer is placed on ventral surface of hand just distal to wrist. (Location should be marked with a skin pencil and perpendicular distance from radial styloid process measured and recorded so that consistency can be maintained across trials and testing sessions.) Resistance is applied perpendicular to hand in direction of wrist extension and is held for 3 to 5 seconds (Fig. 7-17).

▪ WRIST EXTENSION

EXTENSOR CARPI RADIALIS LONGUS AND BREVIS, EXTENSOR CARPI ULNARIS

Patient position: Seated with forearm in neutral rotation, wrist extended, forearm supported on a flat surface (Fig. 7-18).

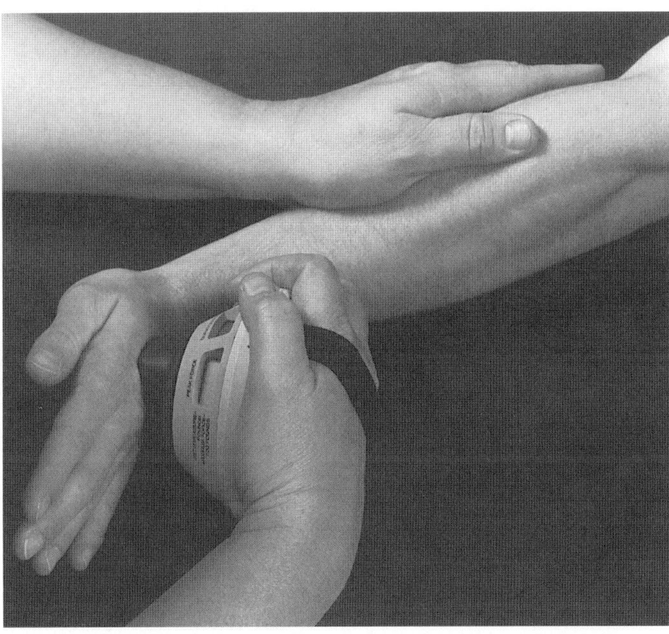

Fig. 7-18.

Stabilization: On radial side of forearm.

Examiner command: "Hold your wrist in this position and don't let me move it."

Dynamometer placement/resistance: Dynamometer is placed on dorsal surface of hand just distal to wrist. (Location should be marked with a skin pencil and perpendicular distance from radial styloid process measured and recorded so that consistency can be maintained across trials and testing sessions.) Resistance is applied perpendicular to hand in direction of wrist flexion and is held for 3 to 5 seconds (Fig. 7-18).

HIP FLEXION

ILIACUS, PSOAS MAJOR

Patient position: Side lying with leg to be tested lowermost. Hip and knee of side to be tested are flexed to 90° (Fig. 7-19).

Fig. 7-19.

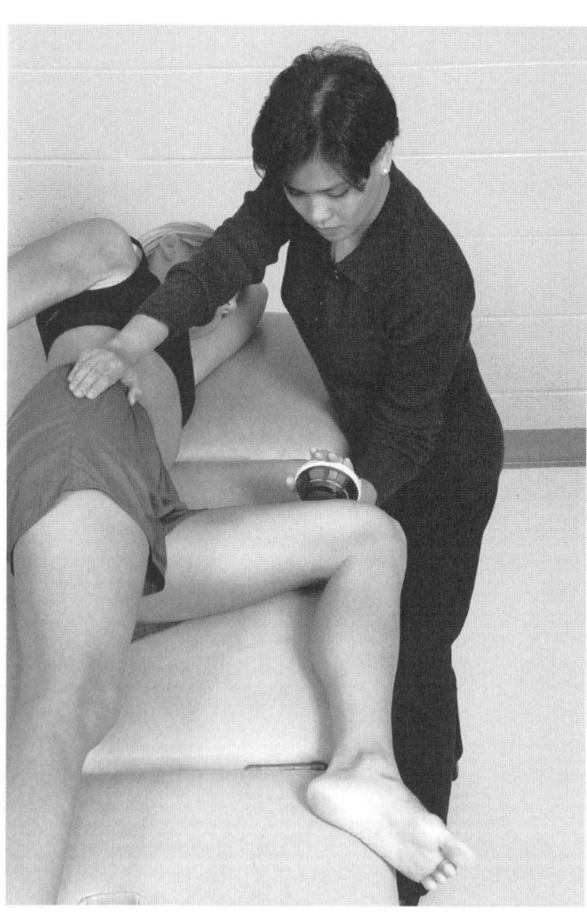

Stabilization: Examiner stabilizes pelvis with one hand (Fig. 7-19).

Examiner command: "Hold your leg in this position and don't let me move it."

Dynamometer placement/resistance: Dynamometer is placed on anterior aspect of distal thigh just proximal to knee. (Location should be marked with a skin pencil and distance from tibial tuberosity measured and recorded so that consistency can be maintained across trials and testing sessions.) Resistance is applied perpendicular to thigh in direction of hip extension and is held for 3 to 5 seconds (Fig. 7-19).

■ HIP EXTENSION

GLUTEUS MAXIMUS

Patient position: Side lying on side of limb to be tested with hip of test limb in extension and knee of limb flexed to 90° (decreases contribution of hamstrings by placing them in a shortened position). Patient should be positioned so that patient's pelvis is close to examiner's trunk for stabilization (Fig. 7-20).

Fig. 7-20.

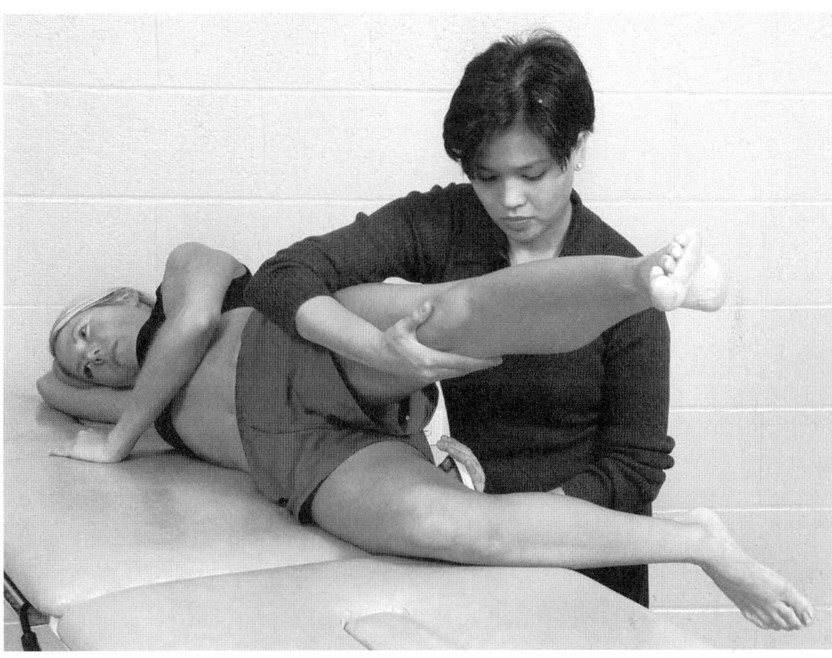

Stabilization: Examiner stands directly behind patient's pelvis and supports uppermost lower extremity while stabilizing pelvis with one hand (Fig. 7-20).

Examiner command: "Hold your leg in this position and don't let me move it."

Dynamometer placement/resistance: Dynamometer is placed on posterior aspect of distal thigh just proximal to knee. (Location should be marked with a skin pencil and distance from ischial tuberosity measured and recorded so that consistency can be maintained across trials and testing sessions.) Resistance is applied perpendicular to thigh in direction of hip flexion and is held for 3 to 5 seconds (Fig. 7-20).

■ HIP ABDUCTION

GLUTEUS MEDIUS AND MINIMUS

Patient position: Supine with hip of limb to be tested abducted and in neutral rotation, knee extended (Fig. 7-21).

Fig. 7-21.

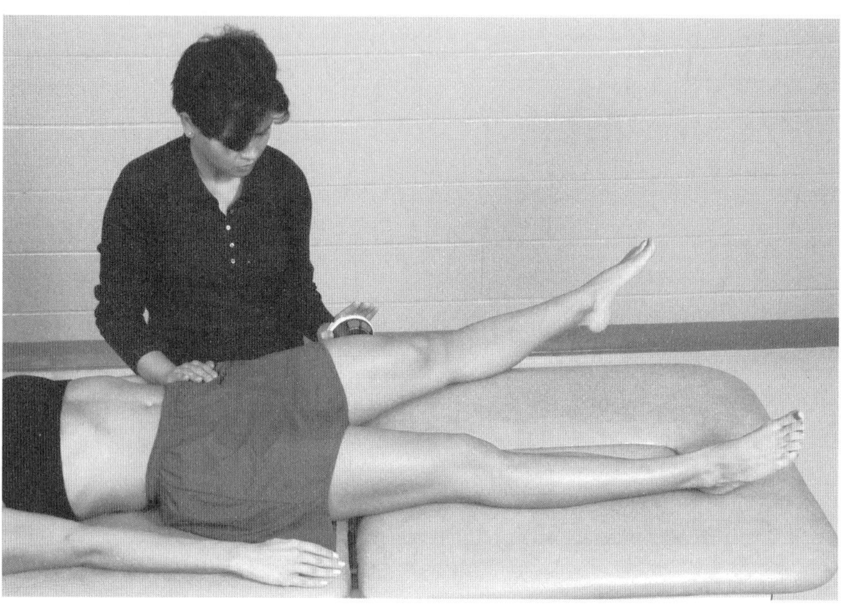

Stabilization: Over anterolateral aspect of ipsilateral pelvis (Fig. 7-21).

Examiner command: "Hold your leg in this position and don't let me move it."

Dynamometer placement/resistance: Dynamometer is placed on lateral aspect of distal thigh just proximal to knee. (Location should be marked with a skin pencil and distance from lateral epicondyle of femur measured and recorded so that consistency can be maintained across trials and testing sessions.) Resistance is applied perpendicular to thigh in direction of hip adduction and is held for 3 to 5 seconds (Fig. 7-21).

HIP ADDUCTION

ADDUCTOR MAGNUS LONGUS AND BREVIS, PECTINEUS, GRACILIS

Patient position: Supine with nontest limb in full abduction, test limb in adduction, pelvis level, knees extended (Fig. 7-22).

Fig. 7-22.

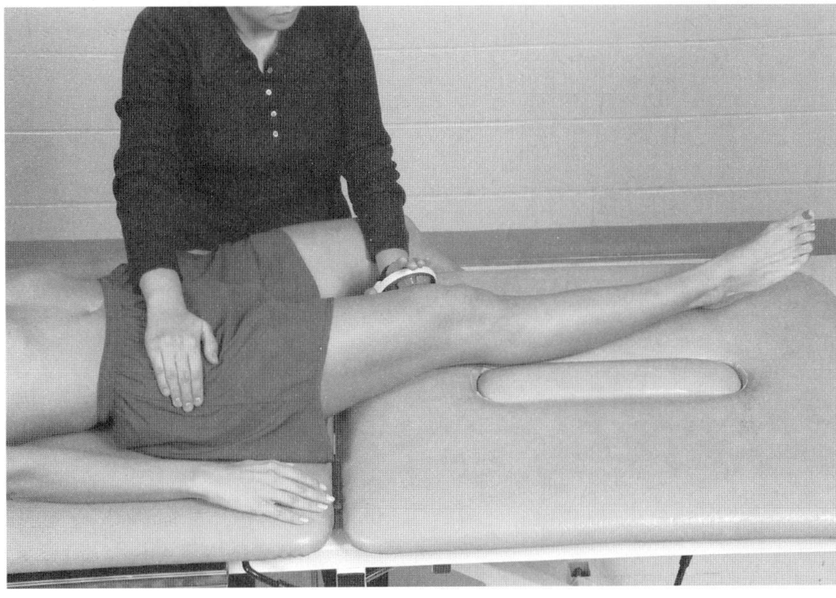

Stabilization: Over anterolateral aspect of ipsilateral pelvis (Fig. 7-22).

Examiner command: "Hold your leg in this position and don't let me move it."

Dynamometer placement/resistance: Dynamometer is placed on medial aspect of distal thigh just proximal to knee. (Location should be marked with a skin pencil and distance from medial epicondyle of femur measured and recorded so that consistency can be maintained across trials and testing sessions.) Resistance is applied perpendicular to thigh in direction of hip abduction and is held for 3 to 5 seconds (Fig. 7-22).

■ HIP MEDIAL ROTATION

TENSOR FASCIA LATA, GLUTEUS MINIMUS AND MEDIUS

Patient position: Supine with hips flexed to 90°, knees flexed to 90°, hip to be tested in neutral rotation (Fig. 7-23).

Fig. 7-23.

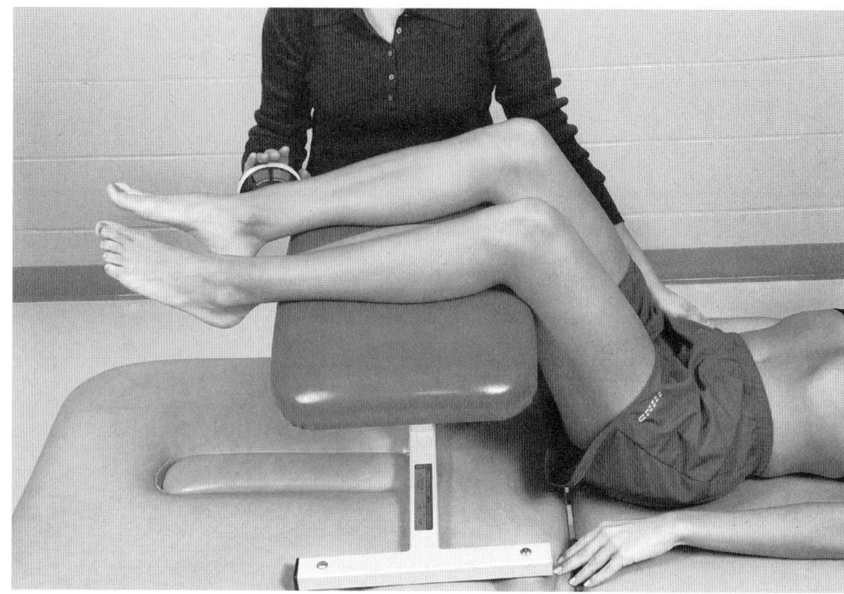

Stabilization: Over anterolateral aspect of ipsilateral pelvis (Fig. 7-23).

Examiner command: "Hold your leg in this position and don't let me move it."

Dynamometer placement/resistance: Dynamometer is placed on lateral aspect of distal leg just proximal to ankle. (Location should be marked with a skin pencil and distance from lateral malleolus measured and recorded so that consistency can be maintained across trials and testing sessions.) Resistance is applied perpendicular to leg in direction of lateral rotation of hip and is held for 3 to 5 seconds (Fig. 7-23).

■ HIP LATERAL ROTATION

PIRIFORMIS, GEMELLUS SUPERIOR AND INFERIOR, OBTURATOR INTERNUS AND EXTERNUS, QUADRATUS FEMORIS

Patient position: Supine with hips flexed to 90°, knees flexed to 90°, hip to be tested in neutral rotation (Fig. 7-24).

Fig. 7-24.

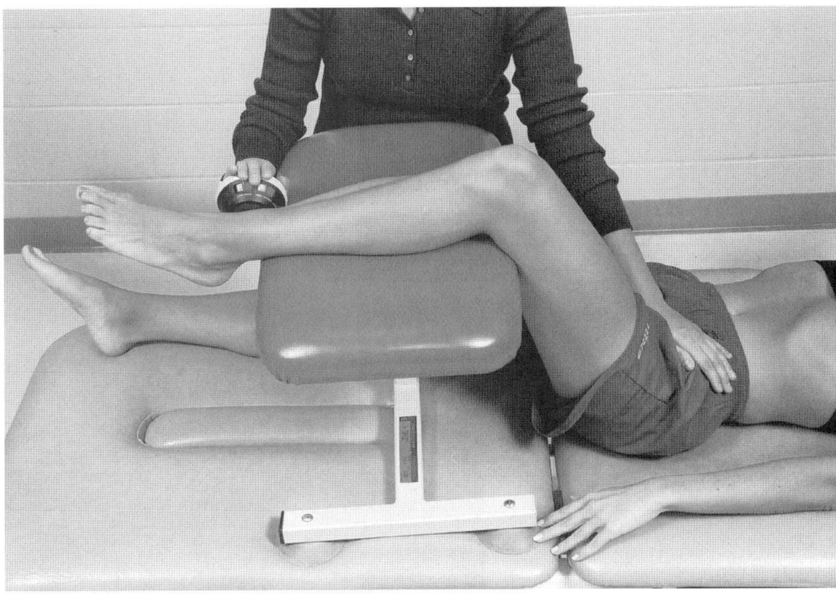

Stabilization: Over anterolateral aspect of ipsilateral pelvis (Fig. 7-24).

Examiner command: "Hold your leg in this position and don't let me move it."

Dynamometer placement/resistance: Dynamometer is placed on medial aspect of distal leg just proximal to ankle. (Location should be marked with a skin pencil and distance from medial malleolus measured and recorded so that consistency can be maintained across trials and testing sessions.) Resistance is applied perpendicular to leg in direction of medial rotation of hip and is held for 3 to 5 seconds (Fig. 7-24).

KNEE EXTENSION

QUADRICEPS FEMORIS

Patient position: Side lying on side to be tested. Hip of lowermost limb is extended, and knee is in approximately 10° flexion (Fig. 7-25). Note: Many patients may be able to generate sufficient force with quadriceps muscles to overcome resistive force generated by examiner. In such instances, patient should be repositioned in sitting and tested as described in Limitations (Figs. 7-2 and 7-3).

Fig. 7-25.

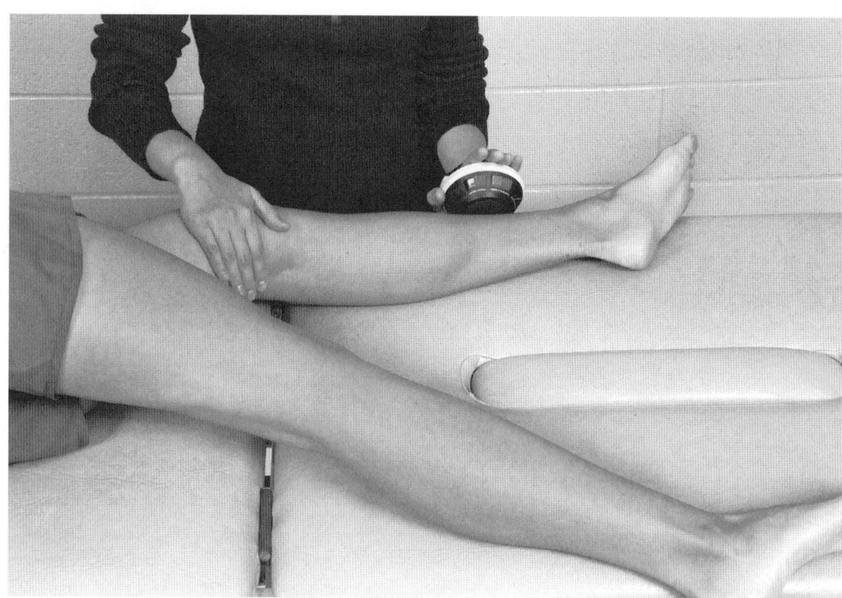

Stabilization: Over medial aspect of femur (Fig. 7-25).

Examiner command: "Hold your leg in this position and don't let me move it."

Dynamometer placement/resistance: Dynamometer is placed on anterior aspect of distal leg just proximal to ankle. (Location should be marked with a skin pencil and distance from tibial tuberosity measured and recorded so that consistency can be maintained across trials and testing sessions.) Resistance is applied perpendicular to leg in direction of knee flexion and is held for 3 to 5 seconds (Fig. 7-25).

■ *KNEE FLEXION*

SEMITENDINOSUS, SEMIMEMBRANOSUS, BICEPS FEMORIS

Patient position: Side lying on side to be tested. Hip of lowermost limb is extended, knee flexed to 90° (Fig. 7-26).

Fig. 7-26.

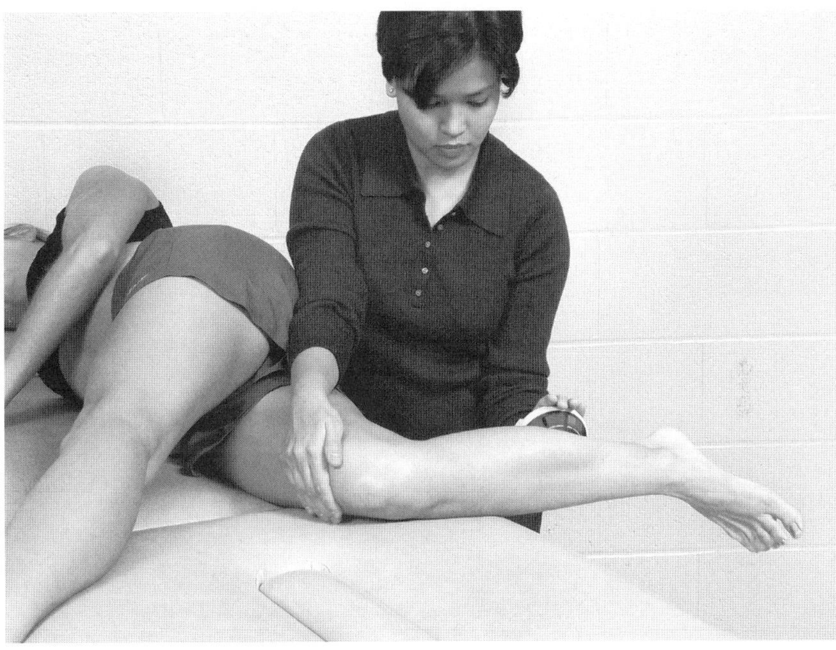

Stabilization: Over medial aspect of femur (Fig. 7-26).

Examiner command: "Hold your leg in this position and don't let me move it."

Dynamometer placement/resistance: Dynamometer is placed on posterior aspect of distal leg just proximal to ankle. (Location should be marked with a skin pencil and perpendicular distance from lateral malleolus measured and recorded so that consistency can be maintained across trials and testing sessions.) Resistance is applied perpendicular to leg in direction of knee extension and is held for 3 to 5 seconds (Fig. 7-26).

■ ANKLE PLANTAR FLEXION

GASTROCNEMIUS, SOLEUS

Patient position: Side lying on side to be tested. Test limb is plantar flexed at ankle (Fig. 7-27).

Fig. 7-27.

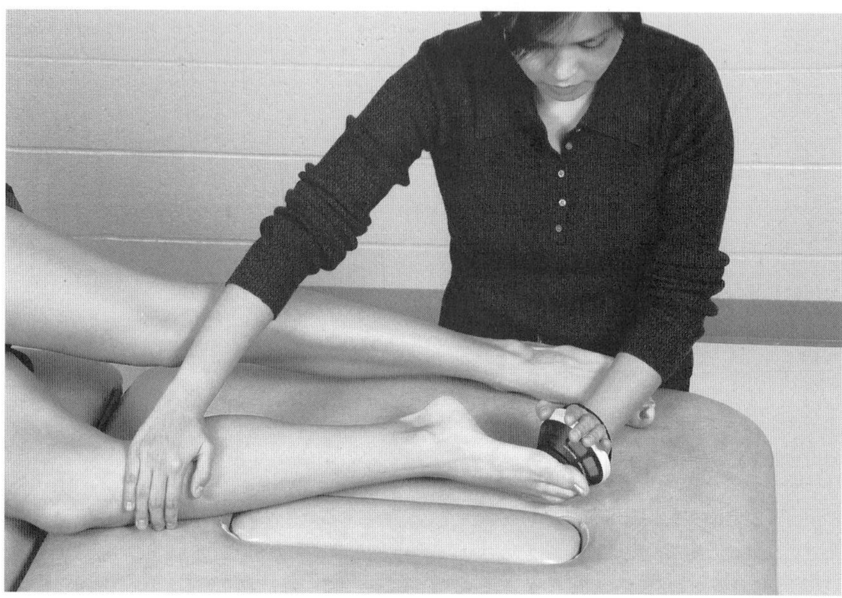

Stabilization: Over anterior aspect of leg (Fig. 7-27).

Examiner command: "Hold your foot in this position and don't let me move it."

Dynamometer placement/resistance: Dynamometer is placed on plantar surface of foot near metatarsal heads. (Location should be marked with a skin pencil and distance from head of first metatarsal measured and recorded so that consistency can be maintained across trials and testing sessions.) Resistance is applied perpendicular to plantar surface of foot in direction of ankle dorsiflexion and is held for 3 to 5 seconds (Fig. 7-27).

ANKLE DORSIFLEXION

TIBIALIS ANTERIOR

Patient position: Side lying on side to be tested. Test limb is dorsiflexed at ankle (Fig. 7-28).

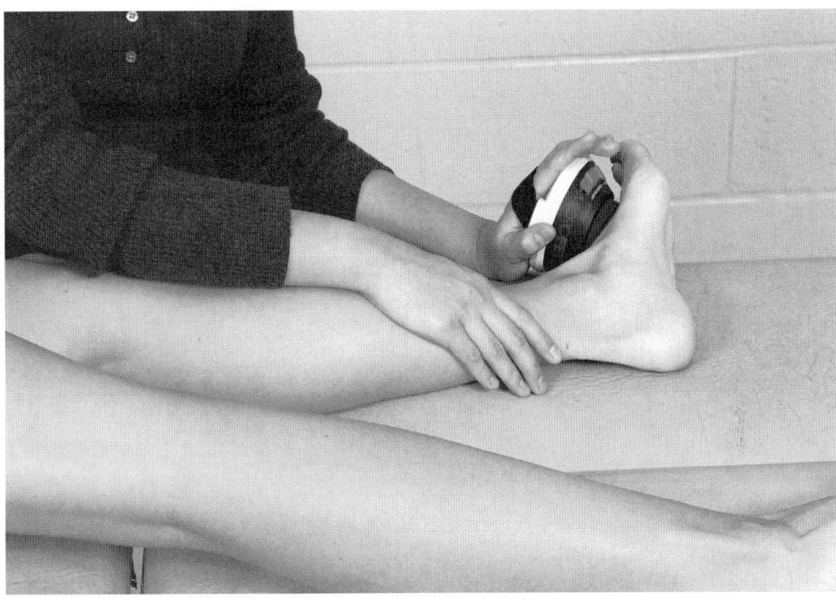

Fig. 7-28.

Stabilization: Over medial aspect of distal leg, avoiding pressure over tibialis anterior (Fig. 7-28).

Examiner command: "Hold your foot in this position and don't let me move it."

Dynamometer placement/resistance: Dynamometer is placed over dorsal aspect of foot near metatarsal heads. (Location should be marked with a skin pencil and distance from medial malleolus measured and recorded so that consistency can be maintained across trials and testing sessions.) Resistance is applied perpendicular to dorsum of foot in direction of ankle plantar flexion and is held for 3 to 5 seconds (Fig. 7-28).

■ SUBTALAR INVERSION

TIBIALIS POSTERIOR

Patient position: Supine with lower extremities extended, ankle of limb to be tested in slight plantar flexion, subtalar joint inverted (Fig. 7-29).

Fig. 7-29.

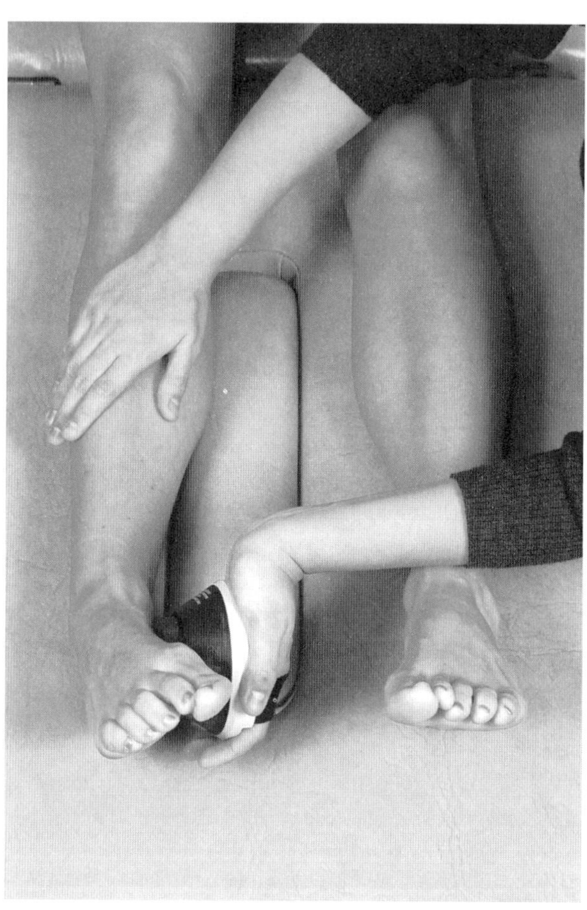

Stabilization: Over anteromedial aspect of tibia (Fig. 7-29).

Examiner command: "Hold your foot in this position and don't let me move it."

Dynamometer placement/resistance: Dynamometer is placed over medial aspect of foot near base of first metatarsal. (Location should be marked with a skin pencil and distance from medial malleolus measured and recorded so that consistency can be maintained across trials and testing sessions.) Resistance is applied perpendicular to medial aspect of foot in direction of subtalar eversion and is held for 3 to 5 seconds (Fig. 7-29).

SUBTALAR EVERSION

PERONEUS LONGUS AND BREVIS

Patient position: Supine with lower extremities extended, ankle of limb to be tested in a neutral position, subtalar joint everted (Fig. 7-30).

Fig. 7-30.

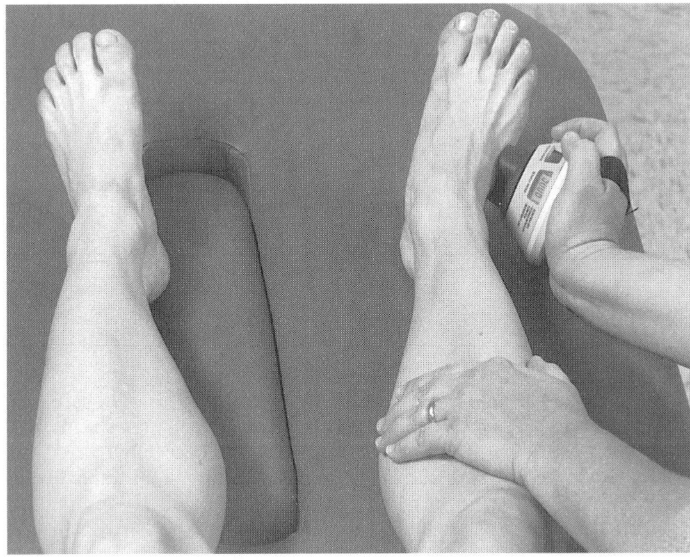

Stabilization: Over medial aspect of distal leg.

Examiner command: "Hold your foot in this position and don't let me move it."

Dynamometer placement/resistance: Dynamometer is placed over lateral aspect of foot just distal to base of fifth metatarsal. (Location should be marked with a skin pencil and distance from lateral malleolus measured and recorded so that consistency can be maintained across trials and testing sessions.) Resistance is applied perpendicular to lateral aspect of foot in direction of subtalar inversion and is held for 3 to 5 seconds (Fig. 7-30).

References

1. Agre JC, Magness JL, Hull SZ, et al. Strength testing with a portable dynamometer: reliability for upper and lower extremities. *Arch Phys Med Rehabil* 1987;68:454–458.
2. Aitkens S, Lord J, Bernauer E, et al. Relationship of manual muscle testing to objective strength measurements. *Muscle Nerve* 1989;12:173–177.
3. Andrews AW. Hand-held dynamometry for measuring muscle strength. *J Hum Muscle Perform* 1991;1:35–50.
4. Andrews AW, Thomas MW, Bohannon RW. Normative values for isometric muscle force measurements obtained with hand-held dynamometers. *Phys Ther* 1996;76:248–259.
5. Appleton RE, Sykanda AM. Objective assessment of muscle strength in chronic relapsing dysimmune polyradiculoneuropathy. *Dev Med Child Neurol* 1988;30:365–369.
6. Askew LJ, An K-N, Morrey BF, et al. Isometric elbow strength in normal individuals. *Clin Orthop* 1987;222:261–266.

7. Bäckman E, Odenrick P, Henriksson KG, et al. Isometric muscle force and anthropometric values in normal children aged between 3.5 and 15 years. *Scand J Rehabil Med* 1989;21:105–114.
8. Bäckman E, Johansson V, Häger B, et al. Isometric muscle strength and muscle endurance in normal persons aged between 17 and 70 years. *Scand J Rehabil Med* 1995;27:109–117.
9. Balogun JA, Powell, Trullender B, et al. Intra- and inter-tester reliability of Nicholas hand-held dynamometer during evaluation of upper extremity isometric muscle strength. *Eur J Phys Med Rehabil* 1998;8:48–53.
10. Beck M, Giess R, Wurffel W, et al. Comparison of maximal voluntary isometric contraction and Drachman's hand-held dynamometry in evaluating patients with amyotrophic lateral sclerosis. *Muscle Nerve* 1999;22:1265–1270.
11. Beenakker EAC, van der Hoeven JH, Fock JM, et al. Reference values of maximum isometric muscle force obtained in 270 children aged 4-16 years by hand-held dynamometry. *Neuromusc Dis* 2001;11:441–446.
12. Beasley WC. Influence of method on estimates of normal knee extensor force among normal and postpolio children. *Phys Ther Rev* 1956;36:21–41.
13. Bohannon RW. Results of resistance exercise on a patient with amyotrophic lateral sclerosis: a case report. *Phys Ther* 1983;63:965–968.
14. Bohannon RW, Dubuc WE. Documentation of resolution of weakness in a patient with Guillain-Barre syndrome: a clinical report. *Phys Ther* 1984;64:388–389.
15. Bohannon RW. Upper extremity strength and strength relationships among young women. *J Ortho Sports Phys Ther* 1986;8:128–133.
16. Bohannon RW. Test-retest reliability of hand-held dynamometry during a single session of strength assessment. *Phys Ther* 1986;66:206–209.
17. Bohannon RW. Manual muscle test scores and dynamometer test scores for knee extension strength. *Arch Phys Med Rehabil* 1986;67:390–392.
18. Bohannon RW. Strength of lower limb related to gait velocity and cadence in stroke patients. *Physiother Can* 1986;38:204–206.
19. Bohannon RW, Jones PL. Results of manual resistance exercise on a manifesting carrier of Duchenne muscular dystrophy: a case report. *Phys Ther* 1986;66:973–975
20. Bohannon RW, Larkin PA, Smith MB, et al. Shoulder pain in hemiplegia: Statistical relationship with five variables. *Arch Phys Med Rehabil* 1986;67:514–516.
21. Bohannon RW. Hand-held dynamometry: stability of muscle strength over multiple measurements. *Clin Biomech* 1987;2:74–77.
22. Bohannon RW. Relationship between static standing capacity and lower limb strength in hemiparetic stroke patients. *Clin Rehabil* 1987;1:287–291.
23. Bohannon RW. Relationship between static strength and various other measures in hemiparetic stroke patients. *Int J Rehabil Med* 1987;8:125–128.
24. Bohannon RW. Differentiation of maximal from submaximal static elbow flexor efforts by measurement variability. *Am J Phys Med* 1987;66:213–218.
25. Bohannon RW. Relationship between strength and movement in plegic lower limb following cerebrovascular accidents. *Int J Rehabil Res* 1987;10:420–422.
26. Bohannon RW. Gait performance of hemiparetic stroke patients: selected variables. *Arch Phys Med Rehabil* 1987;68:777–781.
27. Bohannon RW, Andrews AW. Interrater reliability of hand-held dynamometry. *Phys Ther* 1987;67:931–933.
28. Bohannon RW, Andrews AW. Relative strength of seven upper extremity muscle groups in hemiparetic stroke patients. *J Neurol Rehabil* 1987;1:161–165.
29. Bohannon RW, Larkin RA, Smith MB, et al. Relationship between static muscle strength deficits and spasticity in stroke patients with hemiparesis. *Phys Ther* 1987;67:1068–1071.
30. Bohannon RW, Smith MB. Upper extremity strength deficits in hemiplegic stroke patients: Relationship between admission and discharge assessment and time since onset. *Arch Phys Med Rehabil* 1987;68:155–157.
31. Bohannon RW. Make tests and break tests of elbow flexor muscle strength. *Phys Ther* 1988;68:193–194.
32. Bohannon RW. Determinants of transfer capacity in patients with hemiparesis. *Physiother Can* 1988;40:236–238.
33. Bohannon RW. Knee extension force measurements are reliable and indicative of walking speed in stroke patients. *Int J Rehabil Res* 1989;12:193–194.
34. Bohannon RW, Andrews AW. Accuracy of spring and strain gauge hand-held dynamometers. *J Orthop Sports Phys Ther* 1989;11:323–325.
35. Bohannon RW, Andrews AW. Influence of head-neck rotation on static elbow flexion force of paretic side in patients with hemiparesis. *Phys Ther* 1989;69:135–137.
36. Bohannon RW. Shoulder position influences elbow extension force in healthy individuals. *J Orthop Sports Phys Ther* 1990;12:111–114.
37. Bohannon RW. Make versus break tests for measuring elbow flexor muscle force with a hand-held dynamometer in patients with stroke. *Physiother Can* 1990;42:247–251.

38. Bohannon RW. Knee extension torque in stroke patients: comparison of measurements obtained with a hand-held and a Cybex dynamometer. *Physiother Can* 1990;42:284–287.
39. Bohannon RW. Hand-held compared with isokinetic dynamometry for measurement of static knee extension torque (parallel reliability of dynamometers). *Clin Phys Physiol Meas* 1990; 11:217–222.
40. Bohannon RW. Muscle strength testing with hand-held dynamometers. In: Amundsen LR, ed. *Muscle Strength Testing*. New York: Churchill Livingstone, 1990:69–88.
41. Bohannon RW. Consistency of muscle strength measurements in patient with stroke: Examination from a different perspective. *J Phys Ther Sc*. 1990;2:1–7.
42. Bohannon RW, Saunders N. Hand-held dynamometry: a single trial may be adequate for measuring muscle strength in healthy individuals. *Physiother Can* 1990;42:6–9.
43. Bohannon RW. Relationship between movement deficits and muscle strength and tone at elbow in patients with hemiparesis. *Clin Rehab* 1991;2:110–113.
44. Bohannon RW, Wikholm J. Measurements of knee extension force obtained by two examiners of substantially different experience with a hand-held dynamometer. *Isokinetic Exerc Sci* 1992;2:5–8.
45. Bohannon RW. Comparability of force measurements obtained with different hand-held dynamometers from older adults. *Isokinet Exerc Sci* 1993;3:148–151.
46. Bohannon RW. Comparability of force measurements obtained with different strain gauge hand-held dynamometers. *J Orthop Sports Phys Ther* 1993;18:564–567.
47. Bohannon RW, Smith J, Hull D, et al. Deficits in lower extremity muscle and gait performance among renal transplant candidates. *Arch Phys Med Rehabil* 1995;76:547–551.
48. Bohannon RW. Hand-held dynamometer measurements obtained in a home environment are reliable but not correlated strongly with function. *Int J Rehabil Res* 1996;19:345–347.
49. Bohannon RW. Reference values for extremity muscle strength obtained by hand-held dynamometry from adults aged 20 to 79 years. *Arch Phys Med Rehabil* 1997;78:26–32.
50. Bohannon RW. Alternatives for measuring knee extension strength of elderly at home. *Clin Rehabil* 1998;12:434–440.
51. Bohannon RW. Research incorporating hand-held dynamometry publication trends since 1948. *Percept Mot Skills* 1998;86:1177–1178.
52. Bohannon RW. Intertester reliability of hand-held dynamometry: a concise summary of published research. *Percept Mot Skills* 1999;88:899–902.
53. Bohannon RW. Adoption of hand-held dynamometry. *Percept Mot Skills*. 2001;92:150.
54. Bohannon RW. Measuring knee extensor muscle strength. *Am J Phys Med Rehabil* 2001;80:13–18.
55. Boiteau M, Malouin F, Richards CL. Use of a hand-held dynamometer and a Kin-com dynamometer for evaluating spastic hypertonia in children: a reliability study. *Phys Ther* 1995;74:796–802.
56. Borden R, Colachis SC. Quantitative measurement of good and normal ranges in muscle testing. *Phys Ther* 1968;48:839–843.
57. Brinkman JR. Comparison of a hand-held and fixed dynamometer in measuring strength of patients with neuromuscular disease. *J Orthop Sports Phys Ther* 1994;19;100–104.
58. Byl NN, Richards S, Asturias J. Intrarater and interrater reliability of strength measurements of biceps and deltoid using a hand-held dynamometer. *J Orthop Sports Phys Ther* 1988; 9:399–405.
59. Clarkson HM, Gilewich GB. *Musculoskeletal Assessment: Joint Range of Motion and Manual Muscle Strength*. Baltimore: Williams & Wilkins, 1999.
60. Clause S. Malouin F, Richards CI. Utilisation de la dynamométrie manuelle pour mesurer la spasticité des muscles adducteurs do la hanche. *Annales de Réadaptation en Médecine Physique* 1992;35:17–26.
61. *CompuFET Instruction Manual*. 1995. Draper, UT: Hogan Health.
62. Cook JD, Iannaccone ST, Russman BS, et al. Cooperative study for assessment of therapeutic trials for spinal muscular atrophies: a methodology to measure strength of SMA patients. *Muscle Nerve* 1990;13:S7–S10.
63. Deones VL, Wiley SC, Worrell T. Assessment of quadriceps muscle performance by a hand-held dynamometer and an isokinetic dynamometer. *J Orthop Sports Phys Th*er 1994;20:296–301.
64. Duyff RF, Van den Bosch J, Laman DM, et al. Neuromuscular findings in thyroid dysfunction: a prospective clinical and electrodiagnostic study. *J Neurol Neurosurg Psychiatry* 2000;68: 750–755.
65. Dvir Z, Arbel N, Bar-Haim S. Use of hand-held dynamometry for measuring effect of short-leg tone reducing casts on passive compliance of calf muscles in children with cerebral palsy. *J Neurol Rehabil* 1991;5:229–234.
66. Edwards RHT, McDonnell M. Hand-held dynamometer for evaluating voluntary muscle function. *Lancet* 1974;2:757–758.
67. Emery AEH, Skinner R, Howden LC, et al. Verapamil in Duchenne muscular dystrophy. *Lancet* 1982;1:559.

68. Escolar DM, Henricson EK, Mayhew J, et al. Clinical evaluator reliability for quantitative and manual muscle testing measures of strength in children. *Muscle Nerve* 2001;24:787–793.
69. Finucane SD, Walker ML, Rothstein JM, et al. Reliability of isometric muscle testing of knee flexor and extensor muscles in patients with connective tissue diseases. *Phys Ther* 1988;68:338–343.
70. Frese E, Brown M, Norton BJ. Clinical reliability of manual muscle testing: middle trapezius and gluteus medius muscles. *Phys Ther* 1987;67:1072–1076.
71. Giles C. Modified sphygmomanometer: an instrument to objectively assess muscle strength. *Physiother Can* 1984;36:36–37
72. Goonetilleke A, Modarres-Sadeghi H, Guiloff RJ. Accuracy, reproducibility, and variability of hand-held dynamometry in motor neuron disease. *J Neurol Neurosurg Psychiatry* 1994;57: 326–332.
73. Griffin JW, McClure MH, Bertorini TE. Sequential isokinetic and manual muscle testing in patients with neuromuscular disease. *Phys Ther* 1986;66:32–35.
74. Hayes KW, Falconer J. Reliability of hand-held dynamometry and its relationship with manual muscle testing in patients with osteoarthritis in knee. *J Orthop Sports Phys Ther* 1992;16:145–149.
75. Hedengren E, Knutson LM, Håglund-Akerlind Y, et al. Lower extremity isometric joint torque in children with juvenile chronic arthritis. *Scand J Rheumatol* 2001;30:69–76.
76. Helewa A, Goldsmith C, Smythe H, et al. An evaluation of four different measures of abdominal muscle strength: patient order and instrument variation. *J Rheumatol* 1990:17:965–969.
77. Hinderer KA, Hinderer SR. Muscle strength development and assessment in children and adolescents. In: Ringdahl K, ed. *International Perspectives in Physical Therapy: Muscle Strength.* Edinburgh, UK: Churchill Livingstone, 1993:93–140.
78. Hoogerwaard EM, Bakker E, Ipel PF, et al. Signs and symptoms of Duchenne muscular dystrophy and Becker muscular dystrophy among carriers in Netherlands: a cohort study. *Lancet* 1999;353:2116–2119.
79. Horvat M, Croce, R, Roswal G. Intratester reliability of Nicholas manual muscle tester on individuals with intellectual disabilities by a tester having minimal experience. *Arch Phys Med Rehabil* 1994; 75:808–811.
80. Hosking GP, Bhat US, Dubowitz V, et al. Measurements of muscle strength and performance in children with normal and diseased muscle. *Arch Dis Child* 1976;51:957–963.
81. Hsieh C, Phillips RB. Reliability of manual muscle testing with a computerized dynamometer. *J Manip Physiol Ther* 1990;13:72–82.
82. Hyde SA, Goddard C, Scott O. Myometer: development of a clinical tool. *Physiother* 1983;69:424–427.
83. Iddings DM, Smith LK, Spencer WA. Muscle testing, II: reliability in clinical use. *Phys Ther Rev* 1961;41:249–256.
84. Kaegi C, Thibault MC, Girous F, et al. Interrater reliability of force measurements using a modified sphygmomanometer in elderly subjects. *Phys Ther* 1998;78:1095–1103.
85. Karner PM, Thompson AL, Connelly DM, et al. Strength testing in elderly women using a portable dynamometer. *Physiother Can* 1998;50:35–39.
86. Keating JL, Matyas TA. Influence of subject and test design on dynamometric measurements of extremity muscles. *Phys Ther* 1996;76:866–889.
87. Kilmer DD, McCrary MA, Wright NC, et al. Hand-held dynamometry reliability in persons with neuropathic weakness. *Arch Phys Med Rehabil* 1997;78:1364–1368.
88. Kilmer DD, Aitkens SG, Wright NC et al. Simulated work performance tasks in persons with neuropathic and myopathic weakness. *Arch Phys Med Rehabil* 2000;81:938–943.
89. Kimura IF, Jefferson LM, Gulick DT, et al. Intra- and intertester reliability of Chatillon and MicroFet hand-held dynamometers in measuring force production. *J Sport Rehabil* 1996;5:197–205.
90. Kramer JF, Vaz MD, Vandervoort AA. Reliability of isometric hip abductor torques during examiner and belt-resisted tests. *J Gerontol* 1991;46:M47–M51.
91. Kwoh CK, Petrick MA, Munin MC. Inter-rater reliability for function and strength measurements in acute care hospital after elective hip and knee arthroplasty. *Arthritis Care Res* 1997;10:128–134.
92. Lamontagne A, Malouin F, Richards CL, et al. Evaluation of reflex- and nonreflex-induced muscle resistance to stretch in adults with spinal cord injury using hand-held and isokinetic dynamometry. *Phys Ther* 1998;964–978.
93. Leggin BO, Neuman RM, Iannotti JP, et al. Intrarater and interrater reliability of three isometric dynamometers in assessing shoulder strength. *J Shoulder Elbow Surg* 1996;5:18–24.
94. Lennon SM, Ashburn A. Use of myometry in assessments of neuropathic weakness: testing for reliability in clinical practice. *Clin Rehabil* 1993;7:125–133.
95. Links TP, Zwarts MJ, Oosterhuis HJGH. Improvement in muscle strength in familial hypokalaemic periodic paralysis with acetazolamide. *J Neurol Neurosurg Psychiatry* 1988;51:142–145.

96. Lovett RW, Martin EG. Spring balance muscle test. *Am J Ortho Surg* 1916;14:415–425.
97. Magnussen SP, Gleim GW, Nicholas JA. Shoulder weakness in professional baseball players. *Med Sci Sports Exer* 1994;26:5–9.
98. Malouin F, Boiteau M, Bonneau C, et al. Use of a hand-held dynamometer for evaluation of spasticity in a clinical setting: a reliability study. *Physiother Can* 1989;41:126–134.
99. Malouin F, Bonneau C, Pichard L, et al. Non-reflex mediated changes in plantarflexor muscles early after stroke. *Scand J Rehabil Med* 1997;29:147–153.
100. May LA, Burnham RS, Steadward RD. Assessment of isokinetic and hand-held dynamometer measures of shoulder rotator strength among individuals with spinal cord injury. *Arch Phys Med Rehabil* 1997;78:251–255.
101. Marino M, Nicholas JA, Gleim GW, et al. Efficacy of manual assessment of muscle strength using a new device. *Am J Sports Med* 1982;10:360–364.
102. Mascal CL, Landel R, Powers C. Management of patellofemoral pain targeting hip, pelvis, and trunk muscle function: 2 case reports. *J Orthop Sports Phys Ther* 2003;33:642–660.
103. Mastaglia FL, Knezevic W, Thompson PD. Weakness of head turning in hemiplegia: a quantitative study. *J Neurol Neurosurg Psychiatry* 1986;49:195–197.
104. Mathiowetz V, Kashman N, Volland G, et al. Grip and pinch strength: normative data for adults. *Arch Phys Med Rehabil* 1985;66:69–74.
105. McMahon LM, Burdett RG, Whitney SL. Effects of muscle group and placement site on reliability of hand-held dynamometry strength measurements. *J Orthop Sports Phys Ther* 1992;15:236–242.
106. Mendell JR, Florence J. Manual muscle testing. *Muscle Nerve* 1990;13:S16–S20.
107. Mercer VS, Lewis CL. Hip abductor and knee extensor muscle strength of children with and without Downs syndrome. *Pediatr Phys Ther* 2001;13:18–26.
108. Merlini L, Mazzone ES, Solari AS, et al. Reliability of hand-held dynamometry in spinal muscular atrophy. *Muscle Nerve* 2002;26:64–70.
109. Molnar GE, Alexander J. Objective, quantitative muscle testing in children: a pilot study. *Arch Phys Med Rehabil* 1973;54:224–228.
110. Morris AF, Vaughan SE, Vaccaro P. Measurements of neuromuscular tone and strength in Downs syndrome children. *J Ment Defic Res* 1982;26:41–46.
111. Newman LB. A new device for measuring muscle strength. *Arch Phys Med Rehabil* 1949; 30:234–237.
112. Nicholas J, Sapega A, Kraus H, et al. Factors influencing manual muscle tests in physical therapy. *J Bone Joint Surg* 1978;60A:186–190.
113. Nicklin J, Karni Y, Wiles CM. Shoulder abduction fatiguability. *J Neurol Neurosurg Psychiatry* 1987;50:423–427.
114. Noreau L, Vachon J. Comparison of three methods to assess muscular strength in individuals with spinal cord injury. *Spinal Cord* 1998;36:716–723.
115. Pearn J. Two early dynamometers: an historical account of earliest measurements to study human muscular strength. *J Neurosci* 1978;37:127–134.
116. Pestronk A, Lopate G, Kornberg AJ, et al. Distal lower motor neuron syndrome with high-titer serum IM anti-GM antibodies. *Neurol* 1994;44:2027–2031.
117. Puharic T, Bohannon RW. Measurement of forearm pronation and supination strength with a hand-held dynamometer for wrist flexion and extension. *Isokinet Exerc Sci* 1993;3:202–206.
118. Rabin SI, Post M. A comparative study of clinical muscle testing and Cybex evaluation after shoulder operations. *Clin Orthop* 1990;258:147–156.
119. Rarick L, Gross K, Mohns MJ. Comparison of two methods of measuring strength of selected muscle groups in children. *Res Quart* 1955;26:74–79.
120. Reed RL, Den Hartog R, Yochum K, et al. A comparison of hand-held isometric strength measurement with isokinetic muscle strength measurement in elderly. *J Am Geriatr Soc* 1993; 41:53–56.
121. Reinking MF, Bockrath-Pugliese K, Worrell T, et al. Assessment of quadriceps muscle performance by hand-held, isometric, and isokinetic dynamometry in patients with knee dysfunction. *J Orthop Sports Phys Ther* 1996;24:154–159.
122. Resnick JS, Mammel M, Mundale MO, et al. Muscular strength as an index of response to therapy in childhood dermatomyositis. *Arch Phys Med Rehabil* 1981;62:12–19.
123. Rheault W, Beal JL, Kubik DR, et al. Intertester reliability of hand-held dynamometer for wrist flexion and extension. *Arch Phys Med Rehabil* 1989;70:907–910.
124. Rice CL, Cunningham DA, Paterson DH, et al. Strength in an elderly population. *Arch Phys Med Rehabil* 1989;70:391–297.
125. Richardson J, Stratford P, Cripps D. Assessment of reliability of hand-held dynamometer for measuring strength in healthy older adults. *Physio Theory Practice* 1998;14:49–54.
126. Richardson J, Stratford P, DePaul V, et al. A multirater reliability study of isometric elbow strength in healthy adults. *Physiother Can* 1997;49:178–183.
127. Riddle DL, Finucane SC, Rothstein JL, et al. Intrasession and intersession reliability of hand-held dynamometer measurements taken on brain-damaged patients. *Phys Ther* 1989;69:182–189.

128. Saraniti AJ, Gleim GW, Melvin M, et al. Relationship between subjective and objective measurements of strength. *J Orthop Sports Phys Ther* 1980;2:15–19.
129. Schwartz S, Cohen ME, Berbison GJ, et al. Relationship between two measures of upper extremity strength: manual muscle test compared to hand-held myometry. *Arch Phys Med Rehabil* 1992;73:1063–1068.
130. Schneider-Gold C, Beck M, Wessig C, et al. Creatine monohydrate in DM2/PROMM. *Neurol* 2003;60:500–502.
131. Scott OM, Hyde SA, Goddard C, et al. Quantitation of muscle function in children: a prospective study in Duchenne muscular dystrophy. *Muscle Nerve* 1982;5:291–301.
132. Sexton TC. *Interrater versus intrarater reliability of Microfet manual muscle testing system in assessment of hip flexion* [master's thesis]. Buffalo, NY: D'Youville College, 1994.
133. Shrout PE, Fleiss JL. Intraclass correlations: uses in assessing rater reliability. *Psychol Bull* 1979;86:420–428.
134. Simmonds MJ. Muscle strength. In: Van Deusen J, Brunt D, eds. *Assessment in Occupational Therapy and Physical Therapy*. Philadelphia: WB Saunders, 1996:27–48.
135. Smidt GL. Serial assessment and treatment of a humeral fracture. *J Orthop Sports Phys Ther* 1980;2:25–34.
136. Smidt GL, Albright JP, Deusinger RH. Pre- and postoperative functional changes in total knee patients. *J Orthop Sports Phys Ther* 1984;6:25–29.
137. Smidt WR, Clark CR, Smidt GL. Short-term strength and pain changes in total hip arthroplasty patients. *J Orthop Sports Phys Ther* 1990;12:16–23.
138. Smidt GL, Rodgers MW. Factors contributing to regulation and clinical assessment of muscular strength. *Phys Ther* 1982;62:1283–1290.
139. Soderberg GL. *Kinesiology: Application to Pathological Motion*, 2nd ed. Baltimore: Williams Wilkins, 1997:1–27.
140. Soderberg GL, Robinson S. Letter to editor. *Phys Ther* 2000;80:528.
141. Soderberg GL, Wallentine SW, Knutson LM. Human joint torque: a meta analysis. *Phys Ther*. In review.
142. Soderberg GL, Wallentine SW, Knutson LM. *Clinician's Torque Manual*. Springfield, MO: PTFutures, 2004.
143. Task Force on Standards for Measurement in Physical Therapy. Standards for tests and measurements in physical therapy practice. *Phys Ther* 1991;71:589–622.
144. Stratford DW, Balsor BE. A comparison of make and break tests using a hand-held dynamometer and Kin-Com. *J Orthop Sports Phys Ther* 1993;19:28–32.
145. Stuberg WA, Metcalf WK. Reliability of quantitative muscle testing in healthy children and in children with Duchenne muscular dystrophy using a hand-held dynamometer. *Phys Ther* 1988;68:977–982.
146. Sullivan SJ, Chesley A, Hebert G, et al. Validity and reliability of hand-held dynamometry in assessing isometric external rotator performance. *J Orthop Sports Phys Ther* 1988;10:213–217.
147. Suomi R, Collier D. Effects of arthritis exercise programs on functional fitness and perceived activities of daily living measures in older adults with arthritis. *Arch Phys Med Rehabil* 2003;84:1589–1594.
148. Surberg PR, Suomi R, Poppy WK. Validity and reliability of a hand-held dynamometer applied to adults with mental retardation. *Arch Phys Med Rehabil* 1992;73:535–539.
149. Thuer U, Ingervall B. Pressure from lips on teeth and malocclusion. *Am J Orthod Dentofacial Orthop* 1986;90:234–242.
150. Trudelle-Jackson E, Jackson AW, Frankowski CM, et al. Interdevice reliability and validity assessment of Nicholas hand-held dynamometer. *J Orthop Sports Phys Ther* 1994;20:302–306.
151. Van der Ploeg RJO, Fidler V, Oosterhuis HJGH. Hand-held myometry: reference values. *J Neurol Neurosurg Psychiatry* 1991;54:248–251
152. Van der Ploeg RJO, Oosterhuis HJGH, Reuvekamp J. Measuring muscle strength. *J Neurol* 1984;231:200–203.
153. Wadsworth CT, Krishnan R, Sear M, et al. Intrarater reliability of manual muscle testing and hand-held dynametric muscle testing. *Phys Ther* 1987;67:1342–1347.
154. Wiles CM, Karni Y. Measurement of muscle strength in patients with peripheral neuromuscular disorders. *J Neurol Neurosurg Psychiatry* 1983;46:1006–1013.
155. Wilkolm JB, Bohannon RW. Hand-held dynamometer measurements: tester strength makes a difference. *J Orthop Sports Phys Ther* 1991;13:191–198.

8

TECHNIQUES of the SENSORY EXAMINATION

SENSORY TESTING

One frequently finds that individuals who demonstrate muscle weakness or impairment also have abnormalities of peripheral sensation and other modalities subserved by the nervous system. Chapter 8 presents basic techniques for the clinical examination of sensation throughout the body as well as techniques for examining myotatic or deep tendon reflexes. Chapter 9 expands on Chapter 8 by presenting techniques for the remainder of the neurologic screening examination.

Sensory testing is directed by the patient's history. Rarely is the performance of an entire body sensory examination necessary or efficacious (except in cases such as spinal cord injury). Rather, the examiner is guided toward areas of focus by the patient's response to questioning during history taking and by signs and symptoms that may become apparent during the physical examination. If the patient reports loss of sensation, "numbness," "pins and needles," "tingling," or other subjective feelings associated with possible sensory loss in a particular body area, the examiner should begin the examination in the affected area. Even if the patient reports no sensory changes, other examination findings such as motor loss in a peripheral nerve pattern may cause the examiner to suspect that sensory deficits may be present. Again, the results of the history and physical examination should guide the sensory examination.

The techniques presented in this chapter constitute a method of clinical examination of sensation and provide a means of detecting gross sensory abnormalities in the patient. In general, sensory deficits are detected by comparison of sensation between identical regions of the two sides of the body or between proximal and distal regions of the same side of the body. Differences in the ability to perceive a sensory stimulus between body regions or the patient's failure to detect a stimulus when applied constitute abnormalities in sensation. Clinical sensory testing does not provide for the establishment of sensory thresholds or for the comparison of a patient's response to established standards. For such techniques, one must turn to quantitated sensory testing, the description of which is beyond the scope of this text. For a description of quantitated sensory testing, the reader is referred to the bibliography at the end of this chapter.

GENERAL PRINCIPLES OF SENSORY TESTING

The techniques of clinical sensory examination described in this chapter can be used throughout the body, whether one is examining a peripheral nerve, a nerve root, or a cranial nerve. Several general principles should prove helpful for the examiner during all sensory examinations.

1. **The patient should be positioned comfortably so that all tested areas are accessible.** Supine is the position of choice for most of the tests in this chapter because it allows the easiest accessibility to all tested areas with minimal position changes and allows the easiest comparison to conventional peripheral nerve root and dermatome charts. However, should the supine position not be an option, an alternative position such as prone or side lying is acceptable. Sensation cannot be adequately tested through clothing, so the areas of skin to be tested should be exposed, but in a way that the patient's modesty is maintained. Repositioning of the patient during testing should be kept at a minimum.
2. **The testing procedure should be explained to the patient before beginning the examination.** A clear understanding of what is to happen during the test and what is expected of the patient is essential before beginning the testing. Such an explanation includes a demonstration of the sensory modality to be tested on an area of the patient's skin where the sensation is intact, as well as specific instructions about how the patient is to respond to the stimulus.
3. **The patient's vision should be obscured during the actual sensory testing procedure.** The patient should not be allowed to visualize the testing procedure once the procedure has been sufficiently explained, or the results may be compromised.
4. **The examination should be initiated in areas of impaired or absent sensation and should progress toward areas of normal sensation.** This allows a better visualization of the lines of demarcation between impaired and intact sensation.
5. **Areas of the patient's skin where sensation is normal should be used as a standard.** The examiner should establish an area or areas of the patient's skin where the sensation is intact and use these areas as a reference against which sensation in impaired areas is contrasted. Such an area might be the opposite extremity in cases of unilateral sensory loss or a more proximal part of the body in cases of sensory loss due to spinal cord injury.
6. **Sensory deficits should be carefully noted by the examiner.** Such notation may occur in the form of a written description or a diagram and should be compared with established dermatome and peripheral nerve charts for interpretation of results (Figs. 8-1 to 8-4).
7. **Instruments used to test pain sensation should never be used on more than one patient.** Such instruments should be disposed of in an appropriate (sharps) container after use.

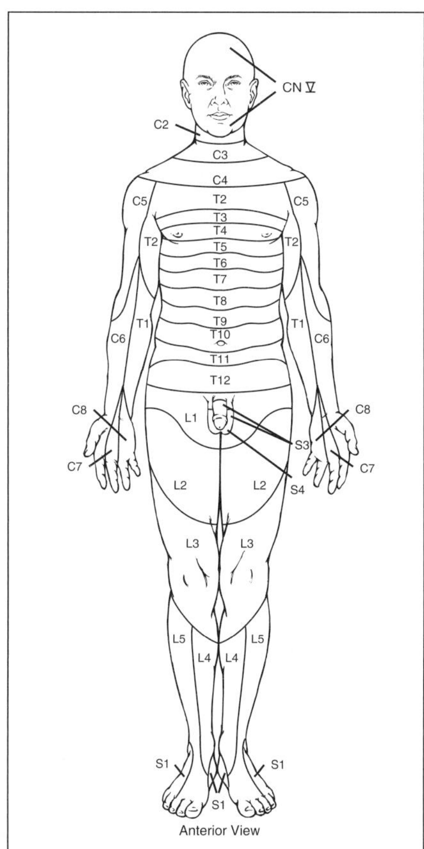

Fig. 8-1. Sensory dermatomes: anterior view.

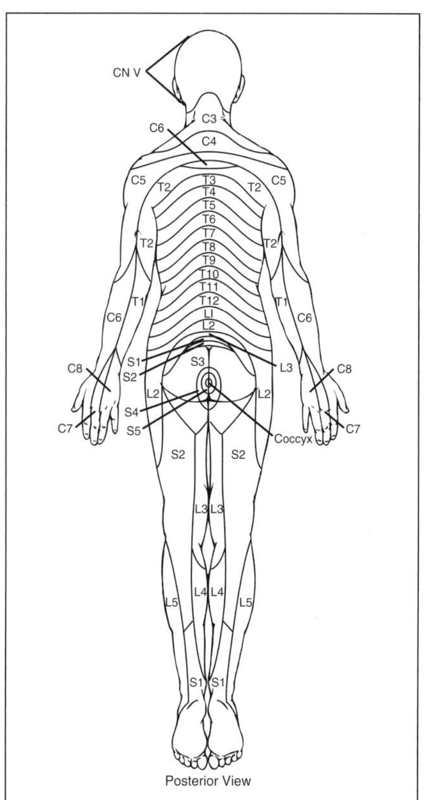

Fig. 8-2. Sensory dermatomes: posterior view.

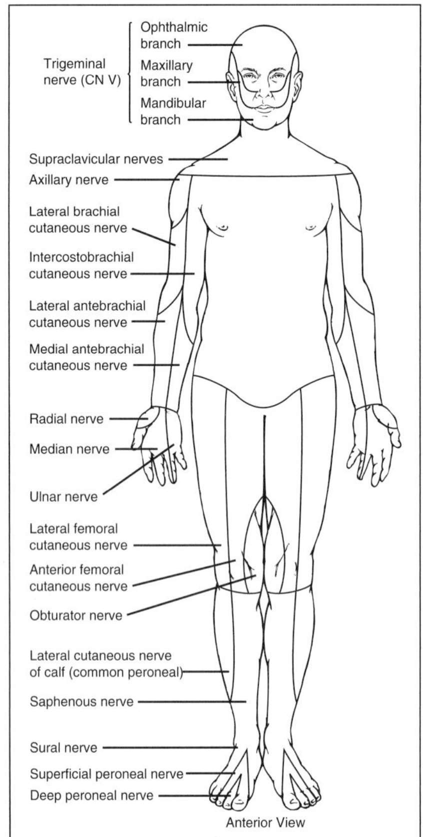

Fig. 8-3. Distribution of peripheral sensory nerves: anterior view.

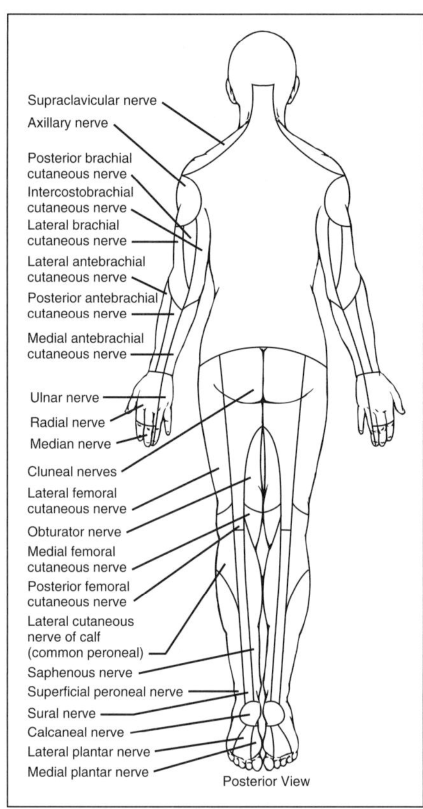

Fig. 8-4. Distribution of peripheral sensory nerves: posterior view.

▪ PAIN

SPINAL CORD TRACT(S)	PERIPHERAL RECEPTORS	FUNCTION	ANATOMY
Anterolateral System	Free nerve endings of Aδ and C fibers	Carries pain sensation from the trunk and extremities	Crosses the spinal cord within 1–2 segments of entry and ascends in the lateral and anterior funiculi on the contralateral side . Terminates in the ventral posterolateral (VPL) nucleus of the thalamus. Information is relayed from the thalamus to the primary somatosensory strip of the cerebral cortex (postcentral gyrus) contralateral to the origin of the pathway.
Ventral trigeminothalamic tract	Free nerve endings of Aδ and C fibers	Carries pain (and other sensations) from the face	Crosses to the opposite side in the medulla. Terminates primarily in the ventral posteromedial (VPM) nucleus of the thalamus. Information is relayed from the thalamus to the face region of the primary somatosensory strip of the cerebral cortex (postcentral gyrus)

■ PAIN

Testing (Figs. 8-5 and 8-6)

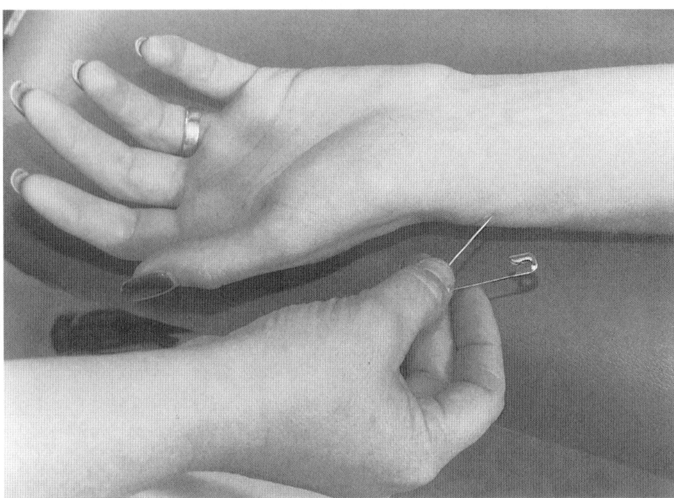

Fig. 8-5. Test for sharp/dull discrimination.

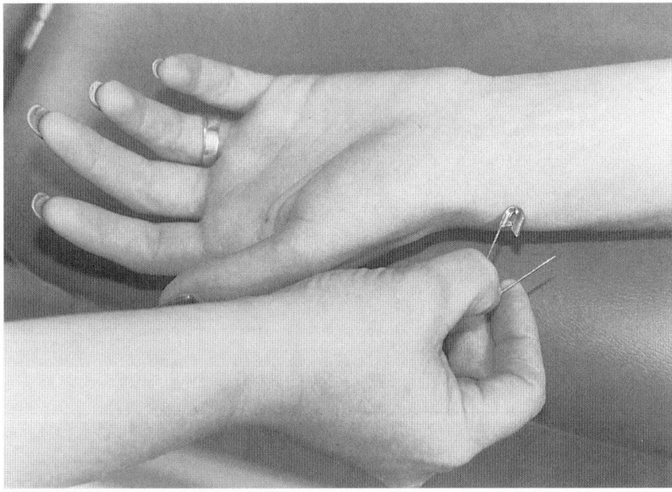

Fig. 8-6. Test for sharp/dull discrimination.

Materials needed: A clean, unused safety pin or a sterile wooden cotton-tipped applicator is used (and then disposed of).

Patient position: Supine with the areas of skin to be tested exposed.

Procedure: Before the examination, the examiner should explain the procedure to the patient, demonstrating the feel of each end of the pin or cotton-tipped applicator in an area where the patient has intact sensation. The neck is an area where sensation is not usually disturbed and may be used for demonstration purposes.

Once the examination begins, the patient's eyes should be closed or covered. Using the safety pin or wooden, cotton-tipped applicator, the examiner touches the patient alternately but in a random order with the sharp or dull end of the pin. (If the wooden applicator is used, the stick of the applicator should be broken to create a "sharp" end, and the cotton-tipped end should be used for the "dull" end.) The force used when touching the patient with the sharp end of the instrument should be sufficient to indent, but not to break, the skin. The patient should be instructed to respond with the words "sharp" or "dull" upon perceiving the stimulus. The examiner should avoid providing any indication, verbal or otherwise, when the patient has been touched during the examination.

When applying the stimulus, the examiner should begin stimulation in areas of the body where the patient has indicated that sensation is impaired, progressing toward areas of intact sensation. Corresponding areas of skin on both sides of the body should be tested for comparison. Once an area of skin is found to have impaired sensation, areas proximal and distal to that area should be tested until areas of normal sensation are found. The examiner should carefully map areas of absent, impaired, and normal sensation and should compare the pattern of sensory loss with established dermatome and peripheral nerve charts for interpretation of results (see Figs. 8-1 to 8-4).

If the patient's responses appear confused or inappropriate at any time during the examination, the examiner should return to the stimulation of the areas of the skin where sensation is known to be intact. In this way, the patient's responses can be checked for accuracy.

Once the examination for pain sensation is completed, the stimulating instrument should be disposed of in the appropriate (sharps) container. Such instruments should never be reused with another patient.

CLINICAL COMMENT: REFERRED PAIN

Patients may feel pain in areas of the body that are physically remote from the site of pathology. Such pain is called referred pain. In many cases, pain is referred to more superficially located structures (skin, muscle) from visceral structures (heart, kidney, gall bladder). For example, most patients are cognizant that pain from the heart commonly is experienced in the left arm and shoulder. The examiner should become familiar with patterns of commonly referred pain, as such knowledge is critical to accurate diagnosis.

■ LIGHT TOUCH

SPINAL CORD TRACT(S)	PERIPHERAL RECEPTORS	FUNCTION	ANATOMY
Anterio-lateral system	Merkel discs, Ruffini endings, hair follicle receptors, free nerve endings (Aβ and Aδ fibers)	Carries non-discriminative touch sensation from the trunk and extremities	Crosses the spinal cord within 1–2 segments of entry and ascends in the lateral and anterior funiculi on the contralateral side. Terminates in the ventral posterolateral (VPL) nucleus of the thalamus. Information is relayed from the thalamus to the primary somatosensory strip of the cerebral cortex (postcentral gyrus) contralateral to the origin of the pathway.
Dorsal column/ medial lemniscus pathway	Merkel discs, Ruffini endings, hair follicle receptors, free nerve endings (Aβ and Aδ fibers)	Carries discriminative touch (and other) sensations from the trunk and extremities	Travels in the fasciculus cuneatus and gracilis in the spinal cord; these 1st order axons terminate in the nucleus cuneatus and gracilis in the medulla. Axons of 2nd order neurons in the medulla cross as internal arcuate fibers (medulla) and ascend the brain stem in the contralateral medial lemniscus; the pathway terminates in the VPL nucleus of the thalamus. Information is relayed from the thalamus to the primary somatosensory strip of the cerebral cortex (postcentral gyrus) contralateral to the origin of the pathway.
Trigeminal lemniscus	Merkel discs, Ruffini endings, hair follicle receptors, free nerve endings (Aβ and Aδ fibers)	Carries discriminative touch (and other) sensations from the face	Mostly contralateral. Terminates in the VPM nucleus of the thalamus. Information is relayed from the thalamus to the face region of the primary somatosensory cortex (postcentral gyrus)

Testing (Fig. 8-7)

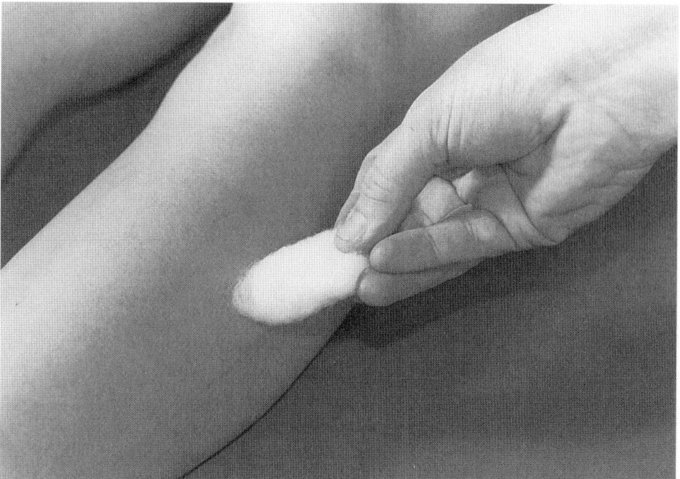

Fig. 8-7. Test for light touch.

Materials needed: A wisp of cotton is used.

Patient position: Supine with the areas of skin to be tested exposed.

Procedure: Before the examination, the examiner should explain the procedure to the patient, demonstrating the feel of the wisp of cotton in an area where the patient has intact sensation.

Once the examination begins, the patient's eyes should be closed or covered. The examiner should instruct the patient to say "yes" as soon as the stimulus is felt and each time the stimulus is felt. Instructions should be given prior to the application of any stimulation. When stimulating the skin with the cotton, the examiner should merely touch the cotton to the skin and should avoid any sort of wiping motion with the cotton. If the cotton is moved over an area of the skin in a wiping motion, the patient will perceive a tickling sensation, which is more closely associated with pain than with light touch.

When applying the stimulus, the examiner should begin stimulation in areas of the body where the patient has indicated that sensation is impaired, progressing toward areas of intact sensation. Corresponding areas of skin on both sides of the body should be tested for comparison. Once an area of skin is found to have impaired sensation, areas proximal and distal to that area should be tested until areas of normal sensation are found. The examiner should carefully map areas of absent, impaired, and normal sensation and should compare the pattern of sensory loss with established dermatome and peripheral nerve charts for interpretation of results (see Figs. 8-1 to 8-4).

If the patient's responses appear confused or inappropriate at any time during the examination, the examiner should return to the stimulation of the areas of the skin where sensation is known to be intact. In this way, the patient's responses can be checked for accuracy.

■ TEMPERATURE

SPINAL CORD TRACT(S)	PERIPHERAL RECEPTORS	FUNCTION	ANATOMY
Antero-lateral system	Thermore-ceptors (Aδ and C fibers)	Carries temperature (and pain) sensation from the trunk and extremities	Crosses the spinal cord within 1–2 segments of entry and ascends in the lateral and anterior funiculi on the contralateral side. Terminates in the ventral posterolateral (VPL) nucleus of the thalamus. Information is relayed from the thalamus to the primary somatosensory strip of the cerebral cortex (postcentral gyrus) contralateral to the origin of the pathway.
Ventral trigemino-thalamic tract	Thermore-ceptors (Aδ and C fibers)	Carries temperature (and other) sensations from the face	Crosses to the opposite side in the medulla. Trigeminothalamic tracts terminate primarily in the VPM nucleus of the thalamus. Information is relayed from the thalamus to the face region of the primary somatosensory strip of the cerebral cortex (postcentral gyrus)

CLINICAL COMMENT: HYPERESTHESIA

Although pathology involving sensory systems can cause decreases or loss of sensation, in some cases, an increased sensitivity to sensory stimulation may be experienced by the patient, particularly when sensory nerves or receptors are irritated. A heightened response to sensory input is known as hyperesthesia and may take the form of hyperpathia (extreme sensitivity to pain), neuralgia (shock-like pain along a dermatome or peripheral nerve distribution), or dysesthesia (numbness, tingling, or burning in the absence of stimulation; frequently also referred to as paresthesia).

Testing (Fig. 8-8)

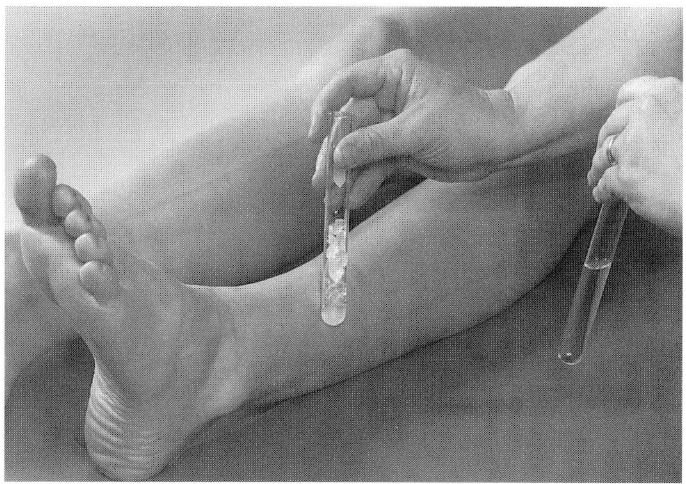

Fig. 8-8. Test for temperature discrimination.

Materials needed:

Two glass test tubes, one filled with crushed ice and water and the other with hot tap water, are used. The temperature of the hot water should not exceed 45° C. At higher temperatures, pain rather than temperature receptors are stimulated, and the patient is at risk for a burn. The outsides of the test tubes should be kept dry.

Patient position:

Supine with the areas of skin to be tested exposed.

Procedure:

Although losses of pain sensibility are generally accompanied by losses of the ability to perceive temperature (because both modalities are carried in the same spinal cord pathway), this is not always the case. Occasionally, a loss of thermal sensation will precede the loss of pain sensation. Testing of thermal sensation is not indicated for all patients, but may be necessary for some.

Before the examination, the examiner should explain the procedure to the patient, demonstrate the feel of each of the two test tubes in an area where the patient has intact sensation, and determine that the patient is able to respond appropriately. The neck is an area where sensation is not usually disturbed and may be used for demonstration purposes.

Once the examination begins, the patient's eyes should be closed or covered. The examiner should instruct the patient to respond with the words "hot" and "cold" in response to being touched with the hot and cold test tubes, respectively. Instructions should be given before the actual testing process. When stimulating the skin with the test tubes, the examiner should apply the tubes in an irregular order and allow each tube to remain in contact with the skin for a minimum of 2 seconds so that the patient has sufficient time to perceive the stimulus.

When applying the stimulus, the examiner should begin stimulation in areas of the body where the patient has indicated that sensation is impaired, progressing toward areas of intact sensation. Corresponding areas of skin on both sides of the body should be tested for comparison. Once an area of skin is found to have impaired sensation, areas proximal and distal to that area should be tested until areas of normal sensation are found. The examiner should return to the area of normal sensation frequently during the examination to ascertain whether a temperature differential still exists when touched by the two test tubes. The examiner should carefully map areas of absent, impaired, and normal sensation and should compare the pattern of sensory loss with established dermatome and peripheral nerve charts for interpretation of results (see Figs. 8-1 to 8-4).

■ *VIBRATION*

SPINAL CORD TRACT(S)	PERIPHERAL RECEPTORS	FUNCTION	ANATOMY
Dorsal column/ medial lemniscus pathway	Meissner and pacinian corpuscles (Aβ fibers)	Carries vibration (and other) sensations from the trunk and extremities	Travels in the fasciculus cuneatus and gracilis in the spinal cord; these 1st order axons terminate in the nucleus cuneatus and gracilis in the medulla. Axons of 2nd order neurons in the medulla cross as internal arcuate fibers (medulla) and ascend the brain stem in the contralateral medial lemniscus; the pathway terminates in the VPL nucleus of the thalamus. Information is relayed from the thalamus to the primary somatosensory strip of the cerebral cortex (postcentral gyrus) contralateral to the origin of the pathway.
Trigeminal lemniscus	Meissner and pacinian corpuscles (Aβ fibers)	Carries vibratory (and other) sensations from the face	Mostly contralateral. Terminates in the VPM nucleus of the thalamus. Information is relayed from the thalamus to the face region of the primary somatosensory cortex (postcentral gyrus)

■ VIBRATION

Testing (Figs. 8-9 and 8-10)

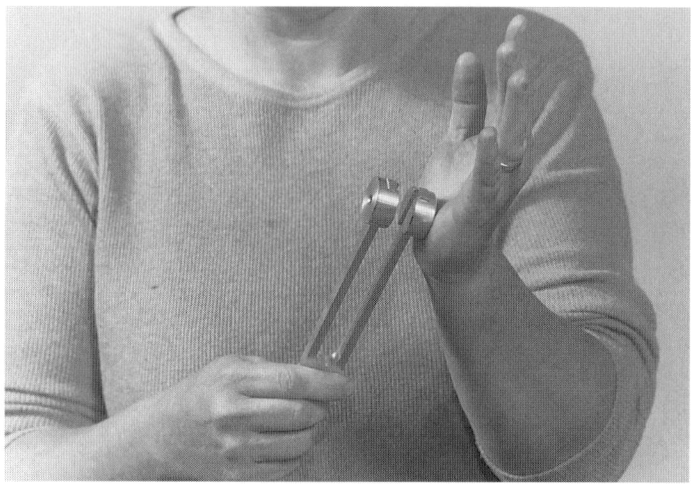

Fig. 8-9. Activation of tuning fork.

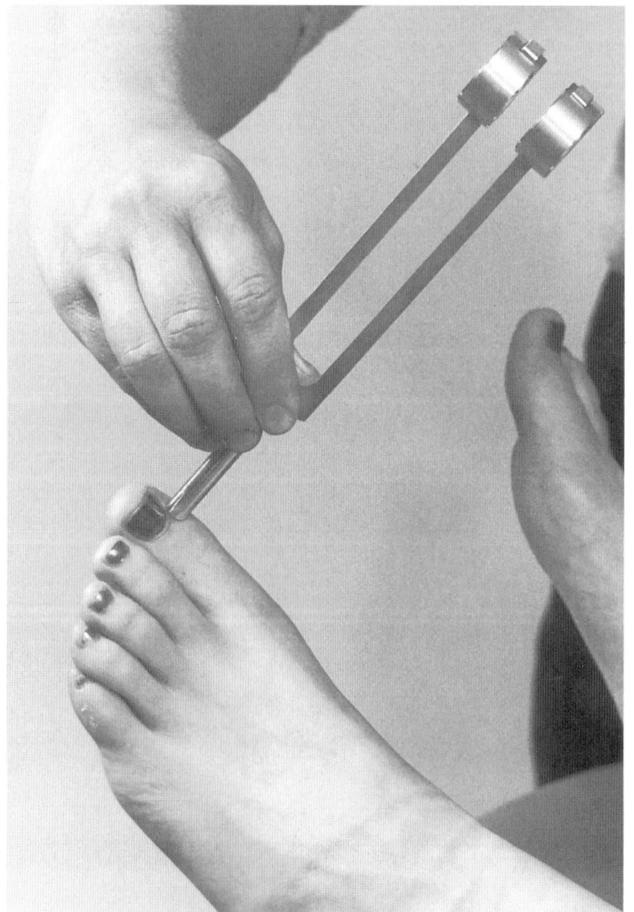

Fig. 8-10. Test for vibratory sensation: great toe.

Materials needed: A 128-Hz tuning fork is used.

Patient position: Supine with the bony prominences to be tested exposed.

Procedure: Before the examination, the examiner should explain the procedure to the patient. The feel of the vibrating tuning fork should be demonstrated over a subcutaneous bony area where sensation is intact. (The sternum or mandible is useful for this purpose.) The patient should be instructed to say "now" or "stopped" the moment the feeling of vibration ceases. By applying both a vibrating and a nonvibrating tuning fork to the patient's sternum or mandible, the examiner can make certain that the patient is responding to the vibration and not to the pressure of the tuning fork.

Once instructions are clearly understood by the patient, the examination may begin. Holding the stem of the tuning fork in one hand, the examiner strikes the tines at their base with the opposite hand to begin the vibration (Fig. 8-9). The stem of the tuning fork is then applied to the bony prominences to be tested and held there until the patient reports that the feeling of vibration has stopped (Fig. 8-10). Once the patient has reported that the sensation of vibration has stopped, the examiner should immediately transfer the tuning fork to the corresponding bony prominence on the opposite extremity. If the patient feels the vibration on the opposite extremity for more than a few seconds, a unilateral sensory deficit should be suspected.

When examining vibratory sensation, the examiner should begin on a distal bony prominence and proceed proximally. In the lower extremity, the testing order could be the distal phalanx of the great toe, the medial malleolus, the knee, the anterior superior iliac spine, and the spinous process of a lumbar vertebra. In the upper extremity, a logical order would be the distal phalanx of the index finger, the ulnar styloid, the olecranon process, the acromion process, and the spinous process of a cervical vertebra.

■ *PROPRIOCEPTION*

SPINAL CORD TRACT(S)	PERIPHERAL RECEPTORS	FUNCTION	ANATOMY
Dorsal column/ medial lemniscus pathway	Meissner and pacinian corpuscles (Aβ fibers)	Carries proprioception (and other) sensations from the trunk and extremities	Travels in the fasciculus cuneatus and gracilis in the spinal cord; these 1st order axons terminate in the nucleus cuneatus and gracilis in the medulla. Axons of 2nd order neurons in the medulla cross as internal arcuate fibers (medulla) and ascend the brain stem in the contralateral medial lemniscus; the pathway terminates in the VPL nucleus of the thalamus. Information is relayed from the thalamus to the primary somatosensory strip of the cerebral cortex (postcentral gyrus) contralateral to the origin of the pathway.
Trigeminal lemniscus	Meissner and pacinian corpuscles (Aβ fibers)	Carries proprioception (and other) sensations from the face	Mostly contralateral. Terminates in the VPM nucleus of the thalamus. Information is relayed from the thalamus to the face region of the primary somatosensory cortex (postcentral gyrus)

Testing (Fig. 8-11)

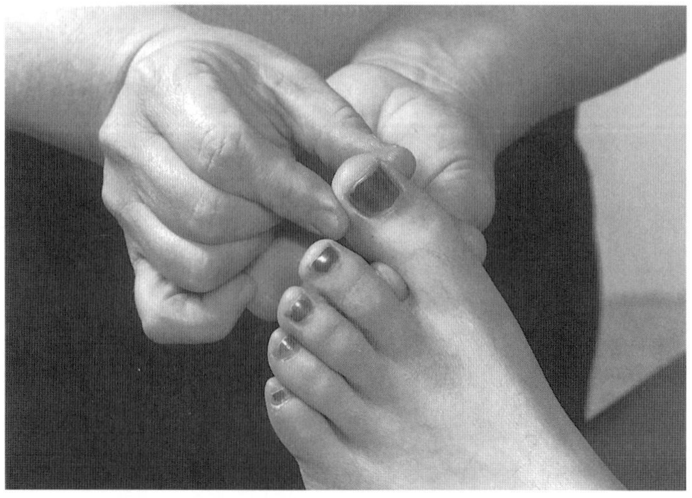

Fig. 8-11. Test for proprioception: first metatarsophalangeal joint.

Materials needed: No materials are needed.

Patient position: Supine with the joints to be tested exposed.

Procedure: Before the examination, the examiner should explain the procedure to the patient. During the explanation, the patient should observe the examiner's movements so that the patient completely understands the procedure to be performed. Once the actual testing begins, the patient's vision should be obscured. Testing is begun with the distal joints of the extremity (toes or fingers) and progresses proximally.

During the explanation, the examiner should begin by grasping the sides of the distal phalanx of the digit to be examined (although the demonstration may be performed on any joint) with one hand and the sides of the more proximal phalanx with the other. The proximal phalanx is stabilized while the distal phalanx is moved slightly into flexion or extension. During this time, the patient's eyes remain uncovered, and the patient is allowed to observe the movement. The examiner instructs the patient to say "up" when the phalanx is moved toward extension and "down" when the phalanx is moved toward flexion.

Once actual testing is begun, the patient's vision is obscured. The examiner then moves the distal phalanx of the digit a few degrees in the direction of flexion or extension and awaits the patient's response. Care should be taken to hold the distal phalanx along its lateral sides, as pressure on the dorsal or ventral surface will cue the patient as to the direction of the movement. The movements are then repeated in a random order in the direction of either flexion or extension, and the patient's responses are noted. The test is performed with the contralateral extremity as well, and the responses for the two sides are compared. If proprioception is intact, the patient's responses should be 100% accurate. Should proprioceptive deficits be suspected, the test should be repeated at progressively more proximal joints until intact proprioception is found. In general, an individual with normal proprioception should be able to detect flexion or extension of 1 to 2° at the interphalangeal joints.

ROMBERG TEST (Figs. 8-12 and 8-13)

Fig. 8-12. Romberg test: eyes open.

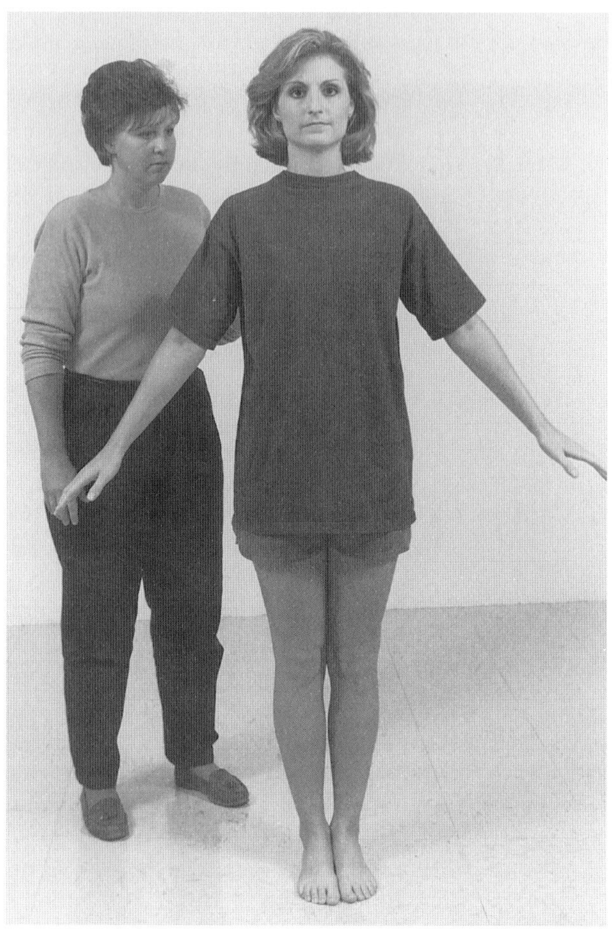

Materials needed: No materials are needed.

Patient position: Standing with the feet as close together as possible.

Procedure: The examiner stands just behind and to the side of the patient and asks the patient to maintain balance while standing with the feet positioned as close together as possible. The test is performed first with the patient's eyes open and then with the eyes closed.

Normal response: The patient should be able to maintain balance in this position both with the eyes open and with the eyes closed. Some small amount of swaying is normal when the eyes are closed, but the patient should not fall.

LESIONS

Patients who are unable to perform the Romberg test with the eyes open should be suspected of having a disease involving the cerebellum, whereas those who fail the test (have a positive Romberg test result) only with the eyes closed most typically possess a proprioceptive deficit (which could be secondary to peripheral nerve disease, posterior column pathology, or cortical sensory loss).

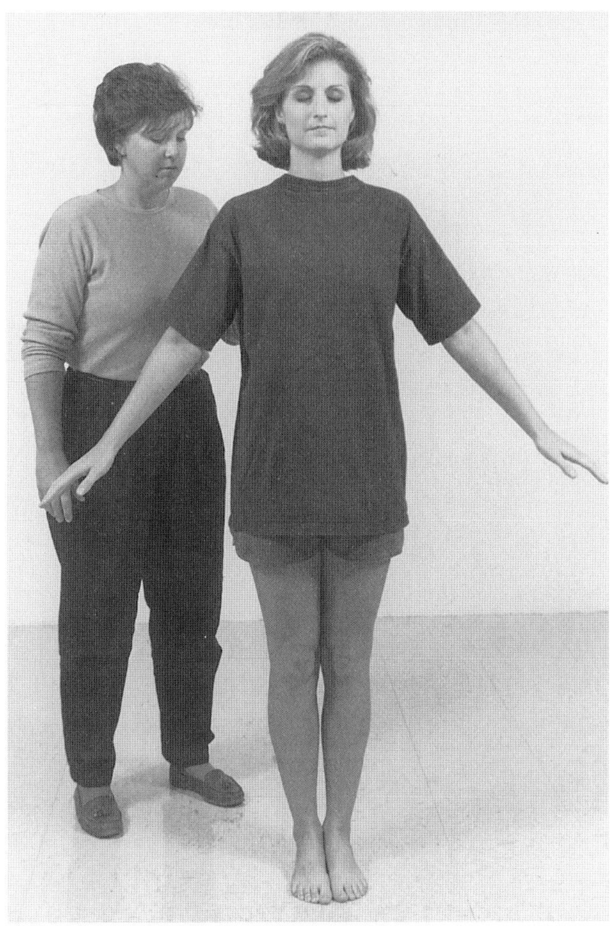

Fig. 8-13. Romberg test: eyes closed.

TANDEM ROMBERG (Figs. 8-14 and 8-15)

Fig. 8-14. Tandem (sharpened) Romberg test: eyes open.

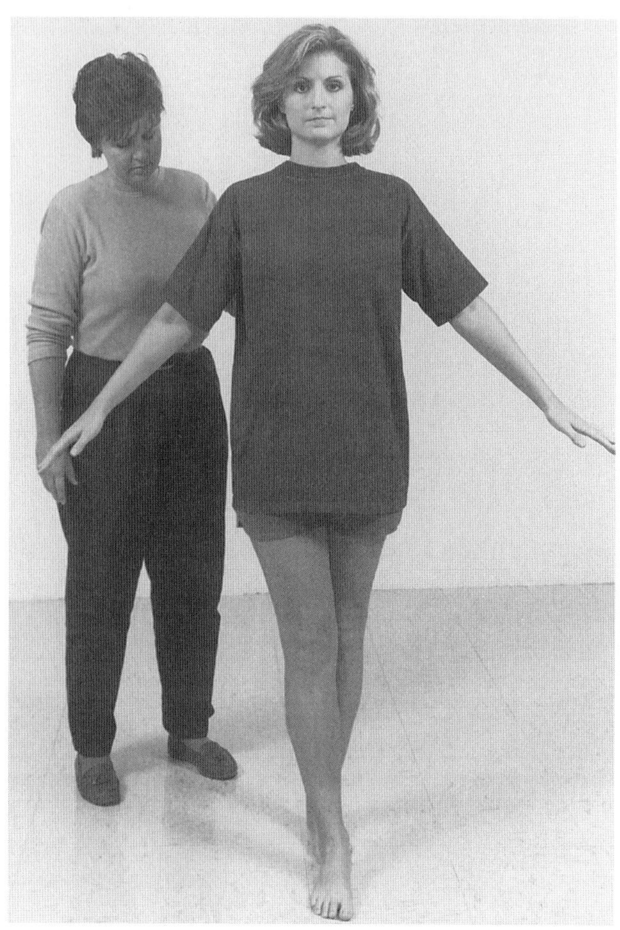

Materials needed: No materials are needed.

Patient position: Standing with the arms at the sides and the feet positioned so that the heel of one foot is directly in front of the toes of the other foot.

Procedure: The examiner asks the patient to stand in this position first with the eyes open and then with the eyes closed.

Normal response: The patient should be able to maintain balance in this position both with the eyes open and with the eyes closed. Some swaying is normal, but excessive swaying should not occur and the patient should not fall.

Note: The tandem Romberg, sometimes called the *sharpened Romberg*, is designed to be used for patients with more subtle balance deficits who are able to complete the basic Romberg test without incident.

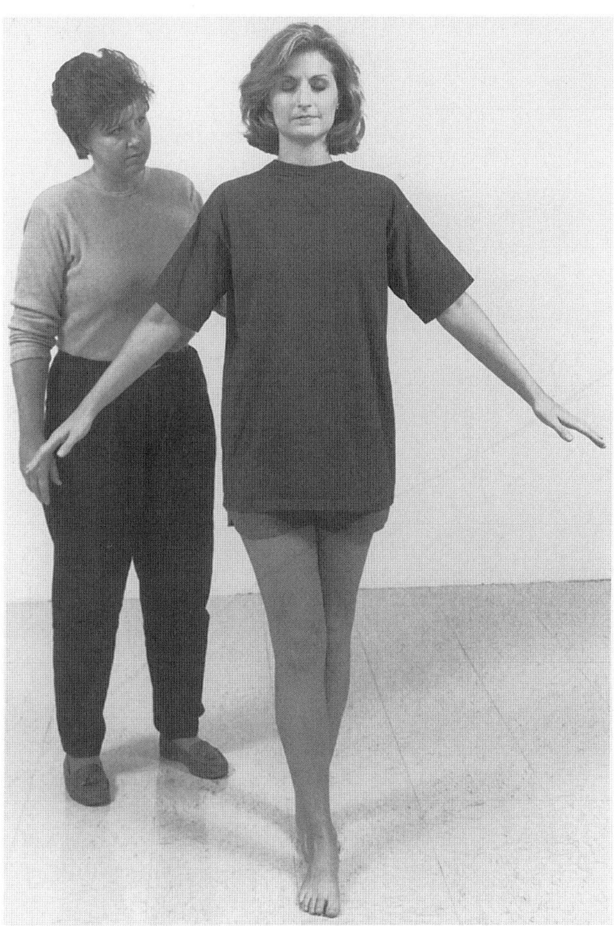

Fig. 8-15. Tandem (sharpened) Romberg test: eyes closed.

CLINICAL COMMENT: ROMBERG TEST

The Romberg test is a test of function of the dorsal column system. Inability to perform the Romberg test with the eyes open may be indicative of cerebellar pathology (see Chapter 9). However, the ability to maintain balance during this test with the eyes open, followed by loss of balance once the eyes are closed, points to a disorder involving proprioceptive systems.

ABNORMAL RESPONSES TO SENSORY TESTING

Correctly interpreting sensory deficits encountered in the patient may seem a daunting task. However, the process is quite straightforward if the examiner possesses the essential tools for solving the problem. A list of such tools and an example of the ways in which they might be used to assist in interpreting sensory deficits follows.

1. **The examiner must possess a working knowledge of the anatomy, physiology, and pathophysiology of the nervous system.** This knowledge forms the basis for an accurate interpretation of the neurologic signs and symptoms presented by the patient.
2. **A conceptual and recorded picture of the patient's sensory deficits must be compiled.** This picture is obtained through the patient history and the results of the sensory examination and is diagrammed or described.
3. **The patient's sensory deficits must be analyzed for the presence of a pattern.** In searching for a pattern, the examiner should ask questions such as "Does the sensory loss occur in only one limb? On only one side of the body? In only one part of a limb?"
4. **Once a pattern is established, the pattern must be interpreted on the basis of the examiner's working knowledge of the nervous system.** For example, the examiner should compare the patient's pattern of sensory loss with established dermatome and peripheral nerve charts to determine if the lesion lies in a peripheral nerve or a nerve root.
5. **After comparing the pattern of sensory deficit with the known anatomy of the nervous system, the examiner must derive one or more possibilities for the location of the lesion(s) causing the deficit.**
6. **Other symptoms of nervous system pathology must be considered.** The patient also may exhibit motor weakness, cranial nerve deficits, motor control problems, or other signs of neurologic involvement that must be taken into account.
7. **Clarification of the location of the lesion should occur.** The consideration of each possible lesion site in light of the nonsensory signs will allow the examiner to arrive at the most likely location for the lesion causing the patient's neurologic signs and symptoms.

The sensory deficits generated by a neurologic lesion depend on the location of that lesion along the neuraxis. While the following guidelines are somewhat simplified and cannot substitute for a thorough understanding of the anatomy and physiology of the nervous system, they provide a basic summary of the pattern of deficits that should be expected on the basis of the location of the neurologic lesion.

Peripheral nerve. Loss of all types of sensation in the distribution of the affected nerve. If more than one nerve is affected, the sensory loss would extend to the territories of all nerves affected. With the exception of polyneuropathy, the sensory loss is typically unilateral. Polyneuropathy frequently causes sensory loss in a "glove and stocking" distribution involving the distal portion of the upper or lower extremities. Irritative lesions of the peripheral nerve may result in pain with or without paresthesias along the nerve's distribution.

Nerve root. Loss of all types of sensation in the dermatome of the affected nerve root. Sensory deficits are typically unilateral. As with peripheral nerves, irritative lesions may result in pain with or without paresthesias along the dermatomal distribution.

Spinal cord. The specific sensory losses observed following lesions of the spinal cord depend on the extent and area of spinal cord damage. If only part of the cord has a lesion, the sensory modality(ies) carried by the damaged tract(s) would be lost. For example, a lesion involving both posterior columns (damaging the dorsal column/medial lemniscus system) would result in bilateral loss of proprioception, vibratory sense, and two-point discrimination below the level of the lesion, whereas a lesion involving one lateral column (damaging the anterolateral system) would cause loss of pain and temperature sensation on the contralateral side of the body beginning about two segments below the level of the lesion. If the damage to the cord is complete, the loss of sensation involves all sensory modalities bilaterally.

Brain stem. Lesions of sensory pathways as they travel through the brain stem generally result in sensory loss in the contralateral side of the body and cranial nerve deficits (if present) on the ipsilateral side. This is because the primary sensory pathways for the trunk and extremities cross to the opposite side either at the level of the spinal cord (anterolateral system) or in the caudal medulla (dorsal column/medial lemniscus system).

Cerebral cortex. Sensory deficits will be experienced in the contralateral limbs. The patient may experience diminished sensory perception or an inability to localize the site of stimulation (atopognosia).

CLINICAL COMMENT: AGNOSIAS

Lesions involving the parietal cortex may produce deficits in associating a sensory stimulus with knowledge or memory of that stimulus. As an example, a patient with auditory agnosia would be able to hear a doorbell ring, but would not associate that noise with the need to answer the door.

Other types of agnosias include:

- Tactile agnosia - inability to recognize objects through the sense of touch
- Agraphagnosia - inability to recognize letters traced on the skin
- Prosopagnosia - inability to recognize faces; usually due to a temporal lobe lesion

DEEP TENDON REFLEX TESTING

Anatomy of the Deep Tendon Reflex

Deep tendon reflexes (also called *myotatic* or *muscle stretch reflexes*) are monosynaptic (one synapse) reflexes. As such, they are composed of an afferent (sensory) limb and an efferent (motor) limb with a synapse between the two limbs in the ventral horn of the spinal cord (Fig. 8-16). The afferent limb of the reflex is composed of a type Ia sensory neuron to the muscle spindle, which responds to a quick stretch of the muscle. When such a quick stretch is applied to the muscle (as in striking the tendon of an already partially stretched muscle with a reflex hammer), many type Ia sensory fibers are activated. These fibers synapse on α motor neurons innervating the stimulated muscle (efferent limb of the reflex), resulting in a contraction of that muscle. Therefore by testing the deep tendon reflexes, one can examine both the afferent and efferent limbs of the spinal nerves that comprise a given reflex.

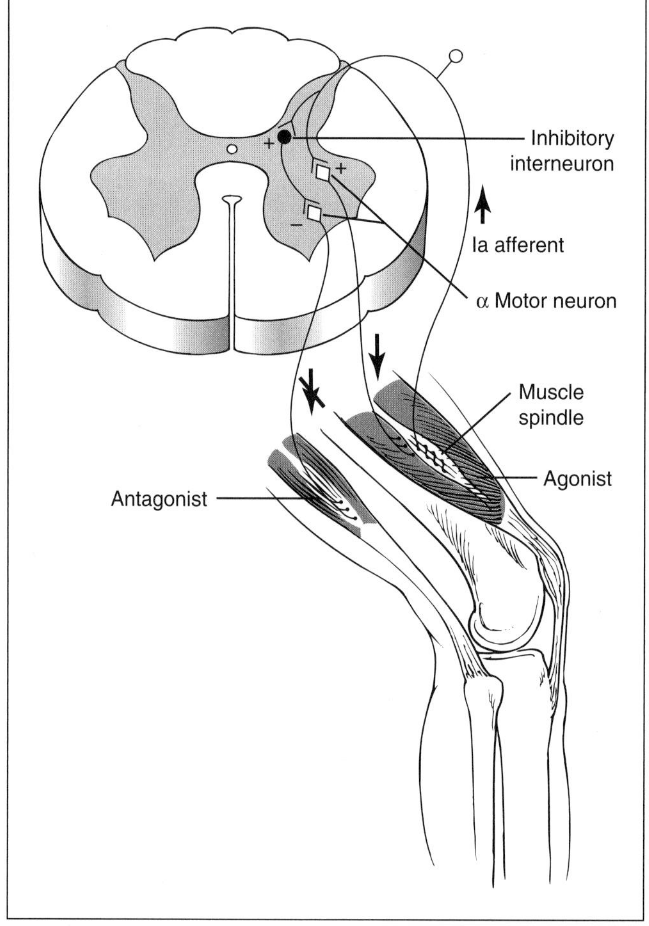

Fig. 8-16. Diagram of deep tendon reflex.

REFLUX	SPINAL SEGMENTS	STIMULATION SITE	RESPONSE
Biceps	C5, C6	Biceps tendon (cubital fossa)	Elbow flexion
Brachioradialis	C5, C6	Brachioradialis tendon (proximal to the radial styloid)	Elbow flexion
Triceps	C6, C7	Triceps tendon (proximal to the olecranon)	Elbow extension
Quadriceps	L2–L4	Patellar tendon (between the patella and tibial tuberosity)	Knee extension
Achilles	S1–S2	Tendo calcaneus (proximal to the calcaneus on the posterior leg)	Ankle plantar flexion

About Testing Deep Tendon Reflexes

Following a few simple guidelines when testing deep tendon reflexes will create a greater chance of successful elicitation of the patient's reflexes and will make testing simpler for the examiner. These guidelines should be followed each time deep tendon reflexes are tested.

1. **Encourage complete relaxation from the patient.** If the patient is tense or uncomfortable, an accurate response cannot be obtained. Part of ensuring patient relaxation is proper support of the tested part. The examiner should provide complete support of the extremity being tested so that no muscle contraction is required by the patient to maintain the test position. If the patient still has difficulty relaxing, the examiner may need to use verbal cues such as "relax your arms" or distraction techniques such as engaging the patient in conversation during testing.
2. **Establish proficiency in using the reflex hammer.** Practice is required before one can become competent at swinging the reflex hammer with the proper force and accuracy. The reflex hammer should be held rather loosely and allowed to swing freely during the testing maneuver. The stimulus should be firm, brisk, and brief and should be applied to the tendon only, avoiding surrounding bony structures.
3. **Use reinforcement techniques if necessary.** Reflexes are more difficult to elicit in some patients than in others. If one is unable to obtain a response even though the stimulus is adequate and accurate, reinforcement techniques should be used. Reinforcement consists of having the patient perform a strong muscle contraction in an area of the body away from the reflex. Such a contraction will heighten the reflex response through an incompletely understood mechanism. The muscle contraction must not involve the extremity being tested, because contraction of the tested muscle will inhibit the reflex. For lower extremity reflexes, the Jendrassik maneuver, in which the patient interlocks the fingers and attempts to pull them apart, is a useful reinforcement technique (Fig. 8-17). For upper extremity reflexes, squeezing the knees together or making a fist with the opposite hand are both good options. Patients who are otherwise motorically impaired may clench their teeth. When reinforcement is used, the patient should be instructed to perform the reinforcement technique just as the examiner strikes the tendon. To ensure that this happens, tell the patient to "squeeze," "pull," and so forth and then immediately strike the tendon with the reflex hammer.

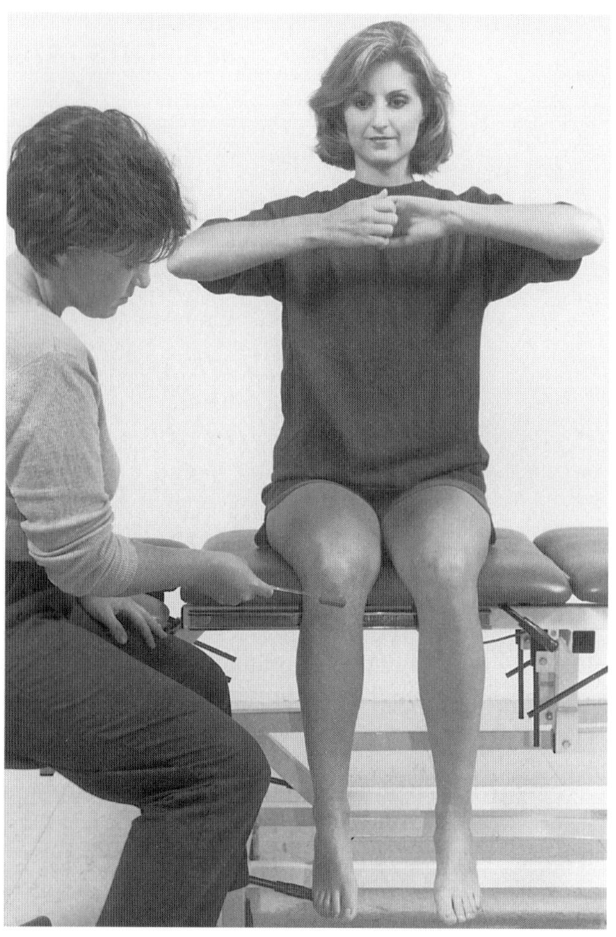

Fig. 8-17. Jendrassik maneuver during patellar reflex testing.

Grading the Reflex Response

Deep tendon reflexes are normally graded on a 0 to 4 scale based on the quality of the response observed. Plus signs are used by convention to the right of all numbers other than 0. The definitions of the various grades are as follows:

0 = No response; muscle contraction is neither palpable nor visible, even with reinforcement.
1+ = Minimal response; generally consisting of slight muscle contraction without joint movement. Reinforcement may be required to produce muscle contraction.
2+ = Normal response; mild muscle contraction is accompanied by minor joint movement.
3+ = Brisk response; moderate to strong muscle contraction occurs with obvious joint movement.
4+ = Hyperactive reflex; very strong brisk muscle contraction is accompanied by exaggerated joint movement, generally associated with clonus.

Grades 0 and 4+ are indicative of pathology. Grades 1+ and 3+ are generally normal unless asymmetric or accompanied by other associated abnormalities.

■ BICEPS REFLEX

Testing (Fig. 8-18)

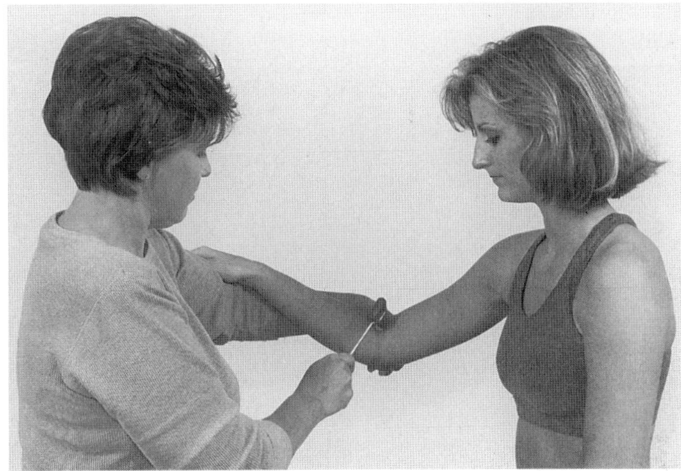

Fig. 8-18. Biceps reflex (C5, C6).

Materials needed: A reflex hammer is used.

Patient position: Seated or standing with the forearm resting on the examiner's forearm. The patient's elbow is flexed with the forearm in supination.

Procedure: The examiner places a thumb over the patient's biceps tendon and strikes the thumbnail with the pointed tip of the reflex hammer.

Normal response: Elbow flexion is the normal response.

■ BRACHIORADIALIS REFLEX

Testing (Fig. 8-19)

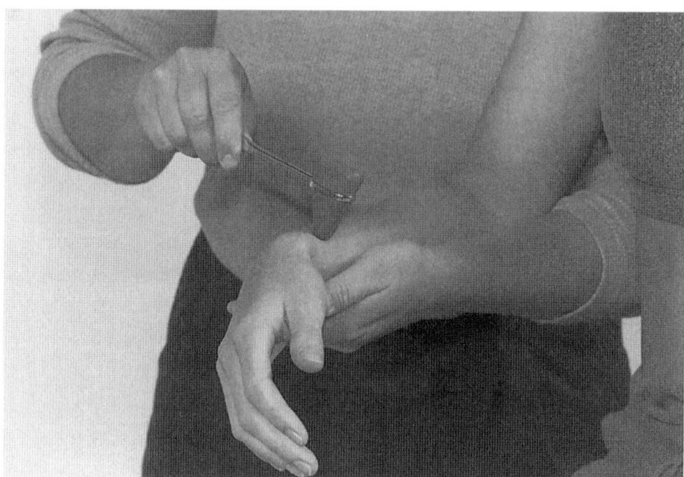

Fig. 8-19. Brachioradialis reflex (C5, C6).

Materials needed: A reflex hammer is used.

Patient position: Seated or standing with the forearm resting on the examiner's forearm. The patient's elbow is flexed, and the forearm is neutral.

Procedure: The examiner strikes the radial side of the patient's forearm with the head of the reflex hammer just proximal to the radial styloid process.

Normal response: Elbow flexion is the normal response.

■ TRICEPS REFLEX

Testing (Fig. 8-20)

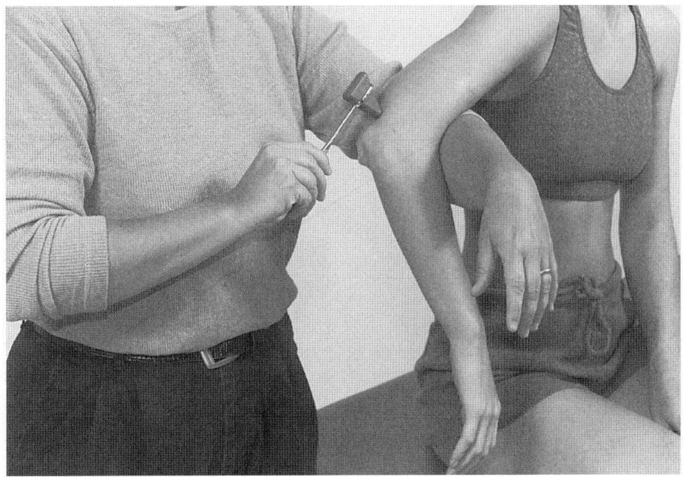

Fig. 8-20. Triceps reflex (C6, C7).

Materials needed: A reflex hammer is used.

Patient position: Seated or standing with the arm supported by the examiner. The patient's arm is abducted and medially rotated, and the elbow is flexed to 90°.

Procedure: The examiner strikes the patient's triceps tendon with the head of the reflex hammer just proximal to the olecranon process.

Normal response: Elbow extension is the normal response.

■ QUADRICEPS REFLEX

Testing (Fig. 8-21)

Fig. 8-21. Quadriceps (patellar) reflex (L2-L4).

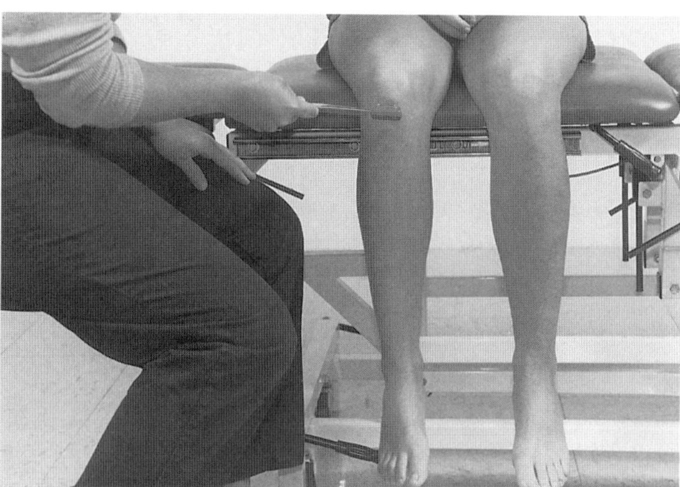

Materials needed: A reflex hammer is used.

Patient position: Seated with the knees flexed to 90°, the legs hanging off the side of the table, and the feet unsupported.

Procedure: The examiner strikes the patient's patellar tendon with the head of the reflex hammer between the patella and the tibial tuberosity.

Normal response: Knee extension is the normal response.

■ ACHILLES REFLEX

Testing (Fig. 8-22)

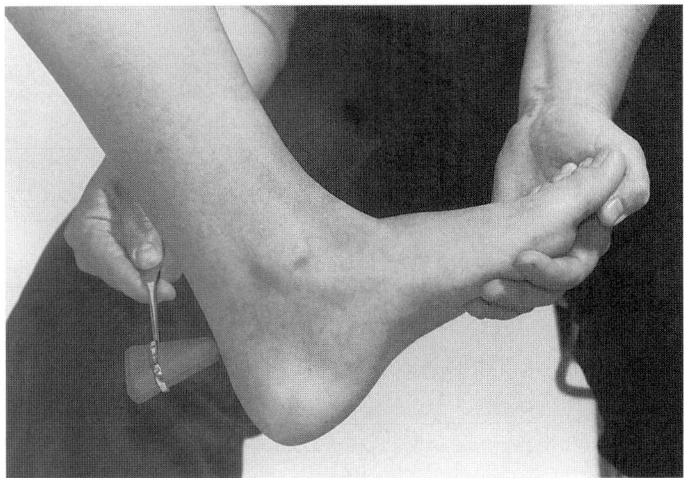

Fig. 8-22. Achilles reflex (S1, S2).

Materials needed: A reflex hammer is used.

Patient position: Seated with the legs hanging off the side of the table, the feet unsupported. (Alternative positions, such as with the patient kneeling or prone, may be used.)

Procedure: The examiner places one hand under the metatarsal heads of the patient's foot, passively bringing the ankle into a neutral position. The examiner then strikes the patient's calcaneal tendon with the head of the reflex hammer while holding the foot in the position described.

Normal response: Ankle plantar flexion is the normal response.

ABNORMAL RESPONSES TO DEEP TENDON REFLEX TESTING

There exists within the general population a wide range of "normal" responses to deep tendon reflex testing. Individuals who exhibit reflex grades of 1+ are generally normal, as are those whose reflexes grade in the 3+ range, particularly in the absence of other neurologic signs or symptoms. In fact, novice examiners should not be overly alarmed when a patient has an apparent grade of 0 on some of the more difficult-to-elicit reflexes (e.g., brachioradialis). A change in technique or examination by a more experienced clinician will generally yield more favorable results in such cases.

However, there are some instances in which the results of reflex testing should lead one to suspect underlying pathology. Among these cases are the following:

1. **Patients with a grade of 0 even when tested by an experienced examiner using reinforcement techniques.** Absent or hypoactive reflexes are generally indicative of lower motor neuron disease, which could occur anywhere from the anterior horn cell to the myoneural junction. Individuals suffering from neural shock (during the first hours to days following a neural insult) also tend to exhibit absent or greatly decreased deep tendon reflexes.
2. **Patients with reflexes that grade 4+.** Hyperactive reflexes are generally indicative of upper motor neuron disease involving the suprasegmental pathways that control the motor neurons of the spinal cord. Such lesions may be localized by examination of other areas of the nervous system (see Chapter 9).
3. **Patients with reflexes that are asymmetric.** A patient who has a right biceps reflex that grades 1+ but a left biceps reflex that grades 3+ should be examined more closely for other neurologic deficits.
4. **Patients whose reflexes change from proximal to distal.** An individual with 2+ patellar tendon reflexes and absent Achilles tendon reflexes may be exhibiting signs of peripheral neuropathy and should be examined further.
5. **Patients with pendular reflexes.** The normal muscular contraction that occurs following a tendon tap is brief and unsustained. Certain individuals exhibit a muscular contraction followed by a continued pendulum-like swinging of the extremity. These so-called pendular reflexes are generally associated with cerebellar disease.

CASE 8-1 SPINAL CORD INJURY (CONTINUED FROM CASE 2-1; CHAPTER 2)

Questions 1 through 6 were answered regarding this case in Chapters 2 and 4. Answer questions 7 through 10 regarding your examination of this patient.

Mr. Q is a 17-year-old male who suffered a fracture of the sixth cervical vertebra during a motor vehicle accident. Due to compression of the spinal cord by the fracture fragments, he sustained an incomplete spinal cord injury at a C7 neurologic level. His fracture site has been completely stabilized, and he has been admitted to the rehabilitation unit at 3 months post injury due to multiple medical complications that delayed his transfer to rehabilitation. As a result of prolonged hospitalization, Mr. Q is unable to tolerate an upright position. You are planning your initial examination in which you must determine his level of motor and sensory functioning.

1. Given that this patient's injury is at the C7 spinal level, which muscles would you expect to be free from motor weakness?
2. How would you need to alter the following muscle tests to accommodate for the patient's inability to maintain an upright position?
   a. Biceps brachii—gravity resisted
   b. Middle deltoid—gravity resisted
   c. Extensor carpi radialis longus and brevis—gravity resisted
   d. Upper trapezius—gravity resisted
   e. Pectoralis major—gravity eliminated
3. How would you alter your documentation to accommodate the changes in patient positioning described in your answer to question number 2?

During a screening examination of Mr. Q's lower extremity function, you observe that Mr. Q has active lower extremity movement that you believe is of sufficient strength in some muscle groups to allow movement against gravity.

4. How would you alter the following lower extremity muscle tests to accommodate for the patient's inability to maintain an upright position?
   a. Rectus femoris—gravity resisted
   b. Tibialis anterior—gravity resisted
   c. Gastroc/soleus—gravity resisted
   d. Medial hip rotators—gravity resisted
5. How would you alter your documentation to accommodate the changes in patient positioning described in your answers to question number 4?
6. How could you organize your muscle tests to minimize changes in patient positioning during the session?

Sensory Examination:

7. List the sensory modalities that need to be tested in this patient and the spinal cord pathway responsible for transmitting each type of modality. Briefly describe the anatomy of each pathway.
8. How would you test each of the sensory modalities listed in your answer to question number 7?
9. Given the patient's level of lesion, describe the areas of skin in which all sensory modalities should be intact.
10. What do you expect this patient's deep tendon (muscle stretch) reflexes to look like? Consider biceps, triceps, brachioradialis, patellar, and Achilles reflexes. Provide a rationale for your answer.

CASE 8-2 PERIPHERAL NERVE INJURY (CONTINUED FROM CASE 2-2; CHAPTER 2)

Questions 1 through 4 were answered in reference to this case in Chapter 2. Answer questions 5 through 9 regarding your examination of this patient (you may want to refer to an anatomy text to assist with your answers).

Dr. J is a 52-year-old dentist who suffered a mid-shaft fracture of the humerus in a motorcycle accident 5 days earlier. Damage to the radial nerve was evident following the fracture, and the fracture site was stabilized with an external fixation device. Dr. J now presents to your clinic for rehabilitation and assistance with activities of daily living (ADLs). He brings no information with him regarding the exact fracture site, and he has not had electrodiagnostic testing to determine the extent of radial nerve damage. You are not completely certain what this patient's functional limitations will be, but have a fairly good idea based on your knowledge of the anatomy of the radial nerve and related structures.

1. Provide a rationale for radial nerve damage in this patient, based on the anatomy of the radial nerve.
2. Which muscles will you need to muscle test in order to determine the level and extent of radial nerve damage?
3. If this patient's radial nerve is functionally severed above the elbow, what muscles would you expect to be weak? Nonfunctional?
4. What movements will the patient be unable to perform due to the muscle weakness/paralysis expected?

Sensory Examination:

5. If this patient's radial nerve is functionally severed above the elbow, will the patient suffer any sensory loss in the upper extremity?
6. How will you test for sensory loss in this patient?
7. What are the cutaneous branches of the radial nerve in the upper extremity?
8. What sensory losses would occur with damage to each of the cutaneous branches described in question number 7?
9. What cutaneous branches of the radial nerve would you expect to be affected in this patient? What pattern of sensory loss would you expect to see as a result of such damage?

CASE 8-3 PERIPHERAL NERVE INJURY (CONTINUED FROM CASE 4-2; CHAPTER 4)

Questions 1 through 7 were answered regarding this case in Chapter 4. Answer questions 8 through 10 regarding your examination of this patient.

Mr. H is a 19-year-old college football player who suffered a peroneal nerve injury following a blow to the lateral side of the right knee from a defensive player's helmet during Saturday evening's game. The patient presents with foot drop and sensory loss in the lower extremity. No fracture occurred during the injury, but there is extensive bruising and swelling involving the lateral side of the knee and proximal calf.

1. Describe the anatomy and course of the common peroneal nerve.
2. Why would the peroneal nerve have been injured as a result of the incident described in the case?
3. What muscle in the *thigh* is innervated by the common peroneal nerve?
4. What named branches of the common peroneal nerve in the *leg* contain motor fibers? Which muscles does each branch innervate?
5. How would you test strength of each of the muscles listed in your answer to question number 4?
6. Explain the mechanism of foot drop in this patient.
7. What muscles, other than those causing the foot drop, might demonstrate weakness in this patient? What functional losses would you expect as a result of such weakness?

Sensory Examination:

8. What named branches of the common peroneal nerve in the leg contain sensory fibers? Are any of these branches purely sensory? If so, which one(s)?
9. Describe the area of skin supplied by each of the branches listed in the answer to question number 8.
10. Given the presence of foot drop in this patient, what sensory loss would you *absolutely expect* to see in this patient? What other sensory loss *might* you see?

Bibliography

Bassetti C, Bogousslavsky J, Regli F. Sensory syndromes in parietal stroke. *Neurology* 1993; 43:1942–1049.

Bell-Krotoski J, Weinstein S, Weinstein C. Testing sensibility, including touch-pressure, two-point discrimination, point localization, and vibration. *J Hand Ther* 1993;6:114–123.

Brown AC. Somatic sensation: peripheral aspects. In: Patton HD, Fuchs AF, Hille B, et al., eds. *Textbook of Physiology,* 21st ed. Philadelphia: WB Saunders, 1989:298–313.

Burgess PR, Wei JY, Clark FJ, et al. Signaling of kinesthetic information by peripheral sensory receptors. *Annu Rev Neurosci* 1982;5:171–187.

Carpenter MB. *Core Text of Neuroanatomy,* 4th ed. Baltimore: Williams & Wilkins, 1991.

Carpenter RHS. *Neurophysiology*. Rockville, MD: Aspen Publishers, 1984.

Deibert E, Kraut M, Kremen S, et al. Neural pathways in tactile object recognition. *Neurology* 1999;52:1413–1417.

Delwaide PJ, Toulouse P. The Jendrassik maneuver: quantitative analysis of reflex reinforcement by remote involuntary muscle contraction. In: Desmedt JE, ed. *Motor Control Mechanisms in Health and Disease*. New York: Raven Press, 1983:661–669.

DeMeyer WE. *Technique of the Neurologic Examination,* 5th ed. New York: McGraw-Hill, 2004.

Duus P. *Topical Diagnosis in Neurology,* 3rd ed. New York: Thieme, 1998.

Dyck PJ, Karnes J, O'Brien PC, et al. Detection thresholds of cutaneous sensation in humans. In: Dyck PI, Thomas PK, eds. *Peripheral Neuropathy,* 3rd ed. Philadelphia: WB Saunders, 1993;706–728.

Dyck PJ, O'Brien PC, Bushek W, et al. Clinical versus quantitative evaluation of cutaneous sensation. *Arch Neurol* 1976;33:651–655.

Fischer A. Pressure threshold meter: its use for quantification of tender spots. *Arch Phys Med Rehabil* 1986;67:836–838.

Fischer A. Tissue compliance meter for objective quantitative assessment of soft tissue consistency and pathology. *Arch Phys Med Rehabil* 1987;68:122–125.

Fruhstorfer H, Lindblum U, Schmidt WG. Method for quantitative estimation of thermal thresholds in patients. *J Neurol Neurosurg Psychiatry* 1976;39:1071–1075.

Gilman S, Newman SW. *Manter and Gatz's Essentials of Clinical Neuroanatomy and Neurophysiology,* 10th ed. Philadelphia: FA Davis, 2003.

Glick TH. *Neurologic Skills: Examination and Diagnosis*. Boston: Blackwell Scientific, 1993.

Goldberg JM, Lindblum U. Standardized method of determining vibratory perception thresholds for diagnosis and screening in neurological investigation. *J Neurol Neurosurg Psychiatry* 1979;42:793–803.

Grigg P, Greenspan BJ. Response of primate joint afferent neurons to mechanical stimulation of knee joint. *J Neurophysiol* 1977;40:1–8.

Haerer AJ. DeJong's: *The Neurological Examination,* 5th ed. Philadelphia: JB Lippincott, 1992.

Haines DE. *Fundamental Neuroscience*. New York: Churchill Livingstone, 1997.

Haines DE. *Neuroanatomy: An Atlas of Structures, Sections, and Systems,* 6th ed. Philadelphia: Lippincott Williams & Wilkins, 2004.

Hallett M. NINDS myotatic reflex scale. *Neurology* 1993;43:2723.

Hansen M, Sindrup SH, Christensen PB, et al. Interobserver variation in the evaluation of neurological signs: observer dependent factors. *Acta Neurol Scand* 1994;90:145–149.

Hansson P, Lindblum U, Lindstrom P. Graded assessment and classification of impaired temperature sensability in patients with diabetic polyneuropathy. *J Neurol Neurosurg Psychiatry* 1991;54:527–530.

Hensel H, Andres KH, von Duering M. Structure and function of cold receptors. *Pflugers Arch* 1974;329:1–8.

Hunt CC. Mammalian muscle spindle: peripheral mechanisms. *Physiol Rev* 1990;70:643–663.

Iggo A. Sensory receptors in the skin of mammals and their sensory function. *Rev Neurol* 1985; 141:599–613.

Kandel ER, Schwartz JH, Jessell TM. *Principles of Neural Science,* 4th ed. New York: McGraw-Hill, 2000.

Kaplan FS, Nixon JE, Reitz M, et al. Age-related changes in proprioception and sensation of joint position. *Acta Orthop Scand* 1985;56:72–74.

Kiernan JA. *Barr's the Human Nervous System: An Anatomical Viewpoint,* 7th ed. Philadelphia: Lippincott Williams & Wilkins, 1998.

Lanska DJ, Goetz CG. Romberg's sign: development, adoption, and adaptation in the 19th century. *Neurology* 2000;55:1201–1206.

Lindblum U, Ochoa J. Somatosensory function and dysfunction. In: Asbury AK, McKhann GM, McDonald WI, eds. *Diseases of the Nervous System*. Philadelphia: WB Saunders, 1992:213–228.

Lindblum U, Tegner R. Quantification of sensibility in mononeuropathy, polyneuropathy, and central lesions. In: Munsat T, ed. *Quantification of Neurological Deficit*. London: Butterworth, 1989:171–185.

Litvan I, Mangone CA, Werden W, et al. Reliability of the NINDS myotatic reflex scale. *Neurology* 1996;47:969–972.

Lundy-Ekman L. *Neuroscience: Fundamentals for Rehabilitation,* 2nd ed. Philadelphia: WB Saunders, 2002.

Matthews PCB. Where does Sherrington's "muscular sense" originate? Muscles, joints, corollary discharges? *Annu Rev Neurosci* 1982;5:189–218.

Nathan PW, Smith MC, Cook AN. Sensory effects in man of lesions of the posterior columns and of some other afferent pathways. *Brain* 1986;109:1003–1041.

Nolan MF. *Introduction to the Neurologic Examination*. Philadelphia: FA Davis, 1996.

Peripheral Neuropathy Association. Quantitative sensory testing. *Neurology* 1993;43:1050– 1052.

Perkins BA, Olaleye D, Zinman B, et al. Simple screening tests for peripheral neuropathy in the diabetes clinic. *Diabetes Care* 2001;24:250–256.

Pressman EK, Zeidman SM, Summers L. Primary care for women: comprehensive assessment of the neurologic system. *J Nurse Midwifery* 1995;40:163–171.

Ross RT. *How to Examine the Nervous System,* 2nd ed. New York: Medical Examination Publishing, 1985.

Schwartzman RJ, Bogdonaff MD. Proprioception and vibration sensibility discrimination in the absence of the posterior columns. *Arch Neurol* 1969;20:349–354.

Sekular R, Nash D, Armstrong R. Sensitive objective procedure for evaluating response to light touch. *Neurology* 1973;23:1282–1291.

Sturmann K. The neurologic examination. *Emerg Med Clin North Am* 1997;15:491–506.

Waxman SG, deGroot J. *Correlative Neuroanatomy,* 22nd ed. Norwalk, CT: Appleton Lange, 1995.

Wolf JK. *Segmental Neurology*. Baltimore: University Park Press, 1981.

9

TECHNIQUES of the REMAINDER of the NEUROLOGIC EXAMINATION: COORDINATION, MENTAL STATUS, CRANIAL NERVES, and SUPERFICIAL REFLEXES

A thorough screening examination of the nervous system does not stop with the examination of the peripheral nerves or dermatomes of the trunk and extremities. Functions subserved by so-called higher levels of the nervous system also must be examined. Accordingly, this chapter addresses the elements of the general neurologic examination that were not covered in the muscle testing and sensory examination chapters of this text.

This chapter provides instruction for the remainder of the general neurologic screening examination. Techniques for examining functions of the cerebral cortex, cerebellum, and cranial nerves are presented as are procedures for the examination of cutaneous reflexes. With practice, the student or practitioner who is familiar with the process should be able to complete a survey examination of the central nervous system without adding more than a few minutes to the total examination time for the patient.

All patients who use your services as their entry point into the health care system for a given problem should be given a neurologic screening examination. Additionally, all patients who report symptoms that could be attributed to pathology within the peripheral or central nervous system should have a thorough, systematic examination of the nervous system. Close attention to the patient's history and list of symptoms is an important part of the neurologic examination, and, although not covered in this text, the taking of a comprehensive patient history is critical in guiding and directing the neurologic examination.

The emphasis in this text is on the neurologic *screening* examination. As such, more in-depth testing procedures that may be warranted for patients in whom neurologic disease is suspected have been omitted. References for such testing procedures may be found under the corresponding screening technique and in the bibliography at the end of the chapter. If practiced and rehearsed, a complete neurologic screening examination may be accomplished in less than 10 minutes.

Not all components of the neurologic examination need be performed with every patient. Taking the patient history can provide an opportunity to observe and examine that patient's neurologic status and serve to clarify the components of the neurologic examination to be tested in that particular patient. Skillful observation of the patient's movement and gait as he or she enters the clinic (see Chapter 10), speech as he or she responds to questions, facial and body symmetry, and behavior can provide a plethora of information regarding nervous system function without requiring additional time for the performance of specific tests. The screening examination then can be geared toward testing of those functions that are less amenable to evaluation by observation alone.

The neurologic examination is based on an understanding of the functioning of the nervous system. Most clinicians would agree that 85% to 90% of all cases of neuropathology can be diagnosed on the basis of the history and physical examination alone, before any laboratory tests are performed. The ability to make such diagnoses is based on the clinician's understanding of the structure and function of the nervous system. Such understanding is critical if the clinician is to make an accurate interpretation of the findings of the neurologic examination. Those who need a review of the anatomy and physiology of the nervous system are referred to standard texts on the subject, such as *Principles of Neural Science*.[4]

CEREBRAL FUNCTION (Fig. 9-1)

A thorough neurologic examination includes a survey of higher cerebral functioning. Individuals who are alert and aware of their surroundings and circumstances; who respond to questions posed during the taking of the medical history in an intelligent, articulate manner; who are able to follow directions during the examination; and who do not exhibit troubling moods or behavior can be assumed to have normal cerebral functioning; and this part of

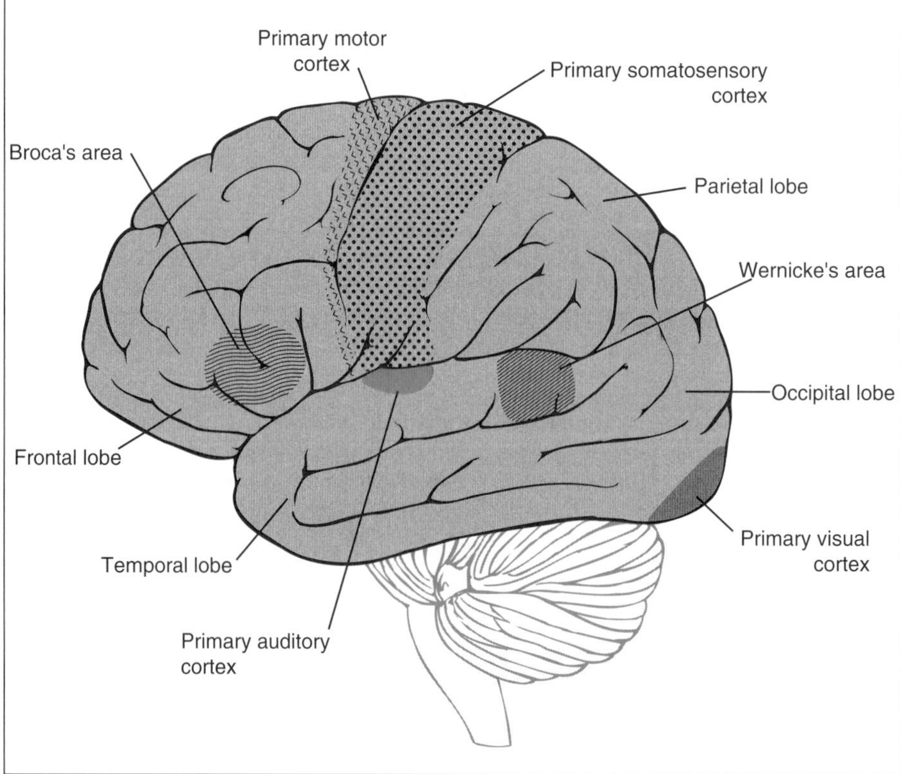

Fig. 9-1. Cerebral cortex (in color) showing the lobes and selected functional areas.

the neurologic examination may be excluded. However, patients who appear unresponsive, confused, or forgetful or for whom you or the family has mental status concerns should be examined more closely as outlined below.

Included in the survey of cerebral function are several areas, which may be remembered with the simple mnemonic *MR. CLOCK*. Examination of each of these areas is described below.

*M*emory
*R*easoning
*C*onsciousness
*L*anguage
*O*rientation
*C*alculation
*K*nowledge

MEMORY

Both short-term and long-term memory should be assessed. Short-term memory allows one to recall information that was acquired seconds to minutes before, whereas long-term memory permits recall of events experienced days, months, or even years earlier. Patients may demonstrate selective loss of short- or long-term memory.

Testing

SHORT-TERM MEMORY

Materials needed: No materials are needed.

Patient position: Seated in a comfortable position.

Procedure: The examiner presents the patient with three or four words that the patient is asked to repeat back to the examiner. The patient is instructed that he or she will be asked to recall those words in a few minutes time. The words presented should be unrelated, such as "book," "automobile," "elephant." After other portions of the examination have been completed, the patient is asked to recall the words.

Normal response: The patient should be able to recall all words presented after about 5 minutes.

LONG-TERM MEMORY

Materials needed: No materials are needed.

Patient position: Seated in a comfortable position.

Procedure: The examiner questions the patient about past events of the patient's own experience that the patient would be expected to remember. Such questions may include "Where and when were you born?" "What are (were) the names of your parents?" "Name several people who have been President of the United States during your lifetime," and so forth.

Normal response: The patient should be able to answer questions accurately.

REASONING

Abstract reasoning is a function of the frontal lobe, and deficits in the ability to reason abstractly may be indicative of the onset of dementia. Assessment of abstract reasoning generally takes the form of proverb interpretation, and the examiner looks for the ability of the patient to provide an abstract, rather than a literal, interpretation of the proverb.

Testing

Materials needed: No materials are needed.

Patient position: Positioned comfortably.

Procedure: The examiner asks the patient to give the meaning of proverbs such as "a stitch in time saves nine," "a bird in the hand is worth two in the bush," and "the early bird catches the worm."

Normal response: The patient provides an explanation of the proverb that goes beyond the literal interpretation of the words. For example, when asked to interpret "the early bird catches the worm," the patient should respond with "timeliness promotes success" or something similar rather than "the first bird out in the morning will catch the worms."

CONSCIOUSNESS

Assessment of consciousness is dependent on the setting and circumstances. Although assessment of consciousness may not be critical in dealing with a patient who has been comatose for a prolonged period, sudden loss of consciousness in an otherwise healthy individual requires an immediate, skilled response. In an emergency such as that described earlier, the examiner should use emergency first aid techniques (cardiopulmonary resuscitation, etc.) that are beyond the scope of this text. In situations of chronic disturbances of consciousness, the patient's status may be assessed using the Glasgow Coma Scale (Table 9-1). In general, patients may be classified as alert, lethargic or drowsy, obtunded, stuporous (light coma), or comatose (deep coma). The ability of the examiner to arouse the patient becomes more difficult as the stages of consciousness progress toward deep coma (from which the patient is unable to be aroused regardless of the stimulus). Patients who are obtunded are arousable with repeated stimulation, whereas those in a stupor require a painful stimulus for arousal.

Table 9-1. GLASGOW COMA SCALE

	BEST RESPONSE	SCORE*
I. Motor	Obeys	6
	Localizes	5
	Withdraws from pain	4
	Abnormal flexion	3
	Abnormal extension (decerebrate posturing)	2
	None	1
II. Verbal	Oriented	5
	Confused conversation	4
	Inappropriate words	3
	Incomprehensible sounds	2
	None	1
III. Eye opening	Spontaneous	4
	To speech	3
	To pain	2
	None	1

*Coma score = I + II + III:
13–15 = minor
9–13 = moderate
<8 = coma
5–8 = severe coma

Testing

Materials needed: No materials are needed.

Procedure: The patient's level of consciousness may be assessed during the history taking as the patient responds to questions posed by the examiner. A lack of response to verbal questioning should lead the examiner to apply physical stimulation (from gentle shaking to sternal rub) to arouse the patient. The resultant level of consciousness is based on the degree of stimulation needed to arouse the patient.

Normal response: The patient responds promptly to questions by the examiner without the need for excessive repetition of the questions or the use of physical stimulation.

LANGUAGE

Although a comprehensive evaluation of a patient's language skills is best accomplished by a speech-language pathologist, a superficial assessment may be made during the neurologic examination. When the examiner, in the course of history taking, suspects a language deficit, he or she should pursue the matter by further examination. Deficits in the ability to produce or comprehend verbal or written language are called *aphasias,* which differ from *dysarthrias* (problems with speech articulation; e.g., secondary to cerebellar disease) and *dysphonias* (difficulties with sound production; e.g., secondary to problems with cranial nerve X). Many different types of aphasia have been described based on the degree and characteristics of the deficit found, but discussion here is limited to the three most basic types: receptive (Wernicke), expressive (Broca), and global. Descriptions of the more specific types of aphasia can be found in most standard neurologic texts.

Receptive aphasia is characterized by poor comprehension of speech with fluent, although error-filled, language production. The lesion typically causing this type of aphasia is generally located in the posterosuperior aspect of the temporal lobe of the dominant hemisphere. Patients suffering from expressive aphasia will usually have few to no problems with the comprehension of speech but typically have great difficulty in producing spoken language. In this type of aphasia, the lesion is normally located in the inferior aspect of the frontal lobe of the dominant hemisphere, just anterior to the primary motor strip. Global aphasia can be considered a combination of expressive and receptive aphasia in that the patient typically loses the abilities both to produce and to comprehend language.

Testing

Materials needed: Paper, pencil, and miscellaneous objects are used.

Patient position: Positioned comfortably.

Procedure: The examiner should begin by listening to the patient's spontaneous speech while taking the history. Fluency, appropriateness of responses, and quantity of speech should be noted. If the patient appears to have difficulty in the production of speech, further examination should occur, such as asking the patient to repeat a number of phrases, to name miscellaneous objects, and to read written sentences aloud. Speech comprehension can be examined by asking the patient to follow simple commands or to point to named objects.

Normal response: The patient should respond in an appropriate and timely manner to all questions and directions posed by the examiner (within the patient's motor abilities).

Lesions: Patients suspected of having language deficits should be referred to the appropriate health professional for further evaluation.

ORIENTATION

Orientation refers to the patient's knowledge of the present circumstances: who he or she is, where he or she is, and the time in which he or she exists. Such orientation is referred to as *orientation to person, place, and time.* Most of the questions used to determine the patient's orientation (listed below) may be incorporated unobtrusively into the patient history and examination.

Testing

Materials needed: No materials are needed.

Patient position: Positioned comfortably.

Procedure: The examiner asks the patient the following questions:

"What is your full name?"
"In which city/town do you live?"
"What is the name of the building we are in?"
"What is today's day and date?"
"Without looking at a clock or your watch, can you tell me the approximate time?"

Normal response: The patient should be able to answer all questions correctly, being able to approximate the time within about an hour of the actual time.

CALCULATION

The ability to perform mathematic calculations is a function of the cerebral cortex and should be tested in all individuals in whom disordered cortical function is suspected.

Testing

Materials needed: No materials are needed.

Patient position: Positioned comfortably.

Procedure: The examiner asks the patient to perform several simple calculation problems by questioning the patient and then waiting for a response before proceeding to the next problem. The problems posed should not be so complex that the patient is unable to solve them through mental calculation. Examples of appropriate problems include the following:

"What is 30 ÷ 6?"
"What is 9 × 12?"
"How much is 90 – 13?"
"How much is 67 + 18?"

Normal response: The patient provides accurate responses to the problems posed. The responses may be slow but should be correct.

KNOWLEDGE

General knowledge is acquired by the patient over the lifetime and will vary in depth depending on the patient's premorbid intelligence and educational levels. Ideally, questions posed to examine the patient's level of knowledge should reflect the premorbid experience. Such questions should not be based on the patient's personal life experiences as was the case in testing long-term memory, but should come from material learned by the patient (e.g., from formal education or job training) before the onset of the current illness.

Testing

Materials needed: No materials are needed.

Patient position: Positioned comfortably.

Procedure: The examiner should ask the patient a number of questions designed to determine the current level of knowledge. Examples of such questions include the following:

"In which year did World War II end?"
"In which country is the Eiffel Tower?"
"Who wrote *Romeo and Juliet*?"
"Water is made of what chemical elements?"
"What is the name of the substance that causes plants to be green?"

Normal response: The patient should be able to answer most questions accurately, given that they are not beyond the premorbid educational experience.

CEREBELLUM: BALANCE AND COORDINATION (Fig. 9-2)

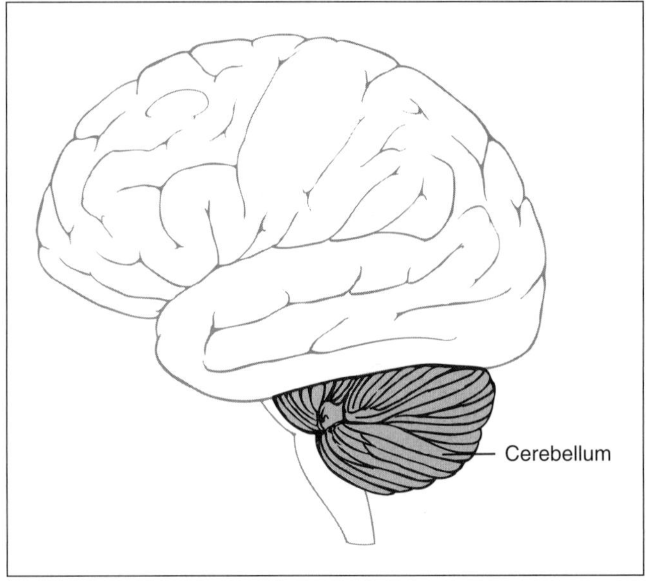

Fig. 9-2. Cerebellum (in color).

The cerebellum is classically believed to function principally in the regulation or coordination of movements, particularly skilled movements, initiated by the cerebral cortex. This regulation is carried out in conjunction with the basal ganglia. The cerebellum also may be necessary for the design of rapid movements before their initiation—movements that are preprogrammed because they are too fast to be regulated by sensory feedback such as fast saccadic eye movements or rapid repetitive hand movements. The cerebellum also functions to maintain posture, muscle tone, and equilibrium.

Pathologies involving the cerebellum include disturbances of voluntary movement, coordination, gait, muscle tone, and equilibrium. Signs and symptoms include hypotonia, muscle fatigability, asynergia (inability to adjust the impulses innervating the various muscles participating in a movement so that the range, direction, and force of movement is altered), nystagmus, gait ataxia, dysarthria, intention tremor, dysdiadochokinesia (impairment of rapid, alternating movements), and disturbances in equilibrium.

Various tests are used to examine the functions of the cerebellum. Care should be taken to examine both the upper and lower extremities of the patient as well as stance and gait. The motor disturbances seen in patients with cerebellar pathology stem from a lack of motor coordination, not from muscular weakness.

Testing: Limb Coordination

FINGER-NOSE TEST (Fig. 9-3)

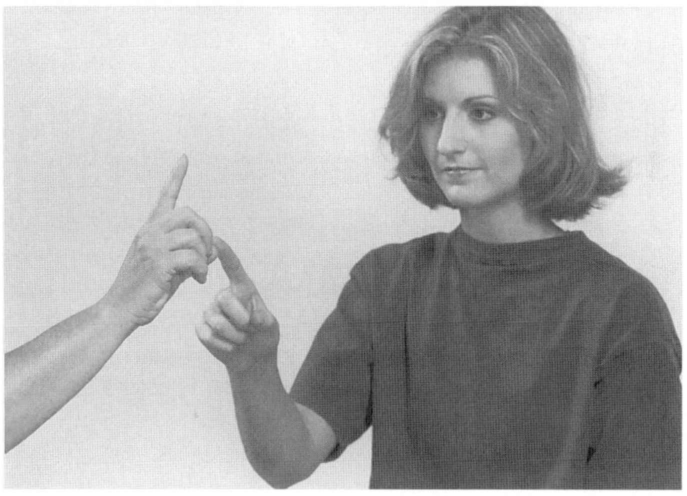

Fig. 9-3. Finger-nose test.

Materials needed: No materials are needed.

Patient position: Seated with the arms at the sides.

Procedure: The examiner holds an index finger vertically slightly more than arm's length away from the patient. The patient is asked to touch, with his or her own index finger, first his or her nose and then the examiner's index finger. The patient is asked to repeat this movement several times as rapidly as possible.

Normal response: Arm movement should be smooth and precise. The patient should be able to alternately touch his nose and the examiner's finger with ease and accuracy.

Lesions: Movements of the upper extremity will be inaccurate. The patient may go past or fail to touch precisely the nose or the examiner's finger (dysmetria). There may be tremorlike movements present, especially as the patient's finger approaches the target (intention tremor). The movement may appear disjointed and will lack the smoothness of normal movement.

HEEL-SHIN TEST (Fig. 9-4)

Fig. 9-4. Heel-shin test (arrow shows direction of movement).

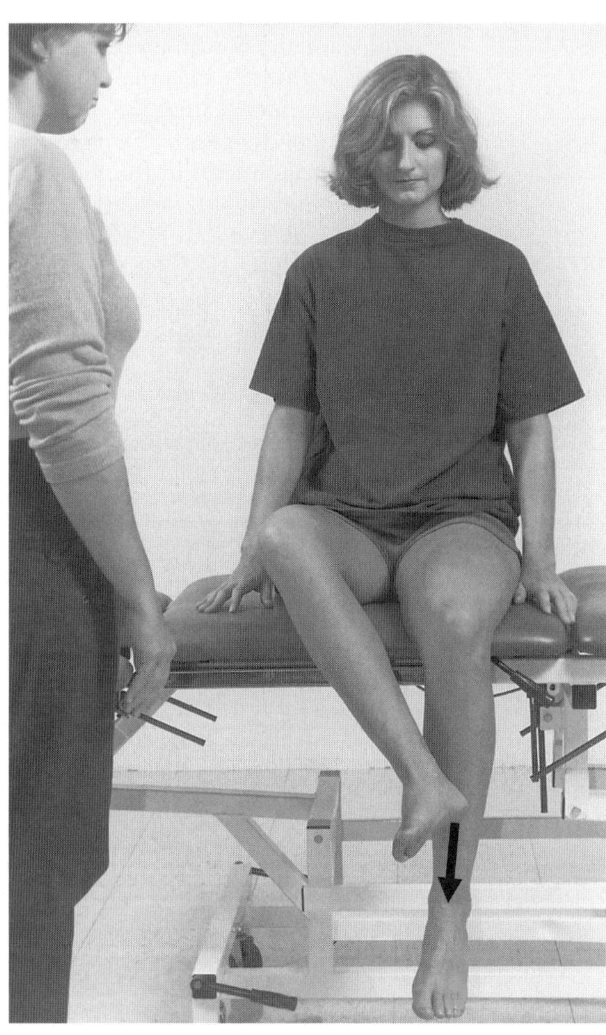

Materials needed: No materials are needed.

Patient position: Seated or supine on an examining table with the shoes removed and the eyes open.

Procedure: The examiner asks the patient to slide the heel of one foot from the knee down toward the great toe of the opposite leg. The test is repeated for the other side.

Normal response: The patient slides the heel smoothly along the shin of the opposite leg, maintaining contact between the heel and the leg.

Lesions: Contact between the heel and shin cannot be maintained, and the movement is jerky and unsteady.

DIADOCHOKINESIA (Figs. 9-5 to 9-8)

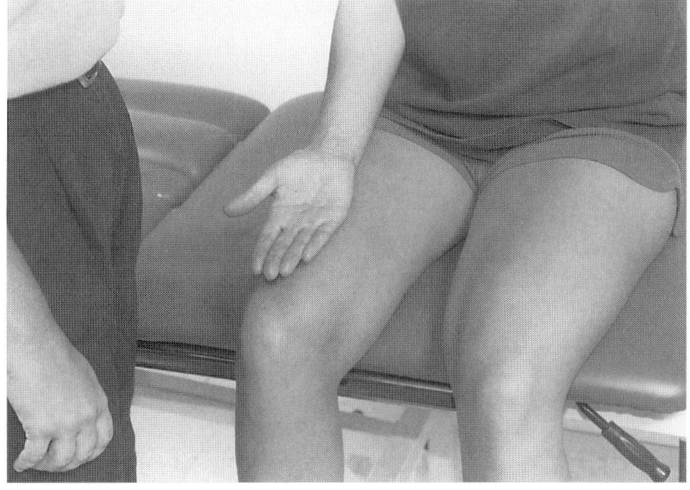

Fig. 9-5. Test for diadochokinesia: rapid hand movement, palm up.

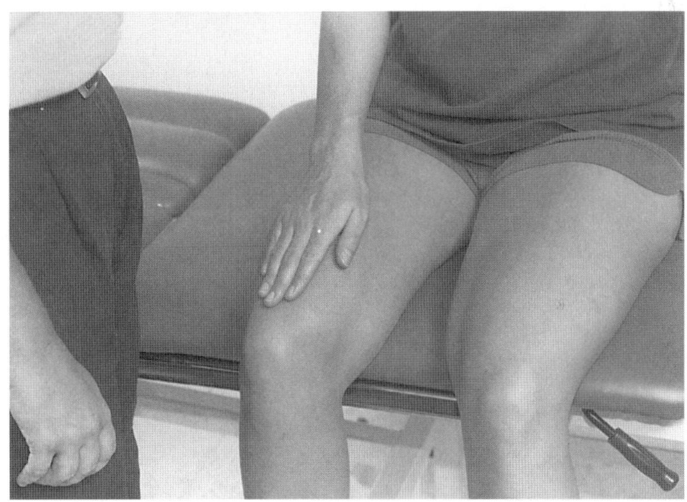

Fig. 9-6. Test for diadochokinesia: rapid hand movement, palm down.

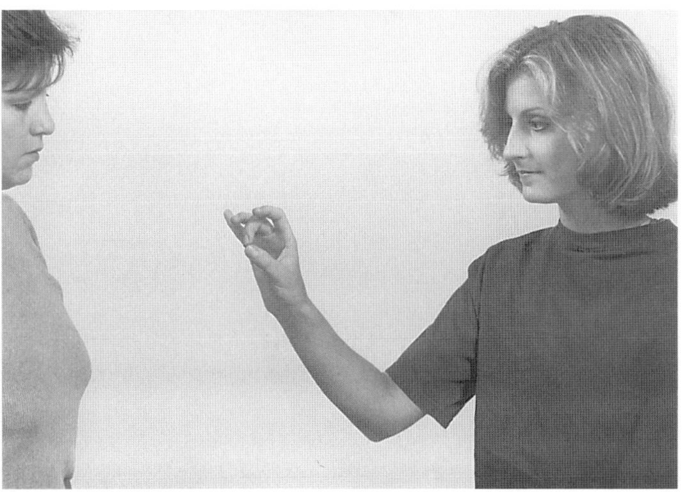

Fig. 9-7. Test for diadochokinesia: rapid finger movement.

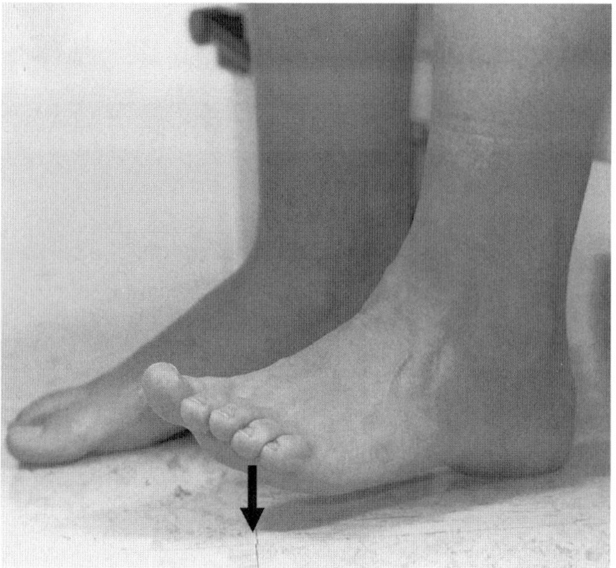

Fig. 9-8. Test for diadochokinesia: rapid toe tapping (arrow shows direction of movement).

Materials needed: No materials are needed.

Patient position: Seated with the hands in the lap.

Procedure: The examiner asks the patient to turn the hands palm up and then palm down as rapidly as possible while resting the hands in the lap. Alternatively, the patient may be asked to tap each of the fingers alternately against the thumb as rapidly as possible. Diadochokinesia should be examined in the lower extremity as well by asking the patient to tap the toes as rapidly as possible.

Normal response: Movements should be rapid and rhythmic bilaterally.

Lesions: The inability to perform rapidly alternating movements of the extremities is termed *dysdiadochokinesia.* Patients who exhibit this problem will perform alternating movements without rhythm or speed.

REBOUND (Fig. 9-9)

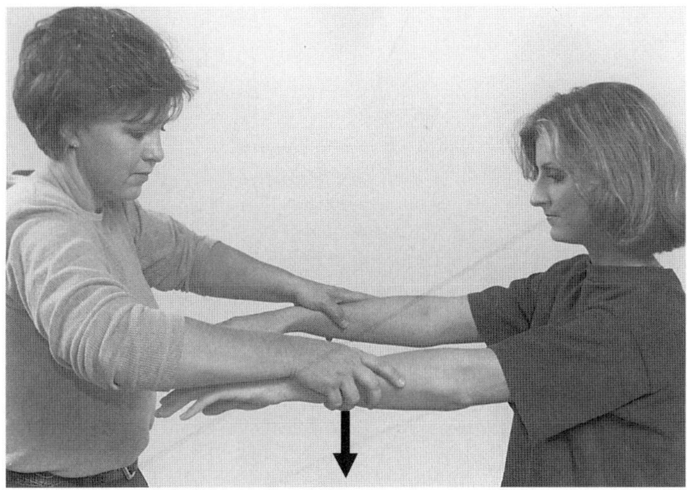

Fig. 9-9. Rebound test (arrow shows direction of resistance by examiner).

Materials needed: No materials are needed.

Patient position: Seated or standing in a comfortable position with the arms held straight out in front.

Procedure: The examiner asks the patient to try as hard as possible to keep the arms level. The examiner then pushes downward on each of the patient's arms with a firm, quick motion to try to displace the arms toward the floor.

Normal response: The patient's arm will move downward toward the floor slightly and then back to a level position without going past the horizontal.

Lesions: Patients with cerebellar pathology will demonstrate *rebounding*, which involves the inability to stop motion quickly. Thus, when the examiner pushes downward on the patient's arm, the arm will move down toward the floor and then back up past the horizontal and downward once again before stopping in the original position. The oscillatory movement may occur more than once prior to the attainment of the original position.

Testing: Stance and Gait

The Romberg, Tandem Romberg, and Tandem Gait tests are used to assess stance and gait. For patients in whom disorders of balance are detected, a more comprehensive assessment is needed. A variety of assessment tools and techniques are available. The reader is referred to Horak,[2] Horak and Nashner,[3] Nashner,[5] Nashner and Peters,[6] and Shumway-Cook and Woollacott[7] for further information.

NARROW-BASED STANCE (Fig. 9-10)

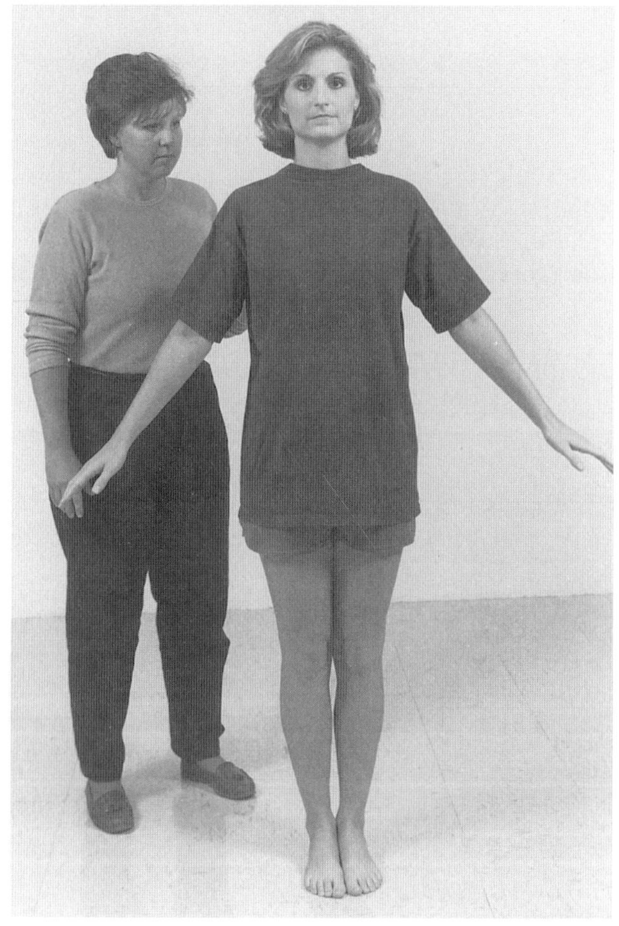

Fig. 9-10. Narrow-based stance.

Materials needed: No materials are needed.

Patient position: Standing with the feet as close together as possible.

Procedure: The examiner stands just behind and to the side of the patient and asks the patient to maintain balance while standing with the feet positioned as close together as possible.

Normal response: The patient should be able to maintain balance in this position.

Lesions: Patients who are unable to perform this test should be investigated further for cerebellar pathology.

CLINICAL COMMENT: ROMBERG TEST

The Narrow-Based Stance Test is identical to the Romberg Test-eyes open (see Chapter 8). The Romberg Test is properly a test for dorsal column functioning, although inability to perform the Romberg test with eyes open is indicative of cerebellar pathology. Failure on the Romberg test-eyes closed points to a disorder of proprioception typical of dorsal column disease.

TANDEM GAIT (Fig. 9-11)

Fig. 9-11. Tandem gait.

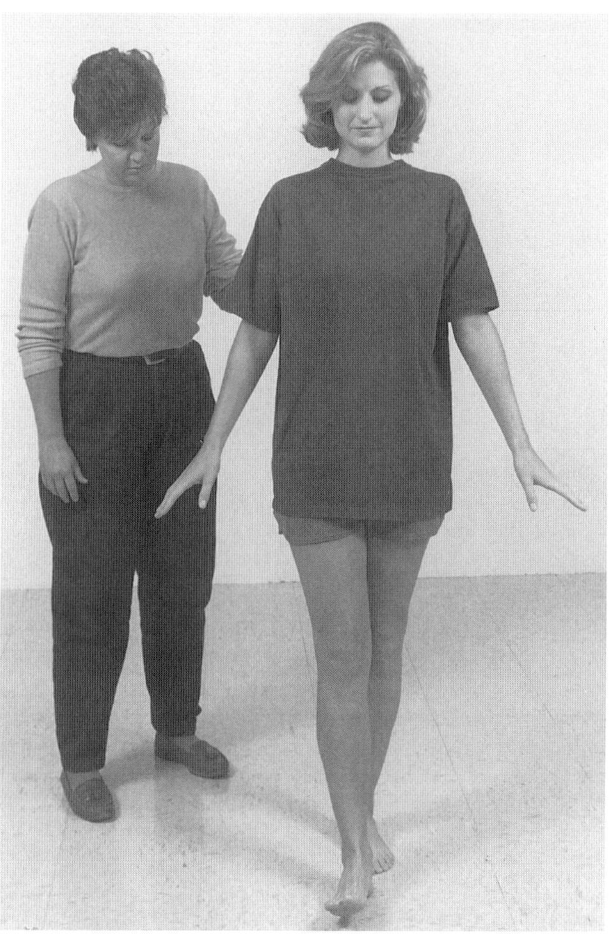

Materials needed: No materials are needed.

Patient position: Standing with the arms at the sides and the feet positioned so that the heel of one foot is directly in front of the toes of the other foot.

Procedure: The examiner asks the patient to walk across the room in tandem fashion, stepping each time so that the heel of the foot is brought down just in front of the toes of the opposite foot.

Normal response: The patient should be able to walk in tandem fashion without excessive sway or loss of balance.

Lesions: Patients with cerebellar disorders will demonstrate loss of balance or excessive arm and trunk movement while attempting tandem gait.

CRANIAL NERVES

A review of the functions of the cranial nerves is essential to any neurologic examination. In general, they are examined in order from I to XII. Not all functions of all cranial nerves are inspected, and many times some cranial nerves (such as the olfactory) are not examined at all. However, in learning to examine the cranial nerves, one should practice examining all 12 so that the techniques will be available when needed.

CRANIAL NERVE I: OLFACTORY

Testing (Fig. 9-12)

CRANIAL NERVE I: OLFACTORY

COMPONENT	ASSOCIATED NUCLEUS	FUNCTION
N/A	Neuronal cell bodies located in the nasal epithelium	Olfaction (smell)

Important points of anatomy: Axons of the olfactory nerve traverse the cribriform plate of the ethmoid bone to synapse in the olfactory bulb (ventral surface of frontal lobe).

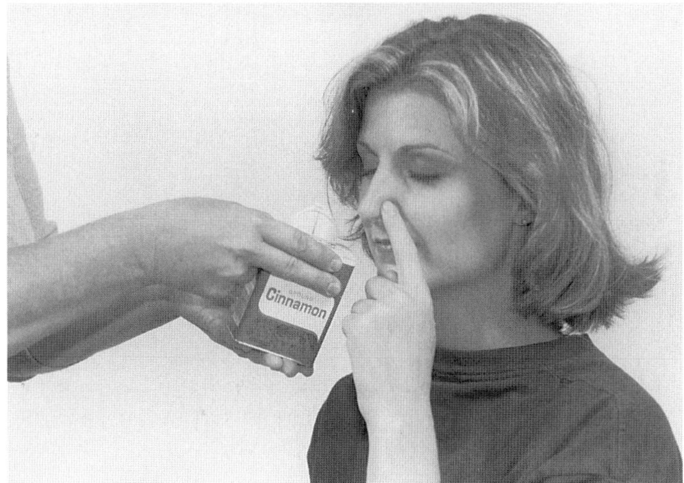

Fig. 9-12. Olfactory testing (cranial nerve I).

Materials needed: Substances with familiar aromatic odors, such as cinnamon, vanilla, orange, and coffee, are used. Noxious stimulants such as alcohol or ammonia should be avoided as these substances may coactivate trigeminal sensory receptors in the nasal mucosa.

Patient position: Seated in a comfortable position with the eyes closed or blindfolded, and one nostril is covered by the patient.

Procedure: The examiner presents the aromatic substances, one at a time, under the open nostril, asking the patient to identify the substance. The test should be repeated for the other nostril.

Normal response: The patient should be able to identify common odors accurately with either nostril.

Lesions: Loss of olfaction is usually unilateral and may occur secondary to such events as trauma (skull fracture, closed head injury), neoplasms (meningioma), or infection. Additionally, increasing age frequently causes a diminution of olfactory sensation.

Note: Testing of the olfactory nerve is frequently omitted in a routine neurologic examination unless the patient complains of problems with smell or taste.

CRANIAL NERVE II: OPTIC

Testing

VISUAL ACUITY (Fig. 9-13)

CRANIAL NERVE II: OPTIC

COMPONENT	ASSOCIATED NUCLEUS	FUNCTION
N/A	Neuronal cell bodies located in retina	Vision

Important points of anatomy: The optic nerve exits the eyeball at the optic disc (blind spot) on its posterior aspect, undergoes a partial decussation (crossing) at the optic chiasm, and then continues posteriorly as the optic tract. Axons in the optic tract terminate in the lateral geniculate body of the thalamus. From the lateral geniculate body, fibers course posteriorly (geniculocalcarine fibers) to terminate in the primary visual cortex of the occipital lobe. During this posterior course, a portion of the fibers loop through the temporal lobe (Meyer's loop) before terminating in the occipital cortex.

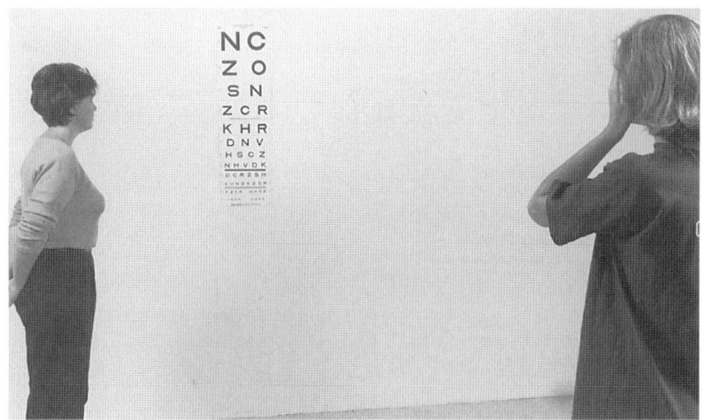

Fig. 9-13. Visual acuity testing using eye chart (cranial nerve II).

Materials needed: An eye chart is used.

Patient position: Seated in a comfortable position with one eye covered.

Procedure: If glasses or contact lenses are normally worn, they should be in place. The examiner places the vision chart the appropriate distance from the patient (as indicated on the chart), and the patient is asked to read the smallest line visible on the chart. The test is repeated for the opposite eye. Note: If a vision chart is unavailable, a crude estimation of visual acuity may be made by asking the patient to read printed material such as a newspaper.

Normal response: Able to read items from the line marked "20 feet" with each eye with the chart positioned at the prescribed distance. However, impaired acuity does not necessarily indicate a cranial nerve lesion.

VISUAL FIELDS (Fig. 9-14)

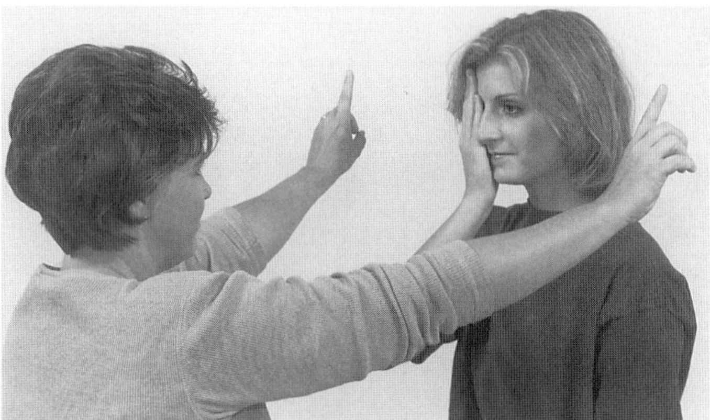

Fig. 9-14. Visual field testing (cranial nerve II).

Materials needed: No materials are needed.

Patient position: Seated in a comfortable position with one eye covered, facing the examiner.

Procedure: The patient is asked to look straight ahead and to focus on the examiner's eye with his or her open eye. The examiner positions one hand on each side of the patient at the periphery of the patient's visual field. The examiner's hands should be positioned above the horizontal to stimulate only the superior visual field. While the patient maintains focus on the examiner's eye, the examiner wiggles the fingers of one hand. The patient is asked to indicate where he or she sees movement. The examiner's hands are moved from above to below the horizontal and back, and the fingers are wiggled at random until all four visual fields in that eye have been tested at least once. The procedure is then repeated for the opposite eye.

Note: The periphery of the visual field may be found by bringing the fingers slowly in from the side and slightly behind the patient until the fingers can be seen by the patient while the patient maintains one eye closed and the other focused forward. The point at which the patient sees the fingers is the periphery of the visual field.

Normal response: The patient should be able to detect movement of the fingers in all four visual fields (superior lateral, superior medial, inferior lateral, and inferior medial) of each eye.

Lesions: See Lesions of the Visual Pathway; p. 580.

PUPILLARY LIGHT REFLEX (CRANIAL NERVES II AND III) (Fig. 9-15)

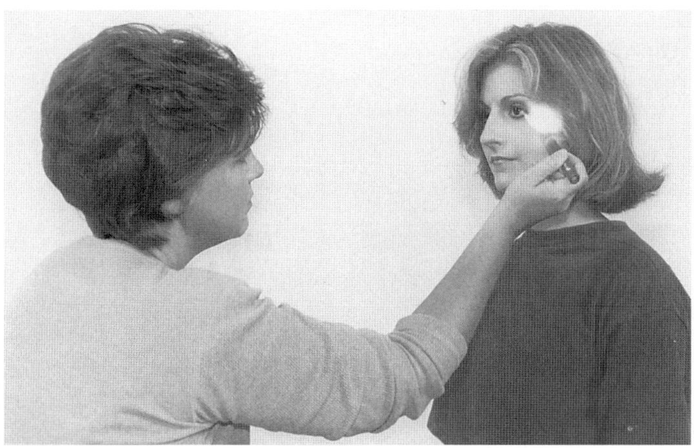

Fig. 9-15. Examination of pupillary light reflex (cranial nerves II and III). The examiner shines a light into the lateral edge of the eye to be tested.

Materials needed: A penlight is used.

Patient position: Seated comfortably in a dimly lit room with the eyes focused on a distant object.

Procedure: The examiner shines a light into one of the patient's eyes from the lateral side. The examiner may place a hand in a position partially covering the patient's opposite eye to block the light from reaching it directly if necessary (not shown in Fig. 9-15). The response to the light is observed in each eye. The eyes are then allowed to dilate, and the test is repeated for the opposite eye.

Normal response: The immediate and simultaneous constriction of both the stimulated pupil (direct light reflex) and unstimulated pupil (consensual light reflex) is normal.

CLINICAL COMMENT: PUPILLARY LIGHT REFLEX

When testing the papillary light reflex, the light should be shone into each eye twice; once to test the direct light reflex (ipsilateral eye) and a second time to test the consensual light reflex (contralateral eye).

ACCOMMODATION REACTION (CRANIAL NERVES II AND III) (Fig. 9-16)

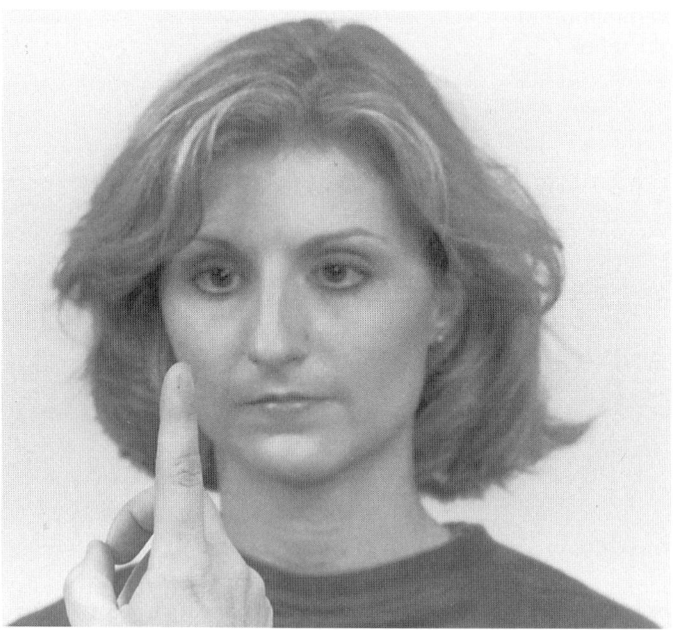

Fig. 9-16. Examination of accommodation reaction (cranial nerves II and III).

Materials needed: No materials are needed.

Patient position: Seated comfortably with the eyes focused forward on a distant object.

Procedure: The examiner places a finger approximately 8 inches from the patient's nose. The patient is then asked to alternately shift his or her focus from the far object to the near (examiner's finger) and back.

Normal response: Focusing on the near object should cause the eyes to converge (adduct) and the pupils to constrict.

LESIONS OF THE VISUAL PATHWAY

The visual loss experienced secondary to a lesion of the visual pathway depends on the location and extent of the damage sustained (Fig. 9-17).

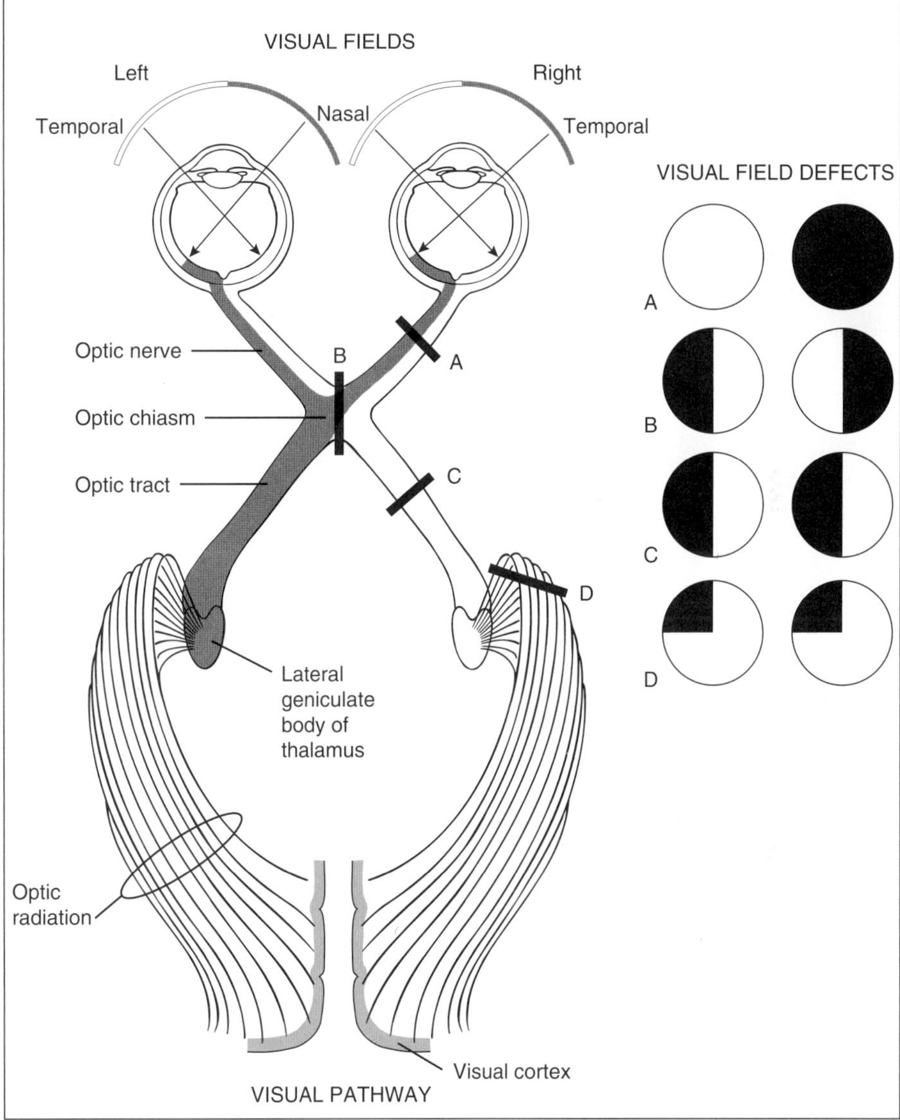

Fig. 9-17. Optic pathway showing selected lesions **(A–D)** and associated visual field defects.

Lesions of the *retina* or *optic nerve* anterior to the chiasm (Fig. 9-17A) result in unilateral visual loss confined to the ipsilateral eye along with an absent direct light reflex in that eye. The consensual light reflex is present in the ipsilateral, but absent in the contralateral, eye.

Lesions of the *optic chiasm* (Fig. 9-17B) may result in bitemporal hemianopia (loss of temporal visual field in both eyes) if the lesion involves the medial aspect of the chiasm (i.e., pituitary tumor) or in the loss of vision in the ipsilateral nasal visual field if the lesion involves the lateral aspect of the chiasm (commonly caused by aneurysm).

Lesions involving the *optic tract, lateral geniculate body* of the thalamus, or *primary visual cortex* (Fig. 9 17C) typically result in homonymous hemianopia (loss of the contralateral visual field in both eyes).

Lesions involving *Meyer's loop* (temporal lobe fibers) (Fig. 9-17D) result in superior homonymous quadrantanopia (loss of the contralateral upper quadrant of the visual field in both eyes).

CRANIAL NERVES III, IV, AND VI (Figs. 9-18 and 9-19)

CRANIAL NERVE III: OCULOMOTOR

COMPONENT	ASSOCIATED NUCLEUS	FUNCTION
Somatic motor	Oculomotor nucleus	Motor to the inferior rectus, rectus medial, superior rectus, inferior oblique, and levator palpebrae superioris muscles of the eye
Visceral motor	Edinger-Westphal nucleus	Parasympathetic innervation to the constrictor pupillae and ciliary muscles of the eye

CRANIAL NERVE IV: TROCHLEAR

COMPONENT	ASSOCIATED NUCLEUS	FUNCTION
Somatic motor	Trochlear	Motor to the superior oblique muscle of the eye

CRANIAL NERVE VI: ABDUCENS

COMPONENT	ASSOCIATED NUCLEUS	FUNCTION
Somatic motor	Abducens	Motor to the lateral rectus muscle of the eye

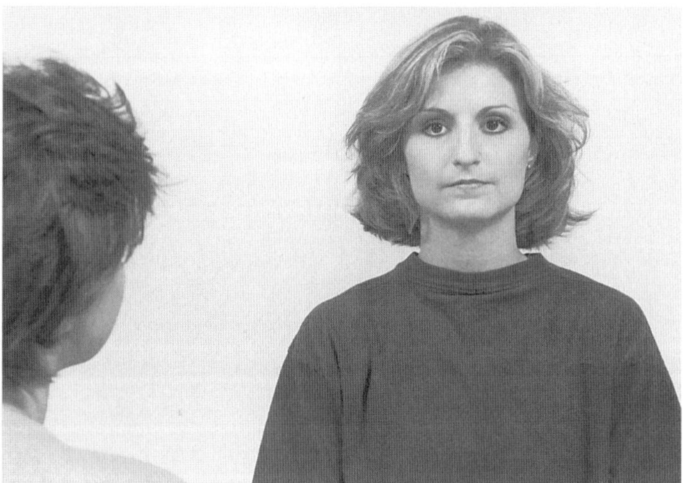

Fig. 9-18. Examination for alignment of eyes and for ptosis.

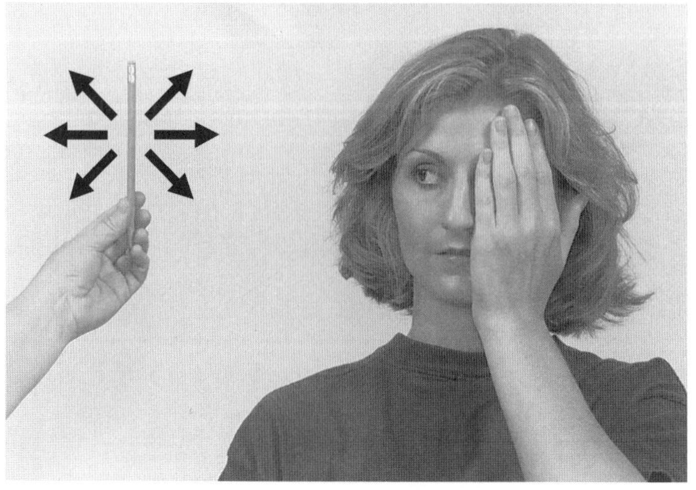

Fig. 9-19. Examination of visual tracking: extraocular muscles (cranial nerves III, IV, and VI). Individual eye testing shown (arrows show direction of pencil movement).

Testing

Materials needed: A pencil or pen is used.

Patient position: Seated comfortably with the eyes focused forward.

Procedure: The examiner begins by observing the alignment of the eyes and checking for ptosis (drooping of the eyelid). The pupils should both be directed straight ahead, the width of the palpebral fissures should be equal bilaterally, and the upper eyelid should cover an equal part of the iris (but none of the pupil) of both eyes.

Examination of the extraocular muscles may be performed initially with both eyes uncovered. The patient is asked to refrain from turning the head during the examination. The examiner holds the pen or pencil approximately an arm's length in front of the patient. The patient is asked to follow the pen with both eyes while it is moved in all directions. The pen should be moved vertically, horizontally, and diagonally across the eyes while the patient tracks the pen visually in all directions.

If weakness of an extraocular muscle is suspected, the examination should be repeated with one eye at a time. The eye to be tested is left open, and the contralateral eye is covered by the patient. Again, the patient is asked to refrain from turning the head during the examination. The examiner moves the pen in all directions as described previously while the patient follows the pen with the open eye. The test is repeated for the opposite eye.

Normal response: The patient should be able to track the pen with each eye in all directions.

Note: Examination of cranial nerve III should include testing the pupillary light reflex and the accommodation reflex. These tests are described in conjunction with cranial nerve II. In cases of a lesion of cranial nerve III, the direct and consensual light reflexes are absent in the ipsilateral eye but are intact in the contralateral eye.

CLINICAL COMMENT: PTOSIS

Lesions of CN III (oculomotor) produce ptosis (drooping of the eyelid) secondary to loss of innervation of the levator palpebrae superioris muscle. Ptosis also is a clinical manifestation of neurologic damage and disorders elsewhere in the nervous system including Horner's syndrome, myasthenia gravis, Bell's palsy, and acute cerebrovascular accident.

CRANIAL NERVE V: TRIGEMINAL (Fig. 9-20)

Fig. 9-20.

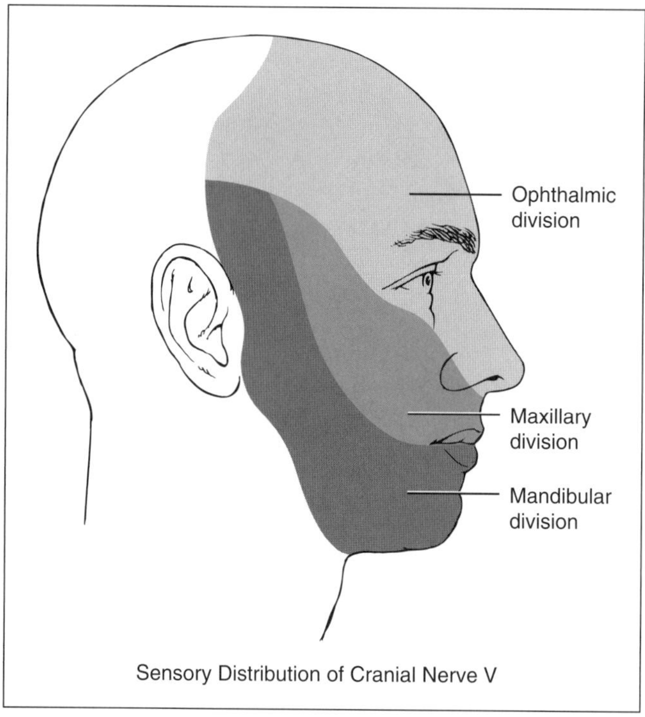

Sensory Distribution of Cranial Nerve V

CRANIAL NERVE V: TRIGEMINAL

COMPONENT	ASSOCIATED NUCLEUS	FUNCTION
Branchial motor	Motor nucleus of cranial nerve V	Motor innervation to the muscles of mastication (masseter, medial pterygoid, lateral pterygoid, temporalis) and the mylohyoid, anterior belly of the diagastric, tensor tympani, and tensor veli palatini
General sensory	Mesencephalic	Proprioceptive information from the muscles of mastication, teeth, and temporomandibular joint
General sensory	Principal nucleus of cranial nerve V	Tactile sensation from the face, oral structures, eye and associated structures, nasal cavity, frontal sinuses, side of the head, and scalp
General sensory	Spinal nucleus of cranial nerve V	Pain and temperature sensation from the face, oral structures, eye and associated structures, nasal cavity, frontal sinuses, side of the head, and scalp

Important points of anatomy: The trigeminal nerve exits the brain stem on the ventral surface of the pons and divides just distal to the trigeminal ganglion into three separate divisions, the ophthalmic, maxillary, and mandibular nerves.

Testing

SENSATION TO THE FACE (Figs. 9-21 to 9-23)

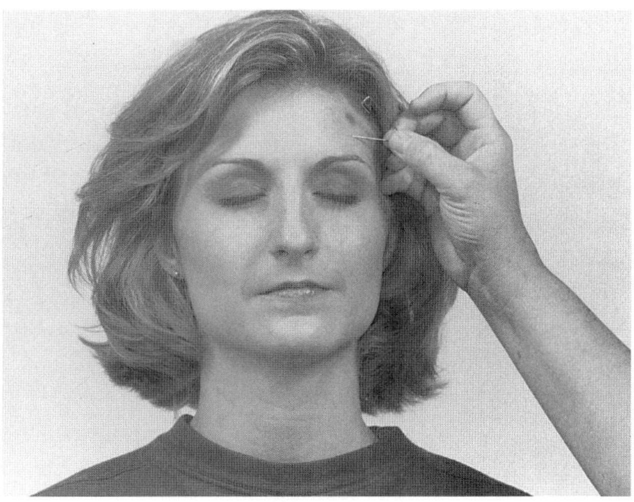

Fig. 9-21. Test for sharp/dull discrimination: ophthalmic division of cranial nerve V.

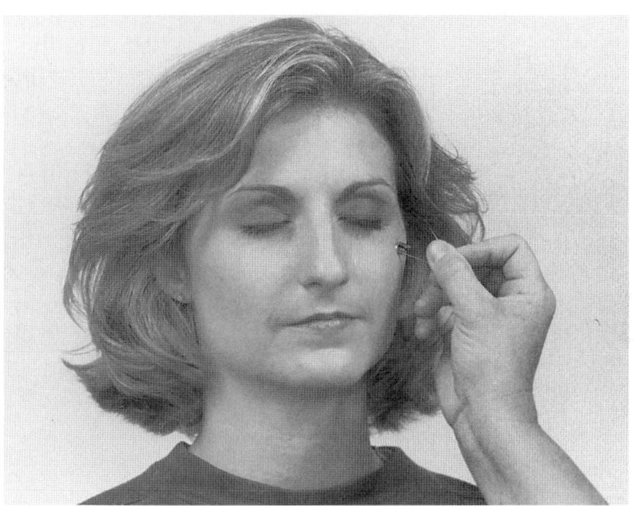

Fig. 9-22. Test for sharp/dull discrimination: maxillary division of cranial nerve V.

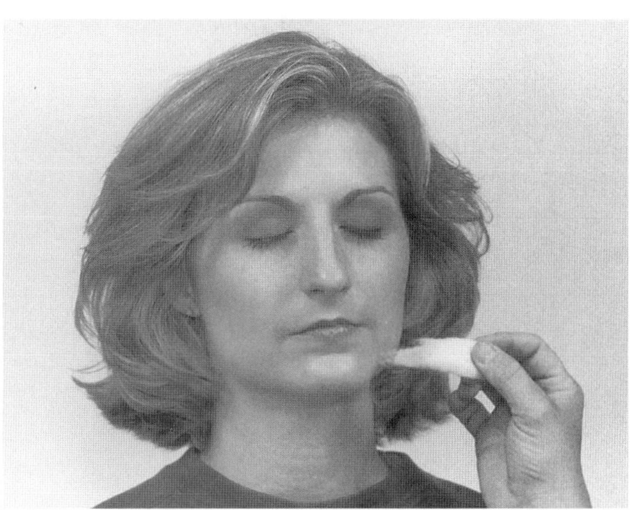

Fig. 9-23. Test for light touch sensation: mandibular division of cranial nerve V.

Materials needed: A clean, unused safety pin or a sterile wooden cotton-tipped applicator is used (and then disposed of).

Patient position: Seated in a comfortable position.

Procedure: Before the examination, the examiner should explain the procedure to the patient, demonstrating the feel of each sensory modality in an area where the patient has intact sensation.

Once the examination begins, the patient's eyes should be closed or covered. Using the safety pin or wooden, cotton-tipped applicator, the examiner touches the patient's face alternately but in a random order with the sharp or dull end. (If the wooden applicator is used, the stick of the applicator should be broken to create a "sharp" end, and the cotton-tipped end should be used for the "dull" end.) The patient should be instructed to respond with the words "sharp" or "dull" upon perceiving the stimulus. The examiner should avoid providing any indication, verbal or otherwise, when the patient is touched during the examination.

The face should be stimulated on both sides, making sure that the areas of all three divisions of cranial nerve V (ophthalmic, maxillary, and mandibular) are covered on each side of the face. The area where there is least overlap between the three divisions is in the central part of the face, so testing is best confined to that area.

Once the examination for pain sensation is complete, the stimulating instrument should be disposed of in the appropriate (sharps) container. Such instruments should never be reused with another patient.

The aforementioned procedure should be repeated with a wisp of cotton to examine light touch sensation. When stimulating the face with the cotton, the examiner should merely touch the cotton to the face and should avoid any sort of wiping motion with the cotton. If the cotton is moved over an area of the face in a wiping motion, the patient will perceive a tickling sensation, which is more closely associated with pain than with light touch.

CORNEAL REFLEX (CRANIAL NERVES V AND VII) (Fig. 9-24)

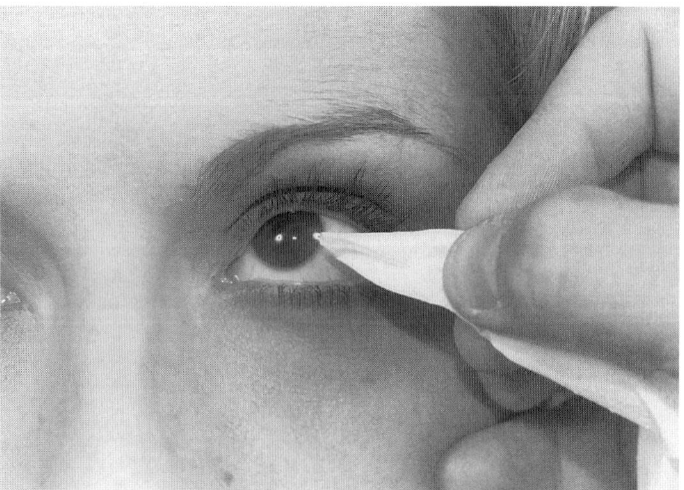

Fig. 9-24. Examination of corneal reflex (cranial nerves V and VII).

Materials needed: A tissue, folded to create a small tip, is used.

Patient position: Supine or seated in a comfortable position.

Procedure: The examiner instructs the patient to look up and away from the examiner. The examiner touches the patient's cornea with the folded tip of the tissue. The tissue should be brought toward the eye from the outer corner of the eye while the patient is looking in the opposite direction. This will prevent the patient from anticipating the touch of the tissue and blinking involuntarily.

Normal response: The patient blinks both eyes rapidly when the cornea is touched.

MUSCLES OF MASTICATION

Materials needed: No materials are needed.

Patient position: Seated in a comfortable position.

Procedure: *Pterygoids:* Ask the patient to open the mouth repeatedly. Observe the jaw for lateral deviation during opening. The pterygoids on one side open the jaw and cause it to deviate to the opposite side. Therefore, if the pterygoids on one side are weak, the mandible will deviate to the weak side upon opening (Fig. 9-25).

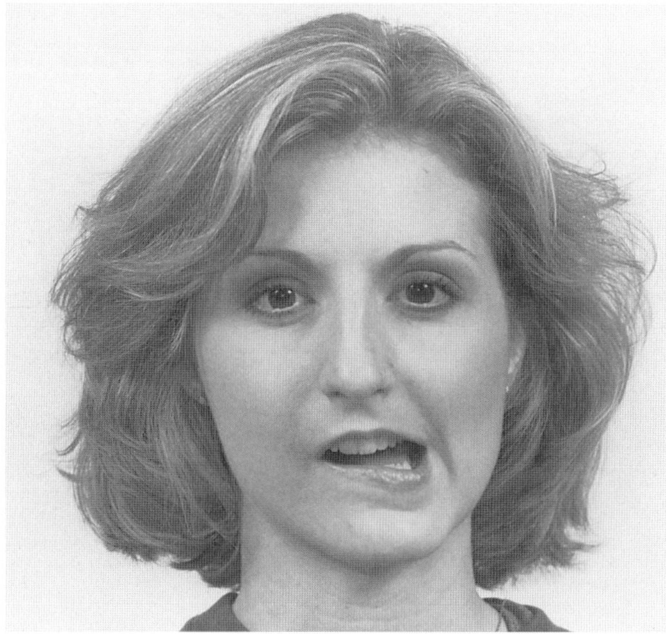

Fig. 9-25. Weakness of the pterygoid muscles on the left causes the jaw to deviate to the left with opening.

Masseter and temporalis: Palpate the masseter muscle on each side simultaneously between the zygomatic arch and the ramus of the mandible. Ask the patient to bite down, and compare the size and strength of contraction of the muscle on the two sides. The temporalis should be examined in a similar manner and can be palpated over the temporal fossa (Figs. 9-26 and 9-27).

Normal response: The mandible should remain in a midline position during opening. The size and strength of contraction of the masseter and temporalis muscles should be identical on both sides.

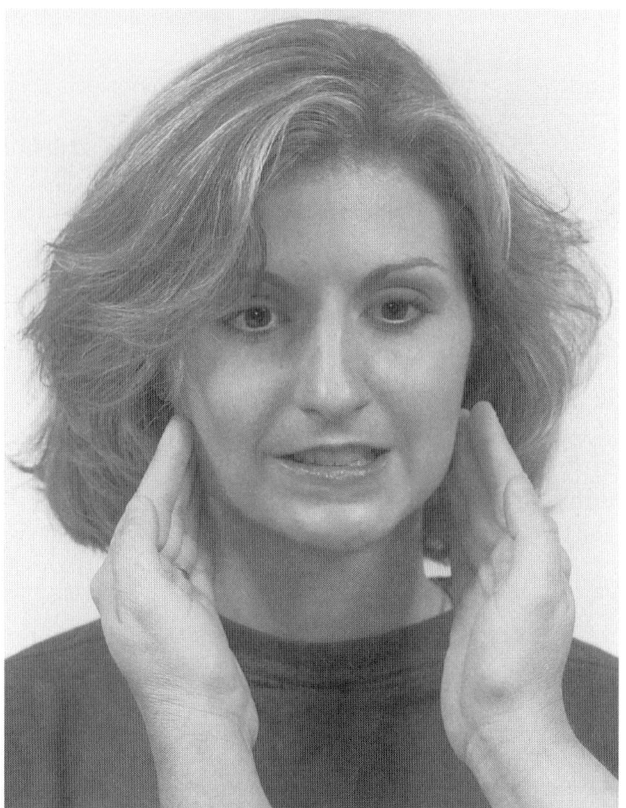

Fig. 9-26. Palpation of the masseter muscles.

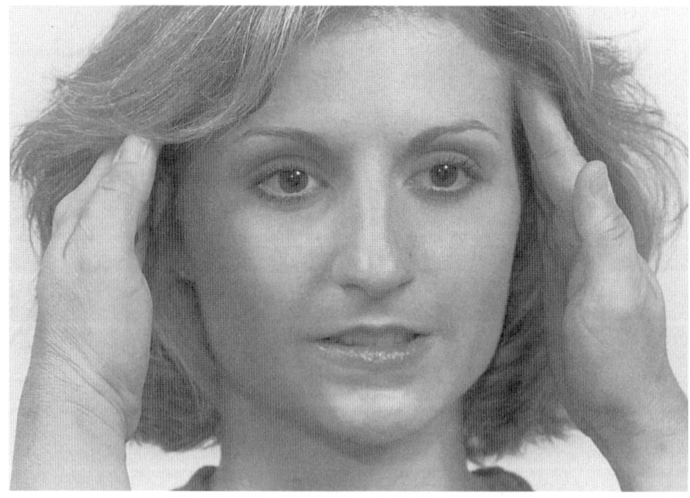

Fig. 9-27. Palpation of the temporalis muscles.

JAW JERK REFLEX (Fig. 9-28)

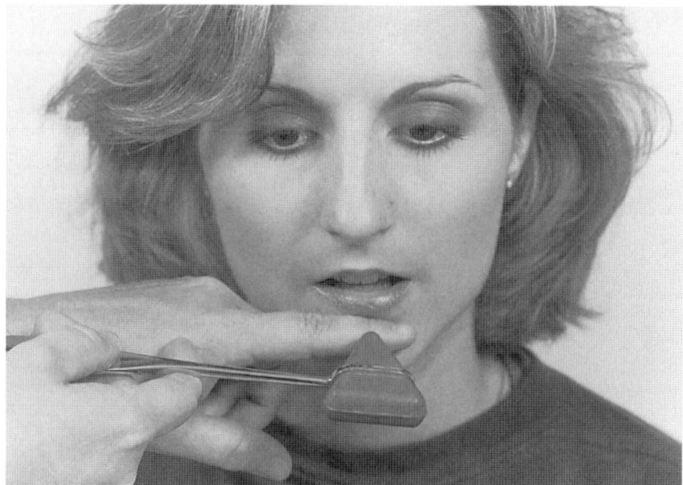

Fig. 9-28. Jaw jerk reflex (cranial nerve V).

Materials needed: A reflex hammer is used.

Patient position: Seated in a comfortable position with the mouth slightly open.

Procedure: The examiner places one finger horizontally on the chin and, with the reflex hammer, taps the horizontal finger.

Normal response: *Slight* closure of the jaw is normal. However, the response is sometimes absent in healthy individuals.

Lesions: An absent response may indicate a lesion of the trigeminal nucleus or nerve. In such cases, additional symptoms of trigeminal neuropathy (facial sensory loss, masticatory muscle weakness) also should be expected to be present. Brisk movement of the mandible is indicative of an upper motor neuron (supranuclear) lesion.

CLINICAL COMMENT: MANDIBULAR MOVEMENT

When assessing movement of the mandible, do not be deceived by deviations of the jaw that are mechanical in origin. Changes in the structure of the temporomandibular joint (TMJ); such as internal derangements, disc displacement, or cartilage remodeling; can cause a variety of mandibular deviations during jaw movement.

CRANIAL NERVE VII: FACIAL

Testing

MUSCLES OF FACIAL EXPRESSION (Figs. 9-29 to 9-33)

CRANIAL NERVE VII: FACIAL

COMPONENT	ASSOCIATED NUCLEUS	FUNCTION
Branchial motor	Motor nucleus of the facial nerve	Motor innervation to the muscles of facial expression, posterior belly of the digastric, stapedius, and stylohyoid
Special sensory	Nucleus solitarius (rostral)	Taste sensation for the anterior ⅔ of the tongue
Visceral motor*	Superior salivatory nucleus	Parasympathetic innervation of the lacrimal, sublingual, and submandibular glands
General sensory*	Spinal nucleus of cranial nerve V	Cutaneous sensation to a small area of skin of and behind the ear

* This component is not tested clinically.

Important points of anatomy: Cranial nerve VII has a close anatomic relationship with the nucleus of cranial nerve VI (in the pons) and with cranial nerve VIII (at the pontocerebellar angle). If symptoms of cranial nerve VI or VIII dysfunction exist simultaneously with cranial nerve VII loss, such symptoms can help to localize the lesion site.

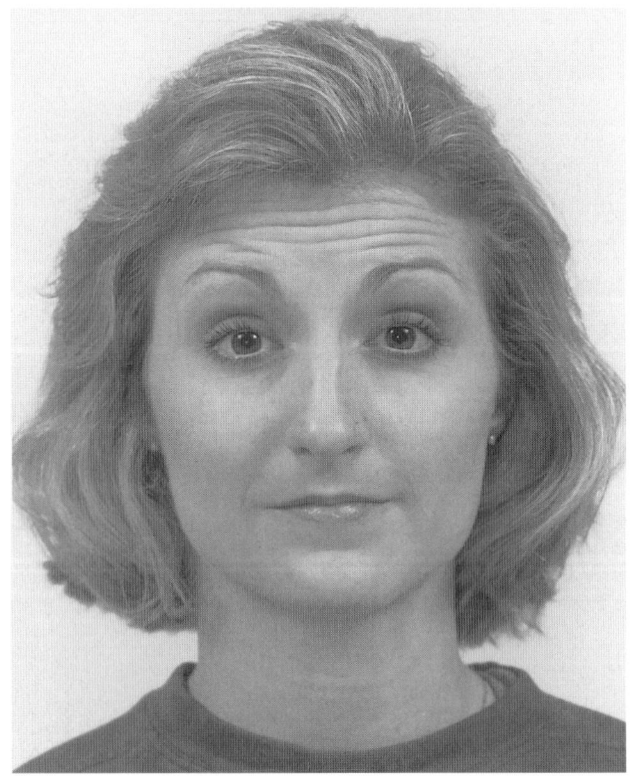

Fig. 9-29. Muscle testing: frontalis (cranial nerve VII).

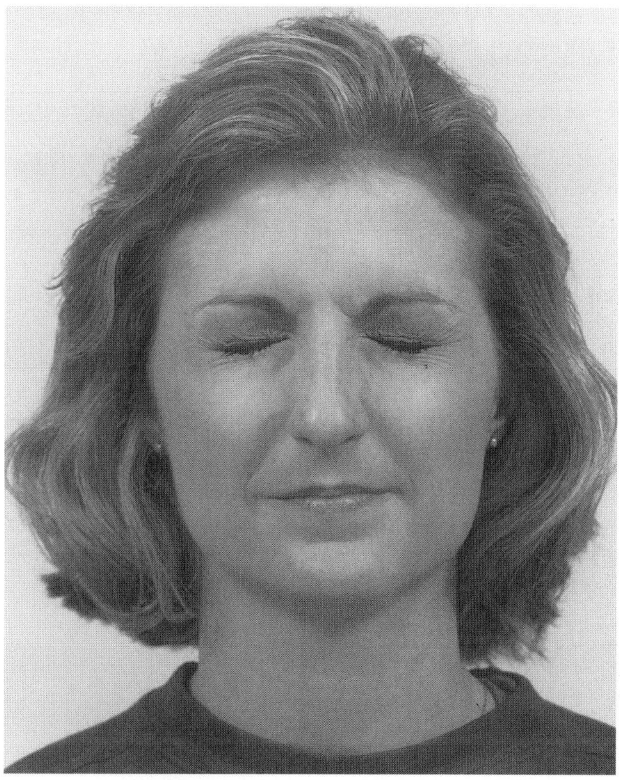

Fig. 9-30. Muscle testing: orbicularis oculi (cranial nerve VII).

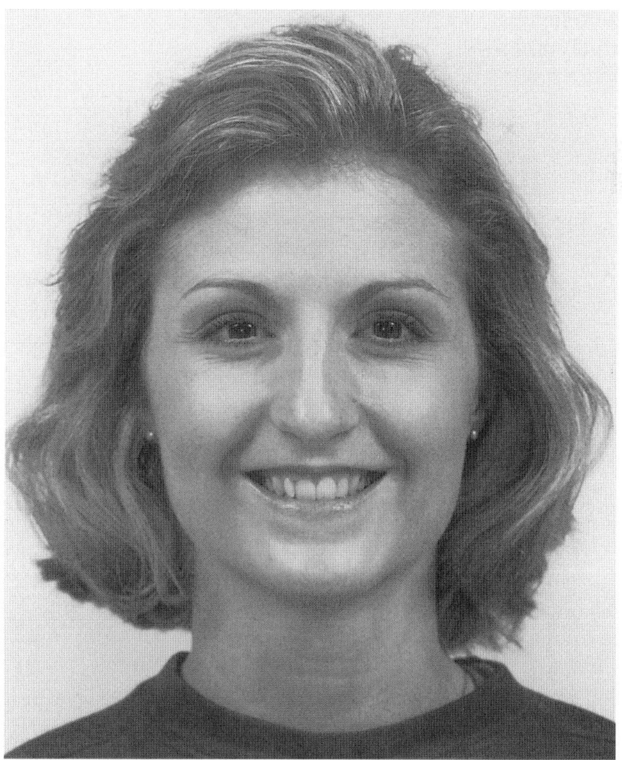

Fig. 9-31. Muscle testing: zygomaticus major (cranial nerve VII).

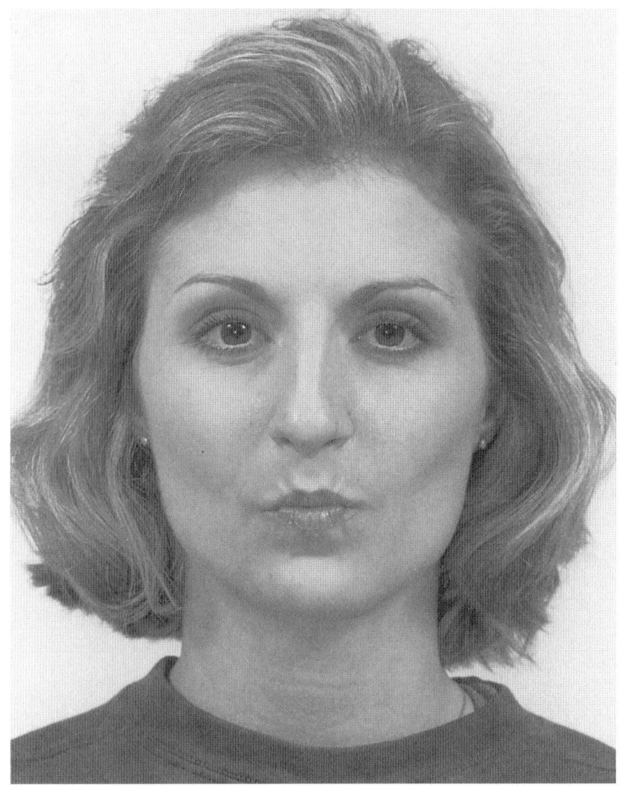

Fig. 9-32. Muscle testing: orbicularis oris (cranial nerve VII).

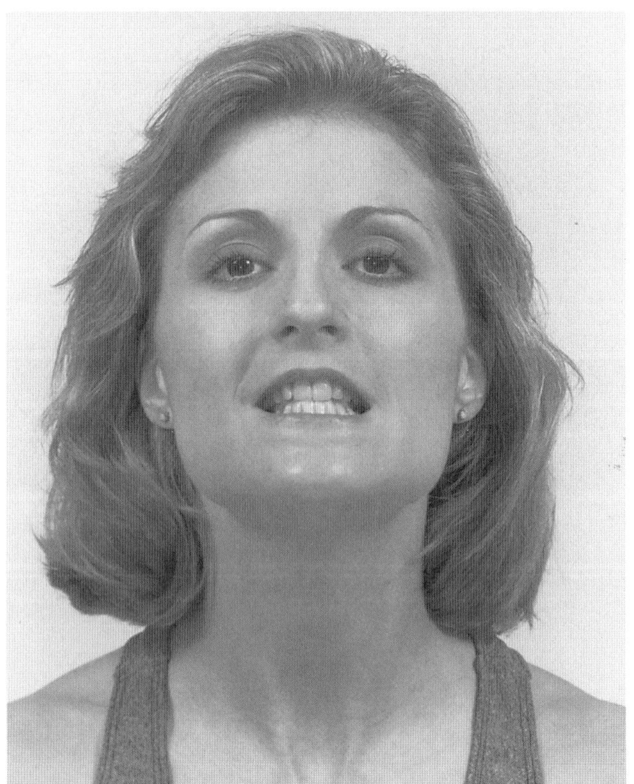

Fig. 9-33. Muscle testing: platysma (cranial nerve VII).

Materials needed: No materials are needed.

Patient position: Seated in a comfortable position.

Procedure: The examiner should perform a manual muscle test of the muscles of facial expression (see Chapter 3). Generally, to eliminate the possibility of facial nerve involvement, not all muscles of facial expression need be tested. At a minimum, the following muscles should be examined: frontalis, orbicularis oculi, zygomaticus major, orbicularis oris, and platysma.

Normal response: The patient should be able to mimic all facial expressions demonstrated by the examiner.

Lesions: Lesions involving the motor component of cranial nerve VII may result from damage to the nucleus or nerve itself (lower motor neuron lesion [LMNL]) or from damage to the corticobulbar fibers innervating the facial motor nucleus (upper motor neuron lesion [UMNL]). Each of these two lesions presents a very different clinical picture (Fig. 9-34).

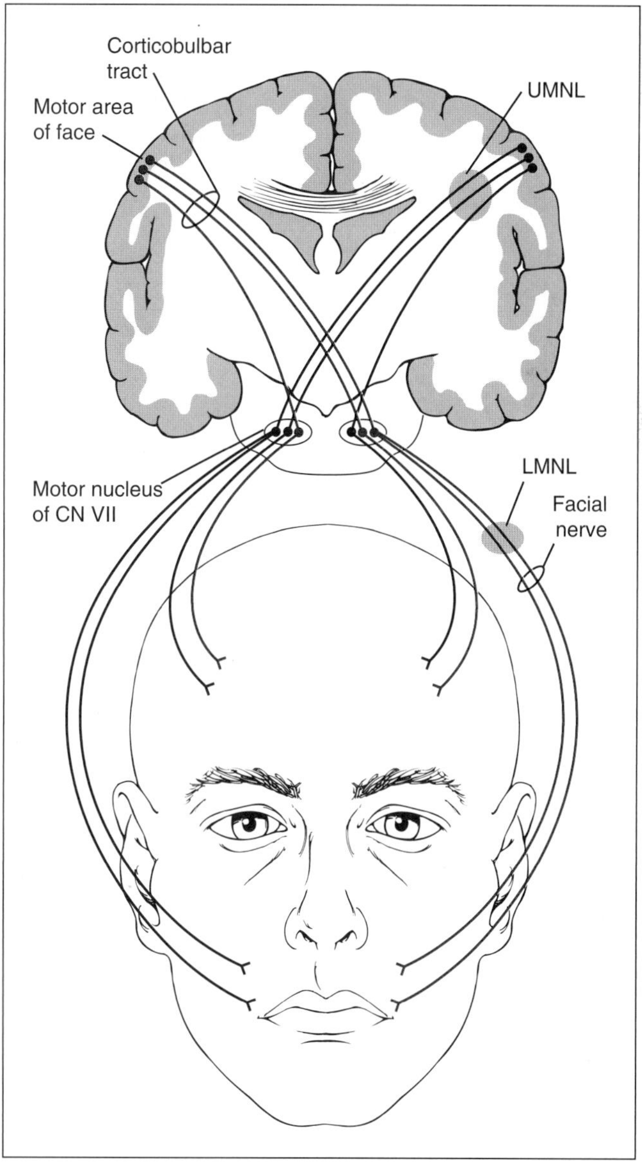

Fig. 9-34. Cortical control of facial nucleus. Note that the upper muscles involved in facial expression receive bilateral cortical control while the lower muscles receive only contralateral control. *UMNL*, upper motor neuron lesion; *LMNL*, lower motor neuron lesion.

LMNL: Lesions involving the facial motor nucleus or facial nerve result in weakness of the muscles of facial expression on the entire side of the face ipsilateral to the lesion.

UMNL: Lesions involving the corticobulbar fibers innervating the facial motor nucleus result in weakness of the muscles of facial expression in the lower half of the face contralateral to the lesion. The apparent lack of involvement of the upper half of the face is because the upper half of the face receives dual innervation from the corticobulbar fibers of both cerebral hemispheres.

CLINICAL COMMENT: FACIAL WEAKNESS

When examining patients with facial weakness, function of the muscles of the forehead should be closely examined. Patients with LMN lesions (ex. Bell's palsy) will be unable to raise the eyebrow on the affected side or to close the eye tightly on that side. A patient with an UMN lesion has no such deficit of forehead movement (can raise both eyebrows). Eye closure ability is variable, as the number of ipsilateral corticobulbar fibers that innervate orbicularis oculi motor neurons is variable from person to person.

TASTE: ANTERIOR TWO THIRDS OF THE TONGUE (Fig. 9-35)

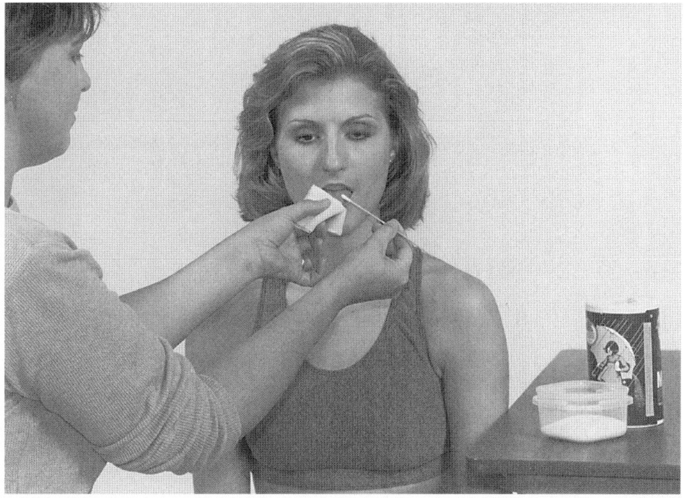

Fig. 9-35. Taste sensation test of the anterior tongue (cranial nerve VII).

Materials needed: Sterile cotton-tipped applicator, salt, sugar, water, sterile gauze squares, and cards on which the words *sweet* and *salty* are written are used.

Patient position: Seated in a comfortable position holding the cards on which the words *sweet* and *salty* are written.

Procedure: The examiner moistens a cotton swab and dips it in either salt or sugar. After grasping the patient's protruded tongue with a gauze square, the examiner applies the substance to one side of the patient's tongue. The examiner continues to grasp the patient's tongue while the patient holds up the card containing the word that describes the substance on the tongue. Repeat the test for the other side of the tongue. If needed, the test may be repeated after the patient has rinsed his or her mouth and a few minutes have elapsed.

Normal response: The patient is able to accurately identify substances placed on each side of the tongue.

CORNEAL REFLEX (CRANIAL NERVES V AND VII)

This reflex is described under testing for cranial nerve V.

CRANIAL NERVE VIII: VESTIBULOCOCHLEAR

Testing: Cochlear Component

GROSS HEARING EXAMINATION (Fig. 9-36)

CRANIAL NERVE VIII: VESTIBULOCOCHLEAR		
COMPONENT	**ASSOCIATED NUCLEUS**	**FUNCTION**
Special sensory	Dorsal and ventral cochlear nuclei	Hearing
Special sensory	Vestibular nuclear complex	Balance

Important points of anatomy: The vestibular and cochlear components of cranial nerve VIII originate in the bony labyrinth and cochlea, respectively, of the inner ear. The cell bodies of the two components of the nerve lie in ganglia within the inner ear (the vestibular and spiral ganglia) and send central processes to synapse on the brain stem nuclei listed in the table.

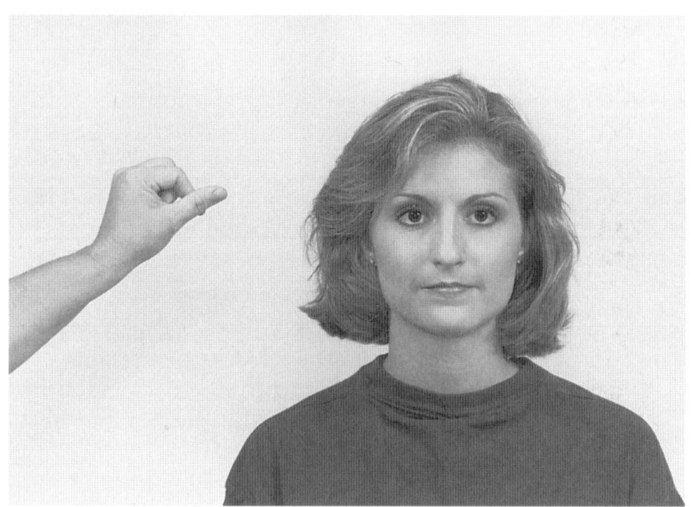

Fig. 9-36. Gross hearing test (cranial nerve VIII). The examiner rubs fingers together lightly at a distance from the patient's ear.

Materials needed: No materials are needed.

Patient position: Seated in a comfortable position in a quiet room.

Procedure: The examiner stands behind and to one side of the patient and makes a faint noise by rubbing the tip of the index finger and thumb together. The examiner's fingers are slowly progressed toward the patient's ear while the noise is continued. The patient is instructed to report the point at which the sound is first heard. The test is repeated for the opposite ear, and the distances at which the sound is first heard for each ear are compared.

Normal response: Patients with normal hearing should be able to hear fingers rubbed together at a distance of about 1.5 to 2 feet. The distance from the ear at which the sound is first heard should be equal bilaterally.

Lesions: A patient who is unable to hear the sound of fingers rubbing together at 1.5 feet or for whom the distance at which the sound is first heard for each ear is unequal should be referred for a more detailed hearing examination.

WEBER TEST (Fig. 9-37)

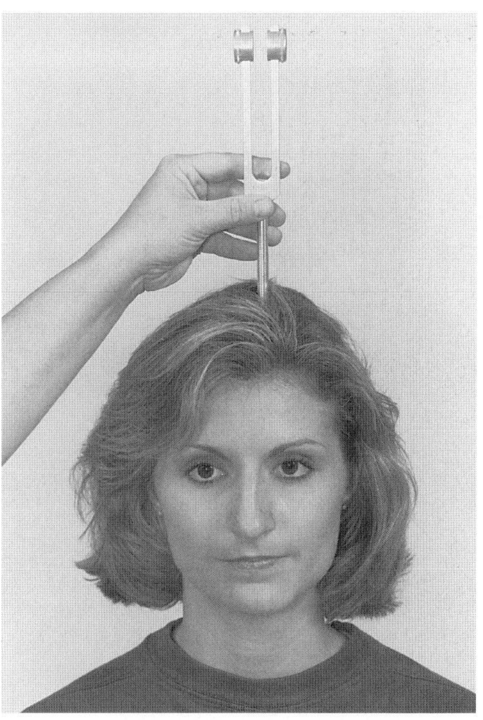

Fig. 9-37. Weber test: tuning fork on the midline of the skull (cranial nerve VIII).

Materials needed: A 256- or 512-Hz tuning fork is used.

Patient position: Seated in a comfortable position in a quiet room.

Procedure: The examiner hits the tines of the tuning fork to begin the vibration. The base of the tuning fork is placed on the midline of the patient's skull, and the patient is asked to tell the examiner where he or she hears the sound.

Normal response: Patients with hearing that is equal in both ears should localize the sound to the inside of the head.

Lesions: See Explanation of Weber and Rinne Tests, p. 598.

RINNE TEST (Figs. 9-38 and 9-39)

Fig. 9-38. Rinne test: tuning fork on the mastoid process (bone conduction; cranial nerve VIII).

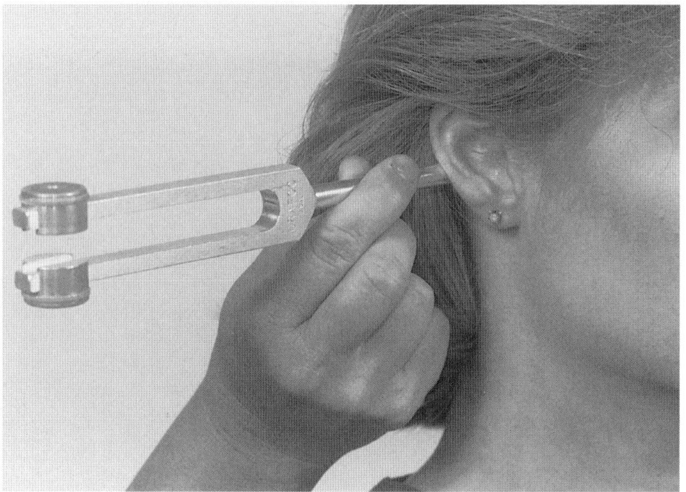

Fig. 9-39. Rinne test: tuning fork near the ear (air conduction; cranial nerve VIII).

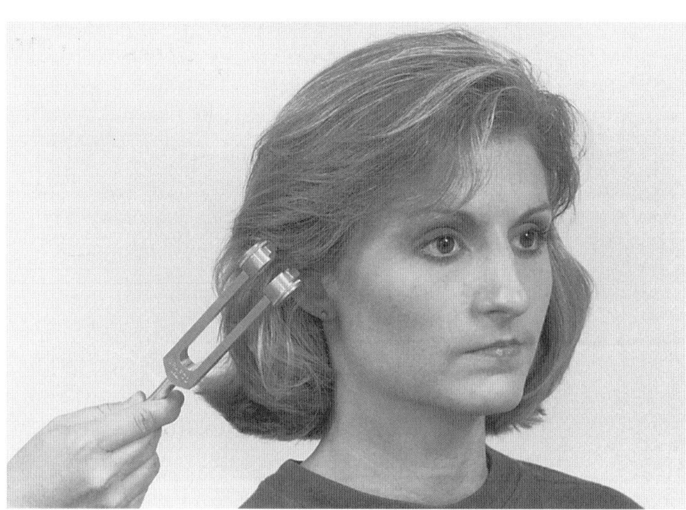

Materials needed: A 256- or 512-Hz tuning fork is used.

Patient position: Seated in a comfortable position in a quiet room.

Procedure: The examiner hits the tines of the tuning fork to begin the vibration. The stem of the tuning fork is placed on one of the patient's mastoid processes. The patient is asked to report the point at which he can no longer hear the sound. Once the sound is no longer heard, the examiner moves the tuning fork close to the ear. The patient is again asked to report the point at which he can no longer hear the sound.

Normal response: The patient should hear the tuning fork outside the ear for at least 15 seconds longer after it is removed from the mastoid process.

Lesions: See Explanation of Weber and Rinne Tests.

EXPLANATION OF WEBER AND RINNE TESTS

The Weber and Rinne tests are simple hearing tests, both of which depend on the differences between air conduction and bone conduction of sound.

When the Weber test is performed and the patient is asked to localize the sound, three possible scenarios can result:

1. Sound is localized to the inside of the head. This occurs when hearing is equal in both ears.
2. Sound is lateralized to the "good" ear. This occurs if the cochlea or auditory nerve is defective, as in sensorineural hearing loss.
3. Sound is lateralized to the "bad" ear. This occurs if the middle ear is defective, as in a conductive hearing loss.

When the Weber test is applied clinically and sound is lateralized to one ear, the examiner cannot, on the basis of the Weber test alone, determine if the ear to which the sound is lateralized is "good" or "bad." To make such a determination, the Rinne test is needed.

The Rinne test is designed to stimulate hearing first via bone and then via air conduction. When the tuning fork is placed on the mastoid process, the cochlea is stimulated by bone conduction. Once the patient can no longer hear the tone via bone conduction, the tuning fork is placed near the ear to stimulate the ear by air conduction. The patient should continue to hear the tone via air conduction for at least 15 more seconds. If the patient cannot hear the tone for an additional 15 seconds, then the *middle ear* is considered dysfunctional. The *cochlea* is considered grossly functional if the patient can hear the tone by bone conduction, but dysfunctional if he or she cannot.

Testing: Vestibular Component

NYSTAGMUS (Fig. 9-40)

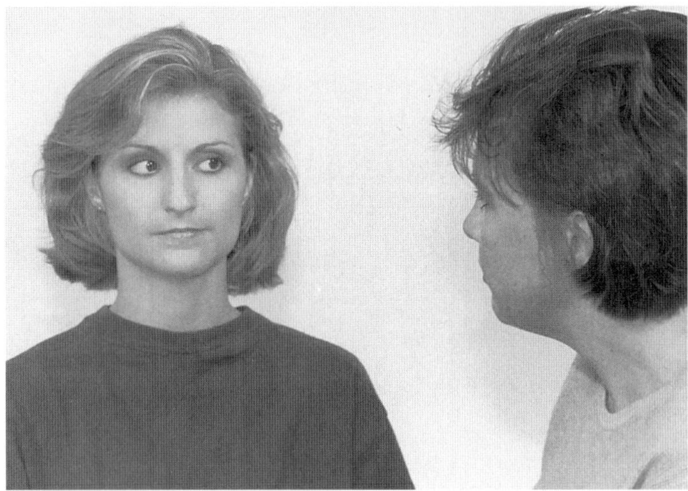

Fig. 9-40. Lateral eye movements to check for presence of nystagmus (cranial nerve VIII).

Materials needed: No materials are needed.

Patient position: Seated in a comfortable position.

Procedure: The examiner asks the patient to look forward, then to the right, then left. The eyes are examined for signs of nystagmus during these maneuvers.

Note: Patients who have been complaining of vertigo may have positional nystagmus in which vertigo and eye movements are noted only when the patient is in a particular position. The Hallpike-Dix maneuver is useful for assessing this situation.[1]

Normal response: The eyes remain steady within the orbit and do not demonstrate the alternating horizontal, vertical, or rotatory movements of nystagmus.

Lesions: Nystagmus (an involuntary oscillation of the eyeball) is noted during the examination.

CLINICAL COMMENT: VERTIGO

Vertigo is a common symptom of vestibular pathology. However, care should be taken to clarify a patient's complaint of "vertigo." True vertigo refers to the specific sensation that the environment is spinning or rotating. Patients who complain of vertigo may in fact be experiencing dizziness, light-headedness, disorientation, or other symptoms of non-vestibular etiology.

PAST POINTING (Figs. 9-41 and 9-42)

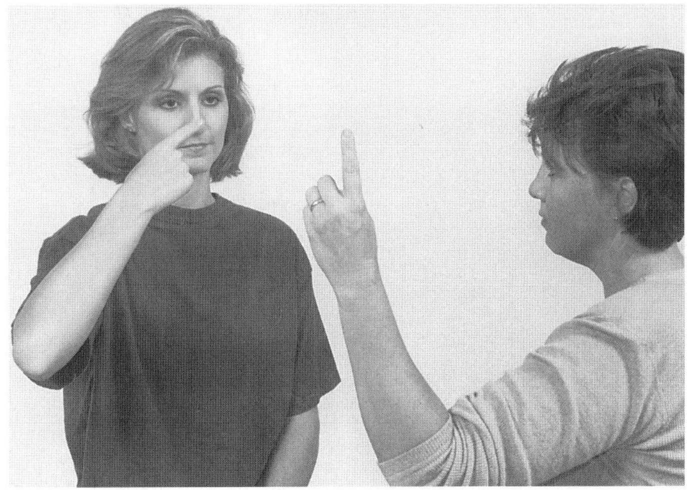

Fig. 9-41. Past pointing test (finger on nose): eyes open (cranial nerve VIII).

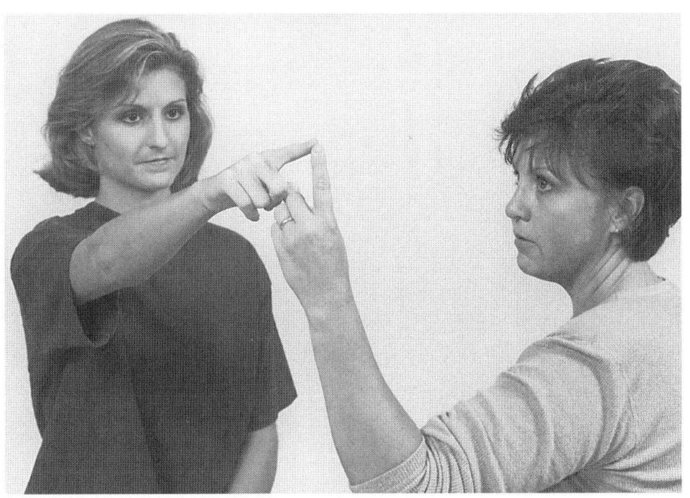

Fig. 9-42. Past pointing test (finger approaching examiner's finger): eyes open (cranial nerve VIII).

Materials needed: No materials are needed.

Patient position: Seated in a comfortable position.

Procedure: The examiner positions a finger slightly more than arm's length away from the patient and asks the patient to alternately touch the patient's nose and reach toward the examiner's finger. The patient is asked to repeat this movement three to four times with the eyes open and then to continue the movement with the eyes closed.

Normal response: The patient should be able to alternately touch his or her nose and then get near the examiner's finger with the eyes closed. Touching the examiner's finger is not necessary.

Lesions: Patients with lesions of the vestibular system will produce drift of the pointing finger to the side of the examiner's finger consistently. With unilateral lesions, the drift will be toward the side of the lesion each time.

Note: This test is very similar to the finger-nose test (see Fig. 9-3) with a few exceptions. The major differences lie in the responses seen with lesions of the vestibular apparatus (drift) versus the cerebellum (tremor, disjointed movement).

CLINICAL COMMENT: CALORIC TESTING

Caloric testing is the classic test for vestibular nerve function, but is generally administered by a physician. Such testing involves the application of hot or cold water to the external auditory canal, resulting in stimulation of the ipsilateral vestibular apparatus. Such stimulation results in a nystagmus whose direction depends on the temperature (hot vs cold) of the water applied. The mnemonic COWS (cold opposite, warm same) describes the expected direction of the fast component of nystagmus following irrigation of the auditory canal. A more comprehensive description of caloric testing can be found in any standard textbook of neurology.

CRANIAL NERVE IX: GLOSSOPHARYNGEAL

Testing

GAG REFLEX (CRANIAL NERVES IX AND X) (Fig. 9-43)

CRANIAL NERVE IX: GLOSSOPHARYNGEAL

COMPONENT	ASSOCIATED NUCLEUS	FUNCTION
General sensory	Spinal nucleus of cranial nerve V	General sensation from the posterior ⅓ of the tongue, the medial surface of the tympanic membrane, and the skin of the external ear
Special sensory*	Nucleus solitarius	Taste from the posterior ⅓ of the tongue
Branchial motor*	Nucleus ambiguus	Motor to the stylopharyngeus
Visceral sensory*	Nucleus solitarius	Sensation from the carotid body and sinus
Visceral motor*	Inferior salivatory nucleus	Parasympathetic innervation to the parotid gland

* This component is generally not tested clinically.

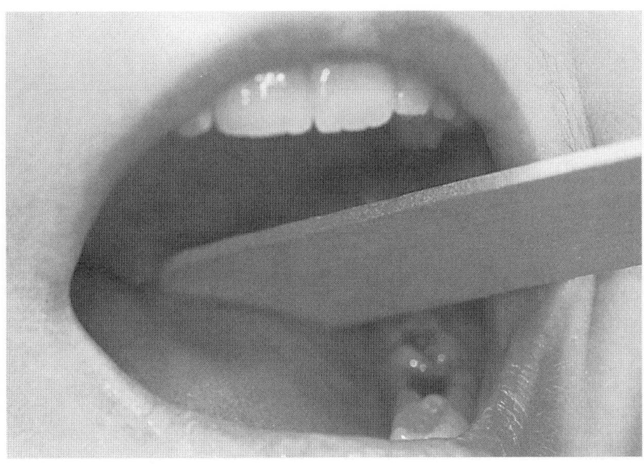

Fig. 9-43. Gag reflex (cranial nerves IX and X).

Materials needed: A sterile tongue depressor or a sterile cotton-tipped applicator is used.

Patient position: Seated in a comfortable position.

Procedure: The examiner touches one side of the pharynx with the tongue depressor or cotton-tipped applicator. After allowing the patient a few seconds rest, the test is repeated for the opposite side of the pharynx.

Normal response: The patient gags when the pharynx is touched with the tongue depressor or cotton-tipped applicator. However, the examiner may be unable to elicit a gag reflex in many healthy individuals. If the gag reflex is absent, the patient should be questioned regarding the ability to feel the tongue depressor touch the back of the throat on each side.

Lesions: A lack of sensation of the pharynx indicates a possible lesion of cranial nerve IX.

CRANIAL NERVE X: VAGUS

Testing

PALATAL ELEVATION (CRANIAL NERVE X) (Fig. 9-44)

CRANIAL NERVE X: VAGUS		
COMPONENT	**ASSOCIATED NUCLEUS**	**FUNCTION**
Branchial motor	Nucleus ambiguus	Motor to the palatoglossus and to the striated muscles of the pharynx and larynx (except the stylopharyngeus [cranial nerve IX] and the tensor veli palatini [cranial nerve V])
General sensory*	Spinal nucleus of cranial nerve V	General sensation from the skin around the ear, external surface of the tympanic membrane, pharynx
Visceral motor*	Dorsal motor nucleus of the vagus nerve	Parasympathetic innervation of the alimentary canal including pharynx, esophagus, trachea, bronchi, stomach, liver, heart, pancreas, small intestine, large intestine to the level of the left colic flexure
Visceral sensory*	Nucleus solitarius	Visceral sensation from the alimentary canal; stretch receptors in aortic arch; chemoreceptors in aortic body

* These components are not generally tested clinically.

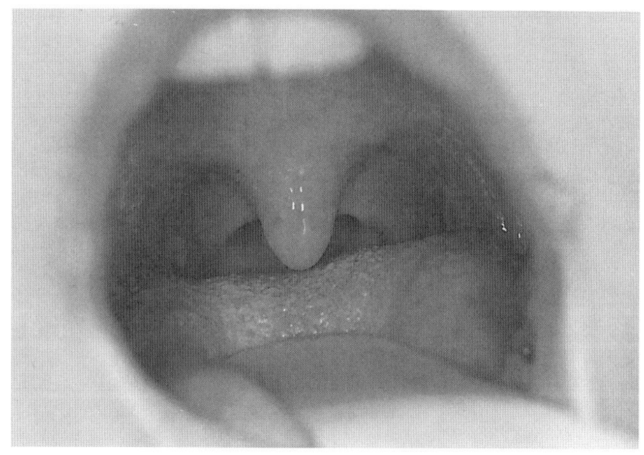

Fig. 9-44. Examination of the movement of the soft palate and uvula (cranial nerve X).

Materials needed: A sterile tongue depressor is used.

Patient position: Seated in a comfortable position.

Procedure: The examiner depresses the patient's tongue with the tongue depressor while asking the patient to say "Ahh." During phonation, the examiner observes the soft palate for elevation and the uvula for movement.

Normal response: The soft palate should elevate symmetrically on both sides.

Lesions: A unilateral lesion of the vagus nerve will result in failure of the soft palate to rise on the side of the lesion and in deviation of the uvula to the opposite side.

CLINICAL COMMENT: SWALLOWING

Normal functioning of cranial nerves IX and X (along with V, VII, and XII) is critical to the act of swallowing. Once a bolus of food has been moved into the region of the soft palate by the tongue (CN XII), sensory fibers in the palate (CN IX) detect the food and cause reflexive contraction of palatal and pharyngeal muscles (CN X) producing swallowing. Jaw and lip closure during the process are accomplished by cranial nerves V and VII respectively. Assessment of swallowing, or questioning the patient about swallowing difficulties, can provide valuable information about several cranial nerves, particularly IX and X. Dysfunction of swallowing is known as dysphagia.

CRANIAL NERVE XI: ACCESSORY

Testing

TRAPEZIUS MUSCLE (UPPER TRAPEZIUS) (Fig. 9-45)

CRANIAL NERVE XI: ACCESSORY		
COMPONENT	ASSOCIATED NUCLEUS	FUNCTION
Branchial motor	Nucleus ambiguus	Motor to the sternocleidomastoid and trapezius

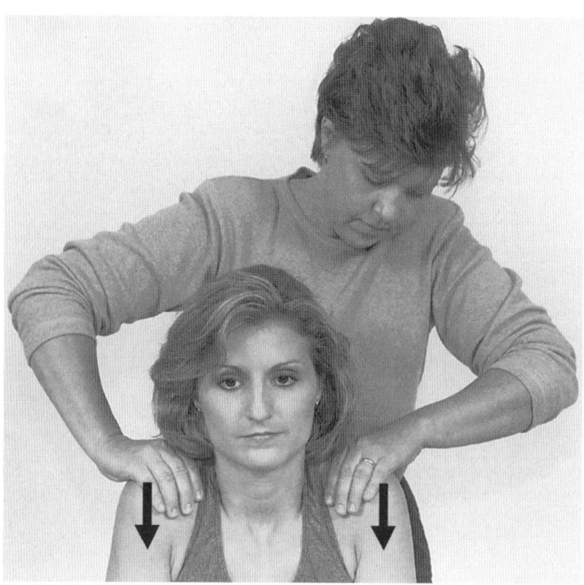

Fig. 9-45. Muscle testing: upper trapezius (cranial nerve XI; arrows show direction of resistance).

Materials needed: No materials are needed.

Patient position: Seated in a comfortable position with the arms at the sides.

Procedure: The examiner asks the patient to shrug the shoulders and to hold against resistance. The examiner applies resistance against the shoulders in the direction of shoulder depression.

Normal response: The patient should be able to hold the shoulders in an elevated position against maximum resistance by the examiner.

Lesion: The patient will be unable to elevate the shoulders or will "give" easily against resistance by the examiner.

STERNOCLEIDOMASTOID (Fig. 9-46)

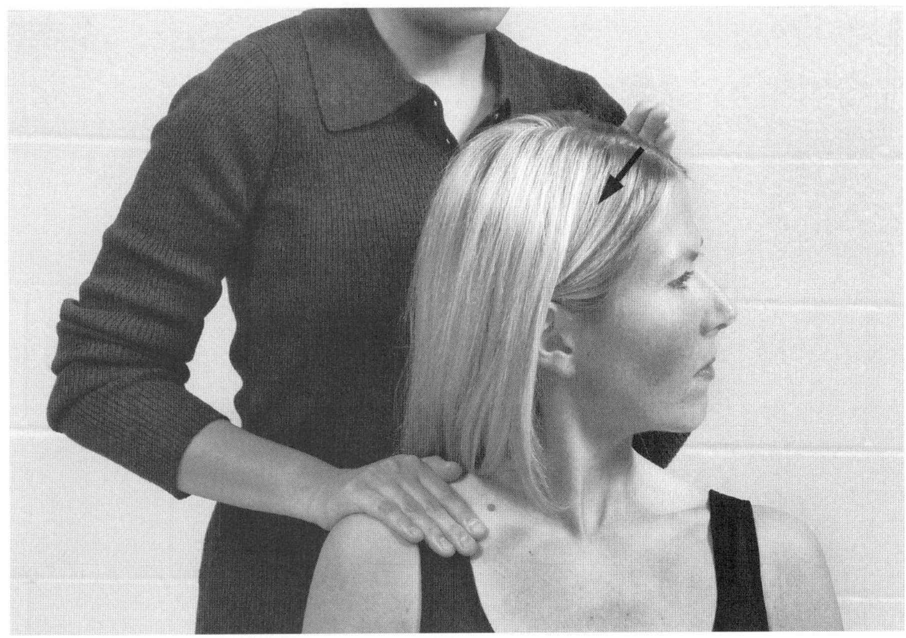

Fig. 9-46. Muscle testing: sternocleidomastoid (cranial nerve XI); arrows show direction of resistance.

Materials needed: No materials are needed.

Patient position: Seated in a comfortable position.

Procedure: The examiner asks the patient to turn the head completely to the left (to test the right sternocleidomastoid [SCM]). The examiner applies resistance against the left side of the patient's skull above the ear in an effort to turn the head back toward the right while the patient resists (Fig 9-46). The examiner is able to visualize the SCM at the same time that strength is being assessed. The test is repeated for the opposite muscle.

Normal response: The patient should be able to keep the head turned against resistance by the examiner.

Lesions: The patient will be unable to maintain rotation of the head in the presence of resistance by the examiner.

Note: A more isolated test of the SCM can be found in Chapter 3. The test described earlier is sufficient for screening purposes.

CRANIAL NERVE XII: HYPOGLOSSAL (Fig. 9-47)

CRANIAL NERVE XII: HYPOGLOSSAL		
COMPONENT	**ASSOCIATED NUCLEUS**	**FUNCTION**
Somatic motor	Hypoglossal nucleus	Motor to the muscles of the tongue (except the palatoglossus)

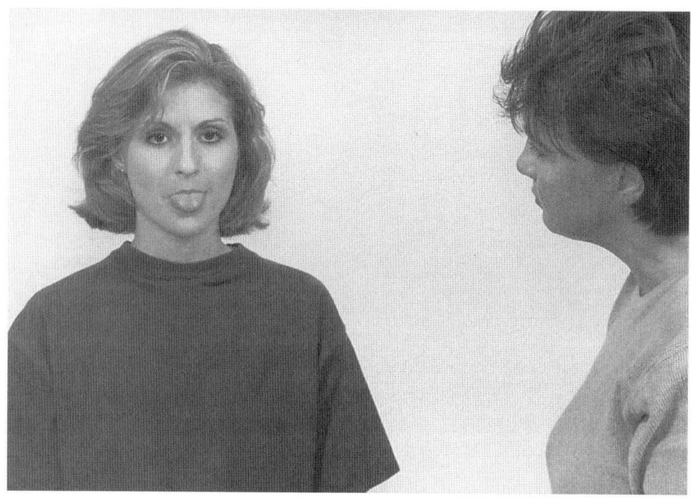

Fig. 9-47. Examination for symmetry of tongue movement (cranial nerve XII).

Testing

Materials needed: No materials are needed.

Patient position: Seated in a comfortable position.

Procedure: The examiner asks the patient to protrude the tongue.

Normal response: The tongue should remain in midline when protruded and should not deviate to either side. The tongue should be symmetric and free of involuntary movements.

Lesions: The tongue deviates to the side of weakness. If weakness is due to an LMNL, the side of the tongue that is involved will demonstrate atrophy (most reliable sign of LMNL), fasciculations, and weakness (the lesion is ipsilateral to the side of weakness). If the lesion is a UMNL, atrophy will not be present, and the weakness of the tongue will not be as unilaterally localized as is present in cases of LMNL.

CLINICAL COMMENT: FASCICULATIONS

A fasciculation is a contraction of an individual motor unit which contains a single motor neuron and anywhere from a few, to several hundred, muscle fibers. Firing of a single motor neuron results in contraction of all its associated muscle fibers- a fasciculation. Fasciculations are visible under the skin and occur in cases of LMN disease, although they also can occur in healthy individuals (ex. eyelid twitching). A fasciculation differs from a fibrillation, which is a spontaneous contraction of an individual denervated muscle fiber. Fibrillations are not visible to the naked eye and always are pathological.

■ CUTANEOUS REFLEXES

The following discussion includes testing techniques for those reflexes not covered in Chapter 8. While the reflex arc of the so-called cutaneous or superficial reflexes is somewhat more complex than that of the deep tendon reflexes discussed in Chapter 8, testing of these reflexes remains useful for determining neuropathology. Indeed, the presence of a Babinski response in an awake adult in and of itself is indicative of pathology within the central nervous system.

Testing

ABDOMINAL REFLEXES (Fig. 9-48)

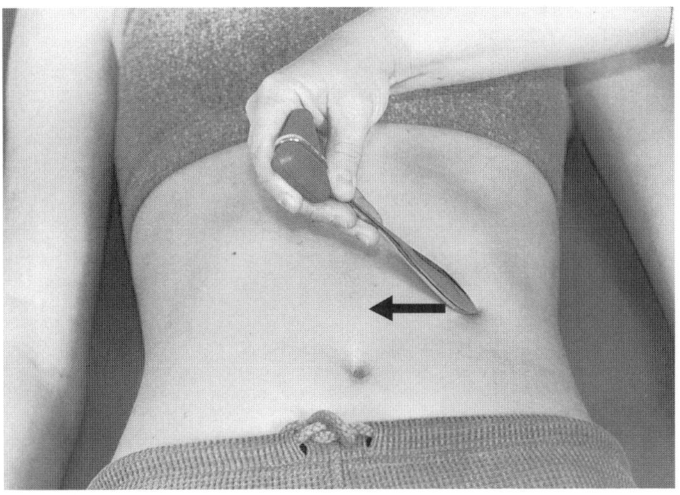

Fig. 9-48. Abdominal reflex test (arrow shows direction of stroking of reflex hammer).

Materials needed: A sharp object such as the pointed end of a reflex hammer is used.

Patient position: Supine with the abdominal muscles relaxed.

Procedure: The skin of the abdominal region is stroked in a lateral to medial direction in one quadrant of the abdomen at a time. The motion used to elicit the reflex should be rapid.

Normal response: Contraction of the abdominal muscle occurs under the segment of skin that was stroked, accompanied by deviation of the umbilicus toward the stimulus.

Lesions: A lack of response may be indicative of interruption of the spinal reflex arc at that level or of suprasegmental damage. Abdominal reflexes also may be absent in infants, in the elderly, or in patients who are obese, who have had abdominal surgery, or who are in the late stages of pregnancy.

CREMASTERIC REFLEX

Materials needed: A sharp object such as the pointed end of a reflex hammer is used.

Patient position: Supine.

Procedure: The examiner strokes the inner aspect of the upper thigh with the sharp end of the reflex hammer.

Normal response: The testicle is elevated on the same side.

Lesions: This reflex is mediated by spinal levels L1 to L2. A lack of response is indicative of interruption of the reflex arc or of suprasegmental pathology. The cremasteric reflex also may be absent in patients with hydrocele, varicocele, orchitis, or epididymitis and in elderly men.

PLANTAR REFLEX (Fig. 9-49)

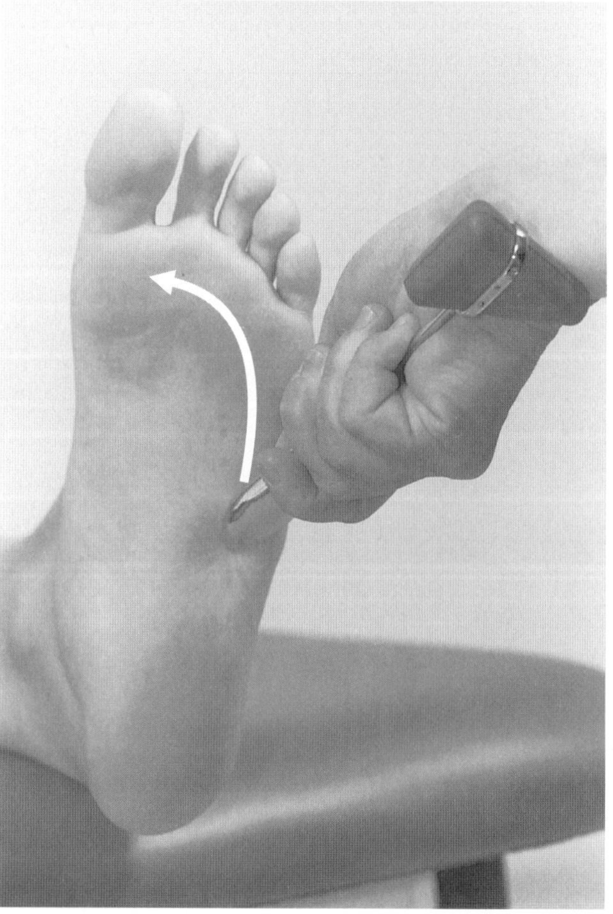

Fig. 9-49. Test for the presence of the Babinski reflex (arrow shows direction of stroking of reflex hammer).

Materials needed: A sharp object such as the pointed end of a reflex hammer is used.

Patient position: Supine.

Procedure: The examiner strokes the plantar surface of the patient's foot with the sharp end of the reflex hammer, beginning at the heel and progressing up the lateral border of the foot and over toward the base of the great toe. The pressure should be firm and even but not painful.

Normal response: Flexion and adduction of the toes occur, often accompanied by flexion of the knee and hip.

Lesions: Lesions of the corticospinal system cause an abnormal plantar reflex known as the *Babinski sign* in which the response to the stimulus is extension (dorsiflexion) of the great toe usually accompanied by flexion of the hip and knee. The lateral four toes may abduct, but extension of the great toe is the most important indicator of a Babinski sign. Note that a Babinski sign is normal in infants and in certain stages of sleep.

CASE 9-1 FACIAL WEAKNESS (CONTINUED FROM CASE 3-2; CHAPTER 3)

Questions 1 through 4 were answered regarding this case in Chapter 3. Answer questions 5 through 9 regarding your examination of this patient.

Mr. S is your 64-year-old neighbor who awoke one morning with weakness and drooping on the right side of his face. His wife, not sure what to do, and knowing you "knew about stuff like that," called and asked you to come see about her husband. She told you little over the telephone, other than her husband "couldn't move his mouth right." Based on the little you know, you believe your neighbor's husband has suffered some pathology either along the facial nerve or in the fibers from the cerebrum that control the facial nucleus.

1. What is the course of the facial nerve within the skull? Where does it exit?
2. After the facial nerve enters the parotid gland, it divides into five main sets of branches. Name these branches and describe their general distribution.
3. How much of the patient's face would demonstrate weakness if the entire facial nerve were damaged during its course through the skull?
4. What is this disorder (described in question number 3) commonly called?

Refer to the section from this chapter regarding examination of the facial nerve in answering the following questions about this case:

5. Name the fibers that originate in the cerebral cortex and provide control of the facial nucleus.
6. How can you differentiate between a lesion of the facial nerve and a lesion of the fibers named in the answer to question number 5?
7. What specific muscles would you need to test to make that differentiation?
8. Describe the patient's functional abilities in regard to facial movements following a lesion of the fibers named in the answer to question number 5.
9. For further exploration: What other kinds of signs and symptoms might a patient with a lesion involving these fibers (question number 5) display?

CASE 9-2 DIZZINESS AND UNILATERAL WEAKNESS

Ms. E is a 24-year-old female patient you have been seeing for rehabilitation of an ankle sprain. After missing an appointment, she arrives one day, complaining of dizziness along with weakness and heaviness on her right side (upper and lower extremities) that has been gradually getting worse over the last week. She indicates that she believes she is "getting the flu." Due to the asymmetry of her symptoms, you are suspicious of her self-diagnosis and decide to perform a few examination techniques to help better define her problem. Your examination reveals generalized weakness on the right, greater in the upper than in the lower extremity. She has a positive plantar reflex on the right and hyperactive deep tendon reflexes in the right extremities compared with the left. Her upper extremity drifts to the right during the past pointing test and she demonstrates unsteadiness during gait with a tendency to fall to the right.

Answer the following questions regarding this patient:

1. What is a plantar reflex and what is its significance?
2. What is the past pointing test?
3. What significance does the patient's direction of upper extremity drift and loss of balance during gait have on the probable location of her lesion?
4. What are the three sensory systems involved in maintenance of balance?
5. What do you believe would happen if you asked the patient to perform the narrow-based stance test with the eyes closed? Why?
6. Why might this patient have hyperactive reflexes on the right side?
7. What should be your next step in managing this patient?

References

1. Herdman SJ. Treatment of benign paroxysmal positional vertigo. *Phys Ther* 1990;70:381–388.
2. Horak FB. Clinical measurement of postural control in adults. *Phys Ther* 1987;67:1881–1885.
3. Horak FB, Nashner LM. Central programming of postural movements: adaptation to altered support surface configurations. *J Neurophysiol* 1986;55:1369–1381.
4. Kandel ER, Schwartz JH, Jessell TM. *Principles of Neural Science,* 4th ed. New York: McGraw-Hill, 2000.
5. Nashner LM. Analysis of movement control in man using the movable platform. In: Desmedt JE, ed. *Motor Control Mechanisms in Health and Disease.* New York: Raven Press, 1983.
6. Nashner LM, Peters JF. Dynamic posturography in the diagnosis and management of dizziness and balance disorders. *Neurol Clin* 1990;8:331–349.
7. Shumway-Cook A, Woollacott M. *Motor Control: Theory and Practical Applications,* 2nd ed. Philadelphia: Lippincott Williams & Wilkins, 2001.

Bibliography

Averbuch-Heller L, Leigh RJ, Mermelstein V, et al. Ptosis in patients with hemispheric stroke. *Neurology* 2002;59:620–624.

Bennett DA, Wilson RS, Schneider JA, et al. Natural history of mild cognitive impairment in older persons. *Neurology* 2002;59:198–205.

Beuttner UW, Zee DS. Vestibular testing in comatose patients. *Arch Neurol* 1989;46:531–563.

Corbett JJ. The bedside and office neuro-ophthalmology examination. *Semin Neurol* 2003;23:63–76.

Darovic G. Assessing pupillary responses. *Nursing* 1997;27:49.

DeMyer WE. *Technique of the Neurologic Examination,* 5th ed. New York: McGraw-Hill, 2004.

Diener HC, Horak FB, Nashner LM. Influence of stimulus parameters on human postural responses. *J Neurophysiol* 1988;59:1888–1905.

Duus P. *Topical Diagnosis in Neurology,* 3rd ed. New York: Thieme, 1998.

Edwards SL. Using the Glasgow Coma Scale: analysis and limitations. *Br J Nurs* 2001;19:92–101.

Fife TD, Tusa RJ, Furman JM, et al. Assessment: vestibular testing techniques in adults and children: report of the therapeutics and technology assessment subcommittee of the American academy of Neurology. *Neurology* 2000;55:1431–1441.

Glick TH. *Neurologic Skills: Examination and Diagnosis.* Boston: Blackwell Scientific, 1993.

Haerer AJ. *DeJong's: The Neurologic Examination,* 5th ed. Philadelphia: JB Lippincott, 1992.

Haines DE. *Neuroanatomy: An Atlas of Structures, Sections, and Systems,* 6th ed. Philadelphia: Lippincott Williams & Wilkins, 2004.

Haines DE. *Fundamental Neuroscience.* New York: Churchill Livingstone, 1997.

Hansen M, Sindrup SH, Christensen PB, et al. Interobserver variation in the evaluation of neurological signs: observer dependent factors. *Acta Neurol Scand* 1994;90:145–149.

Hawkes C. Smart handles and red flags in neurological diagnosis. *Hosp Med* 2002;63:732–742.

Hotson JR, Baloh RW. Acute vestibular syndrome. *N Engl J Med* 1998;339:680–685.

Jennett B, Bond M. Assessment of outcome after severe brain damage: a practical scale. *Lancet* 1975;1:480–484.

Kandel ER, Schwartz JH, Jessell TM. *Principles of Neural Science,* 4th ed. New York: McGraw-Hill, 2000.

Lance JW. The Babinski sign. *J Neurol Neurosurg Psychiatry* 2002;73:360–362.

Lundy-Ekman L. *Neuroscience: Fundamentals for Rehabilitation,* 2nd ed. Philadelphia: WB Saunders, 2002.

MacGregor DL. Vertigo. *Pediatr Rev* 2002;23:10–16.

Malik K, Hess DC. Evaluating the comatose patient: rapid neurologic assessment is key to appropriate management. *Postgrad Med* 2002;111:38–40,43–46,49–50.

McCrea M. Standardized mental status assessment of sports concussion. *Clin J Sport Med* 2001;11:176–181.

Neal L. Is anybody home: basic neurologic assessment of the home care client. *Home Healthc Nurse* 1997;15:156–169.

Nolan MF. *Introduction to the Neurologic Examination.* Philadelphia: F.A. Davis, 1996.

Ohkawa S, Yamasaki H, Osumi Y, et al. Eyebrow lifting test: a novel bedside test for narrowing of the palpebral fissure associated with peripheral facial nerve palsy. *J Neurol Neurosurg Psychiatry* 1997;63:256–257.

Palmer JB, Drennan JC, Baba M. Evaluation and treatment of swallowing impairments. *Am Fam Physician* 2000;61:2453–2462.

Pressman EK, Zeidman SM, Summers L. Primary care for women: comprehensive assessment of the neurologic system. *J Nurse Midwifery* 1995;40:163–171.

Rakel RE. *Saunders Manual of Medical Practice.* Philadelphia: WB Saunders, 1996.

Ross RT. *How to Examine the Nervous System,* 2nd ed. New York: Medical Examination Publishing, 1985.

Smith DV, Margolskee RF. Making sense of taste. *Sci Am* 2001;(March):32–39.

Stolze H, Klebe S, Petersen G, et al. Typical features of cerebellar ataxic gait. *J Neurol Neurosurg Psychiatry* 2002;73:310–312.

Sturmann K. The neurologic examination. *Emerg Med Clin North Am* 1997;15:491–506.

Walshe FMR. The babinski plantar response, its forms and its physiological and pathological significance. *Brain* 1956;79:529–556.

Waxman SG, deGroot J. *Correlative Neuroanatomy,* 22nd ed. Norwalk, CT: Appleton Lange, 1995.

Wijdicks EFM, Kokmen E, O'Brien PC. Measurement of impaired consciousness in the neurological intensive care unit. *J Neurol Neurosurg Psychiatry* 1999;64:117–119.

Wilson-Pauwels L, Akesson Ej, Stewart PA, et al. *Cranial Nerves in Health and Disease.* Philadelphia: BC Decker, 2002.

Zald DH, Pardo JV. The functional neuroanatomy of swallowing. *Ann Neurol* 1999;46:281–286.

10

OBSERVATIONAL GAIT ANALYSIS as a SCREENING TOOL

Observational gait analysis provides a tool whereby one can detect abnormalities in ambulation that may be attributable to muscle weakness, limitations in joint mobility, pain, or disorders of motor control secondary to nervous system lesions. The ability to analyze gait through visual observation allows one to screen patients for possible muscle weakness, particularly of the lower extremities. Such analysis requires considerable practice and a thorough knowledge of the normal gait cycle. A videotape of the patient's gait can be of great assistance in this process; this record can allow one to view the patient's gait pattern repeatedly. Thus the examiner is able to focus on one joint at a time and perform repeated viewings without causing the patient undue fatigue.

This chapter provides an overview of the normal gait cycle, including some common gait deviations and possible causes for each deviation. When muscle weakness is a possible cause, the appropriate muscle test is indicated. With the exception of the hip, gait deviations are restricted at each joint to those occurring in the sagittal plane.

NORMAL GAIT CYCLE

By convention, a single gait cycle begins at initial contact and ends with the next initial contact of the same extremity. Approximately 40% of each gait cycle consists of stance during which the lower extremity is in contact with the supporting surface. During the remaining 60% of the gait cycle, the lower extremity is in a non–weight-bearing posture, and this portion of the gait cycle is referred to as *swing phase.* Both the stance and the swing phases of gait are subdivided into shorter periods for ease of analysis. These periods are listed in the following table by both the conventional and the more current Rancho Los Amigos terminologies. For the remainder of this discussion, only the Rancho Los Amigos terminology is used.

STANCE		SWING	
RANCHO TERMINOLOGY	**CONVENTIONAL TERMINOLOGY**	**RANCHO TERMINOLOGY**	**CONVENTIONAL TERMINOLOGY**
Initial contact	Heel strike	Initial swing	Acceleration
Loading response	Foot flat	Mid-swing	Mid-swing
Mid-stance	Mid-stance	Terminal swing	Deceleration
Terminal stance	Heel off		
Pre-swing	Toe off		

What follows are descriptions of each of the periods of the gait cycle with accompanying photographs that illustrate a point in time during each of the periods. Tables listing common gait deviations for the period are provided after each description. The gait deviations listed in these tables are by no means exhaustive but are meant to provide a starting point from which the examiner can begin to postulate possible etiologies for the patient's gait anomalies.

Initial Contact

Initial contact consists of the instant in time when the lower extremity first makes contact with the supporting surface (Fig. 10-1). As such, initial contact is not a period but an event in the gait cycle. In normal gait, initial contact is made with the heel of the reference limb.

Fig. 10-1. Initial contact

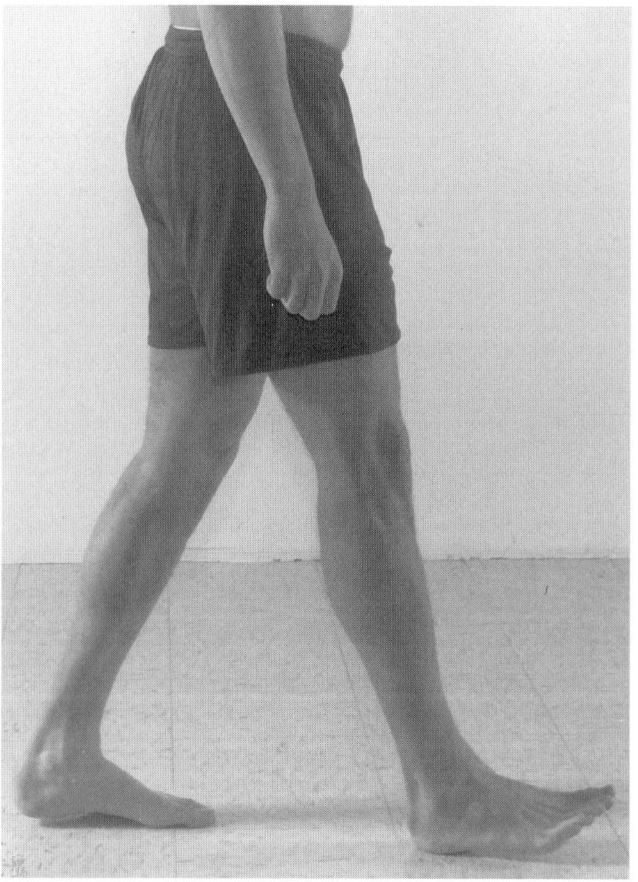

Loading Response

Loading response begins with initial contact of the reference limb and continues until the opposite lower extremity leaves the supporting surface (Fig. 10-2). During this period in which the reference limb is accepting the weight of the head, trunk, and extremities, the knee and ankle undergo controlled flexion (ankle plantar flexion) as a means of shock absorption. Activity of the quadriceps and ankle dorsiflexors is critical to control the knee flexion and ankle plantar flexion, which are occurring during this time.

Fig. 10-2. Loading response

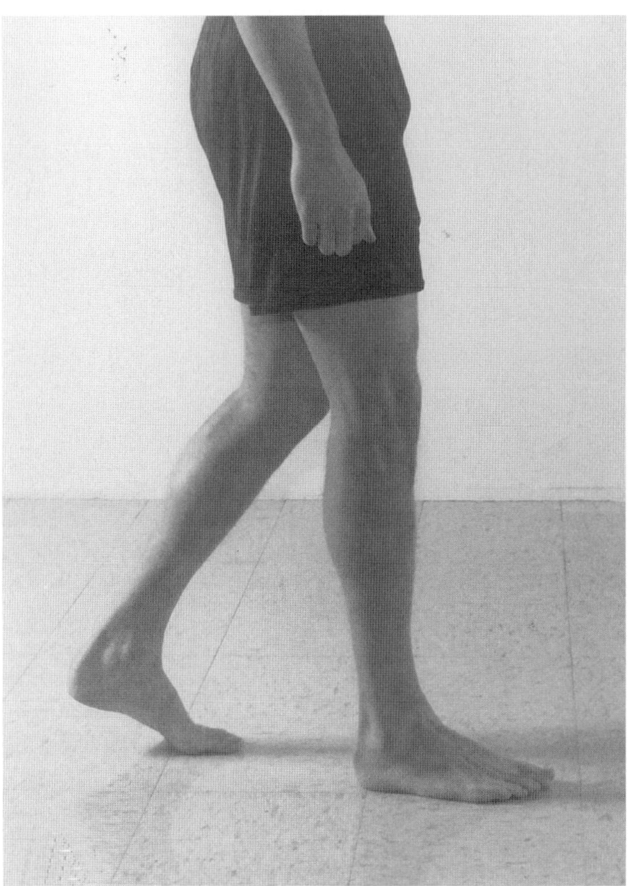

INITIAL CONTACT/LOADING RESPONSE

JOINT	MUSCLES ACTIVE	COMMON GAIT DEVIATIONS	MUSCULAR ETIOLOGY	OTHER POSSIBLE ETIOLOGIES
Hip	Gluteus maximus/ hamstrings/ adductor magnus: Active to control flexion torque at the hip	Anterior pelvic tilt	Weak hip extensors: Perform manual muscle testing (MMT) of the gluteus maximus/ hamstrings to confirm	Hip flexion contracture; hip flexor spasticity
	Gluteus medius/ tensor fasciae latae: Active to counteract hip adduction torque	Backward trunk lean	Weak hip extensors: Perform MMT of the gluteus maximus/ hamstrings to confirm	Hip flexion contracture
Knee	Quadriceps: Active to control flexion of the knee	Insufficient knee flexion, knee hyperextension	Weak knee extensors: Perform MMT of the quadriceps to confirm	Excessive ankle plantar flexion (possibly secondary to spasticity or contracture); knee pain; quadriceps spasticity; knee extension contracture
		Excessive knee flexion	If present during initial contact/ loading response, generally not due to muscle weakness	Knee flexion contracture; hamstring spasticity
Ankle	Pretibial muscles (tibialis anterior, long toe extensors): Active to control ankle plantar flexion	Excessive (or too rapid) ankle plantar flexion	Weak ankle dorsiflexors: Perform MMT of the tibialis anterior and long toe extensors to confirm	Ankle plantar flexor spasticity; ankle plantar flexion contracture

Mid-Stance

Mid-stance occurs from the point at which the opposite lower extremity leaves the supporting surface until the body's weight falls over the forefoot of the supporting extremity (Fig. 10-3). Muscular activity in general decreases during this period as the body's weight becomes more aligned over the supporting limb. One exception occurs at the hip as the center of the body's mass passes medial to the hip joint, resulting in a large adduction torque at the hip. Hip abductors are active during mid stance (and later periods) to counteract this torque.

Fig. 10-3. Mid-stance

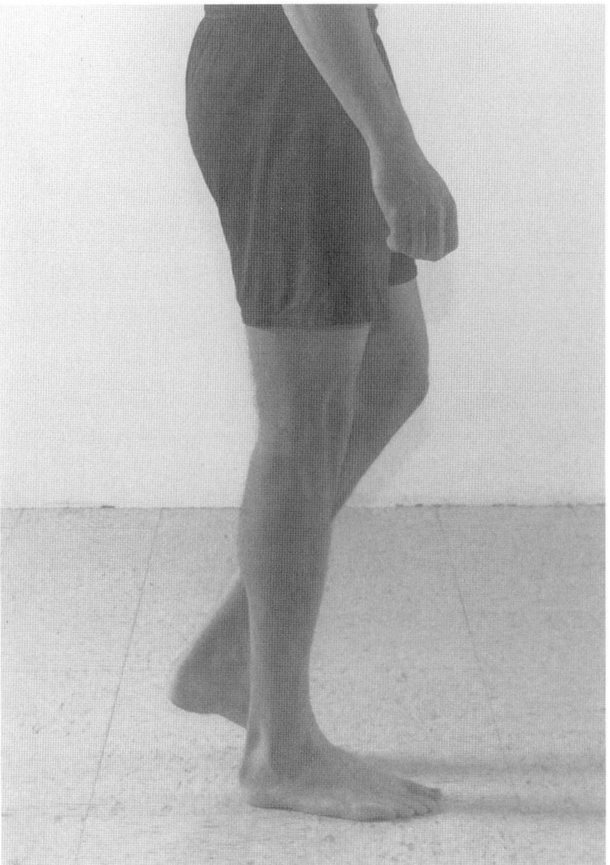

MID-STANCE				
JOINT	**MUSCLES ACTIVE**	**COMMON GAIT DEVIATIONS**	**MUSCULAR ETIOLOGY**	**OTHER POSSIBLE ETIOLOGIES**
Hip	Gluteus medius and minimus/ tensor fasciae latae: Active to counteract hip adduction torque	Contralateral pelvic drop or ipsilateral trunk lean	Weak hip abductors: Perform MMT of the gluteus medius/minimus and tensor fasciae latae to confirm	Hip pain (antalgic gait); ipsilateral hip abduction contracture (causes ipsilateral trunk lean)
		Excessive hip flexion	Generally not caused by muscle weakness	Hip flexion or iliotibial band contracture; spasticity of hip flexors; hip pain
		Backward trunk lean	Weak hip extensors: Perform MMT of the gluteus maximus/ hamstrings to confirm	Hip flexion contracture
Knee	Quadriceps: Active to control knee flexion torque only at the beginning of mid-stance	Knee hyperextension	Weak knee extensors: Perform MMT of the quadriceps to confirm	Excessive ankle plantar flexion (secondary to spasticity or contracture)
		Insufficient knee extension	Soleus weakness (allows uncontrolled anterior advancement of the tibia): Perform MMT of the soleus to confirm	Knee flexion contracture; hamstring spasticity
Ankle	Soleus (and later, gastrocnemius): Active to control anterior advancement of the tibia	Insufficient ankle dorsiflexion	Generally not caused by muscle weakness during this phase of gait	Ankle plantar flexion contracture; ankle plantar flexor spasticity
		Excessive ankle dorsiflexion	Weak soleus: Perform MMT of the soleus to confirm	Flexed knee gait (secondary to, e.g., knee flexion contracture, hamstring spasticity)

Terminal Stance

Terminal stance begins when the heel of the reference limb starts to rise from the supporting surface and ends with initial contact of the opposite lower extremity (Fig. 10-4). During this period, both the knee and hip are extended while the ankle dorsiflexes, and a large dorsiflexion torque develops at the ankle. The plantar flexors of the ankle are active to control the anteriorly progressing tibia and the dorsiflexion torque.

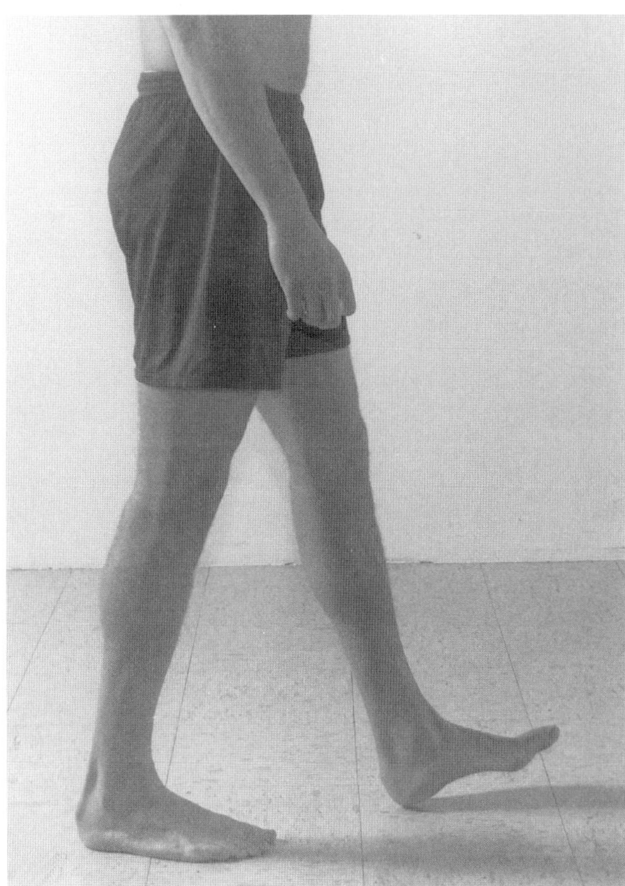

Fig. 10-4. Terminal stance

TERMINAL STANCE				
JOINT	**MUSCLES ACTIVE**	**COMMON GAIT DEVIATIONS**	**MUSCULAR ETIOLOGY**	**OTHER POSSIBLE ETIOLOGIES**
Hip	Anterior fibers of the tensor fasciae latae: Active to control hip extension and counteract the remaining hip adduction torque	Insufficient hip extension	Generally not caused by muscle weakness	Hip flexor contracture; spasticity of hip flexors
		Contralateral pelvic drop or ipsilateral trunk lean	Weak hip abductors: Perform MMT of the gluteus medius/minimus and tensor fasciae latae to confirm	Hip pain (antalgic gait); ipsilateral hip abductor contracture (causes ipsilateral trunk lean)
Knee	Popliteus: Relatively low level of activity to prevent hyperextension of the knee	Knee hyperextension	Weak knee extensors: Perform MMT of the quadriceps to confirm	Excessive ankle plantar flexion (secondary to spasticity or contracture)
		Insufficient knee extension	Soleus weakness: Perform MMT of the soleus to confirm	Knee flexion contracture; hamstring spasticity
Ankle	Soleus gastrocnemius: Active to control dorsiflexion torque at the ankle	Excessive ankle plantar flexion	Generally not caused by muscle weakness during this phase of gait	Ankle plantar flexion contracture; ankle plantar flexor spasticity
		Excessive ankle dorsiflexion	Weak soleus: Perform MMT of the soleus to confirm	Flexed knee gait (secondary to, e.g., knee flexion contracture, hamstring spasticity)

Pre-swing

Pre-swing occurs from the point of initial contact of the opposite limb until the ipsilateral foot leaves the ground (Fig. 10-5). During this period, weight is being unloaded onto the opposite extremity in preparation for the swing phase of the reference limb. Muscular activity to initiate hip and knee flexion and ankle dorsiflexion begins during this time.

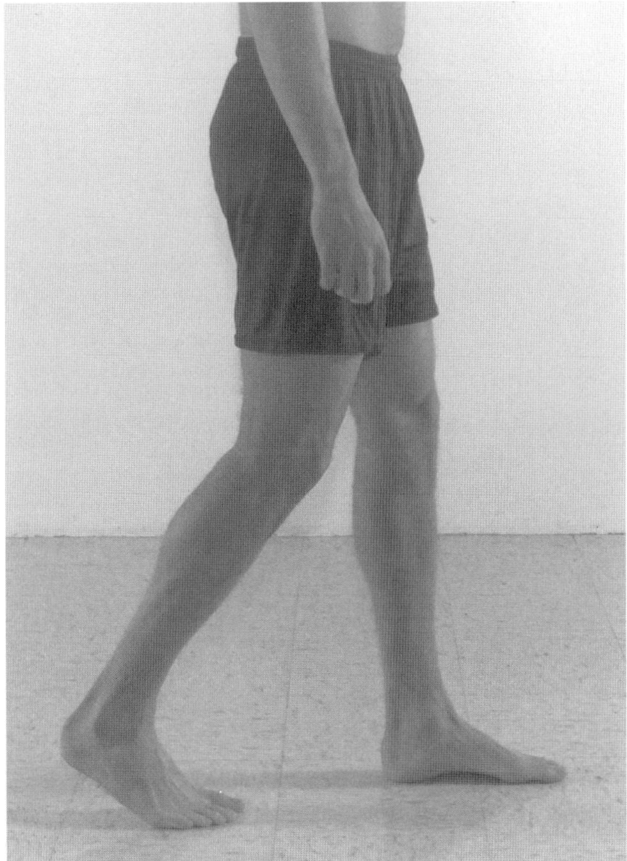

Fig. 10-5. Pre-swing

PRE-SWING				
JOINT	**MUSCLES ACTIVE**	**COMMON GAIT DEVIATIONS**	**MUSCULAR ETIOLOGY**	**OTHER POSSIBLE ETIOLOGIES**
Hip	Adductor longus: Initiates hip flexion and controls abduction of the hip produced by transferring weight to the contralateral lower extremity Rectus femoris: Activity (when present) initiates hip flexion and controls the rate of knee flexion	Excessive hip flexion	Generally not caused by muscle weakness	Hip flexion or iliotibial band contracture; spasticity of hip flexors; hip pain
Knee	Popliteus/gastrocnemius: Initiate knee flexion Rectus femoris: Brief activity to restrain excessive knee flexion if necessary	Insufficient knee flexion	Weak knee extensors: Perform MMT of the quadriceps to confirm	Knee pain; knee extension contracture; quadriceps spasticity
Ankle	Gastrocnemius/soleus: Active in the beginning of pre-swing to provide anterior acceleration of the tibia Tibialis anterior/long toe extensors: Activity initiated at the end of pre-swing to prevent excessive plantar flexion of the ankle	Excessive ankle dorsiflexion	Weak soleus: Perform MMT of the soleus to confirm	AFO with rigid ankle; flexed knee gait (secondary to, e.g., knee flexion contracture, hamstring spasticity)

Initial Swing

Initial swing begins at the point when the ipsilateral foot leaves the ground and continues until the swinging limb is opposite the contralateral extremity (Fig. 10-6). This is a period of acceleration for the swinging limb, and the majority of the muscular activity that occurs is devoted to initiating forward momentum in the limb that will take the extremity through the rest of the swing phase.

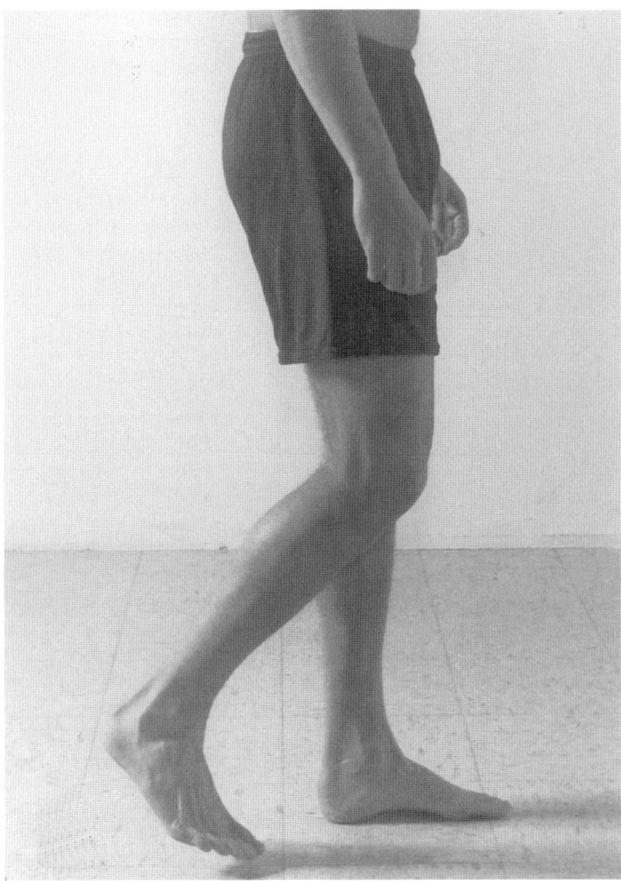

Fig. 10-6. Initial swing

INITIAL SWING				
JOINT	**MUSCLES ACTIVE**	**COMMON GAIT DEVIATIONS**	**MUSCULAR ETIOLOGY**	**OTHER POSSIBLE ETIOLOGIES**
Hip	Iliacus/adductor longus: Flex the hip	Insufficient hip flexion	Hip flexor weakness: Perform MMT of the iliopsoas to confirm	Lack of normal control of hip flexors secondary to central nervous system lesion
	Gracilis/sartorius: Flex the hip and knee	Circumduction of the hip	Hip flexor weakness: Perform MMT of the iliopsoas to confirm	Knee extension contracture; ankle dorsiflexor weak-ness; excessive ankle plantar flexion
		Contralateral trunk lean	Hip flexor weakness: Perform MMT of the iliopsoas to confirm	Weak hip abductors (stance limb); knee extension contracture (swing limb); ankle dorsiflexor weakness (swing limb); excessive ankle plantar flexion (swing limb)
Knee	Biceps femoris (short head): Flexes the knee			
	Gracilis/sartorius: Flex the knee and hip	Insufficient knee flexion	Hip flexor weakness: Perform MMT of the iliopsoas to confirm	Quadriceps spasticity, knee pain, knee extension contracture
Ankle	Tibialis anterior/long toe extensors: Dorsiflex the ankle	Excessive ankle plantar flexion	If significant enough to be noticed during this phase, it is generally due to factors other than muscle weakness	Ankle plantar flexion contracture

Mid-Swing

Mid-swing encompasses the period from when the swinging reference limb falls opposite the stance limb until the tibia of the reference limb attains a vertical position (Fig. 10-7). The swinging limb advances forward during this period primarily under the momentum developed during the initial swing. The ankle dorsiflexors continue their activity to maintain a neutral position of the ankle during swing.

Fig. 10-7. Mid-swing

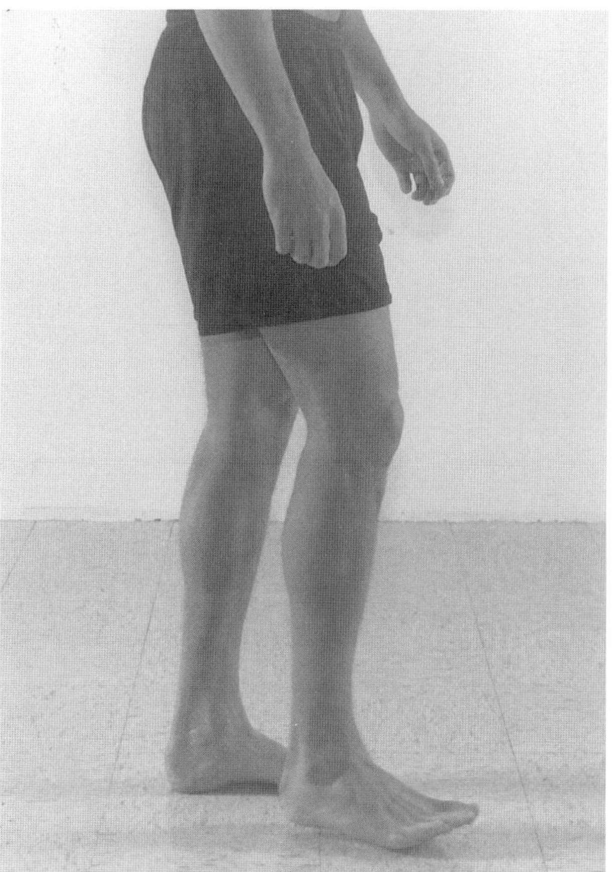

MID-SWING				
JOINT	**MUSCLES ACTIVE**	**COMMON GAIT DEVIATIONS**	**MUSCULAR ETIOLOGY**	**OTHER POSSIBLE ETIOLOGIES**
Hip	Biceps femoris (long head), semimembranosus: Onset of activity late in mid-swing to decelerate the femur	Excessive hip flexion	Weak ankle dorsiflexors (hip flexion increased to clear foot): Perform MMT of the tibialis anterior and long toe extensors to confirm	Hip flexion contracture; excessive ankle plantar flexion (secondary to ankle plantar flexion contracture or spasticity of the plantar flexors)
		Insufficient hip flexion	Weak hip flexors: Perform MMT of the iliopsoas to confirm	Lack of normal control of hip flexors secondary to central nervous system lesion
		Ipsilateral pelvic drop or contralateral trunk lean	Weak hip abductors on stance leg: Perform MMT of the gluteus medius/minimus and tensor fasciae latae to confirm	Hip pain (antalgic gait); contralateral hip abduction contracture (causes contralateral trunk lean)
		Excessive hip adduction	Weak hip flexors (adductors used to substitute): Perform MMT of the iliopsoas to confirm	Hip adductor spasticity
		Circumduction of the hip	Hip flexor weakness: Perform MMT of the iliopsoas to confirm	Knee extension contracture; ankle dorsiflexor weakness; excessive ankle plantar flexion
Knee	Biceps femoris (short head): Controls the rate of knee extension if necessary	Insufficient knee flexion	Weak hip flexors: Perform MMT of the iliopsoas to confirm	Knee extension contracture
Ankle	Tibialis anterior/long toe extensors: Dorsiflex the ankle	Excessive ankle plantar flexion	Weak ankle dorsiflexors: Perform MMT of the tibialis anterior and long toe extensors to confirm	Ankle plantar flexor spasticity; ankle plantar flexion contracture

Terminal Swing

Terminal swing, the final period of the gait cycle, begins from the point at which the tibia attains verticality and ends with initial contact of the swinging limb (Fig. 10-8). Muscular activity during this period is designed to decelerate the forward-moving limb and to provide terminal extension of the knee in preparation for another stance phase.

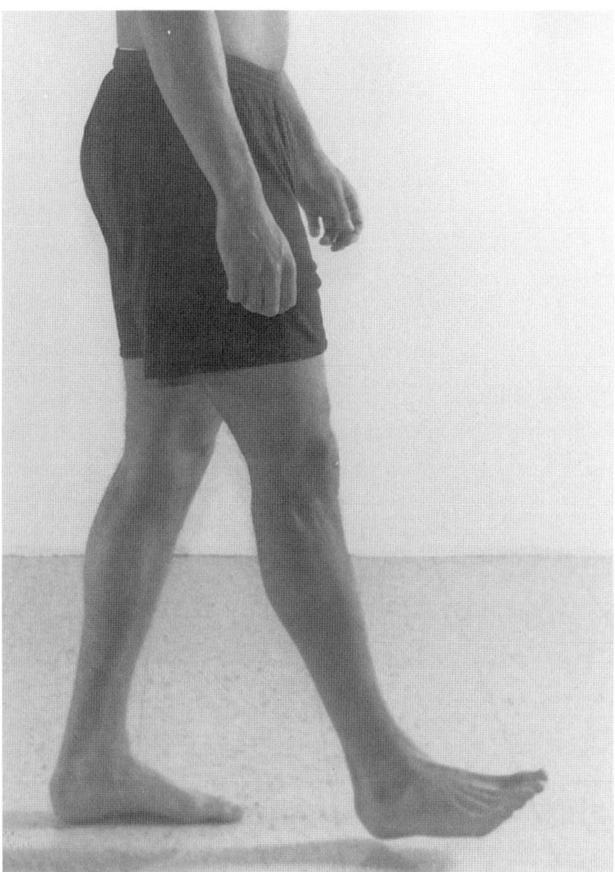

Fig. 10-8. Terminal swing

TERMINAL SWING				
JOINT	**MUSCLES ACTIVE**	**COMMON GAIT DEVIATIONS**	**MUSCULAR ETIOLOGY**	**OTHER POSSIBLE ETIOLOGIES**
Hip	Biceps femoris (long head), semimembranosus, semitendinosus: Deceleration of the femur	Insufficient hip flexion	Weak hip flexors: Perform MMT of the iliopsoas to confirm	Lack of normal control of hip flexors secondary to central nervous system lesion
	Gluteus maximus: Deceleration of the femur	Circumduction of hip	Weak hip flexors: Perform MMT of the iliopsoas to confirm	Knee extension contracture; excessive ankle plantar flexion
		Excessive hip adduction	Weak hip flexors (adductors used to substitute): Perform MMT of the iliopsoas to confirm	Hip adductor spasticity
Knee	Vastus medialis, lateralis, and intermedius: Extend the knee Biceps femoris (long head), semimembranosus, semitendinosus: Control excessive knee extension	Insufficient knee flexion	Weak knee extensors: Perform MMT of the quadriceps to confirm	Hamstring spasticity; Knee flexion contracture
Ankle	Tibialis anterior/long toe extensors: Dorsiflex the ankle	Excessive ankle plantar flexion	Weak ankle dorsiflexors: Perform MMT of the tibialis anterior and long toe extensors to confirm Weak knee extensors: Perform MMT of the quadriceps to confirm	Ankle plantar flexor spasticity; ankle plantar flexion contracture

Bibliography

Alexander NB. Gait disorders in older adults. *J Am Geriatr Soc* 1996;44:434–451.

Brandell BR. Functional roles of the calf and vastus muscles in locomotion. *Am J Phys Med* 1977;56:59–74.

Brinkman JR, Perry J. Rate and range of knee motion during ambulation in healthy and arthritic subjects. *Phys Ther* 1985;65:1055–1060.

Carollo JJ, Mathews D. Strategies for clinical motion analysis based on functional decomposition of the gait cycle. *Phys Med Rehabil Clin N Am* 2002;13:949–977.

Chambers HG, Sutherland DH. A practical guide to gait analysis. *J Am Acad Orthop Surg* 2002;10:222–231.

Coutts F. Gait analysis in the therapeutic environment. *Man Ther* 1999;4:2–10.

Czerniecki JM. Rehabilitation in limb deficiency: gait and motion analysis. *Arch Phys Med Rehabil* 1996;77:S3–S8.

Damiano DL, Kelly LE, Vaughn CL. Effects of quadriceps femoris muscle strengthening on crouch gait in children with spastic diplegia. *Phys Ther* 1995;75:658–667.

Dillingham TR, Lehmann JF, Price R. Effect of lower limb on body propulsion. *Arch Phys Med Rehabil* 1992;73:647–651.

Fisher NM, White SC, Yack HJ, et al. Muscle function and gait in patients with knee osteoarthritis before and after muscle rehabilitation. *Disabil Rehabil* 1997;19:47–55.

Gage JR. An overview of normal walking. *Instr Course Lect* 1990;39:291–303.

Gage JR. Gait analysis: an essential tool in the treatment of cerebral palsy. *Clin Orthop* 1993;288:126–134.

Gyory AN, Chao EY, Stauffer RN. Functional evaluation of normal and pathological knees during gait. *Arch Phys Med Rehabil* 1976;57:571–577.

Harris GF, Wertsch JJ. Procedures for gait analysis. *Arch Phys Med Rehabil* 1994;75:216–225.

Kameyama O, Ogawa R, Okamoto T, et al. Electric discharge patterns of ankle muscle during the normal gait cycle. *Arch Phys Med Rehabil* 1990;71:969–974.

Krawetz P, Nance P. Gait analysis of spinal cord injured subjects: effects of injury level and spasticity. *Arch Phys Med Rehabil* 1996;77:635–638.

Locke M, Perry J, Campbell J, et al. Ankle and subtalar motion during gait in arthritic patients. *Phys Ther* 1984;64:504–509.

Lovejoy CO. Evolution of human walking. *Sci Am* 1988;259:118–125.

Lyons K, Perry J, Gronley JK, et al. Timing and relative intensity of hip extensor and abductor muscle action during level and stair ambulation. *Phys Ther* 1983;63:1597–1605.

Messier SP. Osteoarthritis of the knee and associated factors of age and obesity: effects on gait. *Med Sci Sports Exerc* 1994;26:1446–1451.

Mueller MJ, Minor SD, Sahrmann SA, et al. Differences in the gait characteristics of patients with diabetes and peripheral neuropathy compared with age-matched controls. *Phys Ther* 1994;74:299–308.

Murray MP, Kory RC, Sepic SB. Walking patterns of normal women. *Arch Phys Med Rehabil* 1970;51:637–650.

Ounpuu S. The biomechanics of walking and running. *Clin Sports Med* 1994;13:843–863.

Pazza SJ, Delp SL. The influence of muscles on knee flexion during the swing phase of gait. *J Biomech* 1996;29:723–733.

Perry J. Pathological gait. *Instr Course Lect* 1990;39:325–331.

Perry J. *Gait Analysis: Normal and Pathological Function.* Thorofare, NJ: Slack, 1992.

Perry J, Mulroy SJ, Renwick SE. The relationship of lower extremity strength and gait parameters in patients with post-polio syndrome. *Arch Phys Med Rehabil* 1993;74:165–169.

Powers CM, Perry J, Hsu A, et al. Are patellofemoral pain and quadriceps femoris muscle torque associated with locomotor function? *Phys Ther* 1997;77:1063–1078.

Rancho Los Amigos Medical Center: Observational Gait Analysis. Downey, CA: Los Amigos Research and Education Institute, 2001.

Rose SA, Ounpuu S, DeLuca PA. Strategies for the assessment of pediatric gait in the clinical setting. *Phys Ther* 1991;71:961–980.

Sadeghi H, Allard P, Prince F, et al. Symmetry and limb dominance in able-bodied gait: a review. *Gait Posture* 2000;12:34–45.

Simon SR, Mann RA, Hagy JL, et al. Role of the posterior calf muscles in normal gait. *J Bone Joint Surg* 1978;60A:465–472.

Truckenbrodt H, Hafner R, von Altenbockum C. Functional joint analysis of the foot in juvenile chronic arthritis. *Clin Exp Rheumatol* 1994;12[Suppl 10]:S91–96.

Vasudevan PN, Vaidyalingam KV, Bhaskaran Nair P. Can Trendelenburg's sign be positive if the hip is normal? *J Bone Joint Surg* 1997;79B:462–466.

Wheelwright EF, Minns RA, Law HT, et al. Temporal and spatial parameters of gait in children: normal control data. *Dev Med Child Neurol* 1993;35:102–113.

Wolfson L, Judge J, Whipple R, et al. Strength is a major factor in balance, gait, and the occurrence of falls (special issue). *J Gerontol* 1995;50A:64–67.

Wootten ME, Kadaba MP, Cochran GV. Dynamic electromyography, II. *J Orthop Res* 1990; 8:260–265.

Zatsiorky VM, Werner SL, Kaimin MA. Basic kinematics of walking: step length and step frequency—a review. *J Sports Med* 1994;34:109–134.

APPENDIX A

Table A-1. NORMAL ROM VALUES FOR JOINTS OF THE UPPER EXTREMITY IN ADULTS: VARIOUS SOURCES

JOINT	REESE & BANDY, 2002[4]	AAOS, 1965[1*]	AMA, 1993[3+]
Shoulder			
Flexion	0° - 165°	0° - 180°	0° - 180°
Extension	0° - 60°	0° - 60°	0° - 50°
Abduction	0° - 165°	0° - 180°	0° - 180°
Medial Rotation	0° - 70°	0° - 70°	0° - 90°
Lateral Rotation	0° - 90°	0° - 90°	0° - 90°
Elbow			
Flexion	0° - 140°	0° - 150°	0° - 140°
Extension	0°	0°	0°
Forearm			
Pronation	0° - 80°	0° - 80°	0° - 80°
Supination	0° - 80°	0° - 80°	0° - 80°
Wrist			
Flexion	0° - 80°	0° - 80°	0° - 60°
Extension	0° - 70°	0° - 70°	0° - 60°
Abduction (Radial Deviation)	0° - 20°	0° - 20°	0° - 20°
Adduction (Ulnar Deviation)	0° - 30°	0° - 30°	0° - 30°
1st Carpometacarpal Joint			
Flexion	0° - 15°	0° - 15°	
Extension	0° - 20°	0° - 20°	0° - 50°
Abduction	0° - 70°	0° - 70°	
Metacarpophalangeal Joints			
Flexion			
Thumb	0° - 50°	0° - 50°	0° - 60°
Fingers	0° - 90°	0° - 90°	0° - 90°
Extension			
Thumb	0°	0°	0°
Fingers	0° - 20°	0° - 45°	0° - 20°
Interphalangeal Joints			
Flexion			
IP Joint (Thumb)	0° - 65°	0° - 80°	0° - 80°
PIP Joint (Fingers)	0° - 100°	0° - 100°	0° - 100°
DIP Joint (Fingers)	0° - 70°	0° - 90°	0° - 70°
Extension			
IP Joint (Thumb)	0° - 10° to 20°	0° - 20°	0° - 10°
PIP Joint (Fingers)	0°	0°	0°
DIP Joint (Fingers)	0°	0°	0°

*American Academy of Orthopaedic Surgeons
+American Medical Association
IP, interphalangeal; PIP, proximal interphalangeal; DIP, distal interphalangeal

Table A-2. NORMAL ROM VALUES FOR JOINTS OF THE LOWER EXTREMITY IN ADULTS: VARIOUS SOURCES

JOINT	REESE & BANDY, 2002[4]	AAOS, 1965[1*]	AMA, 1984[2+]
Hip			
Flexion	0° - 120°	0° - 120°	0° - 100°
Extension	0° - 20°	0° - 30°	0° - 30°
Abduction	0° - 40° to 45°	0° - 45°	0° - 40°
Adduction	0° - 25° to 30°	0° - 30°	0° - 20°
Medial Rotation	0° - 35° to 40°	0° - 45°	0° - 50°
Lateral Rotation	0° - 35° to 40°	0° - 45°	0° - 40°
Knee			
Flexion	0° - 140° to 145°	0° - 135°	0° - 150°
Extension	0°	0° - 10°	0°
Ankle/Foot			
Dorsiflexion‡	0° - 15° to 20°	0° - 20°	0° - 20°
Plantarflexion§	0° - 40° to 50°	0° - 50°	0° - 40°
Inversion§	0° - 30° to 35°	0° - 35°	0° - 30°
Eversion‡	0° - 20°	0° - 15°	0° - 20°
1st metatarsophalangeal (MTP) Joint			
Flexion	0° - 20°	0° - 45°	0° - 30°
Extension	0° - 80°	0° - 70°	0° - 50°

*American Academy of Orthodaedic Surgeons
+American Medical Association
‡Component of pronation
§Component of supination

References

1. American Academy of Orthopaedic Surgeons: Joint Motion: Method of Measuring and Recording. Chicago, American Academic of Orthopaedic Surgeons, 1965.
2. American Medical Association: Guides to the Evaluation of Permanent Impairment. 2nd ed. Chicago, 1984.
3. American Medical Association: Guides to the Evaluation of Permanent Impariment, 4th ed. Chicago, 1993.
4. Reese NB, Bandy WB: Joint Range of Motion and Muscle Length Testing. Philadelphia, WB Saunders, Co., 2002.

APPENDIX B

Table B-1. MUSCLE INNERVATIONS BY SPINAL CORD LEVEL

NECK AND UPPER EXTREMITY MUSCLES

Spinal Level	Muscle	
C1	Upper trapezius	Obliquus capitis superior
	Middle trapezius	Rectus capitis posterior major
	Lower trapezius	Rectus capitis posterior minor
	Longus capitis	Semispinalis capitis
	Rectus capitis anterior	
C2	Upper trapezius	Longus colli
	Middle trapezius	Rectus capitis anterior
	Lower trapezius	Sternocleidomastoid
	Longus capitis	Semispinalis capitis
C3	Upper trapezius	Longus colli
	Middle trapezius	Levator scapulae
	Lower trapezius	Sternocleidomastoid
	Longus capitis	Semispinalis capitis
C4	Upper trapezius	Iliocostalis cervicis
	Middle trapezius	Levator scapulae
	Lower trapezius	Sternocleidomastoid
	Longus colli	
C5	Upper trapezius	Pectoralis major
	Middle trapezius	Subscapularis
	Lower trapezius	Infraspinatus
	Longus colli	Teres minor
	Iliocostalis cervicis	Biceps brachii
	Levator scapulae	Brachialis
	Rhomboideus major	Brachioradialis
	Serratus anterior	Anterior Scalene
	Teres major	Semispinalis capitis
	Deltoid	Semispinalis cervicis
	Supraspinatus	
C6	Serratus anterior	Extensor carpi radialis longus
	Coracobrachialis	Extensor carpi radialis brevis
	Latissimus dorsi	Extensor carpi ulnaris
	Deltoid	Extensor digitorum
	Pectoralis major	Extensor indicis
	Subscapularis	Extensor digiti minimi
	Teres major	Extensor pollicis brevis
	Infraspinatus	Extensor pollicis longus
	Biceps brachii	Abductor pollicis longus
	Brachialis	Longus colli
	Brachioradialis	Anterior Scalene
	Supinator	Iliocostalis cervicis
	Pronator teres	Semispinalis capitis
	Flexor carpi radialis	
C7	Serratus anterior	Extensor carpi ulnaris
	Coracobrachialis	Flexor digitorum
	Latissimus dorsi	Extensor digitorum
	Pectoralis major	Extensor indicis
	Triceps brachii	Extensor digiti minimi
	Anconeus	Extensor pollicis brevis
	Pronator teres	Extensor pollicis longus
	Flexor carpi radialis	Abductor pollicis longus
	Extensor carpi radialis longus	Semispinalis cervicis
	Extensor carpi radialis brevis	

Table B-1. MUSCLE INNERVATIONS BY SPINAL CORD LEVEL—cont'd

NECK AND UPPER EXTREMITY MUSCLES

Spinal Level	Muscle	
C8	Latissimus dorsi Pectoralis major Triceps brachii Anconeus Pronator quadratus Flexor carpi ulnaris Extensor carpi ulnaris Lumbricals Palmar interossei Dorsal interossei Flexor digitorum superficialis Flexor digitorum profundus	Extensor digitorum Extensor indicis Extensor digiti minimi Abductor digiti minimi Flexor pollicis brevis Flexor pollicis longus Extensor pollicis longus Abductor pollicis brevis Adductor pollicis Opponens pollicis Semispinalis cervicis
T1	Pectoralis major Pronator quadratus Flexor carpi ulnaris Lumbricals Palmar interossei Dorsal interossei Flexor digitorum superficialis Flexor digitorum profundus	Abductor digiti minimi Flexor pollicis brevis Flexor pollicis longus Abductor pollicis brevis Adductor pollicis Opponens pollicis Opponens digiti minimi

LOWER EXTREMITY MUSCLES

Spinal Level	Muscle	
L2	Sartorius Adductor magnus Adductor longus Adductor brevis Pectineus	Gracilis Rectus femoris Vastus lateralis Vastus medialis Vastus intermedius
L3	Sartorius Adductor magnus Adductor longus Adductor brevis Pectineus	Gracilis Rectus femoris Vastus lateralis Vastus medialis Vastus intermedius
L4	Gluteus medius Gluteus minimus Tensor fascia lata Adductor magnus Adductor longus Adductor brevis Pectineus Gemellus inferior Obturator externus Quadratus femoris	Rectus femoris Vastus lateralis Vastus medialis Vastus intermedius Tibialis anterior Peroneus longus Peroneus brevis Extensor digitorum longus Extensor hallucis longus
L5	Gluteus maximus Semitendinosus Semimembranosus Biceps femoris Gluteus medius Gluteus minimus Tensor fascia lata Gemellus superior Obturator internus Gemellus inferior Obturator externus Quadratus femoris	Tibialis anterior Tibialis posterior Peroneus longus Peroneus brevis 1st Lumbrical Flexor hallucis brevis Flexor digitorum longus Flexor digitorum brevis Flexor hallucis longus Extensor digitorum longus Extensor digitorum brevis Extensor hallucis longus

Continued

Table B-1. MUSCLE INNERVATIONS BY SPINAL CORD LEVEL—cont'd

LOWER EXTREMITY MUSCLES

Spinal Level	Muscle	
S1	Gluteus maximus	Soleus
	Semitendinosus	Tibialis anterior
	Semimembranosus	Tibialis posterior
	Biceps femoris	Peroneus longus
	Gluteus medius	Peroneus brevis
	Gluteus minimus	1st Lumbrical
	Tensor fascia lata	Flexor hallucis brevis
	Piriformis	Flexor digitorum longus
	Gemellus superior	Flexor digitorum brevis
	Obturator internus	Flexor hallucis longus
	Gemellus inferior	Extensor digitorum longus
	Quadratus femoris	Extensor digitorum brevis
	Gastrocnemius	Extensor hallucis longus
S2	Gluteus maximus	Obturator internus
	Semitendinosus	Gastrocnemius
	Semimembranosus	Soleus
	Biceps femoris	Lumbricals (2–4)
	Piriformis	Flexor hallucis longus
	Gemellus superior	
S3	Lumbricals (2–4)	

APPENDIX C

Table C-1. MUSCLE INNERVATIONS BY PERIPHERAL NERVE

UPPER EXTREMITY MUSCLES	
Peripheral Nerve	**Muscle**
Dorsal scapular	Levator scapulae Rhomboideus major Rhomboideus minor
Long thoracic	Serratus anterior
Suprascapular	Supraspinatus Infraspinatus
Medial and lateral pectoral	Pectoralis major
Subscapular	Subscapularis (upper and lower) Teres major (lower)
Thoracodorsal	Latissimus dorsi
Axillary	Deltoid Teres minor
Musculocutaneous	Coracobrachialis Biceps brachii Brachialis
Median	Pronator teres Pronator quadratus Flexor carpi radialis Lumbricals 1 and 2 Flexor digitorum superficialis Flexor digitorum profundus Flexor pollicis brevis Flexor pollicis longus Abductor pollicis brevis Opponens pollicis
Radial	Brachioradialis Triceps brachii Anconeus Supinator Extensor carpi radialis longus Extensor carpi radialis brevis Extensor carpi ulnaris Extensor digitorum Extensor indicis Extensor digiti minimi Extensor pollicis brevis Extensor pollicis longus Abductor pollicis longus
Ulnar	Flexor carpi ulnaris Lumbricals 3 and 4 Palmar interossei Dorsal interossei Flexor digitorum profundus Abductor digiti minimi Flexor pollicis brevis Adductor pollicis Opponens digiti minimi

Continued

Table C-1. MUSCLE INNERVATIONS BY PERIPHERAL NERVE—cont'd

LOWER EXTREMITY MUSCLES

Peripheral Nerve	Muscle
Superior gluteal	Gluteus medius Gluteus minimus Tensor fascia lata
Inferior gluteal	Gluteus maximus
Nerve to the obturator internus	Gemellus superior Obturator internus
Nerve to the quadratus femoris	Quadratus femoris Gemellus inferior
Obturator	Adductor magnus Adductor longus Adductor brevis Gracilis Obturator externus
Femoral	Iliacus Sartorius Pectineus Rectus femoris Vastus medialis Vastus lateralis Vastus intermedius
Sciatic	Semitendinosus (tibial) Semimembranosus (tibial) Biceps femoris—long head (tibial) Biceps femoris—short head (peroneal) Adductor magnus (tibial)
Tibial	Popliteus Gastrocnemius Soleus Plantaris Tibialis posterior Flexor hallucis longus Flexor digitorum longus
Deep peroneal	Tibialis anterior Extensor hallucis longus Extensor digitorum longus Extensor digitorum brevis Superficial peroneal Peroneus longus Peroneus brevis
Medial plantar*	Flexor hallucis brevis Flexor digitorum brevis 1st lumbrical
Lateral plantar*	Lumbricals 2,3,4

*Some of the muscles in the deep layers of the foot have been omitted because they are not generally tested for strength.

SUBJECT INDEX

Page numbers in *italic* indicate figures, page numbers followed by a 't' indicate tables.